Atopic Dermatitis and Eczematous Disorders

Edited by

Donald Rudikoff MD
Chief of Dermatology, Bronx Lebanon Hospital, and Associate Professor of Clinical Medicine (Dermatology), Albert Einstein College of Medicine, Bronx, NY, USA

Steven R. Cohen MD, MPH
Professor and Chief, Division of Dermatology, Albert Einstein College of Medicine, Bronx, NY, USA

Noah Scheinfeld JD, MD
Clinical Assistant Professor of Dermatology, Weill Cornell Medical College, and Adjunct Assistant Clinical Professor of Dermatology, Columbia University College of Physicians and Surgeons, New York, NY, USA

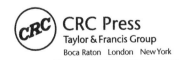
CRC Press
Taylor & Francis Group
Boca Raton London New York

CRC Press is an imprint of the
Taylor & Francis Group, an **informa** business

CRC Press
Taylor & Francis Group
6000 Broken Sound Parkway NW, Suite 300
Boca Raton, FL 33487-2742

© 2014 by Taylor & Francis Group, LLC
CRC Press is an imprint of Taylor & Francis Group, an Informa business

First issued in paperback 2019

No claim to original U.S. Government works

ISBN 13: 978-0-367-45216-2 (pbk)
ISBN 13: 978-1-84076-195-5 (hbk)

Visit the Taylor & Francis Web site at
http://www.taylorandfrancis.com

and the CRC Press Web site at
http://www.crcpress.com

CONTENTS

Contributors   6
Preface   9

CHAPTER 1 THE HISTORY OF ECZEMA AND ATOPIC DERMATITIS   11
Douglas Altchek and Donald Rudikoff
Eczema in history and literature   12
Evolution of the term 'eczema'   13
Infantile eczema   14
Modern dermatologists and early depictions of eczema   15
Should the term 'eczema' be discarded?   21
Treatment   22
Conclusion   24

CHAPTER 2 THE EPIDEMIOLOGY OF ATOPIC DERMATITIS   25
Patrick O. Emanuel, Noah Scheinfeld, and Hywel C. Williams
Introduction   25
Disease classification schemes   27
Descriptive epidemiology of atopic dermatitis   28
Natural history   34
Risk factors   34
The hygiene hypothesis   36
Conclusions   38

CHAPTER 3 CLINICAL ASPECTS AND DIFFERENTIAL DIAGNOSIS OF ATOPIC DERMATITIS   39
Donald Rudikoff, Diana Lee, and Steven R. Cohen
Clinical presentation   39
Differential diagnosis   61
Conclusion   76

CHAPTER 4 INFANTILE ATOPIC DERMATITIS   77
Sadaf H. Hussain, James R. Treat, and Albert C. Yan
Introduction   77
Epidemiology   79
Pathogenesis   81
Clinical characteristics   82
Complications   84
Therapeutic considerations   86
Conclusions   91

CHAPTER 5 PRURITUS IN ATOPIC DERMATITIS: PATHOPHYSIOLOGY AND TREATMENT OPTIONS   93
Tejesh Surendra Patel and Gil Yosipovitch
Pathophysiology of pruritus in atopic dermatitis   93
Mediators of pruritus in atopic dermatitis   96
Crosstalk between cutaneous nerve fibers and the stratum corneum   99
Treatment   99
Conclusion   105

CHAPTER 6 PATHOPHYSIOLOGY OF ATOPIC DERMATITIS AND ATOPIFORM DERMATITIS   107
Donald Rudikoff and Jan D. Bos
Background   107
Aspects of pathogenesis   108
Histopathology and immunohistology   111
T lymphocytes and cytokine milieu   113
Lesion formation in atopic dermatitis   122
The skin barrier in atopic dermatitis   129
Innate immunity and antimicrobial peptides   129
The epidermal barrier to water loss   132
The importance of filaggrin to barrier function and epidermal hydration   134
Lipid and ceramide abnormalities   135
Tight junctions and claudin   136
The acid mantle – skin pH in atopic dermatitis   136
Epicutaneous antigen presentation through an impaired skin barrier   137
The atopy patch test   137
The 500-dalton rule   138
Sweating and sweat antigens   138
S. aureus and other microorganisms   139
Keratinocyte-derived factors   140
Eosinophils   141
Mast cells   142
Histamine   142
Other mast cell mediators   143
Nerves and neurotrophins   143
Conclusion   144

CHAPTER 7 ATOPIC DERMATITIS: THE ALLERGIST'S PERSPECTIVE   145
Mamta Reddy and Yudy K. Persaud
The hygiene hypothesis   145
The atopic march (the correlation of atopic dermatitis and asthma)   146
Intrinsic versus extrinsic atopic dermatitis   148
Allergic immunopathology of atopic skin disease   148
Immunoglobulin E and IgE receptors   149
Identifying allergen triggers   150
Diagnostic testing   150
Prevention   153
Superantigens   156
Association with other disorders of the immune system   157
Conclusions   157

CHAPTER 8 SKIN BARRIER REPAIR IN ATOPIC DERMATITIS THERAPY   159
William Abramovits and Peter Elias
Epidermal barrier function   159
Therapeutic interventions   162
Newer formulations   163
Conclusion   164

CHAPTER 9 THE ROLE OF INFECTIOUS AGENTS IN ATOPIC DERMATITIS — 165

Andrea L. Neimann, Jules Lipoff, Rachel Garner, Anat Lebow, and Steven R. Cohen

Introduction — 165
Staphylococcus aureus in atopic dermatitis — 165
Streptococcal infections — 170
Fungal infections — 170
Dermatophytes — 171
Viral infections — 172
Eczema vaccinatum — 176
Conclusion — 177

CHAPTER 10 TOPICAL TREATMENT OF ATOPIC DERMATITIS — 179

William Abramovits

General treatment measures — 180
Topical corticosteroids — 181
Topical antipruritics and tar — 183
Topical calcineurin inhibitors — 183
Medical devices for the treatment of atopic dermatitis — 184
Topical treatment paradigm — 185

CHAPTER 11 SYSTEMIC AGENTS FOR THE TREATMENT OF ATOPIC DERMATITIS — 187

Arash Akhavan and Donald Rudikoff

Systemic corticosteroids — 187
Cyclosporine and other calcineurin inhibitors — 188
Azathioprine — 190
Mycophenolate mofetil — 190
Methotrexate — 191
Interferon-γ — 193
Immunobiologics — 193
Conclusion — 198

CHAPTER 12 PHOTO(CHEMO)THERAPY OF ATOPIC ECZEMA — 201

Thilo Gambichler, Nordwig S. Tomi, and Stefanie Boms

Ultraviolet A and ultraviolet B — 203
Narrowband ultraviolet B — 203
Ultraviolet A1 — 204
Psoralen and ultraviolet light and extracorporeal photopheresis — 206
Miscellaneous — 207
Conclusions — 209

CHAPTER 13 ECZEMA AND THE EYE — 211

Kevin Stein and Frederick Pereira

Atopic dermatitis — 212
Keratoconjunctivitis — 212
Keratoconus — 213
Cataracts — 214
Retinal detachment — 215
Uveitis — 216
Blepharitis and eyelid dermatitis — 216

CHAPTER 14 HAND DERMATITIS — 223

Nina C. Botto and Erin M. Warshaw

Prevalence — 223
Clinical variants — 224
Contact dermatitis — 224
Clinical features — 226
Occupational concerns — 228
Contact urticaria and evolution to eczematous hand dermatitis — 228
Hand dermatitis risk factors — 233
Therapy — 237
Chronicity, prognosis, and predictive factors — 243
Economics — 244
Conclusions — 244

CHAPTER 15 THE RELATIONSHIP BETWEEN ATOPIC DERMATITIS AND CONTACT DERMATITIS — 247

Sharon Rose, Arash Akhavan, David H. Ciocon, and Steven R. Cohen

Introduction — 247
Pathogenesis — 248
Immunology — 248
Association of AD and ACD — 251
Association of AD and ICD — 252
Diagnosis — 252
Treatment — 252
Conclusions — 254

CHAPTER 16 NUMMULAR DERMATITIS — 255

Noah Scheinfeld and Donald Rudikoff

Background — 255
Epidemiology — 255
Clinical manifestations — 256
Clinical associations — 259
Laboratory and histological findings — 259
Differential diagnosis — 260
Pathogenesis — 263
Treatment — 264
Conclusion — 265

CHAPTER 17 STASIS DERMATITIS — 267

Scott L. Flugman

Background — 267
Clinical features — 267
Clinical complications of stasis dermatitis — 268
Pathophysiology of stasis dermatitis — 271
Diagnosis of stasis dermatitis — 272
Treatment of stasis dermatitis — 273
Conclusion — 274
Acknowledgments — 274

CHAPTER 18 SEBORRHEIC DERMATITIS — 275

Karen Chernoff, Richie Lin, and Steven R. Cohen

Introduction — 275
Definition and classification — 275
Clinical features — 276
Differential diagnosis — 281

Histopathology   283
Causes   283
Treatment   285
Conclusion   287

CHAPTER 19 THE HISTOPATHOLOGY OF ECZEMA   289
Cynthia M. Magro, A. Neil Crowson, Molly E. Dyrsen, and Martin C. Mihm Jr
Introduction   289
General overview of the histomorphology   290
The histomorphology of distinctive forms of eczema   294

CHAPTER 20 ERYTHRODERMIC/EXFOLIATIVE DERMATITIS   309
Daniel Parish, Noah Scheinfeld, and Jane M. Grant-Kels
Pediatric and neonatal erythroderma   314
Malignancies and nondermatological diseases as causes of erythroderma   318
Conclusion   321

CHAPTER 21 PRIMARY IMMUNODEFICIENCY DISEASES   323
Adam Friedman, Manju Chacko Dawkins, and Donald Rudikoff
Introduction   323
Wiskott–Aldrich syndrome   326
Hyper-IgE syndrome (Job syndrome)   329
Omenn syndrome   334
Immune dysregulation, polyendocrinopathy, enteropathy, X-linked syndrome   337
Conclusion   339

CHAPTER 22 HIV INFECTION AND ATOPIC DERMATITIS   341
Adam Friedman, Donald Rudikoff, and Francis Iacobellis
Introduction   341
HIV-associated atopy   342

IgE elevation and eosinophilia in HIV-infected patients   342
Diagnosis   343
Differential diagnosis of HIV-associated atopic dermatitis   344
Therapy   350
Conclusion   350

CHAPTER 23 ICHTHYOSIS VULGARIS   351
Jessica Simon and Robert Buka
Pathophysiology and genetics   351
Epidemiology and clinical manifestations   352
Differential diagnosis   354
Management   356
Conclusion   356

CHAPTER 24 LEGAL ASPECTS OF ATOPIC DERMATITIS   357
Daniel H. Parish and Noah Scheinfeld
Introduction   357
Employment and benefits law   358
Tort law: medical malpractice, product liability, and other injury claims   360
Family and criminal law: pediatrics and child custody, neglect, and abuse   363
Conclusions   364
Table of cases   365

REFERENCES   367

INDEX   435

CONTRIBUTORS

William Abramovits, MD
Assistant Professor of Dermatology, Baylor
University Medical Center, Dallas;
Clinical Assistant Professor, UT Southwestern
Medical School, Dallas, TX, USA

Arash Akhavan, MD
Assistant Clinical Professor of Dermatology, Mount
Sinai School of Medicine, New York, NY, USA

Douglas Altchek, MD
Clinical Professor of Dermatology, Mount Sinai
School of Medicine, New York, NY, USA

Stefanie Boms, MD
Department of Dermatology, Katharinen Hospital,
Unna, Germany

Jan D. Bos, MD, PhD, FRCP
Professor and Chairman, Department of
Dermatology, Academic Medical Center, University
of Amsterdam, Amsterdam, The Netherlands

Nina C. Botto, MD
Department of Dermatology, Tufts University,
Boston, MA, USA

Robert Buka, MD
Assistant Clinical Professor of Dermatology, Mount
Sinai School of Medicine, New York, NY, USA

Manju Chacko Dawkins, MD
Attending Dermatologist, Bronx Lebanon Hospital
Center, Bronx, NY, USA

Karen Chernoff, MD
Weill Medical College of Cornell University,
Department of Dermatology, New York, NY, USA

David H. Ciocon, MD
Clinical Instructor, Department of Medicine
(Dermatology), Albert Einstein College of Medicine,
Bronx, NY, USA

Steven R. Cohen, MD, MPH
Professor and Chief, Division of Dermatology,
Albert Einstein College of Medicine, Bronx,
NY, USA

A. Neil Crowson, MD
Clinical Professor of Dermatology, Pathology,
and Surgery, Director of Dermatopathology,
University of Oklahoma, Regional Medical
Laboratory, Tulsa, OK, USA

Molly E. Dyrsen, MD
Dermpath Diagnostics, Richfield Laboratory
of Dermatopathology, Cincinatti, OH, USA

Peter Elias, MD
Professor of Dermatology, UCSF School of
Medicine, San Francisco, CA, USA

Patrick O. Emanuel, MB,ChB, FRCPA
Dermatopathologist, Associate Professor of
Pathology, University of Auckland, Auckland, New
Zealand

Scott L. Flugman, MD
Consulting Staff, Dermatology Associates of
Huntington PC, Huntington, NY, USA

Adam Friedman, MD
Assistant Professor, Department of Medicine
(Dermatology), Department of Physiology and
Biophysics, Albert Einstein College of Medicine,
Bronx, NY, USA

Thilo Gambichler, MD
Department of Dermatology, Ruhr-University
Bochum, Bochum, Germany

Rachel Garner, MD
Department of Dermatology, University of
Rochester School of Medicine, Rochester, NY, USA

Jane M. Grant-Kels, MD, FAAD
Department Chair and Professor, Department of
Dermatology, University of Connecticut Health
Center, Farmington, CT, USA

Sadaf H. Hussain, MD
Department of Dermatology and Cutaneous
Biology, Jefferson Medical College, Thomas
Jefferson University, Philadelphia, PA, USA

Francis Iacobellis, MD
Clinical Assistant Professor of Dermatology, Weill
Cornell Medical College, New York, NY, USA

Anat Lebow, MD
Clinical Assistant Professor, Department of
Dermatology, NYU Langone Medical Center,
New York, NY, USA

Diana Lee, MD, PhD
Department of Medicine (Dermatology), Albert
Einstein College of Medicine, Bronx, NY, USA

Richie Lin, MD
Dermatology Consultants of Short Hills, LLC,
Short Hills, NJ, USA

Jules Lipoff, MD
Department of Medicine (Dermatology), Albert
Einstein College of Medicine, Bronx, NY, USA

Cynthia M. Magro, MD
Professor of Pathology and Laboratory Medicine,
Professor of Pathology in Dermatology, Weill
Cornell Medical College, New York, NY, USA

Martin C. Mihm Jr, MD, FACP, FRCP
Clinical Professor of Pathology and Dermatology,
Harvard University, Cambridge, MA, USA

Andrea L. Neimann, MD, MPH
Assistant Professor, Department of Dermatology,
NYU Langone Medical Center, New York,
NY, USA

Daniel H. Parish, MD, JD
Department of Dermatology and Cutaneous
Biology, Jefferson Medical College Thomas
Jefferson University, Philadelphia, PA, USA

Tejesh Surendra Patel, MD
Assistant Professor, Department of Dermatology,
University of Tennessee Health Science Center,
Memphis, TN, USA

Frederick Perreira, MD
Clinical Associate Professor of Dermatology, Mount
Sinai School of Medicine; Clinical Instructor in
Dermatology, New York Medical College, New
York, NY, USA

Yudy K. Persaud, MD, MPH
Cheif of Allergy & Immunology, Department
of Pediatrics, Bronx Lebanon Hospital Center;
Assistant Professor of Pediatrics, Albert Einstein
College of Medicine, Bronx, NY, USA

Mamta Reddy, MD
Chief of Allergy and Immunology, Department
of Pediatrics, Bronx Lebanon Hospital Center;
Assistant Professor of Pediatrics, Albert Einstein
College of Medicine, Bronx, NY, USA

Sharon Rose, MD
Department of Anesthesiology, Weill-Cornell
Medical College, New York, NY, USA

Donald Rudikoff, MD
Chief of Dermatology, Bronx Lebanon Hospital
Center; Associate Professor of Clinical Medicine
(Dermatology), Albert Einstein College of Medicine,
Bronx, NY, USA

Noah Scheinfeld, JD, MD
Clinical Assistant Professor of Dermatology, Weill
Cornell Medical College; Adjunct Assistant Clinical
Professor of Dermatology, Columbia University
College of Physicians and Surgeons, New York,
NY, USA

Jessica Simon, MD
Department of Dermatology and Cutaneous
Surgery, University of Miami, Miami, FL, USA

Kevin Stein, MD
The Skin Surgery Center, Winston Salem, NC, USA

Nordwig S. Tomi, MD
Facharzt für Haut und Geschlechtskrankheiten
operative und ästhetische Dermatologie, Frankfurt,
Germany

James R. Treat, MD
Pediatric Dermatology Fellowship Director,
The Children's Hospital of Philadelphia;
Assistant Professor, Pediatrics and Dermatology,
Perelman School of Medicine at the University of
Pennsylvania, Philadelphia, PA, USA

Erin M. Warshaw, MD, MS
Chief of Dermatology, Minneapolis VA Medical
Center; Clinical Associate Professor of Dermatology,
University of Minnesota, Minneapolis, MN, USA

Hywel C. Williams, MSc, PhD, FRCP
Professor of Dermato-Epidemiology, Centre
of Evidence-Based Dermatology, Nottingham
University Hospital NHS Trust, Nottingham, UK

Albert C. Yan, MD
Associate Professor of Pediatrics in Dermatology,
University of Pennsylvania School of Medicine;
Associate Professor of Pediatrics at the Children's
Hospital of Philadelphia, Philadelphia, PA, USA

Gil Yosipovitch, MD
Professor, Department of Dermatology,
Neurobiology & Anatomy, and Regenerative
Medicine, Wake Forest University School of
Medicine, Winston Salem, NC, USA

PREFACE

Atopic dermatitis and eczematous disorders constitute the *bread and butter* of dermatology. They comprise a significant percentage of visits to dermatologists, primary care physicians, and allergists. It is considered that about 15% of the population have atopic dermatitis at some point in their life. In addition, research interest in the disease is at an all-time high. Approximately a third of the 17 000 atopic dermatitis citations in PubMed have been published during the past 5 years, since our text was conceived. Despite the high interest and quality of the literature on this disorder, the pathophysiology and optimum treatment remain uncertain. By comparison the literature related to deconstructing the mysteries of other eczematous disorders is even less well defined. This has been the impetus for crafting a new resource examining the historical and clinical foundations of these important disorders.

Atopic Dermatitis and Eczematous Disorders was created as a comprehensive text exploring the clinical, historical, histopathological, and etiological aspects of atopic dermatitis and other eczema variants, ie, seborrheic dermatitis, nummular eczema, and stasis dermatitis. It also embraces disorders such as exfoliative erythroderma, HIV-related dermatoses, ichthyosis vulgaris, hand dermatitis, and immunodeficiency disorders that occur together with or enter into the differential diagnosis of atopic dermatitis. Complications of atopic dermatitis such as secondary infection and ophthalmic disease, as well as legal aspects, are presented in detail. Most importantly, an abundance of high-quality colored clinical images is provided which convey the subtleties of dermatological diagnosis in relation to the above conditions.

The book serves as a reference for experienced dermatologists and may be used as a comprehensive text by dermatology residents and primary care practitioners with an interest in dermatology. It will also be extremely useful for allergists who may be confronted with atypical dermatological presentations of eczema or simulators of atopic dermatitis. After reading this book the reader should feel knowledgeable in diagnosing the disorders presented herein and in understanding the medical literature on atopic dermatitis and eczematous disorders. The editors are greatly appreciative of the kind participation of our contributors, among whom are international authorities in their respective disciplines.

We have dedicated the book to our teachers, Raúl Fleischmajer, MD, Irwin Kantor, MD, and Morris H. Samitz, MD, who, although no longer with us, remain in our hearts and memories. They taught us clinical dermatology and inspired us throughout our careers.

Raúl Fleischmajer, a remarkable clinician–scientist, was an expert on collagen, the basement membrane, xanthomatosis, and scleroderma. Born in Argentina, he originally trained in psychiatry but went on to become a clinical and research dermatologist. He served as the Chief of Dermatology at Hahnemann Medical College, and then went on to become Chairman of the Department of Dermatology at the Mount Sinai School of Medicine for 17 years. During his tenure he expanded the department and left a legacy of excellence. He authored over 150 papers and book chapters, and wrote or edited several texts.

Irwin Kantor was the *Sage* of the Mount Sinai Dermatology Department who trained generations of residents and students for half a century. An amiable role model and teacher with an irrepressible sense of humor, Dr Kantor imparted to us his profound knowledge of dermatological diagnosis and treatment from years of clinical experience and his voracious reading of the literature. One of us (DR) was lucky enough to share an office with D Kantor for over 10 years and will always cherish his friendship and wisdom.

Morris H. Samitz, father-in-law of one of the editors (SRC), was a beloved Professor of Dermatology at the University of Pennsylvania School of Medicine. A native Philadelphian, Dr Samitz learned the value of hard work early in life through helping his father deliver ice by horse and wagon, and through other jobs. He was a dermatologist with a wide range of interests, especially contact dermatitis and occupational dermatology. He published two books and over 100 papers and was the recipient of many awards including the Clark W. Finnerud Award of the Dermatology Foundation. His profound contribution to dermatological education at the

University of Pennsylvania is memorialized by the M.H. Samitz Lectureship in Cutaneous Medicine.

We also wish to express our gratitude to Michael Fisher, MD, who founded the Division of Dermatology at the Albert Einstein College of Medicine and who served as its chief for 37 years, for his superb clinical teaching, inspiration, and support. We thank Craig Rose and Carl Richmond for their editorial suggestions, Charlotte Cunningham-Rundles, MD, for her critical review and suggestions about congenital immune disorders, and Melvin Rosh, MD, for his review of the chapter on allergy. We are grateful to Warren Heymann, MD, and Alexander Kreuter, MD, for reading the entire text and providing their critical comments and suggestions.

Finally, our profound thanks to Jill Northcott of CRC Press for suggesting this project and for her unwavering support and infinite patience.

Donald Rudikoff, Steven R. Cohen,
and Noah Scheinfeld 2014

CHAPTER 1

THE HISTORY OF ECZEMA AND ATOPIC DERMATITIS

Douglas Altchek and Donald Rudikoff

There was a time when the word 'eczema' was going out of use in England, and it may be that it is coming into favour again because of the inevitable association of the word 'dermatitis' with workmen's compensation (Vickers 1952).

Eczema has been called the keystone of dermatology yet no other disease in the field has provoked such fierce controversy and dissent (Bulkley 1881). Rudolph L. Baer (1955) said that it was a disease 'about which a lively argument can be precipitated at the slightest provocation.' Among nondermatologists, it is a disease often misinterpreted and, among physicians, to quote Sulzberger, it 'serves as a trash basket into which nondescript itching odds and ends are often being thrown even by dermatologists who pride themselves on accuracy in other fields' (Sulzberger and Goodman 1936). He added, 'The subject of eczema is a morass in which many dermatologists are floundering about, and it is not astonishing that some allergists and immunologists who are beginning to attempt to enter here, have already begun to feel the insecurity of the ground beneath their feet.'

The word 'eczema' is used synonymously with 'atopic dermatitis' as well as many other types of dermatitis where nomenclature varies by medical specialty, geographic location, and time periods of history. With a bit of humor and a liberal use of quotes from the great masters of dermatology, this chapter provides the reader with historical sources from which the terms 'eczema' and 'atopic dermatitis' derive.

From the outset, the word *eczema* itself is confusing. Consider at least four different pronunciations: ek´sema, ek´zema, egze´ma, eg´zema. The term is derived from ancient Greek κ ξ ε μ α and literally means *the result of* (-ma) *boiling* (-ze) *out or over* (ec-). The word *atopy*, with which eczema is commonly associated, literally means *no* (a), *place* (top), *ness* (y). Sir Thomas More's name for the ideally perfect place, *utopia*, literally means 'no place' as well, further adding to the confusion.

Despite efforts to expunge eczema from the dermatology lexicon, it has persisted among physicians and the public. Self-help books devoted to the subject invariably use the term 'eczema' in preference to 'atopic dermatitis', a term with its own problems. A search of historical newspaper databases over the past 150 years reveals thousands of classified and display advertisements for patent medicines that claim to be remedies for eczema. The word has even been mistaken for a woman's name, as in the following excerpt from the 1898 *New England Medical Monthly* entitled 'Abortion dangerous in England' which reported:

> A member of a distinguished family in England telegraphed to a no less distinguished dermatologist: 'How can I abort eczema?' The police, getting wind of such a dispatch and thinking 'Eczema' was a woman's name, placed the gentleman under arrest. The tragedy itself was, however, aborted by a prompt explanation that ex-Emma and eczema were not the same (Anonymous 1898).

ECZEMA IN HISTORY AND LITERATURE

Atopic symptoms can be traced back to biblical times. The Hebrew word *tzaárat* was used in the book of Leviticus to describe a skin ailment, generally considered to be leprosy, but which may have been eczema, psoriasis, or other dermatoses. The term 'lepra,' derived from ancient Greek, refers to scaliness and, as Pye-Smith (1893) notes, 'No doubt many other cutaneous affections, obstinate chronic eczema, syphilis, lupus, and perhaps psoriasis were confounded with leprosy in ancient times'.

In the ancient Chinese medical classics, eczema is referred to as *jin yin chuang* (suppurative ulcerative lesion) (Liang 1988). The six external evils are external causes and spleen dampness is its primary internal cause, an obvious reference to the 'outside-in' and 'inside-out' pathogenic mechanisms that are currently in vogue (Elias and Steinhoff 2008). Blood heat and wind heat are secondary causes in the Chinese view.

Historical figures that may have had eczema include the Roman emperor Augustus, the eighteenth-century French physician Jean Paul Marat, Adolf Hitler, and Joseph Stalin (Mier 1975, Dotz and Jean Paul 1979, Montefiore 2005, Kershaw 2008). Mier (1975) quotes the Roman historian Suetonius (AD 69–140) in his description of Augustus: 'His body is said to have been marred by ... a number of hard, dry patches suggesting ringworm, caused by an itching of his skin and a too vigorous use of the scraper at the baths.' Suetonius notes that Augustus was subject to 'certain seasonal disorders: in early spring a tightness of the diaphragm; and when the sirocco blew, catarrh.'

Jean Paul Marat practiced medicine in London before he became a radical voice of the French revolution. He was murdered in 1793 by Charlotte Corday while sitting in his medicinal bath writing down the names of the deputies from Caen whom he intended to send to the guillotine (Mysticus 1920). According to Mysticus (1920), 'Throughout the last year of his life Marat had been suffering from a severe skin disease, *une maladie dartreuse,* which he had contracted during his concealment in the cellars and sewers of Paris. Hints have so often been made that his

complaint was of an unspeakably loathsome nature that the truth should be plainly stated, that he was afflicted with eczema and prurigo.' This retrospective diagnosis is considered to be highly speculative (Dotz and Jean Paul 1979).

The 'summoner' in Chaucer's *Canterbury Tales* is also afflicted with eczema (Chaucer [about 1370] 2006).

A summoner was with us in that place,
Who had a fiery red cherubic face,
For eczema he had; his eyes were narrow,
As hot he was, and lecherous, as a sparrow.

In fourteenth-century England, a summoner was a religious court employee who summoned those suspected of offenses against church law.

Another controversial personage who may have suffered from eczema rubrum was the charlatan and pretender to the throne of France, Eleazar Williams. Williams served as an Episcopal minister to the Oneida and Mohawk Indians in upper New York State.

Alfred Hardy, physician of the Hôpital Saint-Louis in Paris and champion of the diathetic basis of disease, asserted a predisposition to eczema among Jews since biblical times:

It is very frequent among the Jews; and generally of great gravity ... This predisposition seems to me to be inherent in the race, and it is probably for this reason that Moses, that great hygienist, forbade to Israelites the use of pork, which especially favors cutaneous eruptions. (Dickinson 1891).

Even stranger are the bizarre treatments advocated for eczema. Perhaps the strangest example involves a Swedish fisherman who suffered an unbearable itch from eczema. Upon the recommendation of a friend, he smeared fresh pig dung all over his body and, as if that were not enough, the fisherman became so aroused by seeing a sow in heat that his subsequent actions almost landed him in jail for taking animal husbandry a little too far (Rydström 2003).

EVOLUTION OF THE TERM 'ECZEMA'

The word *eczema* was first used by Aetius of Amila (AD 543) to denote 'hot and painful phlyctenae which do not ulcerate' (Wigley 1953). Phlyctenae are small blisters or pustules but as used by Aetius were probably furuncles (Unna 1903, Agnes 2006). The term 'eczema' is nowhere to be found in Daniel Turner's *De Morbis Cutaneis* (1731) or Seguin Henry Jackson's *Dermato-pathologia* published in 1792, and remains absent from the medical literature until Willan's text published in 1797 (Turner 1731, Jackson 1792, Unna 1903). Robert Willan (1757–1812) (**Fig 1.1**) developed a classification of skin disease drawn from a treatise by the Viennese physician Joseph Plenck (Patalay *et al.* 2008). Establishing eight orders of cutaneous disease, the fourth order included seven *vesicular (*or *bullous)* genera – varicella, vaccinia, herpes, rupia, miliaria, eczema, and apthae. Willan's ideas were introduced to the French by Laurent-Theodore Biett (1781–1840), who had visited with Willan's student, Thomas Bateman (1778–1821) at the Public Dispensary in London (Beeson and Pierre 1930, Tilles and Wallach 1999). Except for Alibert, who remained hostile to Willan's ideas, the majority of nineteenth- and twentieth-century French dermatologists embraced his classification. The groundbreaking system of Willan and Bateman, based on primary lesions, rather than symptomatology or clinical course, remains a cornerstone of modern dermatological diagnosis.

Willan and Bateman defined eczema as 'an eruption of *minute vesicles*, non-contagious, crowded together; and which from the absorption of the fluid they contain form into thin flakes or crusts ... the effect of irritation, whether *internally* or externally applied' (Bateman 1836). Lesions had an affinity for the inner thighs, axillae, inframammary area, and anus, lacked surrounding inflammation, and smarted rather than itched.

In a lecture to the Dermatological Society of Great Britain and Ireland in 1902, esteemed German dermatologist Paul Gerson Unna (1850–1929) summarized the history of eczema in the nineteenth century. Unna asserted that Willan's conception of eczema was limited to vesicular sunburn reactions, mercurial dermatitis and eczema impetiginoides, bearing little resemblance to the eczema of his European contemporaries at the turn of the twentieth century (Unna 1903). It was emphasized that Willan used 'internally' to describe the internal administration of mercury; and, areas of predisposition, especially the inner thighs and perianal area, were characteristic of mercurial dermatitis. As Willan stressed the absence of surrounding erythema and smarting rather than itching, Unna concluded that the great British master was not describing the eczema known to European practitioners of 1902. The presence or absence of vesicles was to become a fertile topic of debate in dermatology.

Unna (1903) credited the French physician Pierre Rayer (1793–1867) with the prevailing view of eczema. Born into tempestuous times, Rayer gained renown not only for his prowess in the field of dermatology but also for his work in kidney disease, eventually becoming physician to the king. He lived modestly. When an arrogant financier asked of Rayer, 'Is it true, Doctor, that the Roman physicians were all freed slaves?', he replied, 'Yes, but that was the time when Mercury was the god of bankers and thieves' (Beeson and Pierre 1930). Rayer (1833) wrote, 'Chronic eczema is always dependent on a peculiar

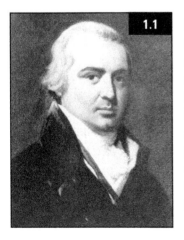

Fig 1.1 Robert Willan: the British physician created a classification of cutaneous disease that formed the basis for diagnosis based on primary lesions. (Reprinted from Crissey and Parish 1998. © 1998 with permission from Elsevier.)

organic disposition, which some pathologists suppose to be an alteration of the humors. This disease may continue for some months or several years' (Rayer 1833). Unna's main criticism of Rayer was the inclusion of Willan's mercurial and solar eczema under the banner of eczema.

With regard to other authors, Unna held Jonathan Green in high regard for building on the work of Rayer, with the addition of a *proper* or *constitutional* eczema (Unna 1903). He credits Devergie with 'having the courage to say, what all dermatologists ... knew ... that Rayer's eczema by no means always commenced with Willan's clear, clustered vesicles on noninflamed bases and ... often did not show vesicles in its whole course.'

If Unna was correct, it would seem ironic that the varieties of eczema discussed nowadays bear little relation to the eczemas of Willan and Bateman, namely mercurial dermatitis, vesicular eruption associated with sunburn, and eczema impetiginoides. In defense of Willan and Bateman, the conditions that we now consider to be eczema/atopic dermatitis were definitely included in their works but in different categories. As for eczema rubrum (darte squameuse humide of Alibert), Bateman clearly states: 'it is often associated with gastrointestinal inflammation, without any mercurial preparation having been taken' (Bateman 1836).

In 1933, the well-known British dermatologist Horatio George Adamson (1866–1955) defended the reputation of the great British masters. Although he thought that Willan's definition of eczema best fit 'dermatitis traumatica v. venenata (contact dermatitis),' Adamson decried the assertion that Willan and Bateman had not recognized what came to be accepted as eczema. According to Adamson, Willan and Bateman used the term 'impetigo' as a surrogate for eczema. Had impetigo not been *appropriated* for bacterial impetigo we would now be calling eczema by Willan's designation of impetigo and contact dermatitis would have retained the name eczema.

Willan and Bateman's impetigo was classified within 'humid or running tetters,' comprising several forms. At the time, a tetter was defined as a skin disease in humans or animals causing itchy or pustular patches, such as eczema or ringworm. Impetigo figurata corresponded to patchy eczema of the limbs (nummular eczema); impetigo sparsa was *dispersed* on the extremities, neck, shoulders, and even on the face, ears, and scalp. This form, they noted, 'in young subjects fixes itself in the flexures of the larger joints and ... is accompanied by intense itching ... .' Bateman described impetigo sparsa as 'not unfrequent in young children in whom it appears to be the sequela of porrigo larvalis, if indeed it be not the same disease ... . It occasionally supervenes to lichen' (Bateman 1836). Thus Bateman alluded to infantile eczema of the face and scalp, as well as its evolution into childhood eczema. Porrigo was a designation of skin diseases of the scalp and larvalis means mask-like.

INFANTILE ECZEMA

Although dermatologists clearly recognized the presence of oozing, crusted eruptions on the face and scalp of infants, they were not categorized as eczema according to Willan and Bateman's classification. Terms such as 'crusta lactea,' 'porrigo larvalis,' 'tinea granulata' (Alibert), and 'strophulus' were used to denote these eruptions. Sir Erasmus Wilson (1809–1884), the revered British dermatologist, Egyptologist, and President of the Biblical Archeology Society, perhaps best remembered for bringing the Egyptian obelisk *Cleopatra's Needle* to London, published the first description of *infantile eczema* (Wilson 1857, 1878, 1881). He recognized the chronicity of infantile eczema into later life. Wilson wrote, 'the crowning suffering of all occurs at night; the child is often frantic with itching, it scratches with all its force, digging its little nails into the flesh, while the blood and ichor run down in streams. At last, worn out with suffering and exhaustion, the child sleeps, probably to be awakened again several times in the night by a repetition of the same agony' and then added, 'it is nevertheless remarkable how little the strength and spirits of the child are affected ... in the morning, after a night of distress, the little thing is fresh and lively, eager for its food, and ready for the battle of the day; while the nurse or mother is languid and powerless, from watching and anxiety.' Of particular interest, Wilson's description of facial involvement mentions a thick discolored scab covering the child's face and he notes:

> This huge, unnatural mask covering the child's face suggested the term *larvalis*, given to one of his species of porrigo by Willan; only that, instead of porrigo larvalis, it should have been *eczema larvalis* or impetigo larvalis (1857).

MODERN DERMATOLOGISTS AND EARLY DEPICTIONS OF ECZEMA

A modern dermatologist attempting to read eighteenth- and nineteenth-century dermatological texts will be adrift in a sea of unfamiliar terminology, rendering unrecognizable conditions that likely existed from time immemorial. Wallach *et al.* (2005), using teledermatology and a consensus method known as the Delphi technique, posted 20 engravings from old texts on an internet site and queried experts in pediatric dermatology regarding images that most closely resembled atopic dermatitis. The experts concluded artistic representations of atopic dermatitis were first described under the names strophulus confertus, lichen agrius, porrigo larvalis, and eczema rubrum (**Fig 1.2**). Strophulus referred

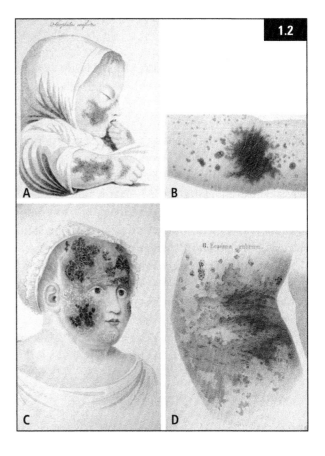

Fig 1.2 First representations of atopic dermatitis. (A) Strophulus confertus (Willan 1808); (B) lichen agrius (Willan 1808); (C) porrigo larvalis (Bateman 1817); and (D) eczema rubrum (Rayer 1835). (Reprinted from Wallach *et al.* 2005. © 2005 with permission from Elsevier.)

to a variety of papular eruptions in infants; lichen is an extensive papular eruption in adults, with lichen agrius being one of the seven types of lichen; porrigo refers to a contagious pustular eruption or in general to scalp eruptions (Wallach *et al.* 2005).

THE HIPPOCRATIC HUMORALIST DOCTRINE

The Hippocratic humoralist doctrine was the prevailing dogma of eighteenth- and nineteenth-century medicine (Farhi *et al.* 2010). It held that external skin disease reflected internal conditions. Hippocrates believed that the body contained four *humors*: the blood, the phlegma (lymph), the yellow bile, and the black bile. Dermatoses resulted from the elimination of noxious humors and were thus beneficial or else reflected a personal diathesis or predisposition to certain maladies. The term 'diathesis' was first identified in the writings of Hippocrates but gained great popularity at the beginning of the nineteenth century, especially in France (Ackerknecht 1982). In an 1812 French medical dictionary by Pariset and Villeneuve, 14 different diatheses are described and the term is defined as 'that state of the body which makes it acquire certain diseases.' The term 'diathesis' of course is still used today, ie, the *atopic diathesis*.

The French dermatologist Alfred Hardy (1811–1893) was the major proponent of the diathetic basis of disease. He applied the term 'dartres' to 'those chronic affections of the skin of "elementary" lesions which are non-contagious, ... are often transmitted hereditarily ... and which present for their principle symptoms, itching, and a disposition to invade new areas' (Hardy and Piffard 1868). Hardy noted that the word 'dartres' was cherished by the public to signify inveterate and constitutional affections of the skin. Accusing Willan and Bateman of having suppressed the term 'dartre,' he championed its continued use. The French physician Charles Caillault also considered that *eczema* and *lichen* were affections of the dartrous state (Caillault and Blake 1861).

The diathetic basis for disease implied to many physicians that topical treatment would 'drive in' the noxious process and cause severe morbidity or death. In Jonathan Turner's *De Morbis Cutaneis* (1731), it is written:

> Children, saith *Sim. Pauli,* are often troubled with an itching Humour, by Reason of their Voraciousness or continual Feeding which if you should go about to heal with Litharge, Quicksilver, Oil of Bays or Brimston, as is the Custom of Empiricks, and idle Women; you may, 'tis certain, quickly cure them of their itch, but you will as certainly put them into hazard of their Lives; because you thereby pollute their Blood and nervous Fluid, by driving back these Excrements into the Vessels, which Nature having separated, is endeavouring to throw forth.

The term 'empiricks' referred to quacks, charlatans, and practitioners who lacked proper qualifications and training (Nolosco 2004). Although physicians disdained empiricks, the populace often made use of their services. Goddard wrote in 1670, 'some Empiricks have stumbled upon very considerable and effectual Medicaments, wherewith, in some particular cases, they have outdone learned Physicians; and, by the Advantage of making their own Medicaments, they bear up, and will do, till they be outdone in the same Kind by such physicians' (Goddard 1670). Of course, considering the remedies mentioned in the above excerpt (litharge = lead, quicksilver = mercury), it is likely the patient would fare much better if nature took its course.

Belief that external treatment would prevent the elimination of the noxious humors, with potentially fatal results to the infant, became known as the *eczema death*. The term extended into the early twentieth century. Van Harlingen, a strong supporter of topical treatment and the use of restraints to prevent scratching, was aghast that some practitioners would allow a severe eczematous reaction to proceed for months without topical applications for fear of *driving it in* (Van Harlingen 1889). He wrote, 'I had thought such excuses were no longer made except by unprincipled quacks.'

NINETEENTH-CENTURY CONTROVERSIES

The nineteenth century witnessed a series of controversies over the concept of eczema and allied conditions. Were vesicles a requirement? Were papules, lichen, squames, and pustules somehow allied with eczematous conditions? Were eczema and dermatitis the same condition?

Willan's requirement for the presence of vesicles was supported by the great Viennese dermatologist Hebra only in cases of acute eczema (Ravogli 1918). Ernest Bazin (1807–1878) of the Hôpital Saint-Louis maintained that, although vesicles might not be visible in acute eczema, they might be detected using a magnifying glass or oblique light. The eminent British dermatologist Tilbury Fox (1836–1879) considered eczema a catarrhal or secretory condition, the special feature of the secretions being that they *stiffened linen* and dried into light yellow crusts. Tilbury Fox believed that there was a tendency to form vesicles (Neligan 1866, Tilbury Fox 1879). Edgar A. Browne, Surgeon to the Liverpool Dispensary for Skin Diseases (1870), wrote:

> The so-called modern school ... composed of the followers of the great Hebra, contend ... that a whole group of affections hitherto carefully differentiated must be regarded as simply varieties of one – Eczema – and ... that it cannot be regarded as essentially vesicular in its nature, inasmuch as examples referrible [sic] under the old classification to the papular, pustular and squamous groups must be admitted.

He envisioned the following scenario:

> For instance, our pity and mirth are alike moved, by learning that when a Willanist, deeply imbued with the belief that Eczema must exhibit vesicles, has a case under his notice, it is quite painful to observe how he strains his eyes in quest of them, when perhaps none are to be found; or how pleased he is if, on a surface ... covered with innumerable papules, one small vesicle is at last detected, or even a papule translucent on its summit, so as to give it the air of a vesicle! Certainly a most misguided man; for, note how he seems to make his diagnosis first and then to search for his favourite lesion, a ... procedure, I admit, sufficient to justify all the scorn that can be heaped upon it.

Ferdinand Hebra (1816–1880) intended to clarify the question of eczema. He and his student Kaposi (1895) considered that eczema was of external origin and merited topical treatment (Farhi *et al.* 2010). After showing that croton oil could induce a reaction indistinguishable from eczema, he concluded that eczema must be externally caused.

The well-regarded New York dermatologist Walter James Highman (1879–1934), who did not have the highest regard for Hebra's talents as a *bacteriologist* and *histologist*, found it odd that the great Viennese master could 'maintain the doctrine of the independence of the skin from the rest of the body' after introducing arsenic, an internal medicine for a type of lichen (Highman 1921). Highman anglicized the spelling of his name from Heimann in 1918 after serving in World War I. He summarized the debate:

> While the Teutons were endeavoring to restrict all dermatoses to the skin, the French had, for nearly a century, been approaching the problem by another avenue. As early as 1777 Lorry, in his *Tractatus de Morbis Cutaneis*, under the Hellenic influence of the humoral causation of disease, sought to explain the etiology of many skin diseases by *arthritism*: the Frankish tendency to correlate all given effects with definite causes, and to find for each an antidote or specific, led the Parisians

and their followers far afield. Thus while the Germans were cataloging dermatoses without reasoning backwards from them, the French were studying etiology without reasoning forwards.

Nevertheless, Hebra (1868) went further. He also recognized lichenoid lesions in eczema but was clear to differentiate the lichenoid papules of eczema from those of lichen planus.

The chief characteristic of the papules of true lichen is … they undergo no transformation to vesicles, pustules or crusts … In eczema, on the contrary, we see its papules always filled with fluid, many even while they still appear hard elevations.

The simmering debate about the nature of eczema finally erupted when Harvard dermatologist, J.C. White (1833–1916) commented on the claim by British dermatologist and founder of St John's Hospital for the Diseases of the Skin, John Laws Milton (1820–1898) that he, Milton, had been the first to assert that eczema was not a vesicular disease even before Hebra. White (1870), in a letter to the *American Journal of Syphilography and Dermatology*, wrote:

When I read in Wilson's Journal Milton's claim to have first defined and published the views of the Vienna school with regard to the pathology of eczema, I looked upon it as an ordinary manifestation of English conceit in such matters.

White added that he had personally heard Hebra express these views in Vienna in 1856 and 1857 and that in fact Hebra had published them in the *Allegemeine Weiner Medizinische Zeitung* for February 8, 1859 (White 1870). The editor of the journal wrote, 'We have yet to learn that Dr White is privileged, or in a position scientifically, to speak of English dermatologists as he does.' Responding to this

in a second letter, White wrote, 'I make no comment on this somewhat superfluous editorial personality, nor do I think it necessary to offer evidence as to the correctness of my judgment in a matter based on historical record. Such claims on the part of English men of science, and especially among medical writers, are too well-known to those familiar with the history of modern inventions and discoveries.' The indefatigable Milton was of course hardly fazed by all of this and went on to publish on various eclectic topics including spermatorrhea, death in the pipe, the stream of life on our globe, and the laws of life and their relation to diseases of the skin (Black 2003).

Walter Heimann (Highman) (1916) commented:

If Willan had lived longer; if Biett and Biett's followers rather than Alibert and Alibert's school had dominated French dermatology; if Hebra and Kaposi had been internists rather than classifiers of dermatoses, and if Unna had never engaged himself with its bacteriological aspect, our understanding of eczema today would be clearer.

But Willan died too soon, Biett's views were heeded too late, Hebra and Kaposi made it their business to ridicule the *Willanists*, and Unna attempted to glorify the pathogenic role, in eczema, of a mythical microorganism – the morococcus. With regard to the 'German School' he wrote:

Among the Teutons, matters were shaping themselves differently from the way they were in France. Hebra and Neumann regarded the disease as purely cutaneous, eliminating with a wave of the hand the remotest possibility of its being in any way related to the general body economy. Unna endeavored to prove that it was caused solely by a bacterium, a view which received but little support in his own country and none at all elsewhere.

Two schools of thought were developing: one asserting that eczema was the same as dermatitis, the other stating that it could exist without external irritation. Sir Malcolm Morris (1847–1924) declared, 'If you know the cause it is not eczema; if you do not know the cause then it is' (Hazen 1915). He added, 'In no subject within the province of dermatology has the loose use of a term given rise to greater confusion than in the description of the various affections of the skin which have, at one time or another, been grouped under the head of *eczema*.' Morris held that vesicles appear in eczematous eruptions but that papules were sometimes the predominant lesion. However, the seemingly papular eruption, if examined closely with a lens, showed that minute vesicles could be seen on the top of each papule (Morris 1898).

In addition to the vesicle controversy and the debate as to whether dermatitis and eczema were the same entity, the notion was arising that papules, lichenification, and prurigo constituted an integral feature of eczema. In the late nineteenth century, descriptions of prurigo, lichenification, neurodermatitis, and chronic eczema would be incorporated into precursors of atopic dermatitis such as disseminated neurodermatitis and prurigo Besnier.

Von Hebra described a chronic, recurrent, highly pruritic skin disorder, beginning in infancy and extending into adulthood, which comprised itchy papules and was covered by a blood-colored crust (Taïeb *et al.* 2006). Lesions favored the extensor surfaces of the extremities and were highly impervious to treatment. Hebra ridiculed the multiplicity of causes championed by previous authors. For example, he regarded as untenable Alibert's attribution of prurigo to a *peculiar perversion of appetite*. In Vienna, Hebra wrote, 'the Tyrolese are great cheese eaters, Slavonians consume enormous quantities of cucumbers, Hungarians flavour everything with Paprika, and Jews are very fond of garlic; but none of these races contribute a larger portion of cases of prurigo to the general hospital than the Italians who live upon sweet meats and polenta' (Hebra 1868).

According to the French dermatologist Louis-Anne-Jean Brocq (1856–1928), this prurigo of Hebra began in infancy with urticaria and papular elevations on the lower extremities, and showed a tendency to become complicated with 'eczematizations, lichenifications and ganglional tumefactions' (Brocq 1896). Brocq considered Hebra's prurigo 'the one dermatosis worthy of the name prurigo' and noted that resistance to that opinion in France, based on the common usage of the word 'prurigo' for other conditions, had caused some to adopt the moniker *prurigo of Hebra* to refer specifically to what Hebra had described. Morris (1912) contended that Hebra's prurigo had already been described previously 'though not clearly discriminated' by Willan under the name *prurigo agria* and by other French writers as *lichen agrius*. With regard to the confusion he wrote, 'As many dermatologists, so many views of prurigo.'

NEURODERMATITIS

Brocq created the concept of 'neurodermatitis' and classified the disease into two forms: localized and disseminated. 'Disseminated neurodermatitis' became a widely accepted name until the concept of 'atopic dermatitis' was introduced by Coca and Sulzberger in 1933.

Brocq and Jacquet, in their original article (1891), theorized that neurodermatitis was a nervous disease in both psychiatric and somatic senses. The following features were considered pathognomonic:

- Nervousness: tendency to furious rages, predisposition to weep, depressions, paraesthesia and hyperesthesia, alcoholism, globus hystericus, hemianesthesias, and attacks of hysterioepilepsy
- Constant itching, always preceding the visible changes of the skin
- Demarcation of the plaque, limited to the area of the preceding itching
- Skin changes in concentric zones
- Complete dryness of the lesions
- Hypertrophy of the papillae of the cutis, and
- Chronicity.

The word *neurodermatitis* was subsequently abused for the following decades.

The terms 'acute neurodermatitis' and 'wet neurodermatitis' were used for years. Another concept was the 'neurodermatitic reaction' which attempted to describe a histological response seen in atopic dermatitis, exudative dermatitis, and lichenoid chronic dermatitis.

Numerous physicians and laymen assumed that neurodermatitis was, indeed, a psychiatric disorder. This was at odds with the awareness of many dermatologists that the disease frequently appeared in people with a history of asthma, allergic rhinitis, and allergic diseases. In 1892, Besnier again called attention to the association of the disease with asthma, hayfever, and gastrointestinal disturbances.

PRURIGO BESNIER

Ernest Besnier's classic description of *prurigos diathésiques* was presented at the *Société Française de Dermatologie et de Syphiligraphie* in 1892 (Besnier 1892). His contribution was praised by the Danish dermatologist Holger Haxthausen (1892–1959) in 1925 when he wrote: 'Besnier was the first to separate the disease from the chaos of the prurigos' (Nexmand 1948). His entity, 'prurigo diathésique eczémato-lichénienne', had as its prime symptom pruritus, 'le symptôme premier et le premier symptôme est ... le prurit intense, rémittent, exacerbant à paroxysmes nocturnes, à rémission et à exacerbations saisonnières.' His description included the frequent onset in infancy with erythematous lesions, the papular and lichenified lesions in older individuals, the chronic course with seasonal fluctuations, and the association with hayfever and asthma (Nexmand 1948).

The association of eczema with asthma was not new. One of the first references to this association was made by Helmont in 1607 (Nexmand 1948). The American dermatologist Lucius Duncan Bulkley wrote in 1882:

Asthma has presented itself to me so frequently in connection with eczema, either in the persons affected or their immediate family, that I have come to look upon the complex state called asthma as in many instances but a condition of the pulmonary mucous tract similar to that found on the skin in eczema ... of the intimate connection between the two conditions.

Although the association of eczema and asthma had been noted by earlier authors, Besnier's conception of a diathetic condition beginning in infancy and continuing often into later life constituted a major synthesis in the field of dermatology. It is difficult to absolutely confirm that Besnier considered infantile eczema as part of the spectrum. He wrote, 'dans le premier age, ce peut être l'une quelconque des nombreuses variétés des erythemes infantiles, des urticaires et des pseuro-lichens, ou l'une des formes d'eczématisation ou de lichénisation de la peau que le vulgaire réunit sous le nom de gourmes.' Crissey and Parrish translate this as: 'In infancy it may be any one of the numerous varieties of infantile erythemas, the urticarias, or pseudolichens, or one of the forms of eczematization or lichenification of the skin commonly known as milk scab' (Crissey and Parish 1981). They considered that he indeed meant infantile eczema. It is curious that he did not specifically mention infantile eczema, which had been clearly defined by Erasmus Wilson, but included several infantile conditions. As Besnier must have been aware of Wilson's work, perhaps he preferred his own terminology.

In the early twentieth century the connection with asthma was gradually regarded as a state of hypersensitiveness known as atopy, a term coined by Coca and Cooke (with the help of the linguist Edward D. Perry of Columbia University) in 1923 (De Benedetto *et al.* 2009). Blackfan (1916) subsequently demonstrated hypersensitivity to proteins in 22 of 27 eczema patients using cutaneous and intracutaneous testing.

Thus the confusing terms of the nineteenth century, such as strophulus confertus, dartre, porrigo larvalis, lichen agrius, and eczema rubrum were replaced by a new set of confusing terms. Besnier spoke of 'prurigo diathésique,' Rost preferred 'exudative eczematoid,' Stokes favored 'hay fever–asthma eczema,' and Blumenthal and Jaffe referred to 'allergic neurodermatitis.'

ATOPIC ECZEMA (DERMATITIS)

In 1933, Wise and Sulzberger (**Fig 1.3**) suggested the name 'atopic dermatitis' which was thought to avoid the confusion between allergic and nonallergic true eczemas. Actually this was not the first use of the term 'atopic' for this condition. Abraham Walzer (1883–1965), a Brooklyn dermatologist discussing a lecture delivered by Arthur F. Coca to the New York Academy of Medicine on December 6, 1928, on the skin as a 'shock organ,' used the term 'atopic eczema' several times in his discussion (Clayton and Coca 1929, Walzer 1929). Even in 1934 Sulzberger and Coca recognized that the stigmata of atopy were not present in every case of atopic dermatitis (Baer 1955). Baer wrote:

> In these cases, which form a small minority, there exists a paradoxical situation: the name atopic dermatitis, which obviously presupposes the presence of *atopy*, has to be used as a morphologic clinical diagnosis despite the fact that none of the other features of atopy can be found.

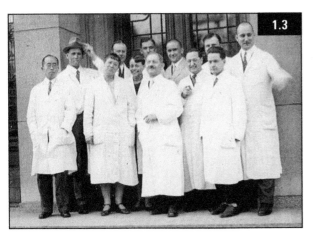

Fig 1.3 Sulzberger (wearing hat), who had done poorly at Harvard, was helped by Dr Bruno Bloch (front, center). (From the collection of Douglas Altchek, MD.)

SHOULD THE TERM 'ECZEMA' BE DISCARDED?

Use of the word 'eczema' has not only persisted but has remained a conundrum in the American dermatological literature. At the turn of the twentieth century, the noted American dermatologist James Nevins Hyde (1840–1910) wrote, 'The word eczema in the mouth of the expert has become a feature of the language of the street, of the advertiser, of the charlatan' (Hyde 1904). In 1935, Sutton (1916) stated, 'It is not possible at this time to formulate a satisfactory definition of this disorder, or to state precisely what the term includes and does not include.' This argument has fueled vocal proponents of eliminating the term altogether (Ackerman and Ragaz 1982). Although some authors agree with this line of reasoning, there are highly regarded dermatologists who oppose this argument. Sulzberger's colleague Rudolf Baer (1982) wrote, 'Rational physicians still use these seemingly irrational and misleading names, because they are universally known and serve a highly useful purpose. Even when better designations become possible, old misleading names are often not discarded for newer better ones because they still serve a purpose and because it is difficult to obtain quickly worldwide acceptance of such improvements'. Morris Leider (1982), the dermatological lexicographer and philologist, wrote, 'There is nothing wrong with the word *eczema*; the wrong is with those who never learned or thought out its meaning.' Sulzberger wrote, 'Eczema is a time-hallowed, fundamental, and broad-based term. Such terms are often the most difficult to define – e.g. love, joy, happiness, truth, good, evil, itch, pain – and today even life or death' (Sulzberger 1982).

Eczema remains, however, a clinical benchmark and a challenge of definition and therapeutics.

TREATMENT

At the annual meeting of the American Medical Association (AMA) in 1881, the previously mentioned Dr J.C. White of Boston presented a paper entitled 'Some of the causes of infantile eczema and the importance of mechanical restraint in its treatment' (Anonymous 1881, White 1881). Based on a large series of patients at the Massachusetts General Hospital he said that the prime factor in the treatment was prevention of scratching. White described a system of swathing in a pillowcase and the 'wonderful results' associated with this *strait-jacket* treatment. He used the AMA platform to advance a preposterous theory that the presence of a grandfather in the house was the first thing that needed to be eliminated. Dr Ulrich of Pennsylvania responded that in a long professional career he had never used a system of restraint in these cases, and that he would prefer to knock the little patient on the head at once rather than submit it to the tortures of Dr White's straitjacket (Anonymous 1881). Yet even in *Kerley's Practice of Pediatrics*, published in 1919, the use of restraint devices is advocated in infants (Kerley 1919) (**Fig 1.4**).

Jay Schamberg (1870–1934), in his text, was enthusiastic about the use of restraints. He wrote in 1908:

> A matter of great importance is the prevention of scratching. When this cannot be accomplished by the use of masks and bandages, it must be effected by some form of physical restraint. Often it will suffice to place padded mittens or bags on the hands; in many instances it will be necessary to place splints upon the arms to prevent the child from scratching its face. The immobilization of the elbows may be conveniently accomplished by bandaging a pasteboard cylinder around the arms.

Historically, countless remedies have been advocated for the treatment of eczema. Older remedies dating to biblical times, such as olive oil and lamb suet, were less scientific than later treatments but probably did less harm. Warm porcine or bovine blood has been recommended for the treatment of eczema in American folk medicine (Hand 1980).

Later remedies such as intravenous calcium gluconate, crude liver extract, bacterial vaccines, and autohemotherapy used through the 1960s were probably counterproductive. Tranquilizers were widely used because it was commonly believed that stress played a major role in the etiology of eczema. Phenobarbital, reserpine, and thorazine were used on a grand scale. Although systemic antibiotics did play a role in some cases of impetiginized eczema, their widespread prophylaxis has remained questionable.

Before the advent of antibiotics and steroids, the mainstay of treatment consisted of internal treatment, diet, and local treatment. This evolved over centuries but was still used until the late 1930s. Purgatives and laxatives, such as calomel, castor oil, rhubarb, and cascara, were routinely given. Vegetarian, elimination, and restrictive diets were used with little uniformity of practice. Roentgenotherapy of the spinal region was advocated in chronic eczema with lichenification. Sulzberger stated with regard to adults, 'Local roentgen therapy is the sovereign remedy and often brings quick results, particularly in the first few attacks' (Sulzberger and Goodman 1936). Local treatments consisting of pastes, ointments, or lotions were used. Their main components were zinc, calamine, rose water, bismuth, tar, lanolin, salicylic

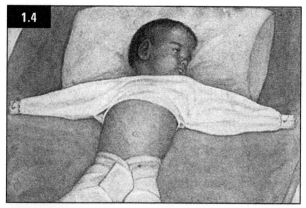

Fig 1.4 Thomas' modified strait-jacket for preventing infants from scratching. (Reprinted from Kerley 1919.)

acid, and sulfur. Compounds were often concocted extemporaneously by dermatologists in a proprietary fashion.

Before the advent of corticosteroids, Sulzberger favored the use of tar ointment as the most effective agent for the treatment of infantile facial eczema (Sulzberger 1939). The tar ointment was recommended for 1–3 days followed by a facemask application of yellow borated petroleum for 24 hours. This procedure was repeated several times as necessary. The efficacy of topical compound F (hydrocortisone) for infantile eczema was first reported by Witten and Sulzberger almost 60 years ago and changed the course of dermatological treatment (Sulzberger and Witten 1952, Witten *et al.* 1954) (**Fig 1.5**).

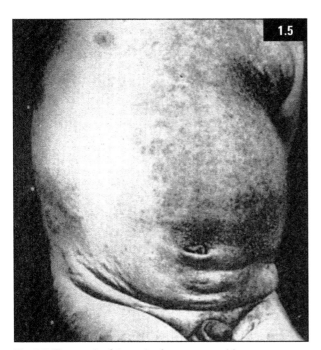

Fig 1.5 The result of 1 week of treatment with hydrocortisone ointment on the right side and the control ointment on the left. The patient originally presented: a generalized erythematous maculopapular eruption with considerable oozing and crusting. (Reprinted from Witten *et al.* 2005. © 1954 American Medical Association. All rights reserved.)

Another issue that has arisen on occasion is: Which specialty is best suited to treat eczema? Citing the importance of digestive issues in many cases of eczema, Fritz Talbot (1918), a pediatrician, wrote:

> Sufficient knowledge of metabolism, digestion, and dietetics in infancy and childhood can only be attained by those who make a special study of the diseases of children, and the knowledge of facts necessary for a complete understanding of the processes of digestion is attained only after many months of study and experience, while the number of external applications which are of any real value in the treatment of eczema in infancy or childhood are so few that they can be learned in a short time … Eczema in infancy and childhood, therefore, is best placed in the specialty of pediatrics.

There are often differences of opinion regarding the role of allergy between dermatologists and allergists. Dermatologists spend hours explaining to parents the importance of bathing practices, use of emollients and topical corticosteroids, avoidance of infection, and stress reduction, and add as an afterthought that in rare instances allergy to foods may play a role, to which parents immediately reply, 'What is he allergic to, Doctor?'

A recent study of 160 patients found that nurse practitioners provided a comparable level of care to that provided by a dermatologist in terms of the improvement in the eczema severity and quality of life outcomes (Schuttelaar *et al.* 2010). Moreover, parents often expressed greater satisfaction with the care provided by a nurse practitioner.

CONCLUSION

Controversy with regard to eczema persists. The concept of intrinsic and extrinsic atopic dermatitis analogous to similar delineations of asthma has brought about a new debate on nomenclature (Bos 2002, Hanifin 2002). This includes intrinsic atopic eczema, extrinsic atopic eczema, nonallergic atopic eczema, nonatopic flexural eczema, and atopic eczema/dermatitis syndrome (AEDS) and atopiform dermatitis. So, for example, when patients have an 'intrinsic' defect causing them to produce allergen-specific IgE, does it make sense to say they have 'extrinsic' atopic eczema (Bos *et al.* 2010)?

Nowadays the debate has shifted from noxious humors to inflammatory cytokines and genetic (diathetic?) barrier defects. We speak of *outside-in* (corneocentric) and *inside-out* (immunocentric) views of atopic dermatitis and various authors advocate barrier repair therapy, whereas others hope for a *magic biological bullet* to reverse the unending inflammation. Arsenic is replaced by cyclosporine (ciclosporin), tar by topical corticosteroids and topical calcineurin inhibitors, and roentgen therapy by narrowband ultraviolet (UV) UVB and UVA1. The term 'eczema' is entrenched in colloquial and medical parlance and is likely to remain so for years to come. We may look back on the great practitioners of dermatology, appalled by their treatments and theories. However, before poking fun at their foibles, it is prudent to remember that these pioneers were devoted to and adored by their patients. One hopes that history will treat us with similar forbearance and respect for accepting the challenges posed by this 'out-of-place' disease.

CHAPTER 2

THE EPIDEMIOLOGY OF ATOPIC DERMATITIS

Patrick O. Emanuel, Noah Scheinfeld, and Hywel C. Williams

INTRODUCTION

The epidemiology of atopic dermatitis (AD) has received less attention than its pathophysiology and treatment. As AD is a dynamic disease with genetic and environmental influences, an understanding of its epidemiology is essential, especially to identify risk factors that, when modified, may ultimately prevent disease. Possibly as a result of an increased incidence of this disease, scientific interest in the epidemiology of AD has increased since the late 1980s (Williams 1992, Williams *et al.* 2008). Quality-of-life issues and the significant financial, social, and personal costs have also elevated the importance of studying AD.

Epidemiology has traditionally focused on the incidence or prevalence of a disease and the relationship of these rates to age, sex, and geography (Holden and Parish 1998). Epidemiology now also focuses on disease risk factors and evaluating the interventions that can prevent and treat the disease (Hennekens and Buring 1987). All of these metrics are important in assessing AD.

As atopic dermatitis is a product of genetic and environmental factors, it is not surprising that estimates of its prevalence vary widely across the world (**Fig 2.1**) (Odhiambo *et al.* 2009). As morphology (varying from acute vesicular to chronic lichenification), body distribution, and the time course of this disease are so variable, AD is also difficult to define. Consequently, comparative estimates of AD prevalence have been difficult to interpret. It is through large collaborative studies such as the International

Study of Asthma and Allergies in Childhood (ISAAC) that we owe much of our knowledge of the global prevalence distribution of AD (Odhiambo *et al.* 2009). It is possible that, as our understanding of the genetics of barrier function and immunological dysfunction is improved, different subtypes of AD will be identified. Continuing epidemiological studies will allow new insights into the causes, prevention, and treatment of these newly recognized variants.

As stated in most texts, a significant challenge to identifying the causes of AD relates to the lack of a standardized disease definition that can be applied over different population surveys. 'Objective' tests, such as the raised total or specific immunoglobulin E (IgE) and skin-prick tests, are often included in stricter definitions of atopic dermatitis, but using these tests may exclude a significant percentage of individuals with the cutaneous phenotype (Schäfer *et al.* 1999, Böhme *et al.* 2001, Flohr *et al.* 2004). Over-reliance on laboratory measures such as IgE in sick, hospitalized individuals may reflect epiphenomena related to severe disease. Restricting the study of community-based cases to only those who are sensitized and therefore have truly 'atopic' dermatitis may be unwise until a clearer understanding of the role of IgE in disease expression becomes clearer and better disease markers are found (Stranegård and Stranegård 1978, Williams and Flohr 2006). Until better objective disease markers are discovered, clinical definitions must be used, however imperfect (Williams 2000b).

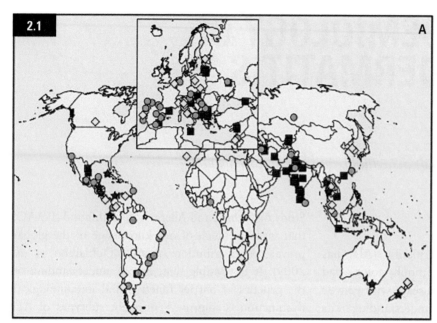

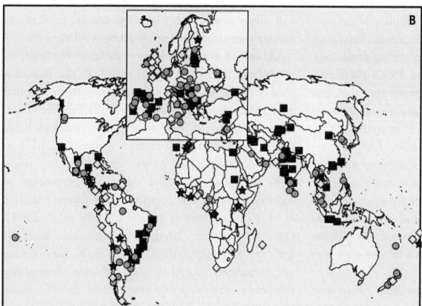

Fig 2.1 World maps showing prevalence of current symptoms of eczema for the age group 6–7 years (A) and 13–14 years (B). Each *symbol* represents a center. *Blue squares* indicate prevalence of <5%, *green circles* indicate prevalence of 5% to <10%, *yellow diamonds* indicate prevalence of 10% to <15%, and *red stars* indicate prevalence of 15% or more. Europe is shown in greater detail in the inset section. (Reprinted from Odhiambo *et al.* 2009. © 2009 with permission from Elsevier.)

Clinical definitions remain inexact. The literature contains various methodologies including questionnaire-based studies (some of which rely on maternal report of 'eczema'), a history of doctor-diagnosed AD, and the results of a doctor's examination (Williams 1999). Others such as the International Study of Asthma and Allergies have opted for symptom-based definitions that avoid disease terms such as AD, the use of which can change according to fashion (Williams *et al.* 2008). Inter- and intraobserver variability in documenting physical signs is another factor that can compromise results. Additional confusion has also resulted from diverse studies using different age groups and varying time periods for reporting symptoms (Williams 2000a).

DISEASE CLASSIFICATION SCHEMES

Different disease classification schemes have been proposed and used in the AD epidemiology literature. The diagnostic criteria of Hanifin and Rajka (1980) for AD represented a milestone in establishing the clinical syndrome of the disorder. Some investigators, however, have questioned the accuracy of these criteria because using them in large-scale population studies is problematic (owing to their complexity and low specificity (Schultz Larsen 1993, Williams 2000b). A UK working party of 16 doctors proposed a minimum list of reliable diagnostic criteria for diagnosing AD based on a refinement of the original Hanifin and Rajka criteria (**Box 2.1**), which have been shown to be valid in both hospital-based and community-based surveys (Brenninkmeijer *et al.* 2008). These UK working party criteria exhibited an acceptable sensitivity (80%) and specificity (97%) when compared with a dermatologist's clinical diagnosis (Williams 2000b). In addition, the UK working party criteria can be applied easily, taking less than 2 minutes to administer. Only one of the UK working party's six criteria – visible flexural dermatitis – required training to ensure accurate assessment. A training protocol with quality control tests has been applied (Williams *et al.* 1995b) and is available free online at www.nottingham.ac.uk/dermatology/eczema/index.html (accessed October 12, 2011). The usefulness of the UK working party criteria has also been confirmed in various geographic settings, including Romania (Popescu *et al.* 1998), China (Gu *et al.* 2001), and Brazil (Yamada *et al.* 2002). One study of a Xhosa-speaking African population showed poor validity when compared with a dermatologist's diagnosis but this may have resulted from difficulties in translation and cultural differences. The one physical sign, visual flexural involvement, however, proved a useful tool, most likely because it is free from any linguistic confusion (Chalmers *et al.* 2007).

Despite the moderate success of the UK working party scheme for capturing prevalence data in diverse populations, there is still debate as to which criteria are the most effective in situations such as case–control or genetic studies. Interestingly, a study

---

Box 2.1   The UK diagnostic criteria for AD for use in epidemiologic studies
Must have:
   An itchy skin condition (or parental report of scratching or rubbing) in the last 12 months
Plus three or more of the following:
- History of involvement of the skin creases (fronts of elbows, behind knees, fronts of ankles, around neck, or around eyes)
- Personal history of asthma or hay fever (or history of atopic disease in a first-degree relative if child aged under 4 years)
- History of a generally dry skin in the last year
- Onset under the age of 2 years (not used if child aged under 4 years)
- Visible flexural dermatitis (this includes dermatitis affecting cheeks or forehead and outer aspects of limbs in children under 4 years)

Table 2.1 Diagnostic criteria for atopic dermatitis

CRITERIA LIST	REQUIREMENTS (NUMBER OF CRITERIA)
Hanifin and Rajka diagnostic criteria, 1980	3 major + 3 minor
Kang and Tian diagnostic criteria, 1989	1 basic + 3 minor
Schultz Larsen criteria, 1994	≥50 points
Lillehammer criteria, 1994	Visible eczema + 4 minor
UK diagnostic criteria, 1994	Pruritus + 3 minor
ISAAC questionnaire, 1995	Score ≥ 3
Japanese Dermatology Association criteria, 1995	All 3 features
Criteria of Diepgen, 1996	≥10 points
Millennium diagnostic criteria, 1998	Allergen-specific IgE + 2 principal
Danish Allergy Research Centre (DARC), 2005	3 features

Adapted from Brenninkmeijer *et al.* (2008) reprinted with permission.

comparing the concordance of the different diagnostic criteria revealed acceptable agreement, except in mild cases. In that study, repeat examinations gave better agreement between the diagnostic criteria than just one examination (Johnke *et al.* 2005). In 23% of the published clinical trials concerning AD, the diagnostic criteria for the diagnosis of the disorder were not specified (Hoare *et al.* 2000). A recent systematic review has summarized the various diagnostic criteria used for AD and the performance of those criteria (Brenninkmeijer *et al.* 2008). The results are summarized in *Table 2.1* (Roguedas *et al.* 2004).

DESCRIPTIVE EPIDEMIOLOGY OF ATOPIC DERMATITIS

PREVALENCE AND INCIDENCE

For most epidemiological studies, measuring the prevalence of 1 year is recommended to account for seasonal and stochastic variation. In the USA, reported AD rates are 17% based on a history of at least one of four eczematous symptoms and 11% in those with empirically defined eczema (Hanifin and Reed 2007). A selection of recent prevalence surveys conducted throughout the world is presented in *Table 2.2*. These

Table 2.2   Worldwide prevalence surveys of atopic dermatitis conducted over the last 12 years

COUNTRY/ REFERENCE	PREVALENCE (%)	NUMBER	DEFINITIONS	AGE (YEARS)	YEAR
Denmark (Mortz et al. 2001)	21.3	1501	Lifetime prevalence based on questionnaire derived from Hanifin and Rajka's criteria and dermatologists' examination	12–16	2001
Brazil (Yamada et al. 2002)	13.2	4127	UK Working Party's diagnostic criteria. Survey of schoolchildren in Sao Paulo	6–7	2002
Germany (Werner et al. 2002)	10.5	4219	Lifetime prevalence based on survey of schoolchildren questionnaire that was developed out of Hanifin and Rajka's diagnostic criteria	5–9	2002
Singapore (Tay et al. 2002)	20.8	12 323	UK Working Party's diagnostic criteria and examination by dermatology nurse	7, 12, 16	2002
Turkey (Kalyoncu et al. 1999)	4.3	738	12-month survey based on questionnaire – doctor diagnosis	6–13	1997
Australia (Marks et al. 1999)	10.8	2491	Point prevalence based on UK Working Party's diagnostic criteria	4–18	1997
Romania (Popescu et al. 1998)	1.8	1114	Point prevalence based on UK Working Party's diagnostic criteria	6–12	1997
USA (Laughter et al. 2000)	17.2	1465	Lifetime prevalence based on questionnaire	5–9	2000
Hong Kong (Fung and Lo 2000)	6.8	1006	Point prevalence based on doctor's examination	6–21	2000
Japan (Yura and Shimizu 2001)	15–22.9	508 490	Lifetime prevalence based on doctor's diagnosis	7–12	2001

(continued)

Table 2.2	Worldwide prevalence surveys of atopic dermatitis conducted over the last 12 years *(continued)*

COUNTRY/ REFERENCE	PREVALENCE (%)	NUMBER	DEFINITIONS	AGE (YEARS)	YEAR
Finland (Lehtonen *et al*. 2003)	16.0	320	Cumulative prevalence (retrospective cohort study of well-baby clinic case records)	0–5	2003
Ethiopia (Haileamlak *et al*. 2005)	1.8	7915	12-month period prevalence UK Working Party diagnostic criteria (questionnaire)	1–5	2005
New Zealand (Purvis *et al*. 2005)	15.8	550	Point prevalence (questionnaire and physical examination) as part of a birth cohort study	At 3.5	2005
Germany (Worm *et al*. 2006)	8.4	1739	Self-reported eczema verified by telephone interview	18–65	2006
Denmark (Halkjaer *et al*. 2006)	44.0	356	Cumulative incidence (Hanifin and Rajka criteria; 6-monthly physical examination) in birth cohort born to mothers with asthma	By age 3	2007
South Africa (Chalmers *et al*. 2007)	1.0	3067	Point prevalence in a rural setting (dermatologist's examination)	3–11	2007
UK (Harris *et al*. 2007)	25.3	593	Cumulative incidence UK Working Party diagnostic criteria (questionnaire and physical examination)	By age 8	2007
25 European countries and USA (Harrop *et al*. 2007)	7.1 (2.2–17.6)	8206	Lifetime prevalence (questionnaire European Community Respiratory Health survey)	27–56	2007
USA (Hanifin and Reed 2007)	6.0	116 202	Empirically defined eczema (self-administered questionnaire)	All ages	2007
Japan (Tanaka K *et al*. 2007)	6.8	23 044	12 months period prevalence (International Study of Asthma and Allergies in Childhood Phase One questionnaire)	6–15	2007

Table 2.2 Worldwide prevalence surveys of atopic dermatitis conducted over the last 12 years *(continued)*

COUNTRY/ REFERENCE	PREVALENCE (%)	NUMBER	DEFINITIONS	AGE (YEARS)	YEAR
Japan (Tanaka K et al. 2007)	6.8	23 044	12 months period prevalence (International Study of Asthma and Allergies in Childhood Phase One questionnaire)	6–15	2007
Australia (Lowe et al. 2007)	28.7	443	Cumulative prevalence (parental recall of doctor diagnosis of eczema in children who also had at least one positive skin-prick test; birth cohort of high-risk children)	By age 2	2007
Taiwan (Lee YL et al. 2007)	6.1 boys 4.9 girls	23 980	12-month period prevalence of flexural eczema (International Study of Asthma and Allergies in Childhood Phase One questionnaire)	6–12	2007
Thailand (Sangsupawanich et al. 2007)	7.4	4021	Cumulative prevalence (questionnaire; population-based birth cohort study)	By age 1	2007
Norway (Smidesang et al. 2008)	15.9	390	UK Working Party Criteria (questionnaire and dermatologist's examination) in a random subsample from a larger cross-sectional study (n = 4784)	2	2008
Taiwan (Lee YL et al. 2008)	1.7	317 926	12-month period prevalence of flexural eczema (International Study of Asthma and Allergies in Childhood Phase One questionnaire)	13–15	2008
Denmark (Kjaer et al. 2008)	14.4	404	12-month period prevalence (Hanifin and Rajka criteria questionnaire and clinical examination) in a birth cohort study	6	2008

studies vary in statistical power and study design. The largest and most comprehensive – which used the same standardized criteria – involved over 700 000 children worldwide (Williams 1999, Odhiambo et al. 2009). These two global surveys, together with many other surveys, suggest that 5–20% of children in developed countries have AD (Kalyoncu et al. 1999, Marks et al. 1999, Popescu et al. 1998, Laughter et al. 2000, Fung and Lo 2000, Yura and Shimizu 2001, Mortz et al. 2001, Tay et al. 2002, Werner et al. 2002, Yamada et al. 2002).

AGE AND SEX

Atopic dermatitis is predominantly a disease of childhood. Although atopy can occur in elderly people, the lifetime prevalence of AD is considerably lower in them compared with prevalence among younger adults, which, in turn, is considerably lower than that seen in children (Wolkewitz et al. 2007). Studies from Norway and the UK suggest that prevalence figures are around 2% in people aged >20 years. Gender probably does not play a major role in disease predisposition. Although a slightly higher incidence in female cases has been previously noted in childhood (Schultz Larsen 1993), this has not been seen in all studies (Schäfer et al. 1999). Overall, the latest ISAAC study of over 700 000 children from 154 centers in 56 countries found that boys were at slightly lower risk of reporting eczema symptoms than girls (odds ratio 0.94 and 0.72 at ages 6–7 and 13–14 years respectively) (Odhiambo et al. 2009). The conventional expectation that up to half the cases of AD will abate with puberty, and that adult AD takes different clinical forms than those seen in childhood, requires more critical research-based support.

SEVERITY/MORBIDITY

Severe cases of AD are costly to treat (Mancini et al. 2008). Therefore the epidemiology of disease that includes an assessment of disease severity offers important data when considering AD public health impact. Studies indicate that severe cases are uncommon (Emerson et al. 1998, Williams and Strachan 1998). One study found that the severity distribution of AD (defined by a dermatologist) in 1760 children living around Nottingham, England, was 84% mild, 14% moderate, and 2% severe (Emerson et al. 2000). Another study showed that eczema severity was related to (1) disease onset during the first year of life, (2) concurrent occurrence of asthma, hayfever, or both, and (3) urban area habitation (Ben-Gashir et al. 2004), ie, factors that can indicate a worse prognosis include severe childhood disease, early onset, and concomitant or family history of asthma/hayfever (Popescu et al. 1998, Marks et al. 1999, Fung and Lo et al. 2000, Laughter et al. 2000, Yura and Shimizu 2001).

Owing to logistics, few studies have quantified the morbidity of AD. Using generic disability morbidity scores, AD was often deemed more severe when compared with other skin diseases in hospital studies (Finlay and Khan 1994). As expected, a negative impact on quality of life is directly related to disease severity (Ben-Gashir et al. 2002). The psychological morbidity associated with a lifetime of scratching, sleep loss, and the stigma of a visible skin disease can also affect both individuals and their families to a considerable degree (Daud et al. 1993, Lawson et al. 1998). Other studies have documented the considerable financial burden of AD (Mancini et al. 2008).

GEOGRAPHIC AND ETHNIC VARIATION

Prevalence figures for AD differ considerably between countries. Up to 20% of children in northern Europe and Australasia have AD, whereas the disorder is rare in some developing countries (Williams et al. 1999, Odhiambo et al. 2009). Some cities from developing countries undergoing rapid demographic transition, however, exhibit high prevalence (see **Fig 2.1**) (Williams et al. 1999, Odhiambo et al. 2009). The relative role of hygiene, climate, or other factors that account for such geographical variation must be more firmly established. Furthermore, there tends to be a gradient between urban and rural areas within the same country. A clear urban/rural gradient has, for instance, been demonstrated in studies conducted in Sweden and the UK (Kjellman *et al.* 1982, NcNally and Phillips 2000). It remains unclear which environmental factors may be responsible for this urban/rural gradient. A recent study showed that the variation is unrelated to mattress mite or cat allergen levels (Harrop *et al.* 2007).

Studies from communities with people of differing ethnic origin have been helpful in assessing ethnicity as a causative factor in AD. African–Caribbean children born in the UK and children of Chinese origin born in the USA and Australia are at an increased risk of developing AD in comparison to their (mainly) white peers in some studies (Worth 1962, Williams *et al.* 1995a, Mar *et al.* 1999). Other studies have failed to show such a strong ethnic variation (Burrel-Morris and Williams 2000).

Migrant studies offer a particularly interesting window into the sizeable role that the environment plays in the pathogenesis of AD and support the notion that urbanization and a 'western' lifestyle affect AD prevalence. Studies of Chinese immigrants in Hawaii, children from Tokelau who migrated to New Zealand, and African–Caribbean children living in London have demonstrated large increases in the prevalence of AD among the migrant children, when compared with similar genetic groups in their country of origin (Worth 1962, Waite *et al.* 1980, Neame *et al.* 1995, Burrel-Morris and Williams 2000). These results are convincing even when accounting for differences in medical practice and referral trends between countries (Neame *et al.* 1995).

SOCIAL CLASS AND FAMILY SIZE

Reported eczema has exhibited a strong positive social class gradient, with prevalence more common in higher socioeconomic groups (Golding and Peters 1987). Adults with more schooling appear to have a higher risk of atopic diseases (Williams *et al.* 1994). Whether this is due to higher reporting of eczema by mothers in advantaged socioeconomic groups or increased labeling by doctors is unclear, although similar trends have been found for children with examined eczema in a UK national birth cohort study for children in the 1970s (Williams *et al.* 1994). Similar trends were shown between increasing prevalence of examined eczema and home ownership.

On the other hand, a reduced risk of AD has been observed for children in larger families, especially if older siblings are present (Williams *et al.* 1992, Karmaus and Botezan 2002). Similar findings have been reported for hayfever, asthma, skin test reactivity, and allergen-specific IgE levels (von Mutius *et al.* 1994). It has been suggested that these observations could be due to a reduction in maternal atopy with pregnancy, possibly secondary to fetomaternal cell trafficking and microchimerism (Williams 1992). It is also possible that this is due to more antigenic exposure when more people live in a household.

SECULAR TRENDS

There is reasonable direct and indirect evidence to suggest that the prevalence of AD has increased two-to-threefold over the last 30 years (Williams 1992). Although some of this increase may be attributable to increased recognition of the disease, a recent global survey that used the same questions about eczema symptoms 5–10 years apart in the same centers found evidence of increasing prevalence, especially in children aged 6–7 years (Williams *et al.* 2008). It is possible that these data reflect a genuine increase in incidence because they have been detected in studies using objective measures such as skin-prick tests. Population-based longitudinal studies in Japan have illustrated an increased incidence and prevalence (Yura and Shimizu 2001).

NATURAL HISTORY

HISTORY OF DISEASE

There have been few studies investigating the history of AD in a longitudinal manner. Even fewer have focused on community-based cases, which can be assumed to be less severe than those studied in a hospital setting (Williams and Wüthrich 2000). Although one study suggests that approximately 90% of children are clear of their AD within 10 years (Vickers 1980), other studies of well-defined populations suggest that AD is a far more chronic condition with a clearance rate of around 60% by age 16 (Rystedt 1980, Williams and Strachan 1998). In the hospital setting, approximately 10% of adults still have AD (Schultz Larsen 1993).

ASSOCIATIONS

Asthma and hayfever (seasonal allergies) are strongly related to AD. Severe AD is more frequently associated with the development of asthma (Schultz Larsen 1993) and, conversely, the presence of asthma confers a poorer prognosis for clearance of AD (Williams and Strachan 1998). This makes sense because AD, asthma, and hayfever constitute the atopic triad. Associations with Crohn disease have been made, although they are controversial (Feeney et al. 2002). Certain forms of cancer have also been noted to be more prevalent in patients with AD, but this could be due to increased xerosis associated with underlying neoplasms (Sanchez-Borges et al. 1986, Kölmel and Compagnone 1988, Montgomery et al. 2002). A recent systematic review found that the incidence of glioma was lower in people with a history of AD (Linos et al. 2007). Other perplexing associations have been made in AD patients and require further investigation to determine their significance, such as an increased susceptibility to mosquito bites (Kölmel and Compagnone 1988), increased urinary tract infections and an increased tendency to headaches (Mortimer et al. 1993). An increased incidence of viral warts has been reported in children with AD; however, this was not supported by evidence gleaned from a large population study (Currie et al. 1971, Williams et al. 1993). Other infections have been associated with AD, perhaps due to impaired epidermal integrity increasing possible portals of entry for infection, including dermatophyte and herpetic infections (Svejgaard 1986).

RISK FACTORS

When discussing risk factors, it is important to distinguish risk factors for disease predisposition (such as filaggrin gene mutations), those for disease occurrence (such as altered gut microflora), and those that exacerbate established AD (such as contact with woolen clothing). Good scientific studies on exacerbating factors for established disease are virtually absent, so the risk factors discussed in this section refer to risk factors for disease occurrence in the main (Langan and Williams 2006).

GENETICS

Family studies, twin studies, and direct genetic analyses have revealed evidence for a genetic component in the pathogenesis of AD (Morar et al. 2006). Recent genetic advances with high-throughput methods for gene identification, such as DNA microarrays and whole-genome genotyping, help to further dissect these complex traits that are emphasized in other chapters. Recently, two loss-of-function mutations (R501X and 2282derl4) in the filaggrin gene (FLG) responsible for ichthyosis vulgaris, one of the most common inherited skin disorders of keratinization, have been reported to be strong predisposing factors for AD. This was subsequently confirmed in two population-based case–control studies and in a prospective birth cohort study (Palmer et al. 2006, Baurecht et al. 2007, Rodriguez et al. 2009). Beside these two most common filaggrin mutations occurring in European patients, diverse filaggrin mutations have been demonstrated in nonEuropean populations (Akiyama 2010, Chen et al. 2011).

FETAL PREDICTORS

As the vast majority of AD presents in the first year of life, and heritability is more strongly linked to the maternal side (Ruiz et al. 1992), it seems logical to hypothesize that environmental influences operating *in utero* or in early infancy may be important in determining disease expression. Preliminary studies have suggested that IgE responsiveness might be related to fetal nutrition (Godfrey et al. 1994), possibly resulting in thymic dysmaturity. Month of birth has been associated with subsequent house dust mite allergy in AD (Beck and Hagdrup 1987), and it has been shown that maternal exposure to allergens during pregnancy can prime T-helper cells *in utero* (Devereux *et al.* 2001). This may predispose to persistent specific allergen sensitivity and AD in the offspring (Warner *et al.* 1994). In addition, decreased interferon (IFN)-γ production is a consistent feature in neonates born to atopic mothers, and this might be the reason why the postnatal immune system of children who later in life develop allergic diseases remains skewed toward a type 2 T-helper cell milieu, predisposing to allergic inflammation (Macaubas *et al.* 2000). Furthermore, exposure to antibiotics *in utero* is associated with an increased risk of atopic dermatitis in a dose-related manner (McKeever *et al.* 2002). Frequent use of antibiotics within the first 2 years of life has a similar promoting effect on the clinical expression of allergic disease (Farooqi and Hopkin 1998, Droste *et al.* 2000).

THE ROLE OF THE GUT MICROFLORA

Commensal microflora of the gut play a major role in educating the immune system of the newborn (Björkstén 1999). Several researchers note that the use of antibiotics both *in utero* and during early life directly influences the composition of the gut microflora. This, in turn, could prevent the normal shift from type 2 T-helper cell dominance at birth toward a type 1 T-helper cell-rich milieu, predisposing to allergic disease (Prescott *et al.* 1998). Indirect evidence comes from studies comparing the gut microflora in children with and without AD. Those without AD have significantly more lactobacilli but fewer enterobacteria than their counterparts with AD, and these changes precede the clinical manifestation of AD (Björkstén 2000). A change in gut microflora composition could not only change the stimulation of the infant's immune system across the intestinal mucosa but also enhance the exposure to allergens, further contributing to the development of allergic disease. Indeed, there is some evidence that the permeability of the gut mucosa is increased in atopic dermatitis (Majamaa and Isolauri 1996).

All of these results, however, need to be interpreted with caution. The normal composition of the gut microflora is still largely unknown, and longitudinal studies that sequentially measure gut microflora composition in people with well-defined disease are needed. The role of the gut microflora is also suggested by the fact that probiotics may prevent or be useful in the treatment of eczema although this remains controversial (Dotterud *et al.* 2001, Lee J *et al.* 2008, Boyle *et al.* 2009).

INFANT FEEDING

Although a history of breastfeeding is associated with a reduced risk of many diseases in infants and mothers, many of the data have been gathered from observational studies, so one should not infer causality based on these findings. Cluster randomized controlled studies done in developing countries on the effectiveness of various breastfeeding promotion interventions will provide a further opportunity to investigate any disparity in health outcomes as a result of the intervention.

Although studies have shown increased risk after exposure to solid foods during the first 4 months of life (Forsyth *et al.* 1993, Fergusson and Horwood 1994), these studies lack clear criteria to determine cases of AD. It has been hypothesized that breastfeeding has a protective effect in the development of AD, but this has not been supported in other studies (Harris *et al.* 2001, Kramer *et al.* 2001, Kull *et al.* 2002, Schoetzau *et al.* 2002, Yang *et al.* 2009). These discrepancies may reflect variations in individual breast milk composition or other factors.

Although longer duration of breastfeeding and later introduction of solid foods are both recommended for preventing asthma and allergic disease, evidence to support these recommendations is controversial. In one study, longer duration of breastfeeding and later introduction of solid foods did not prevent the onset of asthma, eczema, or atopy by age 5 (Mihrshahi *et al.* 2007). Although a large study indicated a history of breastfeeding was associated with a reduction in the risk of developing atopic dermatitis, a more recent study suggested that breastfeeding increased the risk of eczema (Ip *et al.* 2007, Giwercman *et al.* 2010).

THE HYGIENE HYPOTHESIS

Based on the observation that atopic dermatitis is less common among children growing up in larger families and with older siblings, it has been speculated that certain pathogens might protect against atopic dermatitis and other forms of allergic disease (Strachan 1989). This concept has been supported by a reduction in allergic disease through early day care attendance and early regular contact with animals, for example, in children growing up on farms (von Mutius 2002). However, studies on the protective effects of day care focused entirely on respiratory allergies. For exposure to farm environments, statistically significant protective effects were found only for asthma and hayfever, not for AD (Lewis 2000). Whereas common childhood infections and routine immunizations do not appear to exercise a protective effect on allergic disease (Strachan 2000), tuberculosis, hepatitis A, and certain endoparasitic infestations, such as hookworm and schistosomiasis infestation, have been shown to be partly protective against asthma and allergen hypersensitivity measured by skin-prick test (Yazdanbakhsh et al. 2002). Also, an inverse association between domestic exposure to endotoxin and atopy in childhood has been observed (Perzanowski et al. 2006).

These epidemiological findings are supported by results of immunological studies, indicating that anti-inflammatory cytokines, such as interleukin (IL)-10 and transforming growth factor-β, induced by microbial and parasitic disease, can downregulate allergic tissue inflammation as a consequence of an altered balance of type 1, type 2, and regulatory T-helper cells (Strachan 1989). So far, studies have focused on asthma; good data for the potential links between the above infections and atopic dermatitis are lacking (Flohr 2003). Some aspects of the farm environment, not just attributable to contact with livestock, appeared protective for respiratory and allergic conditions among children participating in a 4-H study (Dimich-Ward et al. 2006).

IRRITANTS AND WASHING

Unlike allergic rhinitis, clinically relevant allergens are seldom documented in AD, and irritants may be more prominent in triggering skin inflammation (Hanifin 1992). Low humidity, excessive exposure to soaps and other primary household irritants, and possibly airborne pollution may be important, directly by exacerbating skin disease, and indirectly by increasing vulnerability to sensitization (Riedel 1991). Excessive use of chemical household products and frequent washing were associated with an increase in AD in a UK contemporary pediatric population (Sherriff et al. 2002). The role of irritants might be played out against a background of impaired epidermal integrity, perhaps allowing these two factors together to provide a basis for AD.

INFECTION

The interplay of skin pathogens and inflammatory skin disease has received attention in the past decade. It is possible that skin infection is not just a secondary factor but also a facilitating factor in skin disease. The dry skin so characteristic of AD patients favors colonization by *Staphylococcus aureus*, an organism that is implicated in maintaining cutaneous inflammation, as well as being capable of inciting allergic responses in such individuals (Ong et al. 2002). Some studies suggest a possible role for AD exacerbation by pityrosporum yeasts (Brehler and Luger 2001). Others suggest odontogenic infections as an exacerbating factor in the pathogenesis of some types of AD (Igawa et al. 2007).

ALLERGENS

House dust mite, cat dander, timothy grass, birch pollen, ragweed, and molds such as *Alternaria* spp., have all been implicated in AD exacerbations. Of these, house dust mite allergens seem the most significant. Measures such as eradication of household mite allergens (Friedmann 1999) or removal of patients to allergen-free environments have been associated with clinical improvement in those with

AD (Hoare *et al.* 2000). Cutaneous exposure to house dust mite allergen in individuals with AD has, moreover, produced a flare-up of disease (Norris *et al.* 1988, Tupker *et al.* 1996).

Other evidence to support the role of dust mite allergen in AD patients includes high titers of allergen Der_1-specific IgE antibody in most atopic eczema patients (Colloff 1992), development of eczematous lesions after allergen patch testing, and the presence of mite allergens bound to Langerhans cells and Leu-3a-positive T cells after allergen patch testing AD skin (Tanaka Y *et al.* 1989).

The lack of any clear exposure–disease relationship between allergens early in life and subsequent eczema argues against allergen exposure being a major factor causing AD. Lower levels of eczema in patients exposed to higher levels of house dust mites have been reported, which may imply that interventions aimed at reducing house dust mite in early infancy could paradoxically increase the risk of subsequent eczema (Harris *et al.* 2007).

INGESTED ALLERGENS

Dietary allergens probably have some role in allergic sensitization, especially in early life, and this might contribute to the severity of AD. Approximately a third of children with moderate-to-severe AD have IgE-mediated clinical reactivity to food proteins (Eigenmann *et al.* 1998). Food-specific T cells have been found in inflammatory skin lesions of AD patients (van Reijsen *et al.* 1998), and oral sensitization to certain foods can produce eczematous lesions on oral food challenge in patients with AD (Eigenmann *et al.* 1998). Egg protein is the most common protein involved.

The use of defined criteria of clinical diagnosis for the determination of AD's severity, along with the performance of objective allergometric tests at the time of inclusion, shows that the course of AD is significantly related to egg sensitivity. In addition, the average healing time is higher in egg-sensitive patients who have the most severe form of AD than it is in patients with mild or moderate forms of AD (Ricci *et al.* 2006).

FACTORS THAT ENHANCE VULNERABILITY TO SENSITIZATION

Experimental murine research suggests that exposure to atmospheric pollutants may enhance the IgE immune response (Wüthrich 1989). Passive smoking also has been linked to IgE responsiveness and increased incidence of asthma as a result of chronic airway inflammation and subsequent enhanced sensitization (Kjellman 1981). In fact, smoking may be one of the factors accounting for the increase in asthma seen in recent decades (Burney *et al.* 1990). It is more difficult to attribute atmospheric outdoor pollutants to sensitization and development of AD, as studies have failed to demonstrate a strong association (von Mutius *et al.* 1992, Behrendt *et al.* 1993, Bobak *et al.* 1995). Two studies failed to demonstrate an association between AD prevalence and exposure to outdoor air pollutants such as sulfur dioxide, heavy metals, and traffic (Dotterud *et al.* 2001, Yura *et al.* 2001). Indoor pollutants appear, however, to be risk factors for AD, including certain types of gas heaters and radiators (Schäfer *et al.* 1999) and exposure to tobacco smoke (Schäfer et 1997). Dampness has also been suggested as a risk factor (McNally *et al.* 2001). Given the high potential for confounding factors, difficulty isolating variables of exposure, and the lack of standardized disease definitions in these studies, further investigation is warranted to demonstrate specific pollutants' association with AD. The importance of factors such as water mineral content and pesticide residues (such as organophosphorus compounds that are secreted in breast milk) have yet to be examined fully in AD (Reichtová *et al.* 1999, Karmaus *et al.* 2001). Antioxidants, which have emerged as mediators of aspects of immune regulation, may play a role in the pathogenesis of AD and require further study (Seaton *et al.* 1994, Björkstén 2000). Another interesting potential risk involves parental factors such as oral contraceptive use and increased maternal age (Peters and Golding 1987, Xu *et al.* 1999).

CONCLUSIONS

Given that AD is such a common disease that has been increasing in prevalence, with significant social and economic impact, it is unfortunate that so little is understood about its distribution and causes. The interplay of genetics and multiple environment factors are probably crucial, and the full complexity of AD and its variants will hopefully be revealed with further research. The social class gradient, increasing incidence and increased frequency in genetically similar migrants who move to a developed country, argue strongly that environmental factors are critical in disease expression. Which environmental factors are most important, in what combination and in what order to different populations, is still unclear, but their discovery should lead to effective disease prevention strategies. Now that suitable disease definitions and outcome measures are available (Schmitt *et al.* 2007), further research must focus on identifying specific risk factors for AD and how they interact with each other and predisposing genetic factors. Such discoveries will bring us one step closer to the ultimate goal of preventing disease and reducing the impact of disease in those with established AD.

CHAPTER 3

CLINICAL ASPECTS AND DIFFERENTIAL DIAGNOSIS OF ATOPIC DERMATITIS

Donald Rudikoff, Diana Lee, and Steven R. Cohen

Atopic dermatitis (AD) is a pruritic, chronic, relapsing condition that usually begins in early infancy or childhood. Onset in adulthood is much less common but is reported to be as high as 13.6% in a study from Singapore and 24.5% in Nigeria (Tay *et al.* 1999, Bannister and Freeman 2000, Nnoruka 2004). The term 'atopic dermatitis,' introduced by Wise and Sulzberger (1933), incorporated infantile eczema and so-called generalized neurodermatitis into one clinical syndrome and emphasized the association with allergic rhinitis and asthma, and the presence of the immunoglobulin IgE. There is an active debate over the classification of AD because a minority of cases lack seasonal rhinitis, asthma, and allergen-specific IgE. The AD clinical phenotype described herein is that proposed by Wise and Sulzberger (1933) and later by Hanifin and Rajka (1980). The term 'atopic dermatitis' is used to include both so-called *extrinsic atopic dermatitis* and *intrinsic (atopiform) dermatitis/eczema* (Bos 2002).

CLINICAL PRESENTATION

The vast majority of patients seen in clinical practice are infants, toddlers, and older children. The prerequisite of AD is pruritus. It can be intermittent or constant, may be worse at night, and often interferes with the sleep of both child and family members. The onset of AD usually occurs at about 2 months when the infant develops the necessary coordination to scratch. It is common to see children actively scratching (**Fig 3.1**). On occasion infants may be so agitated from the fierce itch of inaccessible areas that they throw their bodies into contortions, rub against the crib or the person holding them, or even attempt to scratch their backs by hyperextending the neck and using the occiput to rub the affected area. Scratch marks and lichenification provide additional evidence of pruritus.

Fig 3.1 Infants and some adults with atopic dermatitis cannot control the urge to scratch the unremitting itch.

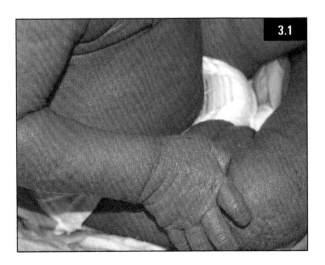

LESION MORPHOLOGY

Patients with AD display a wide range of lesional morphologies. During any stage, one morphology may predominate, but different lesions typically coexist. Early authors described three stages of eczema: the acute, subacute, and chronic.

- Acute eczema is characterized by redness, edema, papules, and/or vesicles (Bulkley 1881) (**Fig 3.2**). A raw, weeping surface may give rise to crusting.
- Subacute eczema shows an excoriated, red surface, sometimes moist, with moderate thickening, scaling, and crusting (**Fig 3.3**). Collarettes of scale suggest previous vesiculation or spongiosis (epidermal edema) (**Fig 3.4**) (Ackerman 1979).

- Chronic eczema appears as red–brown papules and plaques that accentuate skin lines or markings. These changes describe the term 'lichenification' (**Fig 3.5**). Individual lichenoid papules coalesce to form lichenified plaques (**Fig 3.6**).

By comparison, nummular dermatitis describes single or multiple coin-shaped, crusted, eczematous plaques, most commonly on the extremities. This condition may occur as a 'stand-alone' disorder but the nummular morphology sometimes predominates in children with AD (Braun-Falco 2000).

Nummular facial lesions are rare after infancy. **Figure 3.7** illustrates an unusual presentation of oozing and crusting nummular plaques on the face of a 12-year-old boy.

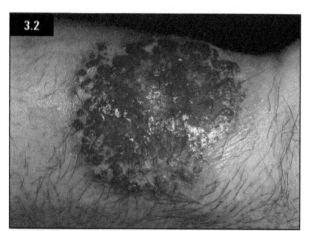

Fig 3.2 Acute eczema displays erythema, oozing, and sometimes vesiculation.

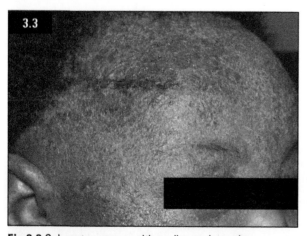

Fig 3.3 Subacute eczema with scaling and crusting.

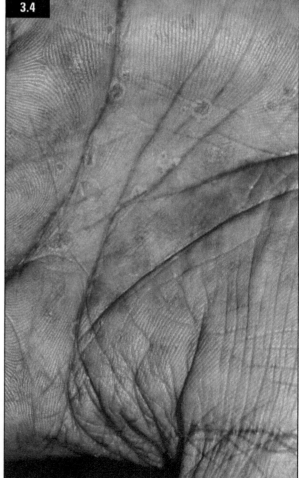

Fig 3.4 Collarettes of scale signify the previous presence of vesiculation or spongiosis.

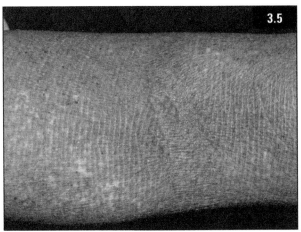

Fig 3.5 Lichenification results from chronic rubbing. Thickened plaques show accentuated skin markings.

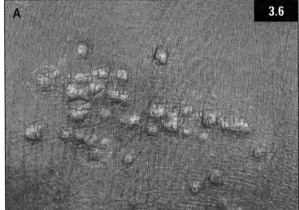

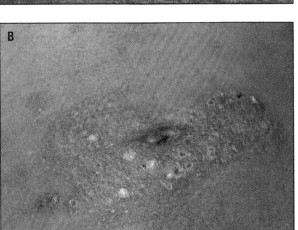

Fig 3.6 (A) In the process of lichenification, lichenoid papules coalesce to plaques. Note collarettes. (B) Excoriated lichenoid papules forming lichenifled plaques.

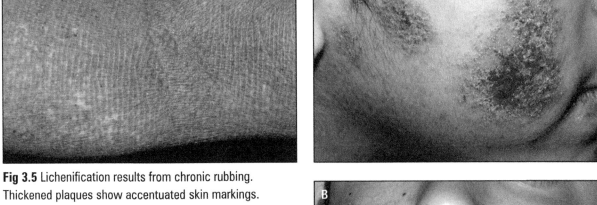

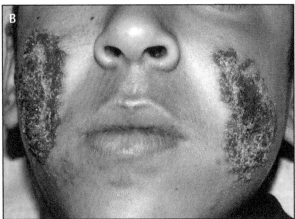

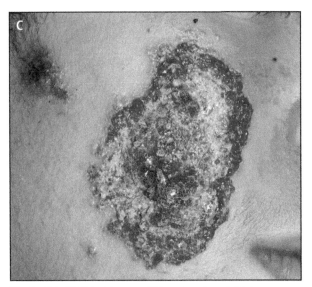

Fig 3.7 (A–C) This 12-year-old boy developed thick plaques on his cheeks with oozing and yellow crusting that responded only to systemic corticosteroids together with antistaphylococcal antibiotics.

Although culture-positive for *Staphylococcus aureus*, the eruption did not respond to intravenous antistaphylococcal antibiotics until systemic corticosteroids were introduced. In our experience, this type of combination therapy is essential for a dominant nummular morphology, independent of bacterial infection.

PHASES OF ATOPIC DERMATITIS

AD has been divided into three clinical phases: the infantile, childhood, and adult phases, each with a typical morphology and distribution; however, it is emphasized that overlap between stages is common.

- The infantile phase of AD (age 2 months to about 2 years) typically displays vesicular and crusted eczematous patches on the scalp and cheeks with scattered patches on the extremities and trunk (Sulzberger 1955) (**Fig 3.8A**).

- The childhood phase spans from 2 years to 11 years of age. The eruption tends to be dryer with a preponderance of papular, prurigo-like, and lichenified lesions. Excoriated papules often predominate on extensor surfaces and flexural involvement is characteristic (**Fig 3.8B**). The sides and back of the neck may show darkening, sometimes called an *atopic dirty neck*, although hands and fingers may also be involved.

- The adolescent and young adult phase extends from ages 12 to 23. Dry, lichenified plaques reflect chronicity. Flexural involvement of the neck, and antecubital and popliteal fossae, exemplify this disease phase (**Fig 3.8C**).

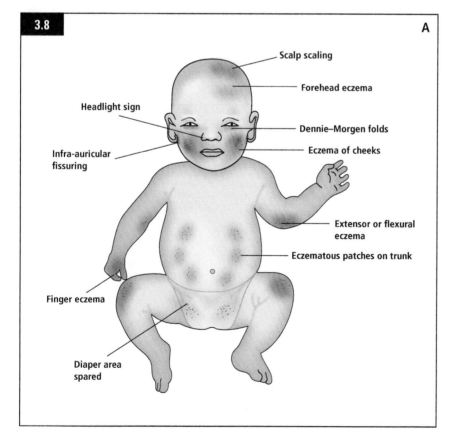

3.8

Scalp scaling

Forehead eczema

Headlight sign

Dennie–Morgen folds

Eczema of cheeks

Infra-auricular fissuring

Extensor or flexural eczema

Eczematous patches on trunk

Finger eczema

Diaper area spared

A

Fig 3.8 (A) The Infantile phase of atopic dermatitis is characterized by oozing, eczematous plaques on the cheeks, forehead, and scalp. Extensor and flexor surfaces of the extremities and trunk may be involved. (B) Childhood eczema often involves the forehead, eyelids, neck, flexures of the arms and legs, wrists, hands, fingers, and ankles. Extensor involvement is also common on the forearms. (C) Typically adults with atopic dermatitis display lichenification and inflammation, often on the flexural areas as well as extensor surfaces. Forehead, eyelids, neck, shoulders, hands, and fingers may be involved. Head and neck involvement, common in adults, has been linked to aeroallergens and *Malassezia sympodialis* yeasts.

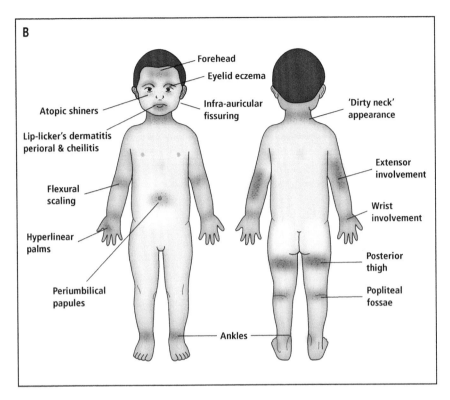

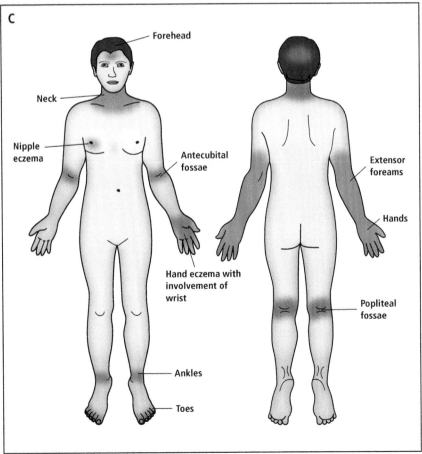

CLINICAL CRITERIA

In 1980, Hanifin and Rajka introduced a number of major and minor diagnostic features of AD (**Box 3.1**). Other groups have created clinical criteria somewhat better suited to clinical studies, including those of the UK Working Party (Williams *et al.* 1994) and the Millennium Criteria (Bos *et al.* 1998).

Box 3.1   Hanifin and Rajka criteria for diagnosis of atopic dermatitis

Panel 1: Major criteria

Must have three or more of:

- Pruritus
- Typical morphology and distribution
- Flexural lichenification or linearity in adults
- Facial and extensor involvement in infants and children
- Chronic or chronically relapsing dermatitis
- Personal or family history of atopy (asthma, allergic rhinitis, atopic dermatitis)

Panel 2: Minor criteria

Should have three or more of:

- Xerosis
- Ichthyosis, palmar hyperlinearity, or keratosis pilaris
- Immediate (type 1) skin-test reactivity
- Raised serum IgE
- Early age of onset
- Tendency toward cutaneous infections (especially *Staphylococcus aureus* and herpes simplex) or impaired cell-mediated immunity
- Tendency toward non-specific hand or foot dermatitis
- Nipple eczema
- Cheilitis
- Recurrent conjunctivitis
- Dennie–Morgan infraorbital fold
- Keratoconus
- Anterior subcapsular cataracts
- Orbital darkening
- Facial pallor or facial erythema
- Pityriasis alba
- Anterior neck folds
- Itch when sweating
- Intolerance to wool and lipid solvents
- Perifollicular accentuation
- Food intolerance
- Course influenced by environmental or emotional factors
- White dermographism or delayed blanch

Many of the minor criteria have been called into question. Some, including ichthyosis, nipple eczema, cheilitis, anterior subcapsular cataracts, keratoconus, anterior neck folds, pityriasis alba, and food intolerance, are not thought to be specific to atopic dermatitis. Infra-auricular fissuring and diffuse scaling of the scalp, although not included in the minor criteria, are commonly seen, especially in severe disease. (Panels 1 and 2 reprinted from Rudikoff and Lebwohl 1998. © 1998 with permission from Elsevier.)

CLINICAL FINDINGS

THE INFANTILE PHASE

The infantile phase of AD is associated with itchy, dry skin that is hyper-reactive to both external and internal stimuli (Hebert and Mays 1996). Acute or subacute eczematous patches occur on the cheeks (**Fig 3.9**) and sometimes on the forehead (**Fig 3.10**).

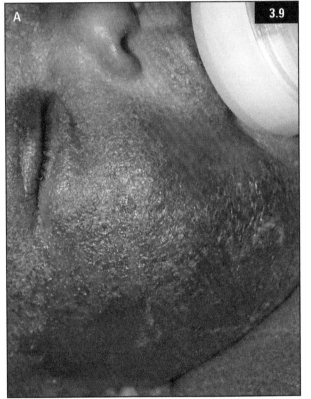

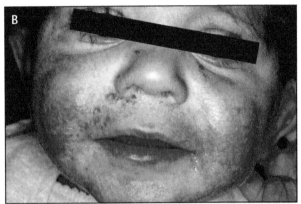

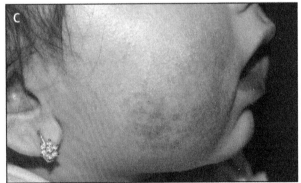

Fig 3.9 Infants with atopic dermatitis may have bright-red erythema of the cheeks with oozing and crusting or they may have dry, erythematous patches. (A) This infant displays subacute eczematous patches on the cheeks, with erythema and crusting but sparing of the nose, melolabial fold, and upper lip. (B) Central pallor of the face ('headlight sign') is noted. Dennie–Morgan folds are also apparent and probably result from eyelid dermatitis. They are not pathognomonic of atopic dermatitis, however, and can be seen as a normal variant. (Reprinted from Rudikoff *et al.* 2003. © 2003 with permission from Elsevier.) (C) Mild eczematous changes on the cheeks of an infant.

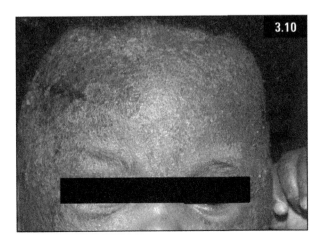

Fig 3.10 Forehead involvement is common in infants.

There may be oozing and crusting, dry scale, and/or papules. In severe cases, erosions can be prominent. Sparing of the nose and paranasal skin gives rise to the so-called *headlight sign* (**Fig 3.9B**). Scalp involvement occurs frequently during infancy, manifest as erythema, scaling, and occasional crusting (**Fig 3.11**).

Excoriations and lichenification after 2 months of age correlate with neuromuscular maturation and coordination that enables scratching. Focal hair loss often results from constant rubbing of the itchy scalp against bedding (**Fig 3.11A,B**). Involvement of the cheeks tends to wane by the first birthday. Infants and young children with AD develop an accentuation of the infraorbital folds or pleats, called *Dennie–Morgan folds*, associated with lower eyelid eczema (**Figs 3.12–3.15**). More than one fold may occur early in life. Redness, scaling, and edema of the eyelids are common (**Fig 3.15B**). Dennie–Morgan folds are not pathognomonic for AD, and may also occur in normal children, especially African–Americans, as well as with contact allergy or other causes (Braun-Falco 2000).

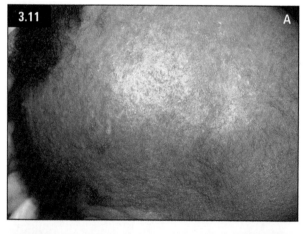

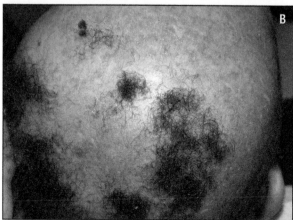

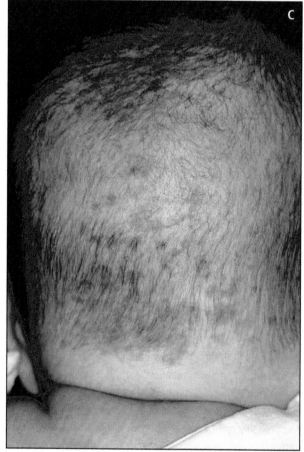

Fig 3.11 Scalp involvement is common in infants with atopic dermatitis. (A, B) Eczema of the scalp with hair loss secondary to rubbing. (C) This child displays erythematous crusted papules on the vertex and nuchal area. (Reprinted from Rudikoff *et al.* 2003. © 2003 with permission from Elsevier.)

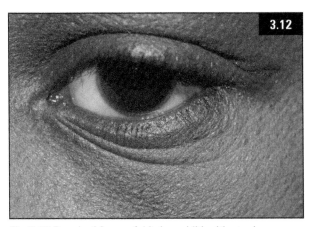

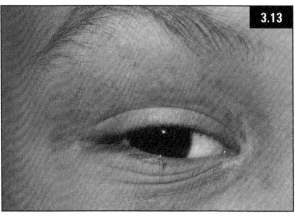

Fig 3.12 Dennie–Morgan folds in a child with atopic dermatitis. They are a reflection of eyelid dermatitis and are not pathognomonic of atopy.

Fig 3.13 Dennie–Morgan folds in a child with dermatomyositis involving the eyelid. Usually related to inflammation, they may be found in normal children.

Fig 3.14 Mild eyelid eczema in a child with atopic dermatitis.

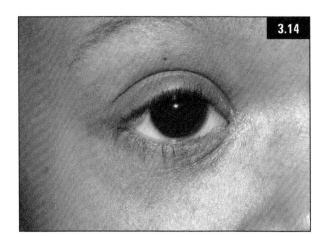

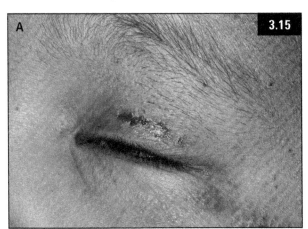

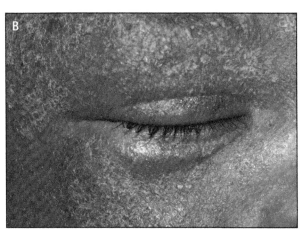

Fig 3.15 Dermatitis affecting both (A) the upper and (B) the lower eyelids of one or both eyes is frequently seen in atopic dermatitis. (Image A reprinted from Rudikoff *et al.* 2003. © 2003 with permission from Elsevier.)

Loss of the lateral eyebrow, *Hertoghe's sign*, is due to chronic rubbing (**Fig 3.16**). Infants and children may also display postauricular and infra-auricular fissuring (**Fig 3.17A,B**).

Eczematous changes and crusting may be present on the upper lip and chin (**Fig 3.18**). Cheilitis derives from habitual lip licking (so-called lip-licker's dermatitis).

A fine papular eruption is often associated with dry skin on the trunk (**Fig 3.19A,B**). More prominent follicular papules with or without patches of lighter skin may result from postinflammatory pigment alteration in infants with darker skins (**Fig 3.19C**). Erythematous scaly patches and occasionally severe diffuse eczematous involvement may occur (**Fig 3.19D,E**). The diaper area is usually spared.

The course of infantile eczema is variable. A German study found a cumulative AD prevalence of 21.5% in the first 2 years of life (Illi *et al.* 2004). A large proportion of the children were in complete remission by age 3 (43.2%); however, intermittent disease still affected 38.3% and more persistent disease was found in 18.7%.

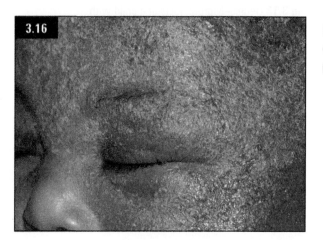

Fig 3.16 Hertoghe's sign: loss of the lateral eyebrow was originally described in patients with hypothyroidism. In patients with atopic dermatitis it results from rubbing.

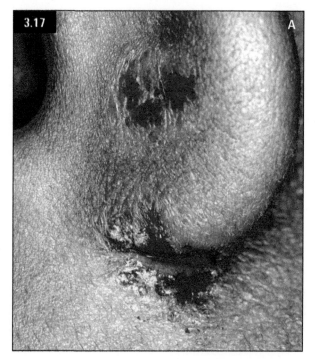

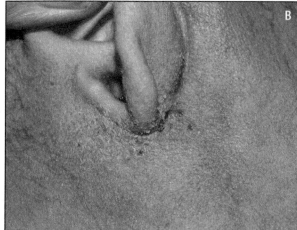

Fig 3.17 (A, B) Although not included in the Hanifin and Rajka criteria for atopic dermatitis, infra-auricular fissuring is so common among patients with atopic dermatitis that many practitioners consider it a reliable diagnostic sign. (Image A reprinted from Rudikoff *et al.* 2003. © 2003 with permission from Elsevier.)

Fig 3.18 Cheilitis and perioral involvement is encountered frequently in children with atopic dermatitis. Lip licking and mouth breathing result in a cycle of wetting and evaporation that promotes chapping and further dermatitis. (Reprinted from Rudikoff *et al.* 2003. © 2003 with permission from Elsevier.)

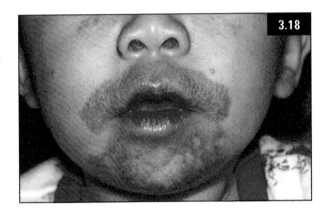

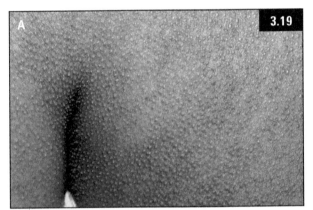

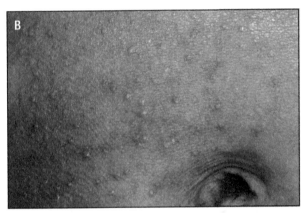

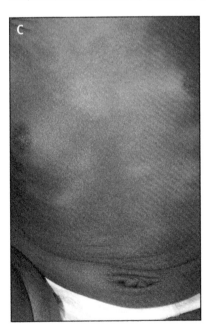

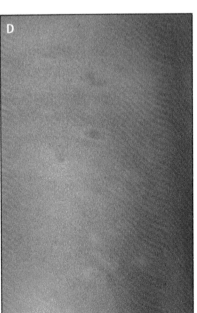

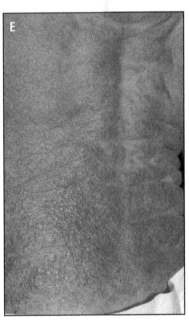

Fig 3.19 Truncal involvement: (A) follicular papules and hypopigmented patches on trunk and arms; (B) lichenoid papules on the abdomen of an infant with atopic dermatitis; (C) papules and dry hypopigmented scaly patches; (D) follicular papules and erythematous scaly plaques; (E) erythematous, infiltrated plaques surmounted by papules on the back of an infant.

Böhme *et al.* (2000) looked at the minor criteria identified by Hanifin and Rajka in children at age 2. They found a high prevalence of xerosis, a clinical course affected by environmental factors, facial erythema, itch associated with sweating, positive skin-prick tests, and hand eczema. A low prevalence (<3%) of Dennie–Morgan infraorbital folds might be attributed to their requirement for a secondary crease in the lower eyelid. Uehara (1981) reported a prevalence of 25% in another population but of greater interest is the finding that infraorbital folds occurred in association with eczematous dermatoses of diverse origin and tendency to skin infection. Mevorah *et al.* (1988) considered Dennie–Morgan folds to be of no diagnostic significance.

THE CHILDHOOD PHASE

This phase of AD may simply be an extension of infantile eczema or a recurrence of previous infantile eczema expressed during the first 2 years of life, or it may appear spontaneously in patients who never had infantile eczema. *Mournful facies* reflecting chronic pruritus and lack of sleep, and/or dark pigmentation under the eyes (*atopic shiners*), may be early cues

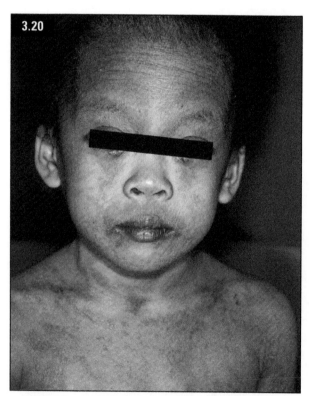

Fig 3.20 Atopic dermatitis in a toddler with eyelid and perioral erythema and scaling as well as extensive involvement of the chest and shoulders. Central pallor and 'mournful facies' are characteristic. The young male patient has not yet developed 'atopic shiners' (darkness around the eyes). (Reprinted from Rudikoff *et al.* 2003. © 2003 with permission from Elsevier.)

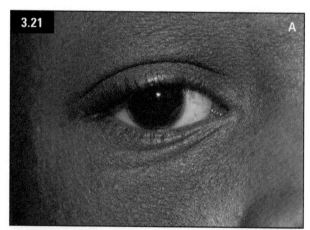

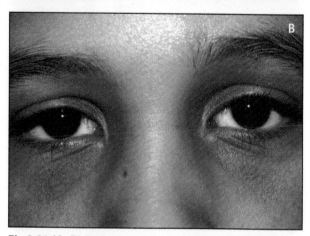

Fig 3.21 (A, B) Darkening of the periorbital skin (*atopic shiners*) and prominent infraorbital pleats in two children with atopic dermatitis.

forecasting skin disease (**Figs 3.20** and **3.21**). Involvement of the cheeks (**Fig 3.22**) is observed less frequently than with infantile eczema. A so-called *dirty neck* is suggested by eczematous lesions (**Fig 3.23**). The childhood eruption tends to be drier than infantile eczema, characterized by papulation rather than vesiculation, exudation, and crusting. Cheilitis and perioral chapping are common, especially in winter months (**Fig 3.24**), and may result from habitual lip licking (lip-licker's dermatitis) (**Fig 3.24A**).

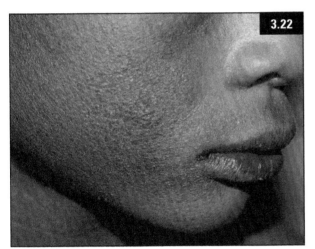

Fig 3.22 Hyperpigmentation and lichenification of the cheeks and neck. Note sparing of the central face.

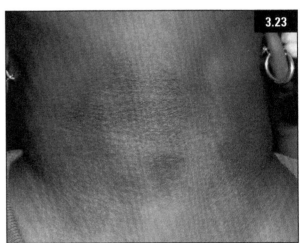

Fig 3.23 Atopic *dirty neck*: eczema and postinflammatory hyperpigmentation give the neck a dirty appearance.

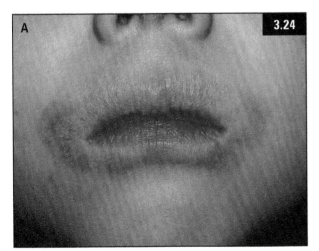

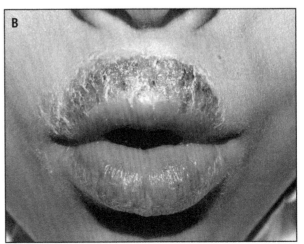

Fig 3.24 (A) Typical *lip-licker's dermatitis* in a child with atopic dermatitis. Repeated licking followed by evaporation leads to chapping and secondary eczematous changes. (B) A young child with crusted, subacute, eczematous lesions on the upper lip.

There may be succulent prurigo papules or lichenified flat-topped papules that coalesce to lichenified plaques favoring the neck, and antecubital and popliteal fossae (**Figs 3.25** and **3.26**). Extensor surfaces may be involved as well (**Fig 3.27**).

Discrete and confluent lichenoid papules have a predilection for the trunk, often localizing to the periumbilical area (**Fig 3.28**). The hands may be dry and chapped or show lichenification and crusting, which includes the volar and dorsal aspects of the wrists (**Fig 3.29**).

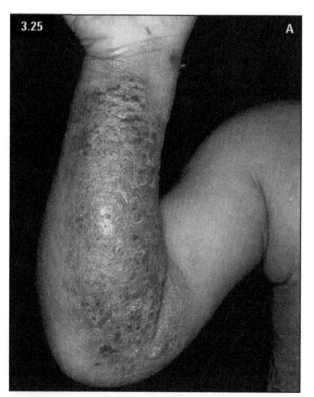

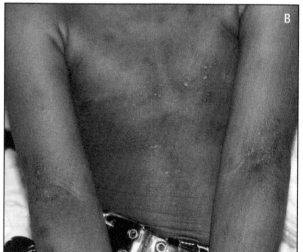

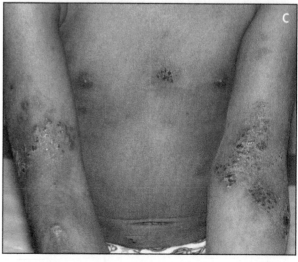

Fig 3.25 (A) Flexural involvement of the wrist, forearm, and arm in a young child with erythematous, scaly, and crusted subacute lesions (Reprinted from Rudikoff *et al.* 2003. © 2003 with permission from Elsevier.) (B) Involvement of the antecubital fossae, chest, and abdomen with hyperpigmented, dry, excoriated papules, and lichenification. (C) Typical childhood flexural involvement with erythematous crusted and eroded plaques and lichenification.

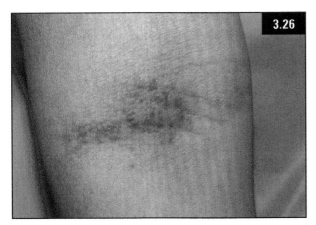

Fig 3.26 Antecubital juicy papules in a child.

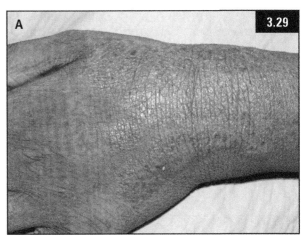

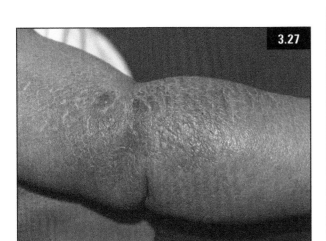

Fig 3.27 Extensor involvement in a toddler: common in infancy and early childhood, then gives way to a pattern of flexural predominance in older children and adolescents.

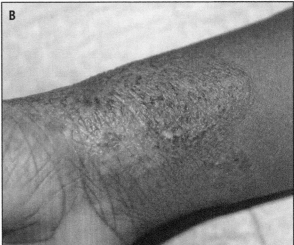

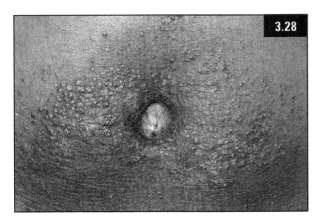

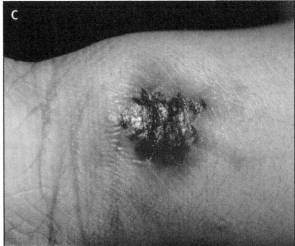

Fig 3.28 Prominent pruritic periumbilical papules provide a clue to childhood atopic dermatitis (Reprinted from Rudikoff *et al.* 2003. © 2003 with permission from Elsevier.)

Fig 3.29 (A) Dorsal and (B) flexural lichenification of the wrists; (C) juicy, erythematous, fissured plaque on the wrist of a young child with atopic dermatitis.

Bilateral involvement of the posterior thighs ('toilet seat dermatitis') or inner thighs is common (**Figs 3.30–3.32**). AD of the posterior thighs should be differentiated from allergic contact dermatitis to nickel in school chairs, the so-called 'school chair sign' (Samimi *et al.* 2004). Genital involvement may cause severe discomfort (**Fig 3.31**). Lichenified lesions may become hyperpigmented, hypopigmented, or frankly depigmented in areas (**Fig 3.33**).

THE ADOLESCENT/YOUNG ADULT PHASE

In this late phase, the major features are pruritus, papulation, scaling, and lichenification usually involving the forehead, eyelids, upper lip (**Figs 3.34–3.36**), flexures of the neck, arms and legs, and the

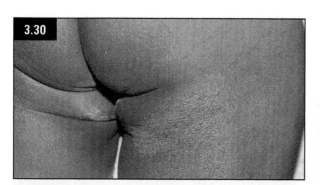

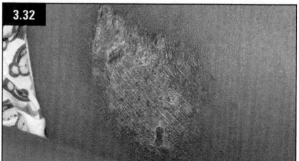

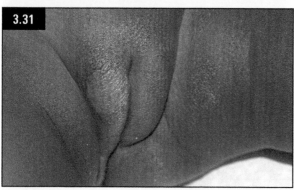

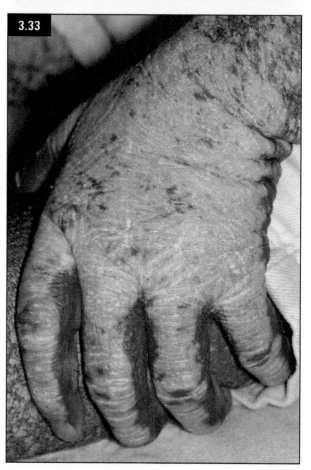

Fig 3.30 Involvement of the posterior thighs below the buttocks, referred to as *toilet seat dermatitis*, may be seen in toddlers and sometimes in older children with atopic dermatitis.

Fig 3.31 Atopic dermatitis involving the inner thighs and vulva in a young girl.

Fig 3.32 Lichenified excoriated erythematous plaque on the inner thigh of a child.

Fig 3.33 Lichenified atopic dermatitis with depigmentation thought at first to be postinflammatory in nature. The patient developed vitiligo and had depigmentation in unrubbed areas as well.

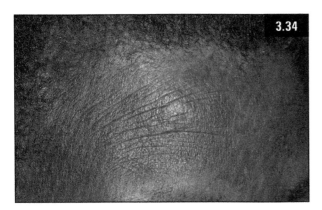

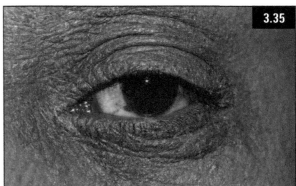

Fig 3.34 Lichenification of the forehead in an adult who never had eczema as a child. It began when she moved to a wooded area with many birch trees.

Fig 3.35 Adult atopic dermatitis of the eyelid: the main differential diagnosis is chronic allergic contact dermatitis.

Fig 3.36 Adult atopic dermatitis with lichenification of the upper lip and nasolabial area.

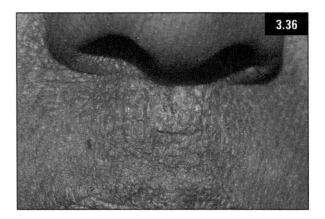

upper trunk (**Fig 3.37**). Dry, thick, extremely pruritic lichenified lesions are characteristic and prurigo nodules may sometimes be seen (**Fig 3.37C**). Poorly demarcated, these lichenified plaques range in color from a bright pinkish-red to a tannish-brown or grayish-brown in white people (**Fig 3.38**). Patients with darker skins may exhibit hyper- and hypopigmentation, as well as focal areas of depigmentation. Generalized xerosis is the rule with variable involvement of extensor surfaces and hands. Older patients may also have extensive head and neck involvement purportedly caused by exposure to aeroallergens and colonization by *Malassezia sympodialis* yeast forms.

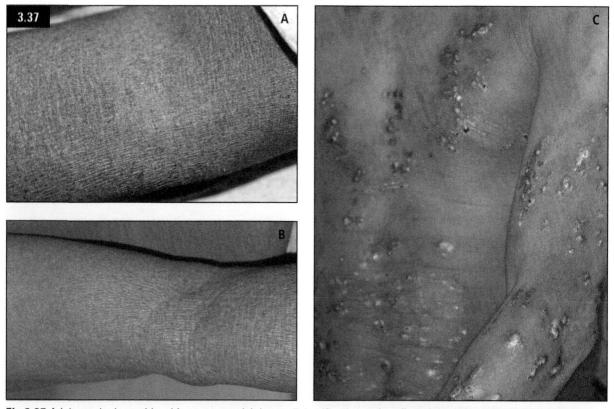

Fig 3.37 Adult atopic dermatitis with severe grayish-brown lichenification and scaling of the (A) antecubital fossa and (B) arm. (C) Lichenified plaques and prurigo nodularis lesions on chest, abdomen, and arms of an adult.

NONESSENTIAL FEATURES

A number of other clinical features may occur in patients with AD.

ATOPIC SHINERS

Orbital darkening refers to asymptomatic bluish-gray or brown hyperpigmentation of the periorbital skin (see **Fig 3.21**). It is thought to result from repetitive rubbing of itchy eyes and possibly impaired venous return from the skin and subcutaneous tissues. *Atopic shiners* are considered a manifestation of atopic rhinitis (Du Toit 2005, Chen *et al.* 2009). The darkness of the shiners correlates with the chronicity of the atopic rhinitis.

The *atopic salute* involves the repetitive vertical rubbing of the nose by the atopic child. The upward folding of the nose with each salute causes an accentuated pale or dark crease on the dorsum of the nose at the junction between the nasal cartilage and bone (Du Toit 2005).

PITYRIASIS ALBA

Hypopigmented or pinkish patches with fine scale usually occur in children, mainly from 6 to 16 years of age (Blessmann Weber *et al.* 2002) (**Fig 3.39**). Pityriasis alba is more common in males and children with darker complexions and higher phototype categories. The frequency of washing/bathing, the presence of dry skin, and sun exposure are thought to contribute.

Fig 3.38 Grayish-brown and pink lichenification of the dorsum of the hand and wrist with fissuring and areas of hypopigmentation.

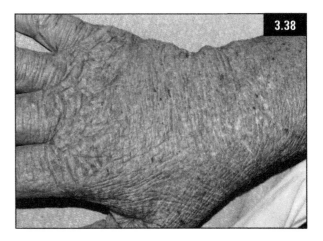

Fig 3.39 Pityriasis alba in an African–American child. Note the smudgy border. On Wood's light examination, this would show only hypopigmentation and not the milky white appearance of vitiligo.

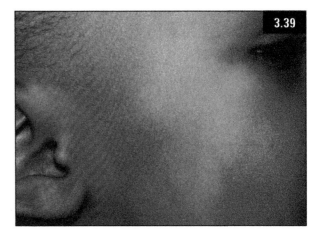

ATOPIC HAND AND FOOT DERMATITIS

Dermatitis of the palms and soles occurs in a significant percentage of children with AD, whereas isolated hand eczema complicated by irritant dermatitis of the hands may be the sole manifestation of AD in adult patients. One study of 2-year-olds with AD revealed hand involvement among 28% (Bohme *et al.* 2000). In a study of predominantly white patients at a tertiary referral center, Simpson *et al.* (2006) found that the overall prevalence of hand eczema was 60% in patients with AD, a trend that crescendoed with age. In this cohort, 43.7% of children up to age 2 experienced hand eczema, 54.1% were affected between ages 3 and 12, and the frequency reached 63.9% in those over 12. Nearly two-thirds of those with AD developed hand eczema within 1 year of diagnosis, and 80% experienced hand involvement during the first 5 years of the disease. Involvement of the dorsal aspect of the hand (89%) was almost three times more frequent than palmar or volar finger involvement (31% and 30% respectively). The study suggested that hand eczema involving the dorsa of hands and fingers with concurrent volar wrist dermatitis was highly suggestive of AD.

By contrast, Lee *et al.* (2001) observed more palmoplantar involvement in 108 children with AD and eczema of the hands and feet between the ages 6 months and 12 years (mean 5.3 years). Concurrent hand and foot dermatitis was present in 44% and isolated hand or foot dermatitis among 13.9% and 42.6%, respectively. Although there is general agreement about the high prevalence of hand and foot eczema in the setting of AD, the predilection for hands versus feet and the distribution of acral disease is poorly understood.

HYPERLINEAR PALMS AND SOLES, ICHTHYOSIS VULGARIS, AND KERATOSIS PILARIS

These features are found in AD patients with filaggrin mutations, which are commonly associated with asthma (**Figs 3.40** and **3.41**). Keratosis pilaris commonly presents as follicular keratotic plugs on the lateral aspect of the arms, on the upper back and on the thighs. We have observed lesions of keratosis pilaris in areas of pre-existing ichthyosis vulgaris on the legs (**Fig 3.41D**).

NIPPLE ECZEMA

Nipple eczema occurs in a minority of women and postpubertal girls, often symmetrically, and may occur in breastfeeding women (Rudzki *et al.* 1994, Amato *et al.* 2005) (**Fig 3.42**). Nevertheless, Paget disease must be considered as a potential cause of longstanding, intractable eczema involving the

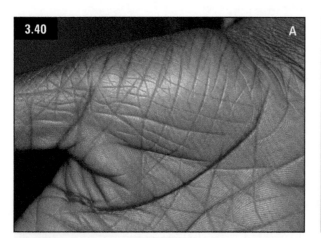 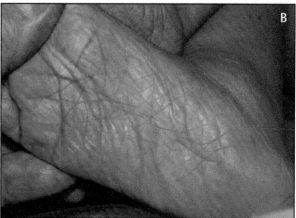

Fig 3.40 Hyperlinear palms (A) and soles (B) in a patient with atopic dermatitis and asthma likely secondary to filaggrin deficiency.

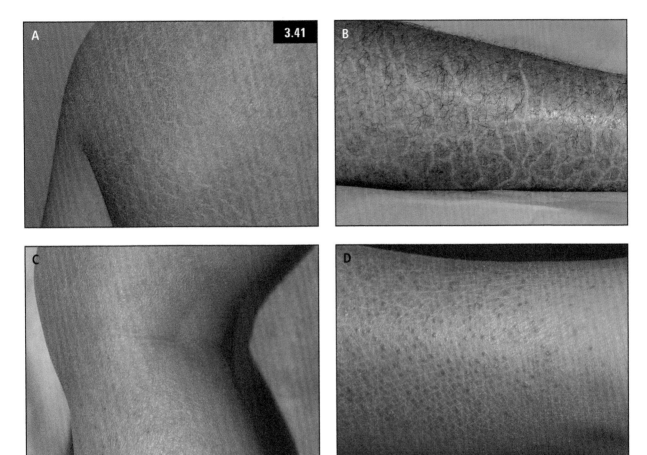

Fig 3.41 Ichthyosis vulgaris of (A) the trunk and (B) the leg; (C) ichthyosis and concomitant eczema of the thigh and leg, sparing the popliteal fossa; (D) keratosis pilaris occurring on the leg of a patient with ichthyosis vulgaris.

Fig 3.42 Erythematous, hyperpigmented, and excoriated plaque of eczema on the nipple and areola of a female with atopic dermatitis. Eczema in this region can be an isolated manifestation of atopic dermatitis. Paget disease of the breast should be considered in cases of persistent nipple eczema and biopsy obtained if there is doubt as to the diagnosis.

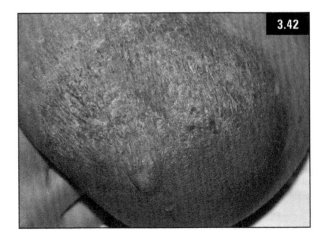

areola, particularly the nipple itself. Nipple eczema may occur in isolation or together with AD of the entire breast (**Fig 3.43**).

Dyshidrotic eczema

Although dyshidrotic eczema typically occurs independently, it may occur in patients with AD. It is characterized by deep-seated vessels on the sides of the fingers and toes, on the palms and on the soles, especially the arches, of the feet (**Fig 3.44**).

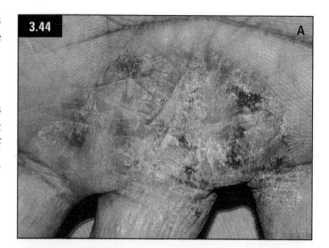

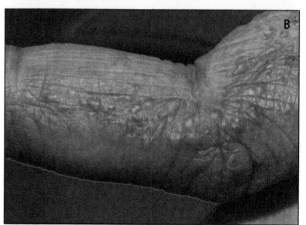

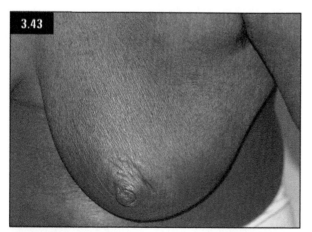

Fig 3.43 Nipple and breast involvement in a female with atopic dermatitis.

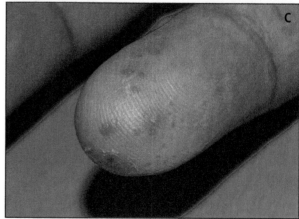

Fig 3.44 Dyshidrotic eczema with blistering, crusting, and scale involving (A) the distal palm and (B) the sides of the fingers. (C) Dyshidrotic eczema with deep-seated blisters on the fingertips.

DIFFERENTIAL DIAGNOSIS

The diagnosis of AD is usually straightforward but atypical features should prompt the clinician to explore alternatives (**Boxes 3.2** and **3.3**).

DIFFERENTIAL DIAGNOSIS OF INFANTILE AND CHILDHOOD ATOPIC DERMATITIS

The most common disorders confused with infantile/childhood AD are infantile seborrheic dermatitis, psoriasis, contact dermatitis, and scabies. Molluscum contagiosum dermatitis and juvenile plantar dermatitis are important considerations in the spectrum of eczematous disorders. Although exceedingly rare, congenital immune deficiency syndromes, acrodermatitis enteropathica, Netherton syndrome, phenylketonuria, pityriasis rubra pilaris, and ichthyosis syndromes can mimic AD; however, syndromic disorders typically have distinctive features.

Box 3.2 Differential diagnosis of atopic dermatitis in infants and children

- Allergic contact dermatitis
- Irritant contact dermatitis
- Seborrheic dermatitis
- Nummular eczema
- Scabies
- Psoriasis
- Dermatophytosis
- Congenital immunodeficiency syndromes
- Wiscott–Aldrich syndrome
- Omenn syndrome
- Hyper-IgE and Job syndrome
- Severe combined immunodeficiency
- Netherton syndrome
- Acrodermatitis enteropathica
- Phenylketonuria
- HTLV-1 infective dermatitis
- Cutaneous T-cell lymphoma
- Ichthyosis vulgaris
- Pityriasis rubra pilaris
- Molluscum dermatitis

Box 3.3 Differential diagnosis of atopic dermatitis in adults

- Allergic contact dermatitis
- Irritant contact dermatitis
- Seborrheic dermatitis
- Nummular eczema
- Scabies
- Dermatophytosis
- Lichen simplex chronicus
- Cutaneous T-cell lymphoma

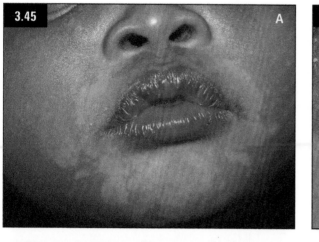

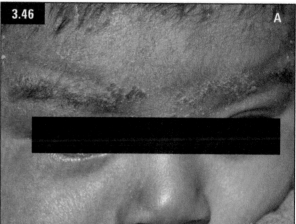

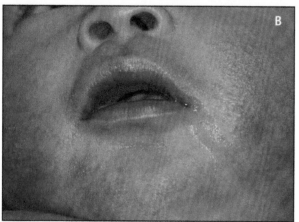

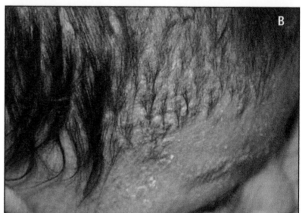

Fig 3.45 (A) Infantile seborrheic dermatitis with mild erythema, hypopigmentation, and slight scale involving melolabial folds and chin, contrasted with (B) atopic dermatitis with central sparing of the face (headlight sign).

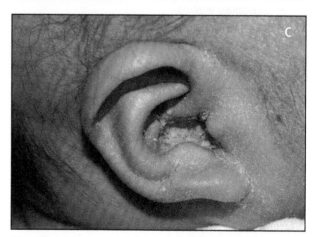

Seborrheic dermatitis

Classic infantile seborrheic dermatitis involves the scalp, face, axillae, and inguinal creases. The nasolabial folds and eyebrows are typically covered with nonpruritic, greasy scale (**Figs 3.45A** and **3.46**), contrasting with central sparing of the face in AD, giving rise to the so-called 'headlight sign' (**Fig 3.45B**). The flexures may be involved in both conditions but AD usually spares the diaper area. Studies of undifferentiated infantile dermatitis expose an ongoing debate about the difficulty in predicting whether the initial presentation will evolve into seborrheic dermatitis, psoriasis, or AD (Neville and Finn 1975, Menni *et al.* 1989, Morris *et al.* 2001).

Fig 3.46 Infantile seborrheic dermatitis with adherent scale in (A) the eyebrows, (B) the scalp, and (C) the conch of the ear analogous to cradle cap.

PSORIASIS

Psoriasis commonly presents in children younger than age 2 as *diaper rash* that may disseminate (Morris *et al.* 2001) (**Fig 3.47**). Beyond infancy, childhood psoriasis involving the face, scalp, palms, and soles may be confused with AD. However, in psoriasis, the lesions are more sharply circumscribed with classic micaceous scales. Examples include facial lesions that commonly occur around or under the eyes (**Fig 3.48**) and sharply demarcated plaques and fissures of the palms and soles (**Fig 3.49**).

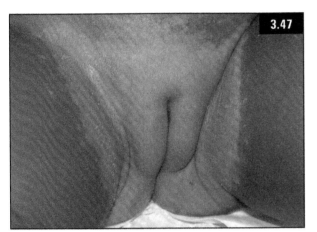

Fig 3.47 Intertriginous sharply demarcated patches in a baby with psoriasis. Although the genitalia may be involved in children with eczema, intertriginous surfaces are usually spared.

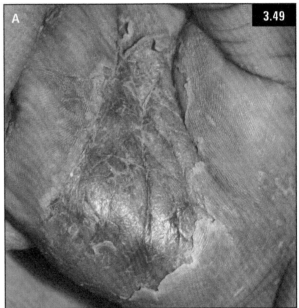

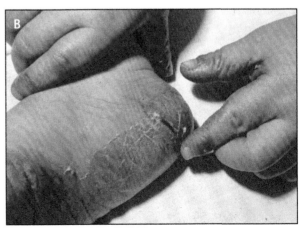

Fig 3.49 Childhood psoriasis with sharply demarcated erythematous plaque on (A) the palms, and (B) fissured plaque on the sole and scaling of the fingers.

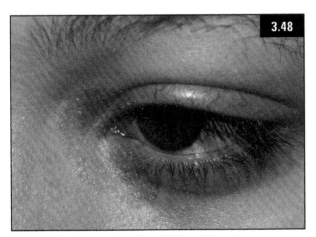

Fig 3.48 Orbital psoriasis in a child involving the inner canthus. The upper and lower eyelids are spared.

NUMMULAR DERMATITIS

Nummular dermatitis consists of coin-shaped eczematous lesions (hence the name) (**Fig 3.50**). In general, it is uncommon to develop nummular dermatitis in the first few years of life. This disorder starts around 5 years of age and the lesions appear as small, pruritic, follicular papules that form large, exudative, crusted plaques. These lesions can be anywhere on the body but facial involvement is unusual. A nummular morphology can be seen in patients with AD but clinical presentations vary. In patients with nummular dermatitis, there is generally no xerosis. Also, the disease rarely persists beyond puberty (Krol and Krafchik 2006).

DERMATOPHYTE INFECTION

Dermatophyte infections can masquerade as AD – especially localized forms (**Figs 3.51** and **3.52**). Dermatophytoses in various distributions, including tinea corporis (affecting the body), tinea capitis (head), tinea pedis (feet), and tinea manuum (hands), can simulate AD. Classic dermatophytosis presents as an annular, sometimes erythematous or hypopigmented, patch or plaque with an advancing, raised peripheral scale and central clearing, referred to as 'ringworm.' *Trichophyton* species are the most frequent causal fungi. Superficial dermatophyte infections may be confirmed by potassium hydroxide (KOH) microscopy or culture (Andrews and Burns 2008).

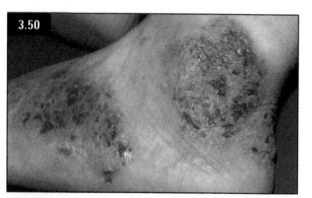

Fig 3.50 Nummular lesions in patients with atopic dermatitis.

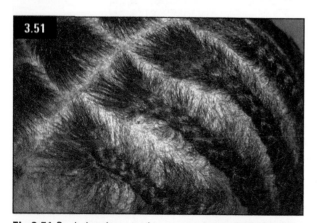

Fig 3.51 Scalp involvement is common in atopic dermatitis and must be differentiated from seborrheic dermatitis, psoriasis, and tinea infection. This child was thought to have scalp psoriasis but biopsy revealed tinea.

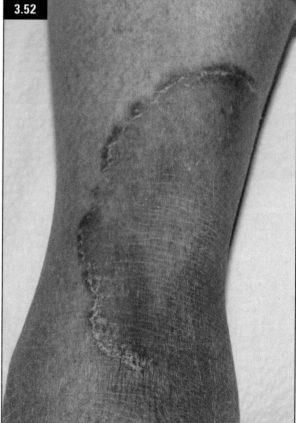

Fig 3.52 Dermatophyte infections usually have a raised, *active* border that may be scaly or vesicular.

CONTACT DERMATITIS

Contact dermatitis is an inflammatory reaction to external agents that may be an irritant or allergen. Irritant contact dermatitis (ICD) is associated with direct chemical or photochemical injury to the skin with activation of innate immunity; the adaptive T-cell response is not involved (Cohen and Heidary 2004). In infants and children ICD often manifests with contact to bodily fluids, including urine or stool in diapers, or with saliva in lip licking, particularly during the winter months.

Allergic contact dermatitis (ACD) involves delayed-type hypersensitivity induced by previous exposure and sensitization. All variants can mimic or complicate AD (**Figs 3.53–3.56**). Sensitization to contact allergens may occur as early as 6 months but

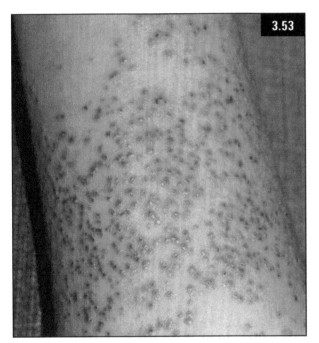

Fig 3.53 Nickel contact dermatitis from bracelets. Note papulation.

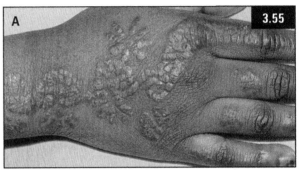

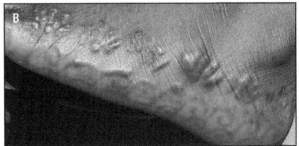

Fig 3.55 Allergic contact dermatitis of (A) the hands and (B) the feet from *p*-phenylenediamine in *black* henna. Red henna does not cause dermatitis.

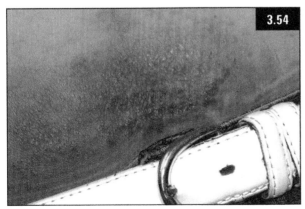

Fig 3.54 Contact dermatitis from a belt buckle containing nickel.

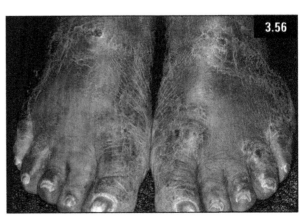

Fig 3.56 Contact dermatitis from leather sandals.

it is rare in the first few months of life, increasing in prevalence with age (Bruckner *et al.* 2000, Militello *et al.* 2006). The most common causes of ACD in children are nickel, topical antibiotics, preservative chemicals, fragrances, and rubber accelerators (Militello *et al.* 2006). Patterns of contact dermatitis may be localized or more generalized depending on the antigen. Allergens must be considered as potential causes of eyelid eczema, atopic cheilitis, hand dermatitis, foot dermatitis, generalized eczema, and even isolated flexural eruptions.

Common allergen sources, such as nickel, may cause earlobe dermatitis from earrings and periumbilical dermatitis from nickel studs in jeans. Sensitization to nickel has also been detected in children and adolescents with cheilitis (Zoli *et al.* 2006). Formaldehyde reactions may occur in children, especially from formaldehyde-releasing preservatives in baby wipes, shampoos, and other personal hygiene products (Jacob and Steele 2007). The preservatives methylchloroisothiazolinone/methylisothiazolinone can be found in baby wipes, emollients such as Eucerin, and other products. Corticosteroid allergy is uncommon in children but should be suspected when an eruption flares or fails to improve with topical corticosteroid therapy (Foti *et al.* 2005).

SCABIES

Scabies is uncommon in infants and young children and may be mistaken for AD (Krol and Krafchik 2006). Infants often display nodules in the axillae, inguinal areas, and penis rather than typical burrows. Infantile scabies may also present as vesicles and pustules on the hands and feet. A family history of other infested individuals should be explored (**Figs 3.57** and **3.58**).

MOLLUSCUM DERMATITIS

The scaly papular dermatitis seen around roughly 10% of molluscum contagiosum lesions may be difficult to distinguish from AD. Alternatively, small papules of molluscum may be overlooked in the setting of atopic dermatitis (**Fig 3.59**). Children with AD may have an increased prevalence of molluscum contagiosum infections and tend to have more widespread disease (Krol and Krafchik 2006, Treadwell 2008).

JUVENILE PLANTAR DERMATITIS

Juvenile plantar dermatitis refers to smooth, shiny, scaly areas on the weight-bearing plantar surfaces in children aged 3–14 (Gibbs 2004) (**Fig 3.60**). It is most prominent on the ball of the foot and the underside of the big toe, or other toes. Painful fissuring may occur.

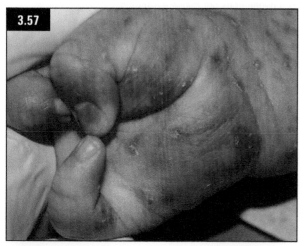

Fig 3.57 Scabies on the hand and wrist of an infant. Note burrows, papules, and vesicles.

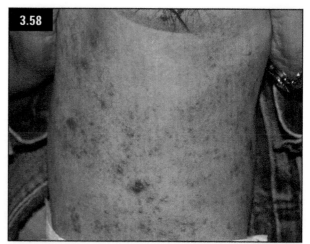

Fig 3.58 Extensive scabetic involvement of the trunk of an infant.

CONGENITAL IMMUNE DEFICIENCY

Several congenital immune deficiencies (discussed in Chapter 21) may cause eczematous lesions that mimic AD. Among these disorders are Wiskott–Aldrich syndrome, Omenn syndrome, and hyper-IgE syndrome (Krol and Krafchik 2006). Immune dysregulation, polyendocrinopathy, enteropathy, X-linked (IPEX) syndrome, and severe combined immunodeficiency (SCID) can also display features of AD or erythroderma (Hunter *et al.* 2008, Halabi-Tawil *et al.* 2009). Wiskott–Aldrich syndrome should be suspected in male children with eczema and features of purpura, bloody diarrhea, hemorrhagic crusting, and bloody excoriations (Krol and Krafchik 2006).

NETHERTON SYNDROME

Eczematous lesions and ichthyosis linearis circumflexa of Netherton syndrome may be confused with AD (**Fig 3.61**).

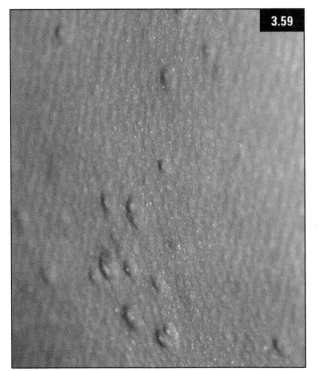

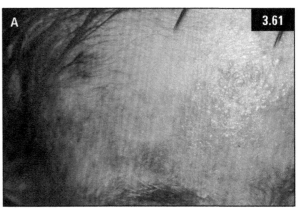

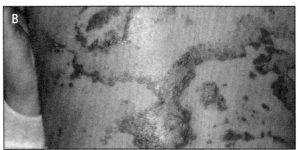

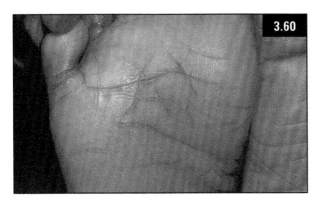

Fig 3.59 Molluscum dermatitis: note the subtle scaling surrounding molluscum lesions.

Fig 3.60 Juvenile plantar dermatitis: note the fissuring under the metatarsals.

Fig 3.61 Netherton syndrome: ichthyosis linearis circumflexa on (A) the forehead and (B) the trunk.

Hair-shaft defects and atopic manifestations, such as elevated IgE levels, food allergy, allergic rhinitis, asthma, and eosinophilia can occur concomitantly in Netherton syndrome. The range of hair and scalp abnormalities includes short, brittle hairs, scaly scalp, and a pathognomonic defect termed 'trichorrhexis invaginata.' Descriptively, trichorrhexis invaginata occurs when the proximal portion of the hair overlaps the distal portion, creating a likeness to intussusception of the bowel or the stalk of bamboo (known as bamboo hair) (Burk *et al.* 2008) (**Fig 3.62**). Dermatoscopic examination of the hair shaft can facilitate early diagnosis (**Fig 3.63**). Powell (2000) has observed that the density of nodes per unit length of hair is 10 times greater in eyebrow hairs than in scalp hairs; eyebrow hairs should be cut, not plucked. Therefore, examining the eyebrows will offer the highest yield of bamboo hairs. Children with Netherton syndrome typically have sparse hair (**Fig 3.64**) but this can be seen as well in some patients with AD. Other hair defects such as trichorrhexis nodosa and pili torti have also been described in these patients. Generalized erythroderma in the first months postpartum can make the diagnosis of Netherton syndrome an enormous challenge. However, within the first year of life, classic lesions of ichthyosis linearis circumflexa appear as distinctive, migratory, polycyclic, erythematous plaques with a double-edged scale (**Fig 3.65** and see **Fig 3.61b**).

PHENYLKETONURIA

The clinical spectrum of phenylketonuria (PKU), an autosomal recessive deficiency of phenylalanine hydroxylase, includes an eczematous condition in 20–40% of untreated patients that resembles AD (with a predilection for flexural creases). It is more common in younger patients and in those with a lower mentality. The dermatitis may improve with dietary intervention. Conversely, it can worsen with a phenylalanine challenge, even in carriers of the recessive gene (Fisch *et al.* 1981).

PITYRIASIS RUBRA PILARIS

Pityriasis rubra pilaris (PRP) is an uncommon dermatosis that often evolves cephalocaudally, progressing from follicular hyperkeratotic papules to a generalized erythroderma with characteristic islands of normal skin. Palmoplantar keratoderma and dystrophic nails are usually present. The disease is often mistaken for the more common erythrodermic AD. Classic juvenile PRP (type III) usually occurs in the late teens, accounting for 10% of all cases and differing only by age of onset from the adult variant (type I) (Griffiths' criteria) (Griffiths 1980, 1992, Allison *et al.* 2002). Curiously, adult-onset PRP may have very atypical features (type II). Circumscribed juvenile PRP (type IV) represents almost 25% of all cases (Allison *et al.* 2002). This form occurs in prepubertal children as sharply demarcated areas

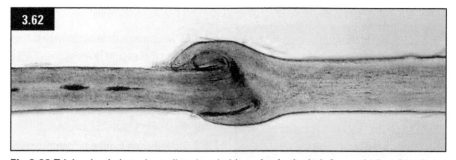

Fig 3.62 Trichorrhexis invaginata (bamboo hair): nodes in the hair form a ball and socket joint that breaks easily, leaving a so-called golf tee hair (de Berker *et al.* 1995). (Reprinted from Werchniak et al. 2004. © 1998 American Medical Association. All rights reserved.)

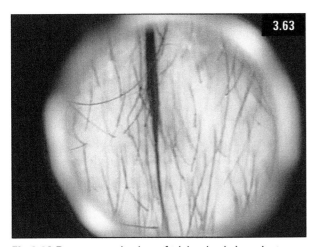

Fig 3.63 Dermatoscopic view of trichorrhexis invaginata. (Reprinted from Burk *et al.* 2008 with permission.)

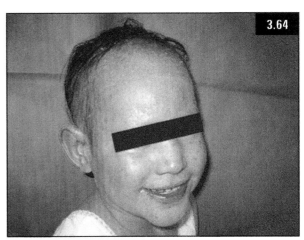

Fig 3.64 (A,B) Short sparse hairs in a patient with Netherton syndrome. (Reprinted from Burk *et al.* 2008 with permission.)

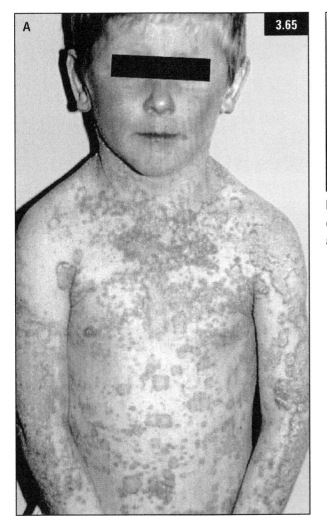

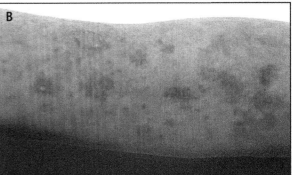

Fig 3.65 (A,B) Netherton syndrome: ichthyosis linearis circumflexa with double-edged scale on the back and arms in a child. (Courtesy Aleksandar Godić, MD.)

of follicular hyperkeratosis, as well as erythema of the knees and the elbows that rarely progresses. In more darkly pigmented children, erythema may not be apparent, obscuring the diagnosis unless hyperpigmented plaques develop with prominent follicular hyperkeratosis on the elbows and knees (**Fig 3.66**).

PITYRIASIS LICHENOIDES CHRONICA

Pityriasis lichenoides chronica is another rare mimicker of AD. In this condition of adolescents and young adults, asymptomatic pink–brown papules occur on the trunk, buttocks, and extremities. When they heal they may leave hypopigmentation likened to a *leopard skin* appearance (**Fig 3.67**).

ICHTHYOSIS VULGARIS

Ichthyosis vulgaris is mistaken for AD because of the overlapping distribution of both conditions. It is the most common variant of ichthyosis, with an incidence of about 1 in 250. The disorder is autosomal dominant, presenting during infancy or childhood, and characterized by fine or centrally adherent scale with superficial fissuring. Unlike AD, there is relative

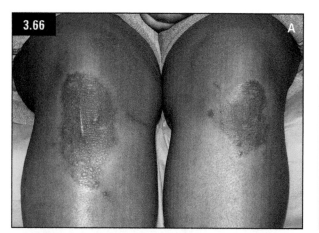
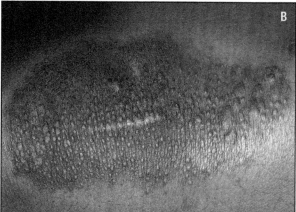

Fig 3.66 Hyperpigmented plaques with follicular prominence on the knees in a child with type IV (localized juvenile) pityriasis rubra pilaris.

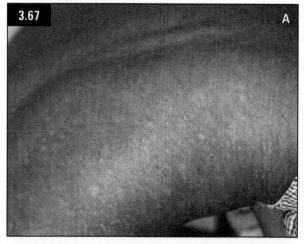
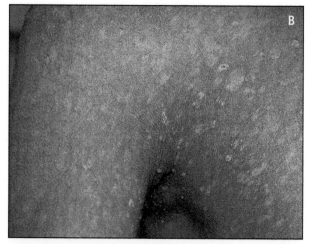

Fig 3.67 Pityriasis lichenoides chronica: this teenager had crusted papules on (A) the trunk, axillae, and (B) extremities for over 5 years. Note the numerous hypopigmented macules giving a *leopard skin* appearance.

flexural sparing and it tends to favor the lower extremities. Hyperlinearity and hyperkeratosis of the palms and soles are common features. This entity can be associated with atopy, as well as keratosis pilaris, and may occur either as a free-standing disorder or together with AD (DiGiovanna and Robinson-Bostom 2003).

ACRODERMATITIS ENTEROPATHICA

Acrodermatitis enteropathica (AE) is a rare autosomal recessive disorder caused by a mutation in the zinc transporter gene, *Zip4*. The scaling red plaques in the perioral and diaper areas can be mistaken for AD but the latter condition usually lacks involvement of the diaper area. The presentation of AE during infancy may appear eczematous with or without vesiculation, bullae, pustules, or desquamation. The distribution focuses on acral aspects of the extremities, the anogenital and periorificial regions. Angular cheilitis (perlèche) and paronychia can been seen. If untreated, these skin lesions can erode

whereas generalized alopecia and diarrhea become increasingly severe (Maverakis *et al.* 2007). As levels of the zinc-dependent enzyme alkaline phosphatase are decreased in zinc deficiency, measurement of alkaline phosphatase can be used as a rapid screening test for zinc deficiency while awaiting serum zinc levels (Weismann and Hoyer 1985).

KWASHIORKOR

Although protein–energy malnutrition (kwashiorkor) is rare in industrialized countries, cases have been reported in the USA as a result of rice beverage-based and other restricted or fad diets (Katz *et al.* 2005). Parents of infants with AD may implement unsupervised elimination diets, leading to nutritional deficiency. Children may present with irritability, lethargy, diarrhea, generalized edema, and characteristic 'flaky paint dermatitis' (**Fig 3.68**). Affected patients should also be screened for zinc, essential fatty acid, and biotin deficiency.

Fig 3.68 Flaky paint dermatitis in a child with kwashiorkor caused by a rice milk diet. (Reprinted from Katz *et al.* 2005 with permission.)

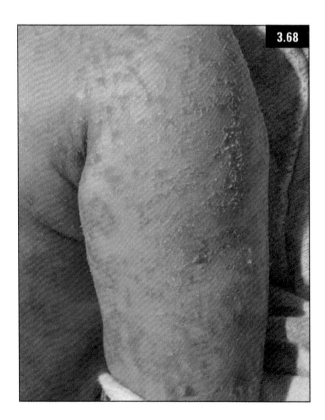

Cutaneous T-cell lymphoma

Mycosis fungoides (MF) is a cutaneous T-cell lymphoma (CTCL) that is rarely seen in children. As it can imitate atopic dermatitis, psoriasis, and dermatophytosis, it is often misdiagnosed initially. The clinical features of early stage MF consist of scaling erythematous patches on the thighs, buttocks, trunk, and extremities. The lesions may be hyperpigmented, ranging from orange to bright red to brown–red, or they may be hypopigmented, resembling generalized pityriasis alba (Nashan *et al.* 2007). Lesions of MF typically have 'smudgy' borders with or without epidermal atrophy (**Fig 3.69**).

HTLV-1 infective dermatitis

T-lymphotropic virus type 1 (HTLV)-associated dermatitis is a severe, chronic, eczematous disorder, associated with exudative, infective dermatitis occurring on the scalp, neck, and ears, which evolves into a generalized fine papular eruption (La Grenade *et al.* 1998, Primo *et al.* 2005) (**Fig 3.70**). It has been described mainly in Jamaica, Trinidad, Colombia, Japan, Brazil, and Senegal (sub-Saharan Africa). La Grenade *et al.* (1998) have described major and minor criteria (**Box 3.4**) to help distinguish this condition from atopic dermatitis.

Miscellaneous conditions

Other conditions that might conceivably be confused with AD include lichen planus, especially if there are larger lesions with lichenification from rubbing, lichen nitidus, and lichen spinulosus. Lichen planus lesions are typically violaceous, polygonal papules that often display the Koebner phenomenon. Lichen nitidus typically presents in children, particularly those of preschool and school age, with numerous, asymptomatic, pinhead-sized papules, often with koebnerization on the abdomen, chest, glans penis,

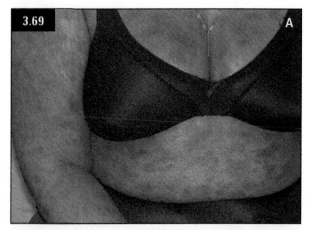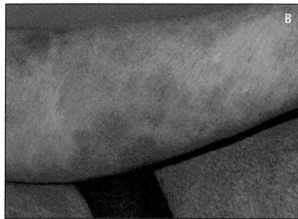

Fig 3.69 (A,B) Mycosis fungoides on the chest, abdomen, and arms with reddish-brown patches with *smudgy borders* and atrophy.

Fig 3.70 HTLV-1 infective dermatitis: (A) widespread superinfected exudative dermatitis of the scalp, nares, ears, and face. (B) Diffuse papular eruption of the trunk, with spontaneous fistulization of a *Staphylococcus aureus* abscess of the groin. (C) Chronic dermatitis of the eyelids, upper lip, and nares. (D) Severe exudative dermatitis of the external ear and neck fold. (E) Erosive dermatitis of the eyebrows, abscess of the scalp, and nasal discharge. (Reprinted from Mahé *et al.* 2004 with permission.)

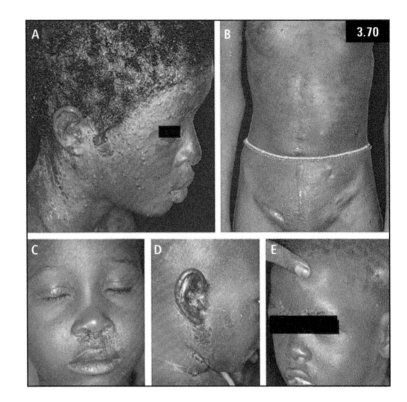

Box 3.4 Characteristics for diagnosis of infective dermatitis

Major[a]
1. Eczema of scalp, axillae, groin, external ear, and retroauricular areas, as well as eyelid margins, paranasal skin, and/or neck
2. Chronic watery nasal discharge without other signs of rhinitis and/or crusting of the anterior nares
3. Chronic relapsing dermatitis with prompt response to appropriate therapy but prompt recurrence on withdrawal of use of antibiotics
4. Usual onset in early childhood
5. Human T-lymphotropic virus type I antibody seropositivity

Minor or less specific
1. Positive cultures for *Staphylococcus aureus* and/or β-hemolytic streptococci from the skin or anterior nares
2. Generalized fine popular rash (in most severe cases)
3. Generalized lymphadenopathy with dermatopathic lymphadenitis
4. Anemia
5. Elevated erythrocyte sedimentation rate
6. Hyperimmunoglobulinemia (IgD and IgE)
7. Elevated CD4 count, CD8 count, and CD4/CD8 ratio

a   Of the five major criteria, four are required for diagnosis with mandatory inclusion of 1, 2, and 5; to fulfil criterion 1, involvement of at least two of the sites is required. (Reprinted from La Grenade *et al.* 1998. © 1998 American Medical Association. All rights reserved.)

and upper extremities (Tilly *et al.* 2004) (**Fig 3.71**). Lichen spinulosus presents as well-delineated patches with multiple keratotic follicular plugs. It may be confused with the patches of eczema in infants with darker skin that display follicular prominence.

DIFFERENTIAL DIAGNOSIS OF ATOPIC DERMATITIS IN ADULTS

In adults, conditions that may be confused with AD are similar to those in infants and children. These include contact dermatitis, seborrheic dermatitis, nummular eczema, dermatophytosis, scabies, and CTCL. Lichen simplex chronicus may resemble AD in adults as well. As childhood forms of these diseases have been described, only the distinctive features in adults are explored here.

Contact dermatitis

Contact dermatitis, of either the allergic or irritant variety, is frequently mistaken for AD. Accounting for roughly 90% of skin disorders acquired in the workplace, contact dermatitis is the most common occupational disease in the USA. Differentiating allergic contact dermatitis from irritant contact reactions can sometimes be quite challenging. Both types are inflammatory but ICD is caused by innate immune mechanisms related to agents that directly damage the skin either acutely or upon repeated contact. ACD is mediated by T-cell-adaptive immunity of the delayed type.

Common agents that cause ICD include water, soaps, detergents, acids, bases, solvents, saliva, urine, and stool. The most prevalent allergens are poison ivy, poison oak, poison sumac, metals, cosmetics, topical medications, foods, rubber products, resins, and adhesives. Patch testing is the 'gold standard' for identifying the cause(s) of allergic contact dermatitis. There is no definitive test for ICD but patch testing is essential to rule out occult allergens.

The prevention of ICD or ACD depends on finding and avoiding the causative agent, whereas treatment of acute disease relies on topical and oral corticosteroids and antipruritic agents (Beltrani and Beltrani 1997, Mark and Slavin 2006, Nichols and Cook-Bolden 2009).

Seborrheic dermatitis

Seborrheic dermatitis in adults is confused with AD far less often than in children. In more severe cases, the mid-chest and back may be involved, with scaly patches occasionally mistaken for atopic dermatitis. Patients with HIV infection may present with severe, extensive seborrheic dermatitis, especially if the CD4 count is less than 400 (Naldi and Rebora 2009).

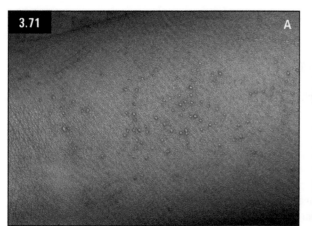
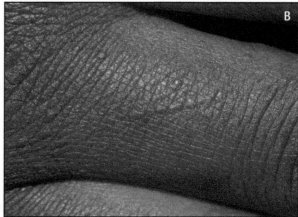

Fig 3.71 (A) Lichen nitidus presents with asymptomatic pinhead-sized papules in children, particularly of preschool and school age, usually on the abdomen, chest, glans penis, and upper extremities. (B) The Koebner phenomenon is almost always present.

Nummular eczema

Nummular eczema can be a 'look-alike' for focal AD. Classic disease predominantly occurs in adults, with a peak incidence during the sixth or seventh decade. The pathogenesis of this disorder is unclear but most patients do not have a personal or family history of atopy. It is noteworthy that nummular plaques are seen in patients with AD. However, the hallmarks of nummular eczema include erythematous papules and vesicles that coalesce into round, coin-shaped plaques with oozing, crusting, and scale. The most common areas of involvement are the upper extremities in females and lower extremities in males (Hellgren and Mobacken 1969, Aoyama *et al.* 1999).

Lichen simplex chronicus

Lichen simplex chronicus (LSC) is a chronic, pruritic disorder characterized by erythematous, scaling, and lichenified plaques with or without overlying excoriation (**Fig 3.72**). The pejorative connotation of older terms such as neurodermatitis circumscripta or circumscribed neurodermatitis has lost favor. LSC occurs either as a primary disease, arising from normal-appearing skin, or secondary to a pre-existing skin disorder such as psoriasis, lichen planus, infection, or neoplasia. As 20–90% of patients with LSC report atopy, a number of investigators consider this a chronic manifestation of AD (Singh 1973, Lynch 2004).

Scabies

The severe pruritus associated with scabetic infestation often evokes a diagnosis of AD, but the two conditions can usually be differentiated based on history and physical examination. Patients with scabies may report itchy contacts or travel to an endemic area. They present with erythematous and scaly, crusted papules, nodules, and burrows that exhibit a predilection for skinfolds. Favored sites include interdigital web spaces, volar surface of the wrists, elbows, periaxillary areas, scrotum, penis, labia, areolae, and lateral aspects of the palms. Face, head, and neck are spared in adults (**Fig 3.73**). Itching is usually worse at night in both conditions. Symptoms are caused by the host immune reaction to burrowed mites and their products. The diagnosis can be confirmed by microscopic identification of mites, eggs, or fecal pellets from skin lesion scrapings (Hicks and Elston 2009).

Dermatophyte infection

As in children, dermatophyte infections in adults mimic AD. Definitive diagnosis can by made by KOH examination of scales from lesional skin (Hainer 2003).

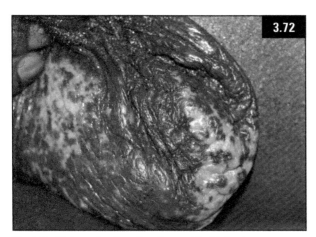

Fig 3.72 Lichen simplex chronicus with thickening, accentuation of skin markings, and depigmentation in a male with no other evidence of atopic dermatitis.

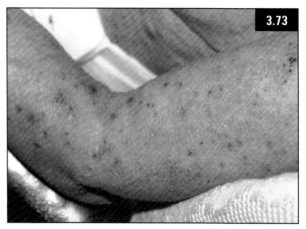

Fig 3.73 Scabies involving the arms and trunk of a nursing-home patient.

CUTANEOUS T-CELL LYMPHOMA

Historically, the prognosis of CTCL was based on 'eczematous,' plaque and tumor morphologies. After more than 200 years since MF was described, the early patch or eczematous lesions still show nonspecific histology that may be confused with a chronic form of AD. More often than not, patients with nondescript *eczematoid* lesions and nonspecific histology on repeated biopsies are followed for years before diagnostic histological features are revealed. Frequently the eruption is suppressed by high-potency topical corticosteroids that can obscure the characteristic histology. Withdrawal of topical corticosteroids is recommended for at least 1 month before obtaining a biopsy of suspected MF. The eruption in adults typically conforms to a *swimsuit* distribution, namely on the abdomen, hips, buttocks, and breasts (Nashan *et al.* 2007). Ultimately, the designation of MF requires the presence of an intractable eczematous eruption in a characteristic distribution supported by diagnostic histological findings.

MISCELLANEOUS ERUPTIONS

Finally, as with children, lichen planus (**Fig 3.74**) and lichen spinulosus (**Fig 3.75**) in adults can also be confused with AD.

CONCLUSION

Atopic dermatitis is a common, inflammatory, skin disease, most common in infancy and childhood, which is usually associated with asthma and allergic rhinitis in the patient or his or her immediate family. Diagnosis is usually straightforward but atypical cases may be confused with a number of other disorders. Not only has atopy increased in frequency in children, but cases starting in adulthood are increasingly reported. Diagnostic accuracy can usually be achieved by appreciation of the typical age-related patterns of distribution, lesional morphology, and family history.

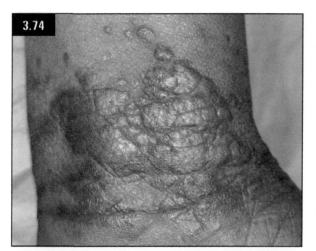

Fig 3.74 Lichen planus with lichenification on the volar aspect of the wrist resembling atopic dermatitis. Note the surrounding smaller papules and slightly violaceous hue.

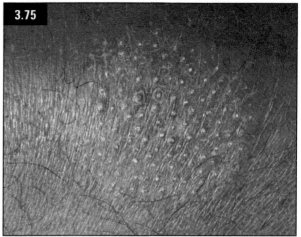

Fig 3.75 Lichen spinulosus in an adult. The cause is unknown but it has been reported in association with alcoholism and Crohn disease.

INFANTILE ATOPIC DERMATITIS

Sadaf H. Hussain, James R. Treat and, Albert C. Yan

INTRODUCTION

Infantile atopic dermatitis describes a subcategory of atopic dermatitis that, as its name implies, affects infants. Most patients with atopic dermatitis exhibit an early onset of their disease, with approximately 60% of those affected showing typical clinical manifestations during the first year of life (Kay *et al.* 1994). Many regard atopic dermatitis principally as a pediatric disorder because 85% of all patients demonstrate clinical findings by 5 years of age.

As with the childhood and adult variants of atopic dermatitis, the infantile form is a syndrome marked by pruritus, a predilection for stereotypical anatomic sites, and a recurrent, relapsing, and remitting course (Eichenfield *et al.* 2003). The diagnosis of infantile atopic dermatitis is made largely on clinical grounds and is based on an age-associated evolution of characteristic historical and physical findings (**Box 4.1**). Less often, corroborating laboratory data are used to establish the diagnosis.

Complications of atopic dermatitis can affect an infant profoundly. Secondary infections in the neonate may require hospitalization and intravenous antibiotic or antiviral therapy owing to the young infant's relatively immature immune system, and the greater likelihood of more significant morbidity and mortality with early onset infections in this age group.

Infantile atopic dermatitis may act as a possible 'gateway disorder' in what has been referred to as

---

Box 4.1   2003 American Academy of Dermatology criteria for the diagnosis of atopic dermatitis

Criteria for the diagnosis of atopic dermatitis include essential, important, and supporting features.

Essential features:
- Chronic relapsing history
- Pruritus
- Eczematous dermatitis with typical morphology and age-specific distribution
- Sparing of intertriginous areas
- Infancy: face, neck, extensor areas
- Any age: flexural involvement

Important features: early age of onset, personal history of atopy, family history of atopy, IgE reactivity

Supporting features: perifollicular accentuation, palmar hyperlinearity, keratosis pilaris, ichthyosis vulgaris, lichenification, prurigo, atypical vascular phenomena (white dermographism, delayed blanch, facial pallor) (Adapted from Eichenfield *et al.* 2003. Reprinted with permission.)

the *atopic march* (Spergel and Paller 2003) (**Fig 4.1**). In infants with atopic dermatitis, the accompanying skin barrier disruption may provide a route for epicutaneous sensitization and result in later childhood-onset asthma and allergic rhinitis, as well as a variety of food and environmental allergies.

In rare cases, infantile atopic dermatitis or atopic dermatitis-like eruptions may also represent an early clinical manifestation that can herald a variety of congenital, metabolic, and immunodeficiency syndromes (**Box 4.2**).

Special considerations must also be taken into account when treating the infant with atopic dermatitis because of differences in body surface area:weight ratios, metabolic variations that may influence responses to medications, and growth and development concerns that must inform any therapeutic decision-making. As atopic dermatitis eventually remits in most patients, use of therapeutic agents in young patients should be balanced against any potential complications that may arise.

Box 4.2   Disorders associated with atopic dermatitis and differential diagnosis of eczematous dermatitis

Disorders with atopic dermatitis as an associated feature
- Chromosome 18q deletion syndrome
- Hyper-IgE syndrome
- Ichthyosis vulgaris
- Wiskott–Aldrich syndrome

Disorders with eczematous skin findings that resemble atopic dermatitis
- Acrodermatitis enteropathica and other necrolytic erythemas
- Ataxia–telangiectasia syndrome
- Congenital ichthyoses (including Netherton syndrome)
- Contact dermatitis (irritant, allergic)
- Cutaneous T-cell lymphoma
- Dermatophytosis
- Gluten-sensitive enteropathy
- Immunodeficiency syndromes (including selective IgA, X-linked agammaglobulinemia, severe combined immunodeficiency, Omenn syndrome)
- Nummular dermatitis
- Langerhans cell histiocytosis
- Lichen simplex chronicus
- Nutritional deficiency syndromes (such as kwashiorkor, hypervitaminosis A)
- Psoriasis (especially partially treated or infantile variants)
- Scabies
- Seborrheic dermatitis
- Syphilis, secondary
- Tinea capitis
- Metabolic disorders (such as biotin deficiency, Hartnup disease, histidinemia, phenylketonuria)
- Sener syndrome (frontonasal dysplasia and dilated Virchow–Robin spaces)
- Smith–Lemli–Opitz syndrome

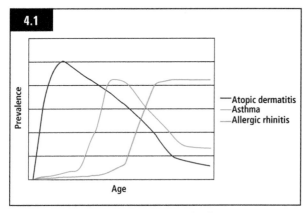

4.1

Fig 4.1 The atopic march: incidence of different types of atopy. Atopic dermatitis peaks in the first years of life and declines after that time. Asthma and allergic rhinitis increase over time as sensitization develops. (Reprinted from Spergel and Paller 2003. © 2003 with permission from Elsevier.)

EPIDEMIOLOGY

The prevalence of atopic dermatitis appears to have increased since the 1970s. Based on a study of Oregon schoolchildren, the current prevalence of atopic dermatitis in the USA is estimated to be approximately 17% (Laughter et al. 2000). By contrast, in studies involving children born before 1960, prevalence rates of atopic dermatitis had ranged from 1.4% to 3.1% (Turner et al. 1974). Although study designs and more standardized definitions of atopic dermatitis may represent some of the reasons for apparent increases in prevalence estimates (Wüthrich 1999), more recent worldwide prevalence surveys have indeed corroborated high lifetime, 12-month, and point prevalence rates of atopic dermatitis, similar to those currently observed in the USA (Flohr and Williams 2006). In western industrialized societies, lifetime prevalence rates have ranged from 10.5% in Germany (Werner et al. 2002) to 21.3% in Denmark (Mortz et al. 2001).

Commonly associated risk factors for atopic dermatitis include sex, geography, socioeconomic status, environmental factors, perinatal influences, and genetics. Although some studies suggest a female predominance for atopic dermatitis, other studies do not corroborate this finding (Schultz Larsen 1993). The prevalence of atopic dermatitis varies based on geography. Point prevalence estimates among rural Tanzanian children aged between 7 and 18 years is quite low (0.73%) when compared with prevalence estimates among western industrialized countries (Henderson 1995). In one inland town in Australia (Wagga Wagga), a point prevalence rate of 31.9% among children aged between 8 and 10 years has been reported (Peat et al. 1994). These geographic factors are likely influenced by a composite of other factors such as ethnic variations, perinatal practices, environmental differences (such as climate and degree of urbanization), socioeconomic factors, and genetics. There are conflicting data on ethnic variation as a factor affecting the prevalence of atopic dermatitis. No significant variation, for instance, is observed among different ethnic groups living in Leicester, England (Neame et al. 1995). Other studies have suggested that those classified as Hispanic, black, or Asian have significantly higher rates of representation among children evaluated for atopic dermatitis in the outpatient setting (Horii et al. 2007). Likewise, when compared with local white cohorts, London-born African–Caribbean and West Indian children had higher prevalence rates of atopic dermatitis (Davis et al. 1961, Williams et al. 1995).

Perinatal practices such as breastfeeding may reduce the risk of atopic dermatitis. However, the data remain somewhat confusing despite large and well-designed studies. Although there are ample data to suggest a benefit of breastfeeding for children of families with a positive family history of atopy, the results of the recent KOALA study indicate that a longer duration of breastfeeding was associated with lower risk of atopic dermatitis in those children who had no atopic family history, but not in those whose families had an atopic background (Gdalevich et al. 2001, Kerkhof et al. 2003, Snijders et al. 2007). KOALA is (in Dutch) an acronym for Child, Parent and Health: Lifestyle and Genetic constitution.

Furthermore, other studies such as the recent German Infant Nutritional Intervention (GINI) Program birth cohort study do not corroborate any benefit for breastfeeding when compared with conventional cows' milk formula (Laubereau et al. 2004). These conflicting data may arise from variations in the definition of atopic dermatitis used in the studies, breast milk composition, duration of breastfeeding, and selection bias (Flohr and Williams 2006). Although cigarette use may not predispose those who smoke to the development of atopic dermatitis, maternal cigarette use may be a risk factor for developing atopic dermatitis in children born to these mothers (Mills et al. 1994, Schäfer et al. 1997). Other perinatal factors that may predispose children to atopic dermatitis include maternal factors (such as maternal oral contraceptive use before pregnancy, or older maternal age at the time of first birth) and infant factors (higher infant birthweight) (Golding and Peters 1987, Peters and Golding 1987, Olesen *et al.* 1997, Braae Olesen and Thestrup-Pedersen 2000).

Environmental factors may influence the development of atopic dermatitis. Urbanization and industrialization and their myriad associations – exposure to pollution, allergens, nutritional diversity, modernized housing – may contribute to the observed increase in prevalence of atopic dermatitis and related disorders (Diepgen 2000). Although many factors appear to predispose to atopic dermatitis, larger family size has been associated with decreased risk of atopic dermatitis, perhaps as a proxy for increased exposure to early childhood infections (Strachan 1989). Rural residence likewise appears to confer a measure of protection against atopic diseases (Bråbäck *et al.* 2004). The increasing prevalence of allergic disorders, the relative decrease in early exposures to childhood infections, and the aforementioned observations form

the basis of the now well-known 'hygiene hypothesis' (Bach 2002) (**Fig 4.2**).

Higher socioeconomic class – itself a potential proxy for smaller family size, increased exposure to medical care, increased immunizations, more allergenic home environments, and greater nutritional variety – also correlates with a predisposition to atopic dermatitis (Williams *et al.* 1994, McNally and Phillips 2000).

The socioeconomic costs of managing atopic dermatitis are also significant. Data from the National Ambulatory Medical Care Survey and National Hospital Ambulatory Medical Care Survey databases indicate that, over an 8-year period, atopic dermatitis is a highly common disorder of childhood and accounted for 7.4 million outpatient visits by children. Approximately 1.1 million or 15% of atopic dermatitis visits involved management specifically of infantile atopic dermatitis (Horii *et al.* 2007). The national cost to healthcare insurers for the care of patients with atopic dermatitis has been estimated as being up to US$3.8 billion annually (Ellis *et al.* 2002).

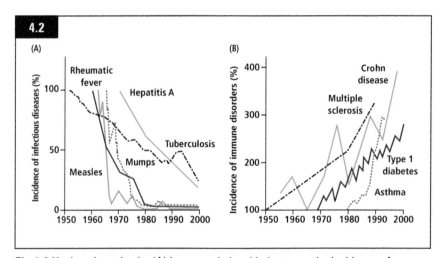

Fig 4.2 Hygiene hypothesis: (A) inverse relationship between the incidence of prototypical infectious diseases and (B) the incidence of immune disorders from 1950 to 2000. (Reprinted with permission from Bach 2002. © 2002 Massachusetts Medical Society. All rights reserved.)

PATHOGENESIS

Emerging evidence indicates that atopic dermatitis is a multifactorial disorder characterized by a genetically determined skin barrier dysfunction, subsequent epicutaneous sensitization, and an associated abnormal immunological response. There is a T-helper cell 2 (Th2)-dominated inflammatory profile in acute atopic dermatitis and a Th1-dominated inflammatory profile in chronic atopic dermatitis.

Mutations in filaggrin, decreased production of natural moisturizing factors, relative ceramide deficiencies, and increased activity of stratum corneum chymotryptic enzymes are among the associated pathomechanisms that contribute to an impaired skin barrier in patients with atopic dermatitis (Higuchi *et al.* 2000, Cork *et al.* 2006, Palmer *et al.* 2006, Kezic *et al.* 2008). The presence of skin barrier dysfunction presumably leads to increased epicutaneous sensitization, as well as predisposing the patient to immunological reactions to environmental allergens (Spergel and Paller 2003) (see **Fig 4.1**).

As the premature infant has an immature skin barrier associated with increased permeability and transepidermal water loss, it might be assumed that premature infants would, in general, be at increased risk of developing atopic dermatitis. Data on this subject remain conflicting. In a review of 443 children with atopic dermatitis, very few were noted as having been born preterm (David and Ewing 1988). A study of 10-year-old Scandinavian children born prematurely with birthweights <1500 g and compared with control children born at term with birthweights >2500 g demonstrated that prematurity was actually associated with a statistically significant reduction in risk of atopic sensitization (Schultz Larsen 1993). Term infants generally had higher total IgE levels and a higher rate of atopy (31% vs 15% in the premature group).

Another Scandinavian study found a correlation between high gestational age, high birthweight, and increased risk of atopic dermatitis (Olesen *et al.* 1997). These findings were contradicted by a study from Denmark indicating that low birthweight and preterm delivery are correlated risk factors predisposing the infant to atopic dermatitis and asthma (Steffensen *et al.* 2000). These studies, as might be expected, are fraught with potential confounding issues, and other influential factors, such as prenatal maternal exposures, preterm nutritional regimens, neonatal skin care regimens, ascertainment bias in the selection of patients or controls, as well as family size and other environmental factors that could affect outcomes.

CLINICAL CHARACTERISTICS

The morphology of the lesions of atopic dermatitis or eczema is similar at any age and is easily recognized by the clinician. As the term 'eczema' implies, skin findings are characterized by erythema, scaling, pruritic patches, plaques, and vesicles which are often coupled with secondary changes of oozing and crusting. Lichenification is less common in infants because infants cannot rub or scratch as aggressively as older children.

Although the morphology of eczema lesions is similar at different ages, the distribution of skin lesions in atopic dermatitis is age dependent. Eczema in infants typically involves the face (**Fig 4.3**) and often demonstrates a more generalized skin eruption with accentuation in the flexural creases of the antecubital and popliteal fossae, wrists, ankles, posterior thighs, and posterior neck areas (**Fig 4.4**). Infants often have their hands in their mouths, and the dorsal aspects of the hands and fingers themselves in children with atopic dermatitis are commonly and more severely involved. Characteristic sparing of the nose and perinasal areas is frequently referred to as the 'headlight sign' and can help differentiate atopic dermatitis from seborrhea and viral eruptions (**Fig 4.5**). Likewise, sparing of the diaper area among children who wear diapers is also highly characteristic and may be a reflection of an occlusive, high-humidity environment. The late pediatrician Walter Tunnessen picturesquely referred to this phenomenon as the *tropical rainforest effect*. The presence of the diaper may also function as a physical barrier against scratching which might explain sparing of the diaper area in infants and recrudescence of eczema in diaper-wearing toddlers, who find the diaper less of a barrier and can find ways around it to scratch the buttocks or perineum.

Atopic dermatitis has been described as *the itch that rashes*, highlighting the development of skin eruptions at sites where the skin is excoriated. A parallel finding is the observation that older infants and young toddlers who spend time crawling on the floor, such as on carpeting and the like, will demonstrate corresponding areas of eczema at sites of friction, namely the extensor surfaces of the arms and legs.

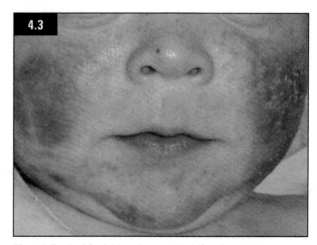

Fig 4.3 Typical facial involvement in infantile atopic dermatitis.

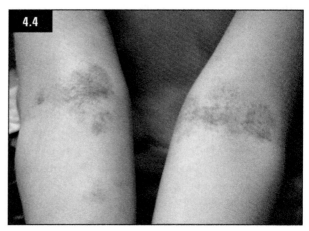

Fig 4.4 Typical morphology and distribution of skin lesions in infantile atopic dermatitis.

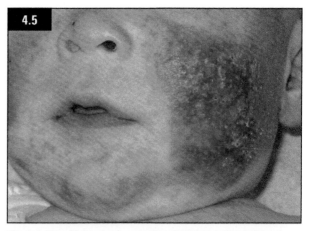

Fig 4.5 'Headlight sign': note the characteristic perinasal sparing in infantile facial atopic dermatitis.

Scalp scaling and erythema are often attributed to seborrheic dermatitis. However, scalp involvement in atopic dermatitis is not uncommon. The findings of infantile seborrheic dermatitis classically manifest as salmon-colored areas of erythema and scaling which may be mildly pruritic (if at all), and are typically concentrated on the scalp, eyebrows, perinasal folds, and intertriginous areas. By contrast, infantile atopic dermatitis is marked by a more intense erythema and characteristic itching, with flexural crease involvement of extremities more typical, along with relative sparing of perinasal and intertriginous areas. As a result of the greater number of skinfolds in infants, it is not unusual to see involvement within multiple skinfolds outside the usual antecubital or popliteal spaces (*Table 4.1*).

In infants, manifestations of atopic and seborrheic dermatitis overlap, giving rise to a kind of hybrid condition, *atoporrheic dermatitis*, for lack of a better term. (This would not be dissimilar to what has been described by some as *PsEma*, an intermediate phenomenon in which features of both psoriasis and eczema coexist (Abramovits *et al.* 2005).)

In older children and adults, atopic dermatitis tends to localize more to skinfolds and often the extremities with less facial involvement. Nummular and more lichenified lesions are also more common in children and adults than in infants.

Other supportive findings on physical examination, which may be seen in children, have been noted by Hanifin and Rajka and include xerosis, ichthyosis vulgaris, keratosis pilaris, palmar hyperlinearity, nipple eczema, atopic pleats (Dennie–Morgan folds), pityriasis alba, anterior neck folds, perifollicular accentuation, orbital darkening (atopic shiners), white dermographism (delayed blanch), and hand and foot dermatitis (Hanifin and Rajka 1980). Lymphadenopathy of the head and neck is likely secondary to inflammation, or sometimes a secondary infection, and also commonly noted in infants with atopic dermatitis.

Infants with atopic dermatitis may be very irritable; both child and parent may suffer disturbances in rest and sleep cycles. Affected infants and children are typically intolerant of wool and other harsh fabrics, which exacerbate pruritus. Poor growth may be the result of an underlying comorbidity such as constitutional growth delay, associated food allergies, eosinophilic gastroenteritis, or an underlying genetic disorder such as Wiskott–Aldrich syndrome.

Table 4.1 Comparison between infantile atopic and seborrheic dermatitis

	INFANTILE ATOPIC DERMATITIS	INFANTILE SEBORRHEIC DERMATITIS
Pruritus	Significant	None to mild
Erythema	Bright pink	Salmon colored
Scalp	Often present	Typically involved
Perinasal areas	Spared	Typically involved
Intertriginous zones	Typically absent	Typically involved

The diagnosis of atopic dermatitis is generally made by careful clinical examination. Consensus clinical criteria have been developed to assist in diagnosis (see **Box 4.1**).

Laboratory studies are not typically helpful for the diagnosis of atopic dermatitis because they are neither sensitive nor specific for the disease. However, an elevated serum IgE and immediate (type 1) skin test reactivity support the diagnosis. Laboratory testing may also be useful in identifying underlying comorbid disorders such as secondary infection, relevant food allergies, or congenital, metabolic, or immunodeficiency disorders. Skin biopsy is often nonspecific, with features of a spongiotic dermatitis with epidermal acanthosis and eosinophils.

In the evaluation of an infant with atopic dermatitis, it is useful to record certain items in the history and to observe them over time at follow-up visits. These include:

- Age of onset
- Frequency and duration of flares
- Typical anatomic sites of involvement
- Degree of pruritus and scratching
- Seasonality
- Bathing practices
- Factors that aggravate or remediate the condition, including pets, foods, weather, illnesses, immunizations, and so on
- History of secondary infections and prior use of antibiotics
- Family history of atopy
- Impact on sleep, diet, growth; for older patients, impact on work, school, and relationships with family and friends
- Therapies used including emollients and pharmacological agents.

COMPLICATIONS

In atopic dermatitis, the defective skin barrier, abnormal immune responses, and associated decreases in production of endogenous antimicrobial peptides all predispose the affected patient to secondary infections (Ong *et al.* 2002). These cutaneous infections may pose a more serious risk to the infant and may at times increase the potential for systemic infection.

Bacterial colonization is common among patients with atopic dermatitis, and these colonized patients are at increased risk for bacterial superinfection (Suh *et al.* 2006). Often, areas of superinfected skin develop oozing, with superimposed crusting that is often yellowish in color (**Fig 4.6**). The most commonly encountered pathogen is *Staphylococcus aureus*, with 93% of atopic dermatitis patients colonized by this organism, although other common skin flora such as group A streptococci may also be involved (Leyden *et al.* 1974, Breuer *et al.* 2002). At the authors' center, approximately 80% of children with atopic dermatitis have evidence of *S. aureus* colonization, and 16% have a meticillin-resistant *S. aureus* (MRSA) strain (Suh *et al.* 2008). Subclinical colonization or overt bacterial infection may manifest as recalcitrant eczema, and may induce apparent tachyphylaxis or steroid resistance (Li *et al.* 2004). Clinical manifestations of *S. aureus* infection may include yellowish crusting and oozing, or frank pustules, abscesses, or cellulitis. Recognizing and treating signs of overcolonization such as widespread erosions and fissuring are also vital to effective therapy. Infection with MRSA species is more commonly associated with abscesses and cellulitis. Streptococcal superinfection may present similarly with pustules and cellulitis, but may also manifest as a foul-smelling intertrigo in infants with or without atopic dermatitis (Honig *et al.* 2003).

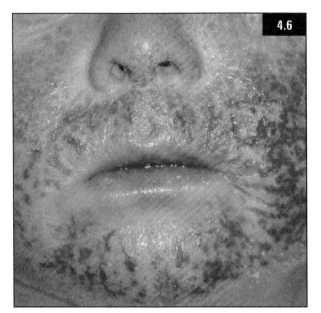

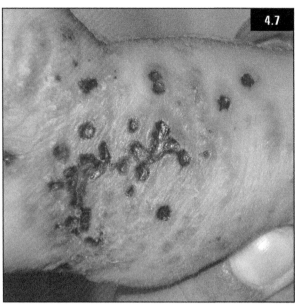

Fig 4.6 Infantile atopic dermatitis with bacterial superinfection.

Fig 4.7 Kaposi varicelliform eruption caused by herpes simplex virus infection (eczema herpeticum).

Kaposi varicelliform eruption represents a viral superinfection of atopic dermatitis. The viruses classically associated include herpes simplex virus (eczema herpeticum), enterovirus, vaccinia (eczema vaccinatum), and variola (smallpox). In the most common form – eczema herpeticum – herpes simplex virus inoculation by direct contact with an infected skin surface or by reactivation from prior infection can result in a sudden, generalized herpes simplex virus infection, characterized by grouped vesicles on an erythematous base, often clustering at sites of atopic dermatitis involvement. This is accompanied by fevers, pruritus, and bacterial superinfection. As the vesicles rupture, punched-out erosions appear at sites of infection (**Fig 4.7**). Eventually, the lesions crust over and leave areas of dyschromia or, less commonly, scarring, but untreated herpes simplex virus infections can lead to keratitis or blindness, or serve as a portal to bacterial sepsis. Eczema herpeticum has been reported in two Japanese neonates who were treated with topical tacrolimus; this agent should be avoided before age 2 (Kimata 2008). Children with eczema herpeticum should be admitted to the hospital and treated with intravenous acyclovir (aciclovir), analgesia, hydration and maintenance of fluid balance, and antibiotic treatment of secondary bacterial infection.

Eczema vaccinatum is a rare, life-threatening reaction occurring in patients with atopic dermatitis who are exposed to the smallpox vaccine virus. Although the prevalence of this condition has decreased since cessation of mandatory vaccinia immunizations, children of military personnel and others receiving the vaccine are still at risk because immunized individuals can shed live virus and inoculate contacts. As a result of the severity of the reaction, immunization of patients with atopic dermatitis or their close contacts is generally contraindicated unless smallpox represents an immediate risk. In the event of eczema vaccinatum, affected patients should be treated promptly with intramuscular vaccinia immune globulin (Centers for Disease Control and Prevention or CDC 2008).

Molluscum contagiosum and warts caused by the human papillomavirus are thought to occur more frequently and extensively in children with atopic dermatitis, owing to the impaired skin barrier. Molluscum contagiosum may be complicated by a benign eczematous 'id' reaction referred to as *molluscum dermatitis*. These eruptions probably signify the development of an immune response to the molluscum virus and impending viral clearance (Netchiporouk and Cohen 2012). A few days of topical corticosteroids may be used if there is significant itching or discomfort, but longer courses should be avoided because local immunosuppression might favor the development of new molluscum lesions. Secondary infections can usually be treated with topical antibiotics such as mupirocin.

Infections with *Malassezia* spp. and other fungi may also contribute to recalcitrant eczematous lesions.

Appropriate management of the id reaction should primarily be focused on educating patients and their families, reassuring them, and encouraging conservative management with topical emollients and antibiotics should the lesions become infected. However, in symptomatic patients, other treatment should be discussed. Short periods of topical steroids may be used for severely pruritic id reactions. However, long-term use of topical steroids or immunomodulating therapies should be discouraged, because it may delay the ultimate resolution of molluscum contagiosum. In addition, the treatment of molluscum contagiosum lesions in rare cases for symptomatic patients may involve local destruction or surgery. However, in cases where patients present with an id reaction to molluscum contagiosum and are otherwise asymptomatic, clinicians should adopt watchful waiting and avoid destructive treatments, because these eruptions signify the development of an immune response to the virus and likely impending viral clearance.

THERAPEUTIC CONSIDERATIONS

Management of infantile atopic dermatitis entails relieving the symptoms and signs of atopic dermatitis, treating associated superinfection, and optimizing epidermal barrier function, while taking into account the safety of the interventions prescribed. Infants have a high surface area:weight ratio compared with older children and adults, and systemic absorption of topically applied medications poses a real risk. Likewise, the degree of skin barrier dysfunction may also exacerbate percutaneous absorption. Metabolic differences must be considered when treating young infants. Antihistamines, for instance, are generally contraindicated for infants younger than 6 months because of unpredictable effects on hepatic metabolism and the risk of apnea. An optimal regimen for treating an infant with atopic dermatitis requires a multimodal plan that begins with appropriate atopic skin care.

ATOPIC SKIN CARE

Atopic skin care is the cornerstone of treatment for patients with infantile atopic dermatitis. Bathing routines should be evaluated at the first visit, as well as at all subsequent visits, because alterations in the duration and frequency of bathing definitely affect the course of atopic dermatitis. As pointed out by Tilles *et al.* (2007), increased bathing, to take advantage of the therapeutic qualities of water, was long ago advised by well-respected dermatologists such as Alibert (1818). During the early twentieth century, advice to decrease bathing and avoid water became more popular (Bulkley 1913). Conflicting advice regarding bathing practices continues today.

Bathing as a means of hydrating the skin has been evaluated in one small pilot study (Chiang and Eichenfield 2006). Five patients with atopic dermatitis and five control patients were randomized to undergo bathing alone, bathing with immediate moisturizer application, bathing with delayed moisturizer application, or no bathing plus use of moisturizer alone. In this pilot study, hygrometer measurements indicated that, although all methods (except bathing alone) increased the water content of the skin, not bathing plus moisturizer application provided the greatest degree of hydration when compared with the alternatives (206% relative to baseline compared with 141–142% for bathing plus moisturizing) (**Fig 4.8**).

Although decreased bathing may increase skin hydration, advocates for bathing suggest that increased bathing can reduce the risk of bacterial skin colonization and infection by removing potential pathogens from the skin. Several studies have documented the utility of using antimicrobial compounds such as iodine or chlorhexidine to reduce bacterial skin colonization. However, two studies of bathing frequency in premature infants failed to show any differences in skin flora type or colony counts when bathing daily was compared to bathing every 4 days (Franck *et al.* 2000, Quinn *et al.* 2005).

Although there is controversy as to whether increased or decreased bathing frequency and duration is more beneficial, the approach should be individualized for each patient. For those who prefer regular bathing, daily short baths may promote bonding between parent and child and allow for hydration, as long as bathing is followed by the application of emollients. For those in whom bathing is painful, unpleasant, or inconvenient, less frequent bathing is preferable along with regular emollient use to help improve hydration.

When bathing infants who have atopic dermatitis, gentle cleansers including syndets (such as Cetaphil or Aveeno) or a gentle fragrance-free pH-balanced soap (such as Dove or Oil of Olay) should be selected over traditional alkaline soaps (such as Ivory). Alkalinization of the skin may increase stratum corneum chymotryptic enzyme activity and further impair already abnormal skin barrier function (Hachem *et al.* 2005).

Topical emollients should be applied liberally on a daily or twice-daily basis, or more frequently as needed. Application of bland emollients is itself therapeutic, and a wide variety of agents are available including petrolatum-based ointments, hydrophilic ointments and creams, as well as newer ceramide-based creams and barrier repair devices (petrolatum, Aquaphor, Eucerin, Cetaphil, Aveeno, Triceram, CeraVe, Epiceram, Atopiclair, Mimyx). As atopic dermatitis is a chronic disorder, consistent use of emollients should be continued even when other topical medications are not being applied. When using emollients together with topical medications, one should preferably wait 30–60 min after application of the medication before applying the emollient. This avoids dilution of the medication and rarely unexpected increased absorption of the medication from stacking the two preparations together (Huang *et al.* 2005).

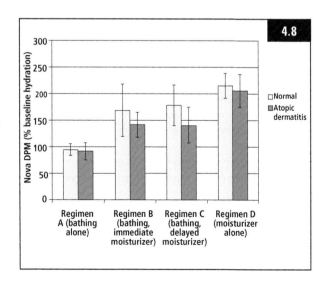

Fig 4.8 Hygrometer measurements indicated show that bathing followed by moisturizing or moisturizing alone increased water content in the skin. Moisturizer application without bathing provided the greatest degree of hydration in patients with atopic dermatitis and in normal individuals when compared with the alternatives (for moisturizing alone skin hydration was 206% above baseline compared with 141–142% for bathing and moisturizing). Bathing without moisturizing resulted in a decrease of hydration below baseline. (Reprinted from Chiang and Eichenfield 2009 with permission from John Wiley & Sons.)

Topical soybean trypsin inhibitors also function as inhibitors of skin serine proteases and their future use in emollients may provide a novel approach to improving skin barrier repair (Isogai *et al.* 2002). Their role in managing infantile atopic dermatitis remains to be determined. Certain emollients, however, should be avoided in infants. Keratolytic moisturizers containing salicylic acid, ammonium lactate, or urea should be used with caution in infants with impaired skin barriers. Not only do they cause stinging and burning, but also systemic absorption of the active ingredients is possible, especially in the context of abnormal skin integrity and increased surface area:weight ratios (Mancini 2004).

Clothing should be soft. Typically 100% cotton fabrics are preferred; wool should be avoided whenever possible. Newer, softer fabrics, such as those made from microfiber polyester yarns or antimicrobial silk, may also provide a suitable alternative for children with sensitive skin. Care should be taken to avoid overdressing the infant, which can cause sweating and overheating. When air-conditioning or dry heating systems are in use, a humidifier in the infant's room can minimize excessive drying of the skin.

Box 4.3   Topical agents for the treatment of atopic dermatitis

- Atopic skin care measures
- Emollients
- Topical corticosteroids
- Topical calcineurin inhibitors
- Pimecrolimus and tacrolimus
- Topical therapeutic emollients/barrier repair agents
- Atopiclair, palmitoylethanolamine (Mimyx)
- Ceramide-based emollients (CeraVe, Epiceram, Triceram)
- Lipid-optimized emollients (Eletone)

TOPICAL PHARMACOLOGICAL AGENTS (BOX 4.3)

As a result of the propensity for systemic absorption of topically applied medications, their attendant risks to the growing infant, and spontaneous improvement that may occur in children over time, the benefits of controlling short-term symptoms should be weighed against the potential for intermediate- and long-term adverse effects.

TOPICAL CORTICOSTEROIDS

Topical corticosteroids, at present, remain the first-line agents recommended for treatment of infantile atopic dermatitis. The specific topical corticosteroid used depends on several factors. Among the more important issues to consider are the infant's age, the anatomic site being treated, the severity of the condition, and the amount of body surface area to be treated.

The vasoconstrictor-based classification of topical corticosteroids has been a useful guide to determining potency and potential adverse effects (McKenzie and Stoughton 1962). Using this system, class 1 indicates super-high potency, 2 and 3 indicate high potency, 4, 5, and 6 indicate intermediate or mid-potency, and 7 indicates low potency. The system is not perfect, and discordances between vasoconstrictor-predicted rankings and clinical outcomes have been observed (Hepburn *et al.* 1996). For example, mometasone furoate ointment (ranked as a class 2 steroid by vasoconstrictor assay) carries an efficacy clinical outcome rating on day 21 of 40.2 whereas mometasone furoate cream (ranked as a class 4 steroid) carries a rating of 65.

An ointment vehicle has traditionally been a rational first choice for infants with atopic dermatitis. Ointments, in general, possess superior occlusive ability, and a decreased propensity to sting, burn, or cause contact sensitization when compared with other conventional vehicles. Their main drawback is lack of cosmetic elegance, as ointments tend to be greasy, sticky, and harder to spread. Newer vehicles including emollient creams, lipidized emulsions, hydrogels, and foams clearly have improved cosmetic elegance, and are more acceptable to older children. This, of course, is less of an issue with infants. The principal drawback of these new vehicles is that they are much more expensive and lack generic substitutes.

Mild-to-moderate infantile atopic dermatitis can usually be successfully managed with a low- or intermediate-potency topical steroid together with optimal atopic skin care. These corticosteroids can be applied over larger body surface areas with less danger of hypothalamic–pituitary–axis (HPA) suppression. The possibility of HPA suppression appears to be low for these classes of corticosteroids in studies provided to the Food and Drug Administration (FDA) (Nonprescription Drugs Advisory Committee and the Dermatologic and Ophthalmic Drugs Advisory Committee 2005a). Currently, the agents that carry an FDA-approved indication for infants aged down to 3 months include fluticasone propionate 0.05% cream, desonide 0.05% hydrogel, desonide 0.05% emulsion foam, and hydrocortisone butyrate 0.1% lotion.

Short-term use of stronger medium- or intermediate-potency corticosteroids (such as class 4 or 5) may be considered when the disease is localized, more severe, and unresponsive to lower-potency agents.

Longer-term intermittent use of topical steroids may be necessary, and nonhalogenated compounds should be preferred, given their shorter half-life and theoretically lower risk of cutaneous atrophy with prolonged use.

Higher-potency topical steroids are not often advised for use in infants because of their generally higher documented rates of HPA suppression (in product information and information provided at FDA advisory committee meetings) and the attendant risks of growth suppression, potential immunosuppression, and cutaneous atrophy (Nonprescription Drugs Advisory Committee and the Dermatologic and Ophthalmic Drugs Advisory Committee 2005b). In addition, only cautious topical steroid use is advised in the diaper area because occlusion of even lower-potency topical corticosteroids applied to perineal and genital skin areas can cause hypopigmentation, telangiectasia, striae, and purpura. A 9-month-old infant was reported to have had topical clobetasol applied to the diaper area for 3 months and developed clinically obvious findings of Cushing syndrome (Siklar et al. 2004).

Once a flare of atopic dermatitis has been brought under better control, topical corticosteroids can be used on an intermittent basis – twice weekly – to reduce the likelihood of repeated flares, especially in patients who flare frequently or who have labile disease. The use of a medium-potency agent, fluticasone cream, twice weekly for up to 16 weeks has resulted in decreased frequency of atopic dermatitis flares and has shown a favorable safety profile (Hanifin et al. 2002, Berth-Jones et al. 2003). Similarly, favorable data are available for methylprednisolone aceponate cream used twice weekly together with an emollient over a 16-week period (Peserico et al. 2008). These studies highlight the utility and safety of intermittent use of a medium-potency topical steroid for maintaining remission of atopic dermatitis in older children. Although not validated in a clinical trial setting, it would seem reasonable to assume that intermittent use of a lower-potency topical corticosteroid for infants in a similar manner could provide a reduction in the frequency of disease relapse.

Most infants, however, benefit from discontinuation of topical steroid therapy once the clinical findings have cleared and are maintained with topical emollients and atopic skin-care measures.

TOPICAL CALCINEURIN INHIBITORS

Currently available topical calcineurin inhibitors, namely pimecrolimus 1% cream and tacrolimus 0.1% ointment, are typically considered second-line agents for the treatment of atopic dermatitis. As high doses of these agents administered either orally or topically in animal studies result in an increased incidence of immunosuppression-related complications of lymphoma and skin malignancies, a boxed warning or so-called black box has been assigned to these drugs, although a causal relationship has not been established:

At concentrations available in the topical formulations, and given the short-term durations anticipated for use, the likelihood of immunosuppression in clinical use is expected to be quite low or clinically insignificant.

Nevertheless, clinical studies have indicated a higher rate of upper respiratory infections in patients treated with these agents compared with those treated with placebo. At the present time, the FDA recommends that clinicians avoid usage of these agents in children younger than 2 years because 'the effect of pimecrolimus and tacrolimus on the developing immune system in infants and children is not known.'

TOPICAL BARRIER REPAIR AGENTS

Several agents have recently been cleared for marketing in the USA as medical devices for the treatment of inflammatory skin conditions such as atopic dermatitis. These include: Atopiclair, palmitoylethanolamine cream, ceramide-based therapeutic emollients, and lipidized emulsions. There are no current age restrictions and they can be used in infants with atopic dermatitis as alternatives to topical corticosteroids. They generally lack the efficacy of more potent topical steroid agents, but may provide a reasonable steroid-sparing alternative for maintenance therapy in infantile atopic dermatitis.

ANTIHISTAMINES

Absorption of orally administered medications and their hepatic metabolism are not entirely predictable in infants. Likewise, use of antihistamines in infants can be associated with paradoxical agitation instead of sedation. Moreover, reports of fatal intoxication with diphenhydramine in young infants (aged 6–12 weeks) have been reported (Baker et al. 2003). As a result, use of antihistamines in young infants (those aged younger than 6 months) for routine management of pruritus is not generally recommended, and alternative topical agents such as topical corticosteroids or emollients are preferred.

Interestingly, in one study of 121 children with atopic dermatitis aged between 1 and 36 months the group receiving ketotifen for 1 year had fewer patients with high IgE compared with those who received placebo (Iikura et al. 1992). In another study of 100 children aged up to 24 months, the group receiving ketotifen had a 25% lower rate of asthma than the control group (Bustos et al. 1995). Finally, in a study of 817 young children aged between 1 and

2 years who received high-dose cetirizine, statistically significant differences in the rates of dust mite-induced asthma (51.5% with cetirizine vs 28.6% with placebo) and grass-associated asthma (58.8% with cetirizine vs 27.8% with placebo) were observed (Diepgen 2002). Although these data are provocative, further studies into the role of antihistamines in the atopic march are needed to validate these initial observations.

ANTIBIOTICS

Antibiotics and antiviral therapies may be needed when infants with atopic dermatitis develop signs and symptoms of superinfection. Given the increasing prevalence of antibiotic-resistant organisms, the choice of an antibiotic for empiric therapy must be informed by regional patterns of antibiotic resistance in the local community. In areas where meticillin resistance among S. aureus remains low, penicillin derivatives such as dicloxacillin as well as cephalosporins and amoxicillin/clavulanate may be reasonable options for empiric therapy. However, in communities where MRSA is common, alternatives such as clindamycin or trimethoprim–sulfamethoxazole may prove to be more effective first-line options. Performing skin cultures is imperative to ensure that the initial antibiotic choice is appropriate.

The optimal management of staphylococcal disease in neonates and infants continues to evolve. Mild, localized infections in neonates and infants may respond to topical therapy whereas multifocal disease, cellulitis, and bacteremia all require appropriate systemic therapy. Invasive bacterial disease warrants hospitalization and systemic therapy with vancomycin, oxacillin, gentamicin, or combination therapy (Fortunov et al. 2007).

An interesting question is whether use of antibiotics, either topically or orally, can favorably affect patients with infantile atopic dermatitis who are simply colonized but not superinfected. Data on this subject are conflicting. Patients with atopic dermatitis can experience a decrease in bacterial colonization by simply treating their eczema with a topical corticosteroid, possibly as a result of improved skin barrier integrity (Gong et al. 2006). At the same time, there is evidence to suggest that the presence of bacterial superantigens may cause steroid resistance or apparent tachyphylaxis, and patients who receive antibiotic therapy may have better responses to therapy; however, there are conflicting data regarding this issue (Leyden *et al.* 1974, Ewing *et al.* 1998, Hauk *et al.* 2000, Li *et al.* 2004).

In the authors' view, children with atopic dermatitis who do not respond sufficiently to atopic skin care measures, topical corticosteroids, topical calcineurin inhibitors, barrier repair agents, and therapeutic emollients may respond to a short 7- to 10-day course of oral antibiotic therapy. In these cases, evaluation of a bacterial culture to identify sensitivities may be helpful in guiding treatment.

SYSTEMIC AGENTS

The vast majority of infants respond well to conventional therapy with topical corticosteroids together with atopic skin care measures. Systemic agents are rarely used to treat atopic dermatitis in infants because of their unfavorable toxicity profiles and the lack of available data on their use in this population. Older children with severe and recalcitrant atopic dermatitis can be treated with ultraviolet light phototherapy and cautiously with systemic agents such as systemic corticosteroids, cyclosporine (ciclosporin), methotrexate, azathioprine, or mycophenolate mofetil.

CONCLUSIONS

Atopic dermatitis often presents during infancy with findings that are often more exuberant – xerosis, erythema, papular and vesicular skin changes, oozing, crusting, and occasionally lichenification – and more generalized in anatomic distribution than what is encountered in older children and adults. Although the diagnosis is typically made on clinical grounds, laboratory data and skin biopsy are occasionally helpful in cases where superinfection or underlying comorbid conditions are suspected. As with older patients, infants with atopic dermatitis frequently become colonized with *S. aureus*, which can predispose them to secondary bacterial infection; they can also occasionally be infected with other organisms such as herpes simplex virus. Pharmacological treatment of infants must take into account the chronic but often self-remitting nature of the disease, the relatively increased ratio of body surface area to weight, and differences between infants and older children in absorption and metabolism of topically and systemically administered medications. Appropriate atopic skin care measures can significantly reduce reliance on prescription medications and limit the frequency and severity of flares. In the end, management of infantile atopic dermatitis should remind the clinician first and foremost of the adage: first, do no harm (*primum non nocere*).

Clinical suggestions

1. First and foremost, infants must not be thought of as 'miniature adults.' Their high surface area:weight ratio, immature skin barrier, and metabolic differences compared with older children and adults put them at real risk of local and systemic adverse effects from topical corticosteroids and other agents. Topical salicylic acid, ammonium lactate, and urea should be avoided and systemic antihistamines should not be used before age 6 months to avoid paradoxical agitation or apnea.

2. On the initial visit and subsequent visits certain factors should be recorded in the history as outlined above. Especially important are anatomic sites, extent and severity of involvement, bathing practices, topical treatment history, exacerbating factors, history of secondary infections, and previous antibiotic treatment. Parents who may attribute their child's eczema to diet or food allergy should be counseled not to change formula or eliminate foods unless so instructed by the dermatologist, pediatrician, or an allergist experienced in the field of food allergy. There are documented cases of malnutrition in children subjected to elimination diets.

(continued)

3. Suggestions for bathing should be individualized. Frequent short baths facilitate parent–child bonding and should be followed by application of bland emollients to damp skin to maintain hydration. Gentle cleansers such as Cetaphil or Aveeno or fragrance-free pH-balanced soap (Dove, Oil of Olay) are preferable to alkaline soaps. Bleach baths, effective in older children, should be avoided in infants. If bathing is uncomfortable or inconvenient, it can be done less frequently, stressing the need for emollients.

4. Daily, twice daily, or more frequent use of emollients is therapeutic and is to be encouraged on a long-term basis. A number of effective, affordable preparations are available such as petrolatum, Aquaphor, Eucerin, Cetaphil, and Aveeno. In addition newer ceramide-based creams and barrier repair agents may be considered, but they are more expensive. If topical medications such as corticosteroids are being used, emollients should be applied 30–60 min after the medication.

5. Cotton clothing is ideal. To avoid sweating and overheating, both of which can exacerbate pruritus, care should be taken to avoid overdressing the infant.

6. Ointment vehicles are recommended in infants to avoid stinging, burning, and contact sensitization. The following agents carry an FDA-approved indication for infants down to age 3 months: fluticasone propionate 0.05% cream; desonide 0.05% hydrogel; desonide 0.05% emulsion foam; and hydrocortisone butyrate 0.1% lotion. In general the use of topical corticosteroids should be discontinued or limited once control of the dermatitis has been achieved. Improvement can be maintained by emollients and 'atopic skin care'.

7. A short course of antibiotics is sometimes useful to control flares caused by staphylococcal infection. Skin culture should be performed and initial antibiotic therapy should be based on local geographic staphylococcal sensitivity patterns.

CHAPTER 5

PRURITUS IN ATOPIC DERMATITIS: PATHOPHYSIOLOGY AND TREATMENT OPTIONS

Tejesh Surendra Patel and Gil Yosipovitch

Pruritus is the cardinal symptom of atopic dermatitis – a diagnosis of active disease cannot be made without a history of itching (Hanifin and Rajka 1980). In fact, pruritus is so central to atopic dermatitis that it has been referred to as *the itch that rashes* (Boguniewicz 2005). The prevalence of itching in atopic dermatitis approaches 100% (Yosipovitch *et al.* 2002, Dawn *et al.* 2009). In addition, pruritus is frequently exacerbated at night and has a profound impact on the quality of life of atopic dermatitis patients (Yosipovitch *et al.* 2002, Dawn *et al.* 2009). Itching not only disturbs sleep but also contributes to depression, agitation, changes in eating habits, and difficulty concentrating. Decreased sexual desire and sexual function have also been reported in patients with atopic dermatitis with itch (Yosipovitch *et al.* 2002, Patel *et al.* 2007b). Scratching leads to increased cutaneous inflammation, which causes further itching and scratching; this is referred to as the *itch–scratch cycle*. Atopic dermatitis patients are often unaware of the extent to which they scratch at night and how this contributes to the severity of their disease (Patel *et al.* 2007b).

Lately the interest of researchers has been piqued by recent insights into the mechanisms underlying both pruritus and atopic dermatitis. Until recently, most research on pruritus focused on its peripheral mechanisms. However, cognitive and affective aspects of the itch experience indicate that central mechanisms are extremely important as well. Indeed, both central and peripheral mediators are now thought to play an important role in the development of itching. This chapter provides an overview of the pathophysiology of pruritus associated with atopic dermatitis and reviews current and emerging treatment options.

PATHOPHYSIOLOGY OF PRURITUS IN ATOPIC DERMATITIS

THE EPIDERMIS AND PRURITUS RECEPTOR UNIT

A unique feature of itch is that it is restricted to the skin, mucous membranes, and cornea – no other tissue experiences pruritus (Charlesworth and Beltrani 2002). Current evidence suggests that the itch sensation emanates from activity in nerve fibers located in the epidermis. Although a specific epidermal itch receptor has not yet been clearly identified, it has been shown that removal of the epidermis abolishes the perception of pruritus (Shelley and Arthur 1957). Recent studies suggest that there are indeed itch-specific receptors in the skin. Certain C-nerve fibers containing Mas-related, G-protein-coupled receptor member A (MRGPRA), a subfamily of G-protein-coupled receptors, have been shown to mediate chloroquine-induced itch (Liu *et al.* 2009). A mutation in the oncostatin M receptor (OSMR) gene has recently been identified in patients with lichen amyloidosis, a localized pruritic condition most common in Hispanic and Asian individuals (Tanaka *et al.* 2009). This gene encodes OSMR-β, an interleukin-31 (IL-31) cytokine receptor. IL-31 is thought to elicit itch in atopic dermatitis and prurigo nodularis patients. Interestingly, keratinocytes express an array of neural mediators and receptors, all of which appear to be involved with the sensation of itch (Denda 2002). These neural mediators include opioids, proteases, substance P, nerve growth factor, neurotrophin-4, and endocannabinoids. Keratinocytes also express voltage-gated ATP channels and adenosine receptor ligands – similar to C-nerve fibers involved in transmission of the perception of pain (Inoue *et al.* 2002). It is thus possible that keratinocytes are involved in generating and transducing the itch sensation through these channels in a manner similar to pain.

Transepidermal water loss reflects epidermal barrier function and has been associated with itch intensity in patients with atopic dermatitis (Lee *et al.* 2006). It is possible that the known barrier defects in atopic dermatitis, which are reflected by a high transepidermal water loss, might permit the entry of irritants and other pruritus-inducing agents. (Cork *et al.* 2006). Interestingly, transepidermal water loss increases at night and could explain nocturnal exacerbations of pruritus commonly occurring in patients with atopic dermatitis (Yosipovitch *et al.* 1998).

THE NEURAL PROCESSING OF PRURITUS

Major advances have been made in the neurophysiology of pruritus in recent years. Histamine-sensitive afferent nerve fibers that convey histamine-induced itch have been identified, suggesting a specialized neuronal pathway for itch processing (Schmelz *et al.* 1997, Schmelz 2001). These histamine-sensitive C-nerve fibers are characterized by low-conduction velocities, large innervation territories, mechanical unresponsiveness, high transcutaneous electrical thresholds, and generation of axon reflex erythema (Schmelz *et al.* 1997, 2000, 2003).

However, antihistamines do not relieve chronic itch in many patients with atopic dermatitis, suggesting that histamine is not the main mediator of pruritus (Klein and Clark 1999, Dawn and Yosipovitch 2006a). Moreover, in both atopic dermatitis patients and healthy individuals, itch can be induced by focal low-intensity, high-frequency electrical stimulation (Ikoma *et al.* 2005). The nerve fibers responsible for this phenomenon are independent of the histamine-sensitive C-fibers, which display a high electrical threshold. Interestingly, this electrically induced itch is not accompanied by axon flare erythema, suggesting that the underlying nerve fibers may be more clinically relevant to pathological itch than those that are histamine-sensitive (Ikoma *et al.* 2005).

Recent studies have revealed a distinct parallel pathway of nonhistaminergic C-nerve fibers that transmit itch in the peripheral nervous system in humans and in the spinothalamic tract of primates (Davidson *et al.* 2007, Johanek *et al.* 2007, Namer *et al.* 2008). These fibers are activated by spicules of the ubiquitous tropical legume cowhage (*Mucuna pruriens*), known to induce an intense sensation of itch when rubbed or inserted into the skin, without inducing a histaminergic axon reflex (Shelley and Arthur 1955a, 1955b). The mechanism by which cowhage induces itch involves the release of an active protease (mucunain), contained in the spicules, which activates protease activated receptor 2 (PAR-2) and PAR-4 present in the skin (Reddy *et al.* 2008). These C-nerve fibers are mechano-heat sensitive and not itch-specific, because they also transmit a burning sensation accompanying the itch. PAR-2 has been shown to have a major role in mediating itch in atopic eczema patients (Steinhoff *et al.* 2003). Nonhistaminergic polymodal C-nerve fibers stimulated by mucunain may therefore have a significant clinical relevance to atopic eczema itch.

The concept of a dedicated neural pathway for itch in the central nervous system (CNS), in addition to the peripheral nervous system, has been an area of recent research interest. There are new data suggesting that neurons expressing gastrin-releasing peptide receptor (GRPR) may transmit only itch but not pain (Sun and Chen 2007). In a mouse model of chronic pruritus and atopic dermatitis-like skin lesions, pretreatment of mice with a GRPR antagonist prevented itch.

Central processing of itch has also been demonstrated using neuroimaging techniques such as positron emission tomography and functional magnetic resonance imaging (fMRI) in healthy humans. In these studies, histamine-induced itch coactivates the anterior cingulate and insular cortex, premotor and supplementary motor areas, cerebellum, primary somatosensory cortex, and thalamus (Hsieh *et al.* 1994, Darsow *et al.* 2000, Drzezga *et al.* 2001, Mochizuki *et al.* 2003, Leknes *et al.* 2007). The multiple brain areas involved with the central processing of pruritus are believed to be reflective of the multidimensional aspects of this distressing symptom (*Table 5.1*). Brain areas activated by pruritus are also involved with the central processing of pain, implying that the neural networks activated by these two sensory stimuli are not distinct but reflect a different but related activation pattern (Paus *et al.* 2006). Interestingly, data from our group based on a new neuroimaging technique (suited to assessing itch) have shown that the central processing of itch in atopic dermatitis patients is different from that in healthy individuals and is associated with disease severity (Ishiuji *et al.* 2007). Using this emerging technique, fMRI with arterial spin labeling, the authors have shown that patients with atopic dermatitis, but not healthy control individuals, demonstrate bilateral activation of the anterior and posterior cingulate cortices and the dorsal lateral prefrontal cortex, which are involved in emotions, reward, and memory of negative experiences (**Fig 5.1**) (Ishiuji *et al.* 2009). In addition, there was a significant correlation between percentage changes of brain activity in the anterior cingulate cortex, insula, and dorsolateral prefrontal cortex with disease severity as assessed by subjective itch intensity and the Eczema Area and Severity Score. These results strongly suggest that the CNS plays a unique role in atopic dermatitis-associated pruritus.

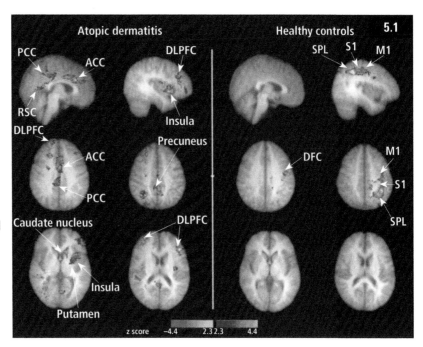

Fig 5.1 Brain activation during histamine stimuli in atopic dermatitis and healthy individuals. In the healthy controls, brain activation was identified contralaterally within the primary motor cortex (M1), primary somatosensory cortex (S1) and superior parietal lobe (SPL). In patients with atopic dermatitis, brain activation was identified bilaterally within the anterior cingulate cortex (ACC), posterior cingulate cortex (PCC), and retrosplenial cingulate cortex (RSC) as well as the dorsolateral prefrontal cortex (DLPFC) and the contralateral caudate nucleus, putamen, and anterior and posterior insular cortices. Red is activation. DFC, dorsofrontal cortex. (Reprinted from Ishiuji *et al.* 2009. © 2009 with permission of John Wiley & Sons.)

Table 5.1   Brain areas involved in the central processing of pruritus and their proposed function with regard to this symptom

BRAIN AREA	PROPOSED FUNCTION RELATING TO PRURITUS
Primary somatosensory cortex	Sensory–discriminative aspects of pruritus Localization of itch
Premotor and supplementary motor area	Motor response of scratching
Anterior cingulate cortex (ACC) and insula	Negative affective aspects of pruritus Rewarding aspects of scratching (ACC)
Posterior cingulate cortex and precuneus	Memory of negative experiences
Dorsal lateral prefrontal cortex	Reward mechanisms and localization of scratching
Prefrontal and orbitofrontal areas	Compulsion to scratch
Cerebellum	Scratch coordination

PERIPHERAL SENSITIZATION

Peripheral mediators of pruritus may acutely sensitize peripheral pruriceptive C-nerve fibers so that their responses to external stimulation are enhanced and/or facilitated (Ikoma *et al.* 2003). Nerve growth factor, a neuropeptide involved with nerve growth and repair, has been shown to play an important role in sustained increased neuronal sensitivity (Shu and Mendell 1999, 2001). This neuropeptide is also increased in chronic localized pain, where there is an augmented sprouting of epidermal nerve fibers and hypersensitivity (Mendell *et al.* 1999, Bohm-Starke *et al.* 2001, Ikoma *et al.* 2003). In atopic dermatitis, expression of nerve growth factor is increased in keratinocytes and mast cells leading to higher serum levels; moreover increased intradermal nerve fiber density has been found (Urashima and Mihara 1998, Toyoda *et al.* 2002, Groneberg *et al.* 2005). These similarities between localized pain and pruritus in atopic dermatitis suggest that similar mechanisms of neuronal sprouting and sensitization may exist for both pain and pruritus on a peripheral level (Ikoma *et al.* 2006).

CENTRAL SENSITIZATION

Central sensitization of itch signaling systems is a key feature of chronic itch states, including atopic dermatitis (Ikoma *et al.* 2004, 2005, 2006). This phenomenon results in sensitization of spinal neurons in the dorsal horn, leading to greater sensitivity to pruritic input. There are two forms of central sensitization that are associated with pruritus:

1. Alloknesis or 'itchy skin' is observed when touch- or brush-evoked itch occurs around an itching site (Simone *et al.* 1991, Heyer *et al.* 1995). This is analogous to the more familiar phenomenon of allodynia in chronic pain, where inflamed skin reacts to gentle mechanical stimuli causing the perception of pain. Similar to allodynia, alloknesis requires ongoing activity in primary afferents and is elicited by low-threshold mechanoreceptor Aβ fibers (Ikoma *et al.* 2006). Alloknesis is commonly encountered in atopic dermatitis, explaining patients' complaints of severe pruritus associated with sweating, sudden changes in temperature, dressing, and undressing.

2. Punctuate hyperknesis, in which a needle prick induces intense itch sensation in the area surrounding histamine induction, is similar to the phenomenon in chronic pain termed 'punctuate hyperalgesia.'

Painful stimuli, including scratching, have been shown normally to inhibit pruritus in psychophysical studies (Ward *et al.* 1996, Yosipovitch *et al.* 2007). However, painful electrical stimuli elicit itch in atopic dermatitis patients, indicating central sensitization (Nilsson and Schouenborg 1999, Ikoma *et al.* 2004, Ishiuji *et al.* 2007). Serotonin and bradykinin, both classic endogenous algogens, have been shown to act as potent histamine-independent pruritogens in lesional atopic dermatitis skin. Both sensitization of local nerve endings in lesional skin and sensitization of spinal processing have been postulated to explain these observations (Hosogi *et al.* 2006). Moreover, acetylcholine (a neuromediator that normally induces pain) provokes itch in atopic dermatitis patients, indicating that inhibition of itch through pain may be altered in these patients (Rukwied and Heyer 1999, Ikoma *et al.* 2006).

MEDIATORS OF PRURITUS IN ATOPIC DERMATITIS

Many peripheral and central mediators play an important role in pruritus. They act either directly on free nerve endings and keratinocytes or indirectly

---

Box 5.1   Summary of possible mediators of pruritus in atopic dermatitis

- Proteases
- Histamine
- Interleukins
- Neurotrophins
- Opioids
- Acetylcholine
- Prostanoids

by inducing the release of mast cell content or by potentiation of other mediators. Although several mediators exist for pruritus, only those that pertain to atopic dermatitis are discussed here (**Box 5.1**).

PROTEASES AND CATHEPSINS

Certain proteases such as papain and mucanain have been known for years to induce itching (Shelley and Arthur 1955b, Rajka 1969). They interact with the peripheral nervous system by activating PAR-2, which is abundantly expressed on nerve fibers (Stefansson *et al.* 2008). Proteases play a major role in neurogenic inflammation, pain perception, secretory and motor functions, and the response to nerve injury (Vergnolle *et al.* 2003).

In patients with atopic dermatitis PAR-2 is upregulated in epidermal nerves, keratinocytes, and endothelium, indicating increased signaling (Steinhoff *et al.* 2003). In addition, the concentration of mast cell tryptase, an endogenous PAR-2 agonist, is increased whereas concentrations of histamine are unaltered. There is also enhanced responsiveness to PAR-2 agonists in inducing pruritus in these patients (Steinhoff *et al.* 2003). These data suggest that proteases, via activation of PAR-2, play an important role in mediating pruritus in atopic dermatitis. In addition, common allergens, such as house dust mites and staphylococci colonizing atopic dermatitis lesional skin, also have protease activity and this may explain their role in aggravating atopic dermatitis and its associated pruritus (Grobe *et al.* 2002). A recent study identified an endogenous itch-producing cysteine protease, cathepsin S, which may be involved in atopic dermatitis pruritus as well (Reddy *et al.* 2010).

HISTAMINE

Many attempts have been made to control the pruritus of atopic dermatitis by targeting histamine, a classic mediator of itch. Histamine is released from activated mast cells and epidermal keratinocytes (Biró *et al.* 2007). Of the four histamine receptors identified to date, H_1-receptors have been most commonly implicated in histamine-induced pruritus. Although H_1-receptor antagonists relieve itch in chronic urticaria and mastocytosis, they are ineffective in the vast majority of chronic pruritic diseases including atopic dermatitis.

On the other hand, histamine H_4- and H_3-receptors have recently been shown to have a role in pruritic responses in mice (Bell *et al.* 2004, Sugimoto *et al.* 2004, Dunford *et al.* 2007). Functionally active H_4-receptors (H_4R) have been identified on inflammatory dendritic epidermal cells, important antigen-presenting cells in atopic dermatitis and human CD4(+) T cells where they are upregulated under T-helper cell 2 (Th2) conditions (Dijkstra *et al.* 2008, Gutzmer *et al.* 2009). Stimulation of the Th2 H_4R leads to induction of IL-31, an important cytokine in the induction of itch. Moreover, certain polymorphisms in the H_4R gene have been found to be associated with atopic dermatitis (Yu *et al.* 2010).

Novel pharmacological agents that target these receptors (especially H_4-receptor antagonists) may provide alternative and effective therapies to treat pruritus in skin diseases such as atopic dermatitis. A recent small study demonstrated that epinastine, an H_1-receptor, antagonist that may have cross-reactivity with the H_4-receptor was shown to decrease serum IL-31 levels and itching assessed by a visual analog scale (Otsuka *et al.* 2011).

INTERLEUKINS

Interleukins may directly affect nerve fibers to cause itch. IL-2, a product of T-lymphocyte activation, has been suggested as one cause of pruritus in atopic dermatitis, and inhibition of IL-2 production forms the basis for treatment of atopic dermatitis with systemic and topical immunosuppressants such as cyclosporine (ciclosporin) and topical calcineurin inhibitors. Whether this effect is directly mediated via receptors or is an indirect effect (eg, through mast cells) is still unresolved.

Recent studies have also implicated IL-8 as a mediator of pruritus in atopic dermatitis but this is unlikely because prick testing with IL-8 does not induce pruritus or erythema (Steinhoff *et al.* 2006). On the other hand, the recent discovery of IL-31 as an inducer of itch and dermatitis in mice, as well as overexpression of IL-31 in keratinocytes in atopic dermatitis, suggests a specific role for this cytokine in pruritus associated with this disease process (Dillon *et al.* 2004, Sonkoly *et al.* 2006). Elevation of serum IL-31 levels has been correlated with the severity of atopic dermatitis (Raap *et al.* 2008).

Another important cytokine, interferon-γ appears to have a beneficial effect on pruritus in atopic dermatitis, although the mode of action is unknown (Stevens *et al.* 1998).

NEUROTROPHINS

Nerve growth factor (NGF), a neurotrophin that modulates cutaneous innervation, has been suggested as playing an important role in the pathophysiology of pruritus. In addition to its possible role in peripheral itch sensitization, serum NGF levels have been correlated with disease severity in atopic dermatitis patients (Toyoda *et al.* 2002). The most sensitive marker of pruritus was the presence of increased levels of NGF receptor in the urine. However, other studies, including data from the authors' group, do not support the findings of serum NGF or cutaneous NGF levels (measured using skin microdialysis) correlating with disease severity in patients with atopic dermatitis (Schulte-Herbrüggen *et al.* 2007, Wang *et al.* 2010).

Interestingly, the sources of increased serum NGF in these patients have been shown to be mainly keratinocytes, mast cells, and skin fibroblasts, which can be further stimulated by histamine. Moreover, receptors for NGF are upregulated in the skin of atopic dermatitis (Groneberg *et al.* 2005, Dou *et al.* 2006). Other neurotrophins have also been implicated in the pathophysiology of pruritus associated with atopic dermatitis. Expression of neurotrophin-4 in keratinocytes was found to be enhanced in atopic dermatitis whereas brain-derived neurotrophic factor has been shown to induce chemotaxis of eosinophils in these patients (Grewe *et al.* 2000, Raap *et al.* 2005).

OPIOIDS

The opioidergic system has recently received attention with regard to its possible role in the pathophysiology of pruritus and in chronic pruritic conditions. Opioid-induced pruritus is a well-known adverse effect of treatment with morphine and other μ-opioid receptor agonists. In actuality, different opioid receptors have contrasting effects on pruritus. Both μ-opioid receptor agonists and κ-opioid receptor antagonists can induce itch, whereas μ-receptor antagonists and κ-receptor agonists can reduce it (**Fig 5.2**) (Ikoma *et al.* 2006, Steinhoff *et al.* 2006). Patients with atopic dermatitis have a significantly increased concentration of serum β-endorphin (a μ-opioid receptor agonist) compared with controls, and these increased concentrations are correlated with both itch intensity and disease severity (Lee *et al.* 2006). Interestingly, there is significant downregulation of the κ-opioid system in the epidermis of atopic dermatitis patients (Tominaga, *et al.* 2007).

There is ongoing discussion as to whether opioids act centrally or peripherally in their modulation of pruritus. Opioid receptor antagonists that do and do not cross the blood–brain barrier have been reported to decrease pruritus in atopic dermatitis patients (Metze *et al.* 1999, Bigliardi *et al.* 2007). Of note, opioids have been shown to induce histamine release from cutaneous mast cells as well as to have a direct peripheral pruritogenic effect (Bernstein and Swift 1979, Fjellner and Hägermark 1982, 1984, Hägermark 1992).

ACETYLCHOLINE

Acetylcholine, one of the major neurotransmitters of the autonomic nervous system, has been implicated as

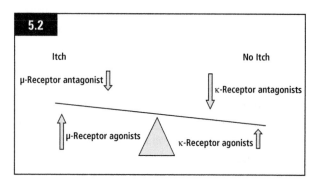

Fig 5.2 The contrasting effects of different opioids upon pruritus. Shown is the proposed imbalance of opioids in the pathophysiology of pruritus.

a possible mediator of pruritus in patients with atopic dermatitis. Intradermal injection of acetylcholine has been shown to elicit pruritus instead of pain in atopic dermatitis patients through a histamine-independent mechanism (Vogelsang *et al.* 1995, Heyer *et al.* 1997, Rukwied and Heyer 1999). In addition, vagal nerve stimulation inhibits experimentally induced itch (Kirchner *et al.* 2002). Acetylcholine is the primary neurotransmitter that activates eccrine sweat glands via muscarinic receptors. Interestingly, pruritus, in a subset of atopic dermatitis patients, is associated with perspiration, a response under autonomic control (Yosipovitch *et al.* 2002). Of note, keratinocytes express muscarinic receptors and they synthesize, store, release, and degrade acetylcholine *in vitro* (Grando *et al.* 1993).

A recent study demonstrated that atopic dermatitis is a stress-responsive disorder with autonomic nervous system involvement (Tran *et al.* 2010). Atopic individuals showed an overactive sympathetic response to itch and scratching, whereas the parasympathetic tone, which responded swiftly to itch and scratching in healthy control individuals, was persistently and rigidly elevated, showing a blunted response to stress.

PROSTANOIDS

Prostanoids, encompassing the prostaglandins and the thromboxanes, are the cyclooxygenase products of arachidonic acid. Prostaglandins were initially thought to potentiate histamine-induced itch (Hägermark *et al.* 1977). However, it was later demonstrated that certain prostaglandins, such as prostaglandin E_2, have a direct low-level pruritogenic effect without inducing protein extravasation in normal individuals and atopic dermatitis patients (Neisius *et al.* 2002). More recently, thromboxane A_2 has been shown to induce itch-associated responses through its thromboxane protein (TP) receptors located on keratinocytes and murine cutaneous nerve fibers. This response was abolished by deficiency of the TP receptor and a TP receptor antagonist (Andoh *et al.* 2007). It has also been shown that prostaglandin D_2 inhibits itching in negative control/ nucleotide group (NC/NG) mice with atopic-like dermatitis. Repeated scratching in this model further reduced levels of prostaglandin D_2 suggesting that the

itch–scratch cycle may be associated with low levels of prostaglandin D_2 (Sugimoto *et al.* 2007).

CROSSTALK BETWEEN CUTANEOUS NERVE FIBERS AND THE STRATUM CORNEUM

Itch associated with impaired barrier function in atopic dermatitis might be explained by crosstalk between cutaneous nerve fibers and the stratum corneum, eg, damage to the stratum corneum barrier is known to cause neuromediator release by keratinocytes and nerve fiber sprouting in the epidermis (Yosipovitch 2004). In a murine model of atopic dermatitis, the increased scratching associated with barrier damage was significantly diminished upon barrier repair (Miyamoto *et al.* 2002). As described previously, proteases may serve as important mediators of itch in atopic dermatitis. An alkaline environment enhances protease activity and, thus, an elevated stratum corneum pH may increase the perception of itch (Hachem *et al.* 2005).

TREATMENT

Management of pruritus in atopic dermatitis can be challenging. As a result of the poorly understood pathophysiology, development of effective treatments for pruritus has been particularly difficult. At present, there are no general-purpose antipruritic drugs. Instead, therapy for pruritus in atopic dermatitis must be tailored to the individual patient. Of prime importance is acquiring a detailed history, including the precise quality, timing, and distribution of itch, so that a more focused treatment plan can be instituted. The following text addresses treatment of pruritus as a symptom, not the treatment of atopic dermatitis as such.

GENERAL MEASURES

Patient education is central to managing pruritus in atopic dermatitis; identifying and removing aggravating factors or agents is often the first step in effective treatment. Breaking the itch–scratch cycle is also critical, and patients should be made aware that scratching leads to increased cutaneous inflammation.

Simple measures such as keeping fingernails short may help interrupt this cycle. The sensation of pruritus is often heightened by warmth; thus, measures should be taken to keep the skin cool with tepid showering, light clothing, and air conditioning where appropriate. Keeping the skin moisturized also may help reduce pruritus. **Box 5.2** provides some preventive measures to reduce itch.

TOPICAL ANTIPRURITIC TREATMENTS (TABLE 5.2)
MOISTURIZERS AND EMOLLIENTS

As increased transepidermal water loss is correlated with itch intensity in patients with atopic dermatitis, moisturizers and emollients play a central role in treating pruritus in those affected (Lee *et al.* 2006). Not only can some of these preparations increase skin moisture, but also some produce an occlusive film that limits evaporation of water. Moisturizers with a low pH may be especially useful in optimizing the skin barrier function via their maintenance of the normal acidic pH of the skin surface. Low-pH moisturizers may be of further benefit via their reduction of tryptase activity, which is known to activate PAR-2 in skin nerve fibers (Steinhoff *et al.* 2003).

Of note, stratum corneum ceramide deficiency is believed to be a putative cause of atopic dermatitis barrier abnormality. As a result, a ceramide-dominant, barrier-repair, lipid-based emollient was studied in patients with severe atopic dermatitis and shown to decrease overall severity of the disease (Chamlin *et al.* 2002). Emollients or moisturizers should be applied to all pruritic areas in atopic dermatitis at least twice daily; six times a day is recommended for more effective results.

TOPICAL CORTICOSTEROIDS

Topical corticosteroids remain the cornerstone of therapy of atopic dermatitis. These agents have anti-inflammatory, antiproliferative, and immunosuppressive properties but are not directly antipruritic; they exert a beneficial effect on pruritus in atopic dermatitis by their reduction of skin inflammation. Given the adverse effects associated with topical corticosteroids (skin atrophy, bruising, telangiectasia, and stretch marks), their use should be recommended only in itchy, inflammatory, atopic dermatitis lesions for short periods (up to 2 or 3 weeks). Although higher strengths of corticosteroid have greater effectiveness, there is also an increased incidence of adverse effects. Combinations of topical steroids and emollients as well as keratolytics are particularly effective in treating atopic dermatitis.

TOPICAL CALCINEURIN INHIBITORS

The topical calcineurin inhibitors, tacrolimus and pimecrolimus, have been shown to be effective and safe treatments for atopic dermatitis. Both agents ameliorate pruritus in affected patients, possibly via a direct effect on nerve fibers in addition to their anti-inflammatory effects (Senba *et al.* 2004, Kaufmann *et al.* 2006, Hon *et al.* 2007). The most common adverse effect associated with these agents is transient burning and stinging at the application site when treatment is first initiated. These adverse sensations

---

Box 5.2　Some preventive measures to reduce itch

- Apply moisturizers immediately after bathing to ensure high retention of moisture
- Keep fingernails short
- Wear light and loose-fitting clothing that absorbs sweat
- Avoid wearing wool or tight clothing
- Restrict time in the shower or bathtub
- Shower/bathe in cool or lukewarm water – hot water can be drying
- Avoid cleaners containing alcohol

usually subside within the first few days of therapy, and effective suppression of inflammation and pruritus ensues. Interestingly, the temporary burning and stinging may be related to the activation of transient receptor potential cation channel subfamily V member 1 (TRPV1) receptors and/or the transient release of neuropeptides and mast cell degranulation caused by topical calcineurin inhibitors (Stände and Luger 2003, Pereira *et al.* 2010).

TOPICAL ANTIHISTAMINES

Doxepin, a tricyclic antidepressant, is a potent H_1- and H_2-receptor antagonist with significant atropine-like (anticholinergic) properties. In a large, placebo-controlled, double-blind study, doxepin 5% cream significantly reduced pruritus in patients with atopic dermatitis (Drake *et al.* 1994). However, drowsiness, through percutaneous absorption of doxepin, occurs in approximately 25% of patients, limiting its use, especially in children. It should never be used in infants. Localized cutaneous burning and allergic contact dermatitis are other common adverse effects of this treatment.

MENTHOL

Menthol, a naturally occurring cyclic terpene alcohol of plant origin, is frequently used alone or in combination as a topical antipruritic. Menthol elicits the same cool sensation as ambient low temperature through the TRP subfamily M member 8 (TRPM8) receptor, which is a member of the TRP family of excitatory ion channels (Patel *et al.* 2007a). The

Table 5.2 Topical antipruritics for atopic dermatitis

TOPICAL ANTIPRURITIC	DOSE	COMMENTS
Emollients and moisturizers	Frequent application	Low-pH products may be particularly helpful
Topical steroids	Product/agent dependent	Not directly antipruritic, reduces cutaneous inflammation
Topical calcineurin inhibitors	Tacrolimus 0.03% and 0.1% ointment Pimecrolimus 1% cream	Common adverse effects include burning and stinging
Doxepin	5% cream	Drowsiness in 25% of patients
Menthol	1% cream	May be particularly useful in patients for whom cool temperatures relieve itch
Pramoxine	1–2.5%	Particularly effective for pruritus affecting the face
Polidocanol	5% urea and 3% polidocanol	Both moisturizing and anesthetic properties
Topical salicylates	2–6%	Cannot be applied in acute inflammatory skin processes Should not be applied in young children Effective for lichenified hyperkeratotic plaques and scalp
Wet-wrap dressings	Not applicable	Increased absorption of topical steroids if used

mechanism by which menthol alleviates pruritus is unknown, although it has been suggested that the activation of Aδ fibers by menthol centrally inhibits itch (Bromm *et al.* 1995). Menthol at concentrations of 1–3% commonly relieves pruritus, whereas higher doses can induce irritation. Of note, a subset of people with atopic dermatitis frequently report a reduction in itch associated with cold showers (Yosipovitch *et al.* 2002). The cooling sensation that menthol imparts to the skin is particularly useful in reducing itch perception in such patients.

Pramoxine

Pramoxine, a local anesthetic, reduces itch, especially when applied to the face, by interfering with transmission of impulses along sensory nerve fibers. A double-blind study has shown that pramoxine inhibits histamine-induced itch in humans (Yosipovitch and Maibach 1997).

Polidocanol

Pilodocanol is a nonionic surfactant with moisturizing and local anesthetic properties. In an open-label study, a topical preparation containing 5% urea and 3% pilodocanol significantly reduced pruritus in atopic dermatitis as well as in psoriasis and contact dermatitis (Freitag and Höppner 1997).

Topical salicylates

Topical aspirin has been shown to significantly reduce pruritus in patients with lichen simplex chronicus (Yosipovitch *et al.* 2001). Lichen simplex chronicus is a form of chronic localized itch which in some cases can be associated with atopic dermatitis. Use of topical salicylates may benefit atopic dermatitis patients with lichenified plaques. It is possible that the antipruritic actions of topical salicylates may be explained not only by their keratolytic effects but also, in part, by their inhibitory effects on prostanoids. They should not be used in children.

WET WRAP DRESSINGS

The use of wet-wrap dressings with diluted steroids and/or emollients is a well-established occlusive therapy in managing severe and/or refractory atopic dermatitis (Oranje *et al.* 2006). The therapeutic effects of topical steroids and emollients can be further enhanced by the occlusive nature of wet wrapping. A treatment of 1–3 days is highly effective for acute flare-ups of atopic dermatitis; use of this treatment is considered safe up to 14 days (Devillers and Oranje 2006, Oranje *et al.* 2006). The advantages of this treatment modality include a rapid response to therapy as well as a decrease in pruritus and sleep disturbance. Adverse effects of wet-wrap dressings include bacterial folliculitis and chilling. If topical corticosteroids are used, their absorption and adverse effects may be increased (Oranje *et al.* 2006). Lowering the absolute amount of topical applied corticosteroids to once daily, and further dilution of the product, can reduce the systemic absorption of corticosteroids (Devillers and Oranje 2006).

SYSTEMIC ANTIPRURITIC TREATMENTS (TABLE 5.3)

Oral antihistamines

Oral antihistamines have traditionally been the cornerstone of pruritus treatment in atopic dermatitis. Although sedating antihistamines may have a role in treating nocturnal itch through their soporific effects, there is little objective evidence that nonsedating antihistamines relieve itch in this disease process (Herman and Vender 2003).

Oral corticosteroids

In severe flares of atopic dermatitis, a short course of prednisone 1 mg/kg tapered during 2–3 weeks may be beneficial in reducing itch.

Cyclosporine (ciclosporin)

The T-cell immunosuppressant, cyclosporine, has been used extensively in organ transplantation and autoimmunity. In addition, clinical studies in atopic dermatitis have shown significant benefit from oral cyclosporine therapy with decreased itching and disease severity (Wahlgren *et al.* 1990, Wahlgren 1991). Although the effects of oral cyclosporine are rapid, they are not long-lasting and relapses are frequent. This agent can also cause significant hypertension, elevated creatinine and blood urea nitrogen levels, immunosuppression, and renal toxicity (Munro *et al.* 1994, Lee *et al.* 2004, Schmitt

Table 5.3 Systemic antipruritics for atopic dermatitis

SYSTEMIC ANTIPRURITIC	DOSE	COMMENTS
Oral sedating antihistamines	Agent dependent	No evidence of direct antipruritic effect
Oral corticosteroids	Prednisolone 1 mg/kg per day orally	Acute flares of atopic dermatitis taper down within 2–3 weeks
Cyclosporine (ciclosporin)	2.5–5 mg/kg per day orally	Can cause significant hypertension, elevated creatinine and blood urea nitrogen levels, immunosuppression, and renal toxicity Consider in those who have failed conventional therapy
Azathioprine	2.5 mg/kg per day orally	Pretreatment measurement of erythrocyte thiopurine methyltransferase levels helps identify those at risk of myelosuppression Consider in those who have failed conventional therapy
Mycophenolate mofetil		
Children	30–50 mg/kg per day orally	Consider in children aged >2 years who have failed conventional therapy
Adults	2 g per day	
Methotrexate		
Children	7.5 mg per week orally in 3 divided doses with 12h intervals	Folic acid supplementation to reduce risk of myelosuppression and gastrointestinal toxicity
Adults	10-22.5 mg per week orally	Consider in those who have failed conventional therapy
Mirtazapine	15 mg per night orally	Particularly useful in patients with nocturnal pruritus
Butorphanol	1–4 mg per night inhaled intranasally	Consider in those who have failed conventional therapy – intractable itch Adverse effects include somnolence, dizziness, nausea, and vomiting

et al. 2007). Therefore, oral cyclosporine should be used only in the short term for patients who have failed conventional therapy. Patients should be monitored carefully for hypertension and elevated creatinine. The long-term effectiveness and safety of cyclosporine in patients with atopic dermatitis is unknown (Schmitt et al. 2007).

AZATHIOPRINE

The immunosuppressant, azathioprine, inhibits T-lymphocyte and B-lymphocyte proliferation by interference with purine synthesis. In a double-blind, placebo-controlled study, monotherapy with oral azathioprine in refractory moderate-to-severe atopic dermatitis resulted in significant improvements in itch score, disease activity, and quality of life (Meggitt et al. 2006). A not uncommon, serious, adverse effect of azathioprine is, however, dose-dependent myelotoxicity. The susceptibility of individuals to myelosuppression induced by azathioprine is known to be related to the activity of thiopurine methyltransferase, a key enzyme in azathioprine metabolism. Of note, African–American individuals are more susceptible to low levels of this enzyme. Measurement of erythrocyte thiopurine methyltransferase activity before initiation of therapy helps identify those patients at high risk of this serious adverse effect (Meggitt and Reynolds 2001). In addition, thiopurine methyltransferase activity also may be useful in determining dosing strategies for azathioprine (Meggitt et al. 2006).

MYCOPHENOLATE MOFETIL

Mycophenolate mofetil (MMF) has been successfully used to treat severe atopic eczema in children (age range 2–16) at a dose of 30–50 mg/kg. The medication was well tolerated in all patients, with no infectious complications or development of leukopenia, anemia, thrombocytopenia, or elevated aminotransferases. The response to this therapy is of a longer duration when compared with cyclosporine (Heller et al. 2007).

METHOTREXATE

The antimetabolite methotrexate is used in a variety of dermatological conditions. It has been shown to reduce disease severity and pruritis in adults with severe atopic dermatitis when administered at a dose of between 10 to 22.5 mg per week orally (Schram et al. 2011). In addition, methotrexate has been shown to reduce the overall severity of atopic dermatitis including pruritis in children with severe disease at a dose of 7.5 mg per week orally in 3 divided doses with 12 h intervals (El-Khalawany et al. 2013).

Patients receiving methotrexate should be monitored for gastrointestinal, hepatic and pulmonary toxicity as well as myelosuppression.

ANTIDEPRESSANTS

Mirtazapine, an oral antidepressant, has been shown to reduce itch – especially nocturnal itch – in patients with chronic pruritus due to both inflammatory skin and systemic disorders (Hundley and Yosipovitch 2004). This antidepressant acts as an antagonist at noradrenergic α2-receptors and 5-HT2 and 5-HT3 serotonin (5-hydroxytryptamine) receptors, increasing central noradrenergic and serotoninergic neurotransmission. It also has a sedative effect through its H1-receptor antihistamine properties. Which of these mechanisms mediates the antipruritic properties of mirtazapine remains unclear, but it has been suggested that the α_2-adrenergic antagonism acts centrally to reduce pruritus. Mirtazapine is safe and without the serious adverse effects often associated with antidepressant agents such as cardiotoxicity and decreased seizure threshold (Hartmann 1999). It may be particularly useful in reducing the nocturnal pruritus often associated with atopic dermatitis. The authors have used this drug with excellent results in children aged over 10 years and in adults with severe nocturnal itch in a dose of 7.5 mg up to 15 mg at bedtime. Other oral antidepressants do not appear to be effective for pruritus in this setting.

OPIOID AGONISTS AND ANTAGONISTS

As mentioned previously, the opioidergic system may play an important role in the pathophysiology of pruritus in atopic dermatitis. Butorphanol, a κ-opioid receptor agonist and μ-receptor antagonist, has been reported to be effective in treating opioid-induced itch as well as chronic intractable itch due to either systemic or inflammatory skin diseases (Dunteman et al. 1996, Dawn and Yosipovitch 2006b). In clinical trials of intranasal butorphanol, the most frequently reported adverse effects were somnolence (43%), dizziness (19%), and nausea or vomiting (13%). Sedation has been noted at doses of 0.5 mg or more and, thus, this agent may be particularly useful for nocturnal pruritus (Dawn and Yosipovitch 2006b).

Naltrexone, a μ-receptor antagonist, has also been reported to relieve pruritus in atopic dermatitis, but such agents may be associated with significant adverse effects such as nausea, vomiting, diarrhea, fatigue, and, at higher doses, hepatotoxicity (Metze *et al.* 1999, Malekzad *et al.* 2009, Phan *et al.* 2010).

NONPHARMACOLOGICAL ANTIPRURITIC TREATMENTS
PHOTOTHERAPY
Ultraviolet (UV)-based therapy has been used to treat various pruritic conditions including atopic dermatitis. UVA, broadband UVB (BB-UVB), narrowband UVB (NB-UVB), and psoralen plus UVA (PUVA), as well as a combination of these, have been used to treat pruritus associated with atopic dermatitis (Rivard and Lim 2005). In addition to the reduction of proinflammatory cytokines, phototherapy may also mediate its beneficial effects in pruritus by inducing mast cell apoptosis (Szepietowski *et al.* 2002). Remissions may last up to 18 months.

PSYCHOLOGICAL APPROACHES
Stress can clearly induce or aggravate itch in atopic dermatitis (Yosipovitch *et al.* 2002). Studies have shown that behavioral therapy reduces itch intensity in this disease process (Shenefelt 2003). Furthermore, group psychotherapy and behavioral therapy directed toward stopping scratching may also be useful. Recent studies suggest that acupuncture has a significant anti-pruritic effect and reduces type 1 hypersensitivity in atopic dermatitis patients (Pfab *et al.* 2009).

CONCLUSION

Despite advances in the pathophysiology of pruritus in atopic dermatitis, treatment of this distressing symptom continues to be challenging for clinicians. Each patient should be considered unique and treatment tailored individually. Improved understanding of the mechanisms that underlie pruritus will facilitate developing better therapies in the future.

Clinical suggestions

1. Take measures to prevent itching and scratching such as application of moisturizers immediately after bathing, keeping fingernails short, wearing light and loose-fitting clothing, avoiding wool, bathing in cool or lukewarm water, and avoiding cleansers containing alcohol or other irritants.
2. Besides topical emollients, topical corticosteroids, and calcineurin inhibitors, other topical agents such as doxepin 5% cream, menthol 1% cream, or topical pramoxine 1% or 2.5% may be helpful in reducing pruritus.
3. Oral antihistamines do not directly reduce pruritus but may be useful for their sedative effect, especially when sleep is interrupted by scratching.
4. Oral corticosteroids and immunosuppressive agents such as cyclosporine (ciclosporin), methotrexate, azathioprine, and mycophenolate may be useful in patients who have failed conventional topical therapy or phototherapy.
5. Oral mirtazapine and intranasal butorphanol may be useful in adult patients with intractable nocturnal pruritus.

CHAPTER 6

PATHOPHYSIOLOGY OF ATOPIC DERMATITIS AND ATOPIFORM DERMATITIS

Donald Rudikoff and Jan D. Bos

BACKGROUND

Atopic dermatitis (AD) is a common, relapsing, inflammatory skin disease that has been the subject of debate since its earliest description. Although there has been a significant increase in the incidence of AD in recent years and an exponential rise in research as to its causes, it continues to provoke controversy.

The term 'atopic dermatitis,' popularized by Wise and Sulzberger, replaced the labels *generalized neurodermatitis of Brocq and Jacquet* and *prurigo Besnier*. It was defined as 'those inflammatory dermatoses … associated with other atopic stigmata in the affected person and/or his family … including … asthma; hay fever; sensitization by … protein allergens, and urticarial reactions to skin tests with these; Prausnitz–Kuestner antibodies (IgE); and eosinophilia' (Sulzberger 1955). Sulzberger admitted, however, his 'own uncertainty regarding the relative importance of allergic mechanisms' and emphasized the association with generalized dry skin, follicular hyperkeratosis, and disturbances in sweating. He reported 'histologically demonstrable obstruction of the sweat ducts' which he envisioned gave rise 'to millions of minute injections of sweat with its solutes and suspended materials' acting as the stimulus to itching.

Some authors considered 'atopic dermatitis' an unfortunate term, because it implied that the skin lesions were the cutaneous equivalents of asthma and hay fever. They believed that the primary defect was underlying pruritus in a genetically predisposed or *diathetic* individual and preferred terms such as 'generalized neurodermatitis' or 'diathetic dermatitis.'

Despite extensive research and numerous advances in our knowledge about AD, its pathogenesis still provokes controversy, mostly centered on the relative importance of compromised barrier function, inherent perturbations of innate and acquired immunity, aeroallergen exposure, food allergy, and staphylococcal colonization in its etiopathogenesis.

It is accepted that AD has a strong genetic component with high concordance rates among monozygotic twins (sevenfold increase in monozygotic twins versus threefold increase in dizygotic twins) and the identification of associated genes, but epidemiological studies suggest strong environmental influences as well (Thomsen *et al.* 2007).

ASPECTS OF PATHOGENESIS

A number of clinical, histological, and immunological phenomena must be considered when attempting to explain the pathogenesis of AD. Acute lesions with oozing, crusting, and *Staphylococcus aureus* colonization coexist with lichenified plaques caused by rubbing and scratching. These dry, thickened lesions entail additional and/or distinct pathogenic mechanisms from acute or subacute eczema.

Questions that must be considered include:

- Why do patients with AD have dry skin colonized with *S. aureus* and why the apparent propensity to viral infections such as warts, molluscum contagiosum and eczema herpeticum?
- Why does eczema clear with age in some and persist in others?
- What causes the increased levels of total and allergen-specific IgE associated with eosinophilia?
- Are these central to pathogenesis or merely epiphenomena?
- Is AD merely *glorified* allergic protein-contact dermatitis caused by aeroallergens penetrating a genetically compromised skin barrier?

Theories of pathogenesis should address the well-known, age-related patterns of lesional distribution and sites of predilection.

- Why, for example, do infants display eczematous changes on the cheeks, sparing the central face, which tend to resolve by 1 year of age?
- Is the typical extensor involvement of early childhood connected with crawling behavior or patterns of scratching?
- Is the flexural involvement, typical of older children and young adults, related to areas of sweating?
- Does perspiration in flexural areas cause a subclinical miliaria, allow deposition of sweat-containing antigens, enhance penetration of external antigens, alter local pH, or simply serve as an irritant?

Recently, loss-of-function mutations of the filaggrin gene have been strongly associated with ichthyosis vulgaris and AD; yet in ichthyosis vulgaris, the flexures are characteristically spared, whereas they are typically involved in patients with AD, and many patients with ichthyosis vulgaris never develop eczema.

Finally, and perhaps most importantly, why does AD itch so much? Anyone who has treated toddlers with AD has witnessed their inability to stop scratching.

Another important aspect is that up to 20 percent of patients with a typical AD skin phenotype based on the popular Hanifin and Rajka diagnostic criteria, do not have a personal or family history of atopy, elevated total IgE, or specific IgE for common food allergens or aeroallergens. Recently, investigators have drawn a distinction between so-called 'extrinsic atopic dermatitis' (EAD) and 'atopiform dermatitis,' or so-called 'intrinsic atopic dermatitis,' based on the presence or absence of these indicators of atopy. But this distinction is not universally accepted (Bos 2002, Williams and Johansson 2005).

Besnier's description of AD, which he termed 'prurigo diathésique,' emphasized the intense unremitting pruritus with nocturnal paroxysms of uncontrollable itch typified by seasonal remissions and exacerbations (Shelley and Crissey 2003). This early concept of a *diathetic* tendency to intrinsic, unremitting itch (*the itch that rashes*) giving rise to scratching and lichenification has, in part, given way to newer theories (**Box 6.1**).

One theory, for example, holds that genetically induced epidermal barrier defects allowing facilitated antigen penetration of the skin is the primary defect (*outside–inside hypothesis*). This *corneocentric* view presupposes a damaged skin barrier caused by malfunction of the corneal layer from filaggrin mutations, degradation of corneodesmosomes by endogenous and exogenous proteases from dust mites such as Der p 1 and Der f 1, and perturbations in the epidermal tight junctions located in the granular layer (De Benedetto *et al.* 2010) (**Fig 6.1**). As a consequence, antigens derived from parts of aeroallergens, and microbial antigens, penetrate a compromised skin barrier, bind to IgE on antigen-presenting cells, and are internalized and presented to antigen-specific T cells. A deficiency in endogenous protease inhibitors is an additional factor postulated by this view (Komatsu *et al.* 2007, Vasilopoulos *et al.* 2007, Bos *et al.* 2010).

Box 6.1 Theories of atopic dermatitis pathogenesis

1. The *Itch that rashes*: lesion formation is secondary to scratching in predisposed *diathetic* individuals with tendency to intense pruritus
2. Allergic: skin lesions result from immediate hypersensitivity to food allergens and aeroallergens
3. Inside–outside: genetically determined abnormalities of immune cells and cytokine milieu give rise to inflammation and secondary eczematous change
4. Outside–inside: primary genetic defects in the skin barrier facilitate antigen presentation through the skin initiating an inflammatory cascade
5. Outside–inside–outside: epidermal barrier defects cause enhanced antigen presentation resulting in inflammation and lesion formation. In addition, immunological and other processes impede barrier recovery, resulting in a *vicious cycle* of epidermal damage and further inflammation
6. Autoimmune: self-antigens drive inflammation

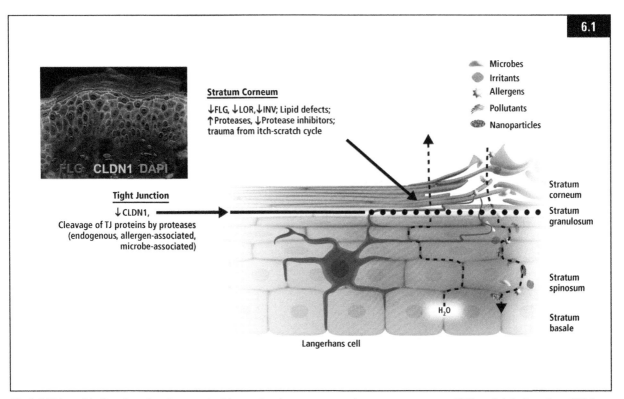

Fig 6.1 Skin epithelium is uniquely armed with two barrier structures: the stratum corneum (SC) and tight junctions (TJs). The SC is the outermost structure, consisting of multiple layers of enucleated keratinocytes called corneocytes. The SC barrier is maintained by the complex interaction of the cornified envelope, intracytoplasmic moisturizing factors, and a complex lipid mixture in the extracellular space. TJs are located just below the SC at the level of the stratum granulosum and might be compromised in patients with AD due to reductions in claudin-1 levels. (Reprinted from De Benedetto *et al.* 2010. © 2010 with permission from Elsevier.)

The so-called *inside–outside hypothesis* holds that intrinsic, genetically determined, immunological alterations are responsible for the dermatitis and barrier dysfunction. As mentioned, many patients with filaggrin mutation-associated ichthyosis and barrier defect do not develop AD. Are they missing some immunological propensity to develop eczema? So, for example, Hanifin (1990) and coworkers (Hanifin and Chan 1995) suggest that there is an intrinsic abnormality in AD leukocytes (monocytes and Langerhans cells) with elevated cyclic AMP phosphodiesterase and resultant reduction in intracellular cAMP, and increased prostaglandin E_2 production that inhibits T-helper type 1 cell (Th1) responses (Hanifin 1990, Hanifin and Chan 1995).

The *outside–inside–outside hypothesis* recognizes the effects of barrier defects, and intrinsic immunological mechanisms, adding additional mechanisms that result in compromised barrier repair and a vicious cycle perpetuating inflammation and further barrier disruption (Ogawa and Yoshiike 1993, Elias and Schmuth 2009).

Ogawa and Yoshiike (1993) conceptualized AD as a volcano with two magma cores: the first comprises immune-mediated inflammation and the second involves barrier dysfunction, which *simultaneously explode into a number of eruptions* (**Fig 6.2**). They posited that a mucocutaneous barrier defect allowed penetration of multiple antigens, which caused allergic inflammation. The allergic inflammation stemming from immunological abnormalities would enhance breakdown of barrier function. This sequence, in their view, resulted in a 'vicious circle' and answered the question as to why patients with AD demonstrate IgE production and hypersensitivity to various antigens (Ogawa and Yoshiike 1993).

It will become apparent that AD is an exceedingly complex disease with both genetic and environmental aspects, including the participation of a variety of cell types, cytokines, chemokines, lipids, structural proteins, proteolytic enzymes, neural elements, and bacterial products. The text starts with the histopathology and immunohistology, and then discusses aspects of adaptive and innate immunity, the role of epidermal barrier defects, aspects of lesion formation, neural mechanisms, and the role of eosinophils and mast cells, to provide the reader with the tools to understand and interpret critically the current literature on AD pathophysiology.

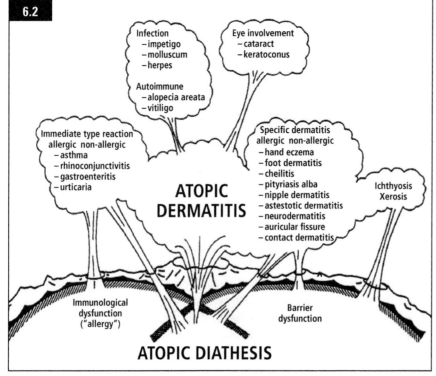

Fig 6.2 Atopic volcano: when two abnormalities, dry skin/ barrier dysfunction and allergy/ immunological dysfunction, are considered as the underlying major defects in atopic dermatitis (AD), the wide range of clinical manifestations of AD are easily comprehended. It is like a volcano with two magma cores that simultaneously explode into a number of eruptions. (Reprinted from Ogawa and Yoshiike 1993. © 1993 with permission from Elsevier.)

HISTOPATHOLOGY AND IMMUNOHISTOLOGY

The histopathology of eczema is reviewed in Chapter 19. Acute lesions of AD demonstrate varying degrees of epidermal spongiosis, epidermal exocytosis, and perivascular infiltrates of lymphocytes and macrophages (Mihm *et al.* 1976). Chronic lesions show increased numbers of lymphocytes, macrophages, and mast cells accompanied by epidermal hyperplasia which varies with the stage of the disease. The histological picture is more reminiscent of a type IV (delayed-type) hypersensitivity reaction akin to allergic contact dermatitis than of a type 1 (urticarial) reaction.

As AD has been linked to mutations in the filaggrin gene, it might be expected, similar to ichthyosis vulgaris, to have a diminished, absent, or altered stratum granulosum. Prose and Sedlis (1960), examining skin biopsy specimens of children with AD, predominantly infants and very young children, reported that the granular cell layer was usually prominent in the diseased skin. Another study of the stratum granulosum in biopsy skin from the upper outer buttock of children with AD and/or ichthyosis vulgaris found only a slight decrease in the stratum granulosum thickness in those with AD, and a marked decrease in patients with ichthyosis vulgaris compared with normal individuals (Erickson and Kahn 1970). Looking at the dry, noneczematous skin of patients with AD, Finlay *et al.* (1980) found slight hypergranulosis in most biopsies and, occasionally, slight patchy vacuolation of the granular layer in some specimens. Although the Erickson study shows a decrease in the granular layer in AD patients, as might be expected, the other two studies failed to confirm this.

The mononuclear infiltrate in AD has been found to contain mostly CD4+ T lymphocytes but also CD8+ lymphocytes and increased numbers of Langerhans cells (LCs) (Braathen *et al.* 1979, Uno and Hanifin 1980, Sillevis Smitt *et al.* 1986).

Subsequent investigations revealed positive staining for IgE in the dermis and epidermis localized to LCs and *inflammatory dendritic epidermal cells* (IDECs) (Bruynzeel-Koomen *et al.* 1986, Barker *et al.* 1988, Wollenberg *et al.* 1996) (**Fig 6.3**). This suggested

Fig 6.3 Lesional skin from an atopic dermatitis patient, labeled with anti-IgE, visualized by immunofluorescence reaction. Dendritic morphology of positively labeled cells can be seen in both the dermis (a) and epidermis (b). Magnification × 200. (Reprinted by permission from Barker *et al.* 1988. © 1988 Macmillan Publishers Ltd.)

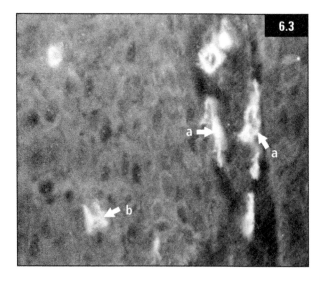

that allergens conjugated to IgE may be internalized by dendritic cells and presented to T lymphocytes, thus initiating the inflammatory process (**Fig 6.4**).

Several lines of evidence suggested an altered cytokine milieu in AD so that, although the histology resembles allergic contact dermatitis, the cytokine milieu, at least in early lesions, shows a T-helper type 2 (Th2) cytokine predominance. Studies of chronic AD lesions suggest a re-emergence of Th1 cytokine expression in later lesions. The validity of this purported *Th2 to Th1 switch* has been questioned (Bos *et al.* 2010). It has also been suggested that this later Th1 response, if genuine, might represent a homeostatic mechanism to restore normal cytokine balance, but this has not been established (Thepen *et al.* 1996). Increased levels of the pluripotential cytokine, macrophage migration inhibitory factor (MIF), in AD skin are thought to play an important role in the Th1–Th2 imbalance (Shimizu *et al.* 1997).

In the context of IgE-mediated antigen presentation and Th1–Th2 imbalance, effector lymphocytes are thought to ultimately produce epidermal spongiosis resulting in acute eczema. The types of antigens thought to be involved include aeroallergens, food allergens, autoantigens, and bacterial products. Although aeroallergens and food allergens are purported to exacerbate AD, the latter mostly in young children, there is still controversy as to the relative importance of these allergens in initiating and maintaining the disease state (Sampson and Jolie 1984, Suh 2010), eg, despite reports of improvement of AD with dust mite elimination or immunotherapy, such treatment approaches still lack rigorous corroboration. There is, in addition, evidence of autoantigens in patients with AD, raising the possibility that it may in part be an autoimmune disease (Mittermann *et al.* 2004). This view suggests that allergen-specific IgE responses are gradually replaced by autoantigen-specific IgE responses in AD skin (Valenta *et al.* 1996, Aichberger *et al.* 2005). More than 140 IgE-binding self-antigens that may promote and/or perpetuate skin inflammation have been associated with AD (Zeller *et al.* 2009).

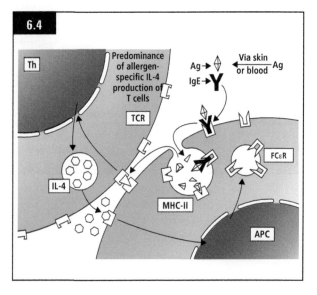

Fig 6.4 Schematic representation of what may occur within the skin in atopic eczema. Increased systemic allergen-specific interleukin 4 (IL-4) levels lead to increased levels of circulating allergen-specific IgE. Langerhans cells are then enabled to process allergens that are bound via allergen-specific IgE in IgE receptors. Within involved skin, allergen-specific T cells are enabled to proliferate on recognition of processed allergens, leading to IL-4 production *in situ* and further enhancement of allergen-specific immune reactivity. Th, T-helper cell; TCR, T-cell receptor; FcεR, receptor for the Fc part of IgE; MHC, major histocompatibility complex; APC, antigen-presenting cell. (Adapted from Van der Heijden *et al.* 1991 with permission of the publishers. Reprinted from Bos *et al.* 1992. © 1992 American Medical Association. All rights reserved.)

T LYMPHOCYTES AND CYTOKINE MILIEU

T-CELL INVOLVEMENT IN ATOPIC DERMATITIS

Abundant evidence suggests an important role for T lymphocytes in the pathogenesis of AD. Case reports have documented the transfer of atopy, including eczema, to nonatopic recipients of bone marrow transplants from atopic donors and resolution of AD after transplantation of nonatopic marrow to an atopic recipient (Koharazawa *et al.* 2005). Congenital immune deficiencies often manifest eczema and patients with the acquired immune deficiency syndrome (AIDS), many with no prior history of eczema, develop xerotic skin and on occasion lichenified lesions associated with eosinophilia. In addition, the efficacy in treating AD with drugs such as cyclosporine (ciclosporin), mycophenolate, pimecrolimus, and tacrolimus, which primarily affect T cells, is compelling evidence of involvement of these cells in pathogenesis (Cooper 1994).

Activated lymphocytes, predominantly CD4 helper cells, occur in lesional and uninvolved skin of AD patients and allergen-specific T lymphocytes can be cloned from AD lesional skin. A proportion of these lesional cells derive from circulating antigen-specific effector T cells that express cutaneous lymphocyte antigen (CLA), the 'skin-homing' receptor. However, some studies suggest that only a small minority of skin-infiltrating T cells in AD are antigen specific (Werfel *et al.* 1996).

The heightened activation status of AD lesional T cells is reflected by their expression of HLA-DR and elevated levels of the secretory Interleukin (IL)-2 receptor (sIL-2R) (Piletta *et al.* 1996). The majority show an altered cytokine secretion and, although many express the skin-homing receptor, CLA, a significant number do not express this marker but rather the gut-homing receptor αE β7 recognized by the monoclonal antibody HML-1 (de Vries *et al.* 1997). This suggests that an additional 'bystander' response of nonspecific T cells that lack CLA receptors might follow the purported initial antigen-specific T-cell response.

THE THYMUS

T-lymphocyte precursors arise in the bone marrow and migrate to the thymus where they undergo proliferation, maturation, differentiation, and selection. Thymic epithelial cells are essential for positive selection of T lymphocytes able to recognize foreign antigens presented by antigen-presenting cells (APCs) in the periphery. Interestingly, children with AD have a larger thymic volume than their nonatopic counterparts (Olesen *et al.* 2005). In addition, CD4+ CD8+ (thymocyte-like) lymphocytes have been demonstrated in the skin and blood of patients with AD, suggesting a possible disturbance of T-cell maturation in this disease. Interestingly, filaggrin referred to previously is also expressed in Hassall corpuscles of the thymus (Favre 1989).

Hassall corpuscles are collections of epithelial cells within the thymic medulla. They express thymic stromal lymphopoietin (TSLP) and instruct thymic dendritic cells to induce CD4+ CD25+ FoxP3+ regulatory T cells (Watanabe *et al.* 2005). This same protein, TSLP, is strongly expressed in AD lesional skin and is thought to play an important role in establishing a Th2 milieu. This raises the question of whether filaggrin mutations, aside from causing stratum corneum barrier defects, might have a more central role in T-cell regulation in patients with AD. Perhaps decreased or absent filaggrin in the thymus alters TSLP expression and affects T-cell maturation, along with regulatory cell formation.

THE TH1–TH2 PARADIGM

Murine and human CD4 helper lymphocytes have been characterized on the basis of their cytokine secretion profiles. In this discussion, the authors use the terminology Th1 and Th2 *cells* and *cytokines* to indicate these cytokine patterns, but CD8 cells demonstrate similar polarization, so it is probably more correct to refer to these profiles as type 1 (Tc1) and type 2 (Tc2). More recently an additional subclass of T lymphocytes, Th17 cells, have been described based on their distinctive cytokine repertoire (Miossec *et al.* 2009). Cytokines involved in the pathogenesis of AD are summarized in *Table 6.1*.

Table 6.1 Important cytokines and molecules in the pathophysiology of atopic dermatitis (AD)

CYTOKINE OR MOLECULE	SOURCE	ACTIONS
Interleukin (IL)-4	T-helper type 2 (Th2) lymphocytes (CD4, CD8) Mast cells Natural killer (NK) T cells Percutaneous sensitization with allergens through barrier-disrupted skin elicits Th2 response with IL-4	Promotes Th cell differentiation to the Th2 type Triggers B cells to produce IgE although IL-13 more important in AD IgE production. IL-4 induces the intracellular expression of α-chain of the high-affinity IgE receptor (FcϵR1) in DCs (Geiger *et al.* 2000) Reduces keratinocyte filaggrin and antimicrobial peptide expression (Howell *et al.* 2007) Linkage association of IL-4 and IL-4 receptor gene polymorphisms with AD in Japanese families Supports staphylococcal superantigen TSST-1-induced IgE production by PBMC (Hofer *et al.* 1999)
IL-5	Th2 cells Mast cells Eosinophils IL-4 and IL-5 ↑ in patients with EAD, but patients with IAD show ↑ IL-5 with low IL-4 levels (Kägi *et al.* 1994)	Controls the production, activation, survival and migration of eosinophils
IL-10	Th1 and Th2 cells Tr1-regulatory cells NK cells Tissue 'mononuclear cells' in AD B cells derived from peripheral blood monocytes in patients with AD	Modulates production of multiple cytokines ↑ IL-10 expression in AD may contribute to upregulation of humoral responses and the downregulation of interferon (IFN)-γ/Th1 responses (Ohmen *et al.* 1995) Early impaired production of IL-10 in response to environmental stimuli (foods, intestinal flora, *Staphylococcus aureus*, vaccines) may be associated with ↑↑ propensity for Th2 responses in children with AD (Dunstan *et al.* 2005) IL-10 promoter polymorphisms associated with AD phenotypes in children (Sohn *et al.* 2007) Severe AD is associated with a reduced frequency of IL-10-producing allergen-specific CD4+ T cells (Seneviratne *et al.* 2006). ↑ levels of IL-10 may contribute to the AMP deficiency in both IAD and EAD (Howell *et al.* 2005)
IL-12	Macrophages Monocytes Eosinophils (Grewe *et al.* 1998b) IDECs	The relative increase in IL-12 mRNA-positive cells in chronic AD lesions may reflect the ability of macrophages, eosinophils, and IDECs to regulate the polarity and control the inflammatory response in AD IL-12 has the ability to suppress IgE production *in vitro* by both IFN-γ-dependent and IFN-γ-independent mechanisms and can switch Th0 cells to a Th1-like phenotype

Table 6.1 Important cytokines and molecules in the pathophysiology of atopic dermatitis (AD) *(continued)*

CYTOKINE OR MOLECULE	SOURCE	ACTIONS
IL-13	IL-13 is produced mainly by activated T cells of the Th2 subset Mast cells Basophils Skin-derived T cells from patients with EAD displayed an increased IL-13 production, whereas lower levels of IL-13 were observed in T cells from patients with IAD (Akdis *et al.* 1999b)	Shares many biologic properties with IL-4, including ability to act as a switch factor inducing production of IgE Downregulates production of IL-12 and IFN-γ and may explain relative paucity of IL-12 mRNA-positive cells in acute AD (Hamid *et al.* 1996)
IL-18	IDECs, keratinocytes increased in the serum of AD patients and in AD lesional skin	Serum levels correlate with disease activity IL-18 together with IL-12 may lead to switch of initial T(h)2-type immune response into a response of the T(h)1 type in AD (Novak *et al.* 2004) Enhances eosinophil recruitment Induces increased IFN-γ production Affects IL-13 production
IL-22	Th-17 cells, Th-22 cells, CD-8 cells	Progressive activation of IL-22 occurs from acute to chronic lesions. IL-22 may be involved in AD epidermal hyperplasia
IL-25 (aka IL-17E)	Keratinocytes, Th2 cells, mast cells, DCs in dermis, lung epithelial cells	Induces Th2 responses Decreases filaggrin synthesis in cultured keratinocytes (Hvid *et al.* 2011)
IL-31	IL-31 is produced by activated T lymphocytes, preferentially by Th2 cells and is associated with infiltrating CLA+ cells in AD Circulating IL-31 levels are increased in AD, correlate with disease activity and are reduced by cyclosporine (ciclosporin) treatment IL-31RA expression at higher levels on epidermal keratinocytes in AD	Associated with expression of the Th2 cytokines IL-4 and IL-13 in AD and ACD (Neis *et al.* 2006) Induces pruritus via the IL-31 receptor on sensory nerve cells (Leung *et al.* 2004, Sonkoly *et al.* 2006) Induces proinflammatory cytokines in human monocytes and macrophages after stimulation with staphylococcal exotoxins (Kasraie *et al.* 2010)
IFN-γ	CD4 and CD8 cells	Inhibits IL-4-induced IgE and IgG4 when added for the first 24 h or 48 h but had no effect when added on day 4 or 5

(continued)

Table 6.1   Important cytokines and molecules in the pathophysiology of atopic dermatitis (AD) *(continued)*

CYTOKINE OR MOLECULE	SOURCE	ACTIONS
FcεR1	Langerhans cells IDECs Mast cells Basophils	Internalization of IgE-associated antigens into dendritic cells for presentation to T cells CD1a+ epidermal DCs and monocytes in EAD patients showed increased FcεRI surface expression compared with IAD patients
Thymus- and activation-regulated chemokine (TARC)	Thymus-constitutive expression in AD: Keratinocytes	Induces selective migration of lymphocytes, especially Th2 cells (Sandoval-Lopez and Teran 2001) Induces integrin-dependent adhesion to ICAM-1 of skin memory T cells
CCL17	Dermal infiltrating cells including CD3 lymphocytes CD1a DCs Endothelial cells	No significant difference in CCL17 expression in PBMCs, sera, and lesional skin of patients with IAD and EAD (Park *et al.* 2008)
CCL18	High FcεR1 surface-expressing DCs, Langerhans cells and IDECs, are the major source of CCL18 Monocytes	Role in mediating migration of memory cells CCL18 expression did not differ in PBMCs, sera and LC-like DCs from the two subgroups, but strong CCL18 expression was observed in lesional skins and IDEC-like DCs in patients with EAD Chemokine micromilieu, especially the prominent CCL18, is different between EAD and IAD patients
CLA	Skin-infiltrating memory T cells	Binds E-selectin Mediates homing of CD4 and CD8 lymphocytes to the skin

ACD, allergic contact dermatitis; CLA, cutaneous lymphocyte antigen; DC, dendritic cell; EAD, extrinsic atopic dermatitis; IAD, intrinsic atopic dermatitis; IDEC, inflammatory dendritic epidermal cell; PBMC, peripheral blood mononuclear cell.

Th1 lymphocytes produce interferon-γ (IFN-γ), lymphotoxin, and tumor necrosis factor-α (TNF-α) but not IL-4, -5, and -13, and are involved in so-called 'cellular immunity.' Th2 cells secrete IL-4, -5, and -13. Certain Th1 or Th2 cytokines can further polarize immune responses by their effect on precursor T cells. Thus IFN-γ can inhibit differentiation of Th2 cells and IL-4 can inhibit Th1 polarization (**Fig 6.5**). Many circulating lymphocytes in humans express a combination of Th1 and Th2 cytokines and are referred to as Th0 cells.

IS ATOPIC DERMATITIS A TH2 DISEASE?

The concept that polarized Th1 and Th2 cells and cytokines dominate certain illnesses provided new insights into the pathophysiology of disease. This was especially true for infectious processes such as leprosy, in which the Th1–Th2 paradigm could explain the dichotomous nature of the condition. Likewise, this paradigm shed new light on the pathogenesis of AD.

It was well known that patients with AD often displayed peripheral eosinophilia and elevated circulating levels of IgE. This suggested that Th2

Fig 6.5 T-helper type 1 (Th1) cells produce interferon-γ (IFN)-γ and interleukin (IL)-2. They are activated by IL-12 and inhibited by IL-4. Th2 cells express IL-4, -5, and -13. They are stimulated by IL-4 and inhibited by IL-12.

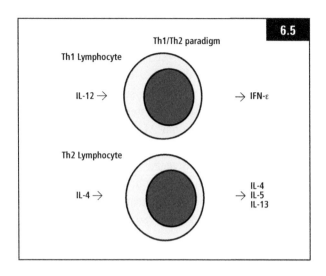

cytokines, specifically IL-4, -5, and -13, might be relevant. IL-5 is important for the activation and survival of eosinophils. IL-4 and -13 are able to induce IgE production by B cells (de Vries *et al.* 1993). A study utilizing *in situ* hybridization showed increased expression of IL-4 mRNA in cells infiltrating the epidermis and upper dermis in the acute phase of AD (Hamid *et al.* 1994). Chronic AD lesions also expressed IL-4 mRNA but had significantly fewer IL-4 mRNA+ cells than acute lesions. In an atopic dermatitis model, the atopy patch test (APT), aeroallergen-specific T-cell clones producing IL-4 were isolated from eczematous patch test sites 24 h after allergen application to the skin (van Reijsen *et al.* 1992). Moreover, increased expression of mRNA of the IL-4 receptor α-subunit was detected only in acute lesions of AD (Taha *et al.* 1998).

Thus IL-4, the prototypic Th2 cytokine, seemed to play a major role. This also proved to be true for other Th2 cytokines such as IL-5 and IL-13. Whereas IL-4 mRNA was prominent in acute AD lesions, chronic AD skin lesions had significantly fewer IL-4 mRNA-expressing cells but significantly greater IL-5 mRNA expression, most of it by T cells (Hamid *et al.* 1994). Thus, initiation of acute skin inflammation seemed to be associated with a predominance of IL-4 expression whereas maintenance of chronic inflammation was mostly associated with increased IL-5 expression and eosinophil infiltration (Hamid

et al. 1994). Interestingly, recent work in a mouse model of AD suggests that accumulation of IL-5-producing Th2 cells and eosinophilic infiltration of the skin is mediated by interactions between the chemokine receptor CCR8 and its ligands (Debes and Diehl 2011, Islam *et al.* 2011).

Another Th2 cytokine, IL-13, plays an important role in regulating IgE synthesis in AD (Katagiri *et al.* 1997). Peripheral blood mononuclear cells of AD patients showed increased concentrations of IL-13 mRNA but not IL-4 mRNA. Acute lesions of truly ('extrinsic') AD show a marked increase in IL-13 mRNA expression demonstrated by *in situ* hybridization (Hamid *et al.* 1996). Upregulation of IL-13 mRNA, moreover, far exceeds the scant expression of IL-4 mRNA in subacute and chronic lesions of AD (Tazawa *et al.* 2004).

The aforementioned Th-2 predominance in AD was shown to be possibly due to preferential activation-induced cell death of memory/effector Th1 cells (Akdis *et al.* 2003). Patients with atopiform ('intrinsic atopic') dermatitis showed no evidence for enhanced T-cell apoptosis.

These studies suggested that atopic dermatitis was indeed a Th2 disease, but, as is so often the case in medicine, this proved to be an oversimplification. A number of studies suggested that Th1 cytokines such as IL-12 and IFN-γ also played a major role in AD.

Grewe *et al.* (1994) demonstrated a key role for Th1 cytokines in AD lesional skin. IFN-γ mRNA and protein were highly expressed in lesional skin of 80% of AD patients, and decreased to levels comparable to those in normal skin after successful treatment. Thepen *et al.* (1996) demonstrated a predominance of IFN-γ over IL-4 in lesional AD skin (morphology or chronicity of lesions not described) but of IL-4 over IFN-γ at 24 h in positive APTs. They also showed increasing expression of IFN-γ in APTs and suggested a biphasic response to allergens in AD. Chronic lichenified lesions of AD showed greater IL-13 mRNA expression than uninvolved skin, but importantly showed significant expression of IL-12 mRNA. Interestingly, in a mouse model, scratching was shown to modulate the immune response from a Th2-biased response to Th1 with significant expression of IFN-γ but not IL-13 (Matsushima *et al.* 2003).

As a result of these data, a biphasic model of AD was introduced in which Th2 responses predominated in early, acute lesions whereas Th1 responses became prominent in chronic lesions (Grewe *et al.* 1998a) (**Fig 6.6** and **Box 6.2**).

6.6

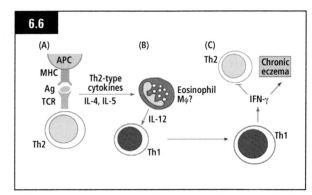

Fig 6.6 The biphasic model of atopic dermatitis (AD). The late T-helper type 1 (Th1) environment in this model follows stimulation of lymphocytes by interleukin IL-12 presumed to be derived from eosinophils and possibly macrophages. An as yet unknown genetic predisposition leads to an imbalance of the immune system favoring Th2-type immunological characteristics such as enhanced IgE levels, blood eosinophilia, and increased numbers of Th2 cells. (A) The initiation phase of AD is driven by cytokines derived from activated, allergen-specific Th2 cells. (B) Skin-invading cells, such as macrophages (Mφ) or eosinophils attracted and activated by Th2 cytokines, produce IL-12, which leads to activation of allergen-specific and nonspecific Th1 and Th0 cells. (C) The predominance of IFN-γ-producing T cells is responsible for chronicity of AD lesions and determines severity of the disease. Ag, antigen; APC, antigen-presenting cell; MHC, major histocompatibility complex; TCR, T-cell receptor. (Reprinted from Grewe *et al.* 1998a. © 1998, with permission from Elsevier.)

Box 6.2 Acute and chronic phases of atopic dermatitis

Acute phase
- ↑ interleukin (IL)-4 mRNA in cells infiltrating the epidermis and upper dermis
- Aeroallergen-specific IL-4-producing T-cell clones isolated from patch test sites 24 h after allergen application
- ↑ IL-13 mRNA expression
- ↑ IL-4 receptor high-affinity α-subunit (IL-4α) mRNA

Chronic phase
- IL-4 mRNA present but fewer IL-4 mRNA-expressing cells than acute lesions
- ↑ IL-5 mRNA expression compared with acute lesions
- ↑ expression of IL-12 mRNA
- ↑ IFN-γ expression
- ↑ expression of granulocyte–macrophage colony-stimulating factor (GM-CSFRα) and IL-5Rα mRNA (predominantly increased in chronic lesions and to lesser extent in acute lesions)

Recent work suggests that so-called *super-Th1* cells, which produce IFN-γ and IL-13 on stimulation with keratinocyte-derived IL-18, play an important role in inducing a Th1 cytokine milieu (discussed below) (Ikezawa *et al.* 2010).

ROLE OF CD8 CELLS

Not only are CD4+ Th2 cells present, but also significant numbers of IFN-γ-expressing CD4+ and CD8+ T cells in acute lesions of AD and in a model (APT) (Simon *et al.* 2006). Werfel *et al.* (1996) demonstrated that 15% of allergen-specific T cells in chronic AD lesions were CD8+. It is thought that CD8+ cells are essential for the formation of primary spongiotic changes in acute AD. Epidermal spongiosis in AD and allergic contact dermatitis results from keratinocyte apoptosis caused by FasL-expressing T cells infiltrating the epidermis (Trautmann *et al.* 2000).

In a mouse model of allergen (Der f)-induced skin inflammation resembling AD, IFN-γ-producing CD8+ T cells infiltrated the skin a few hours after allergen exposure in sensitized mice and initiated a mixed Th1–Th2 (Tc1–Tc2) inflammatory reaction (Hennino *et al.* 2007).

REGULATORY T CELLS, IL-10, AND TRANSFORMING GROWTH FACTOR α

As mentioned previously, AD is characterized by hyperstimulatory T-cell responses. One possible explanation for this might be defective negative feedback mechanisms affecting T-cell function. For this reason, there has been renewed interest in T-suppressor cells, now referred to as T-regulatory cells, and their possible role in AD. Regulatory T cells modulate immune reactions through release of anti-inflammatory cytokines or by cell-to-cell contact-dependent mechanisms (Cavani *et al.* 2003). So-called Th3 cells secrete transforming growth factor β (TGF-β), and Tr1 cells secrete IL-10. Human (Tr1) cells, their suppressive cytokines IL-10 and TGF-β, and their respective receptors have been demonstrated in lesional AD skin (Verhagen *et al.* 2006).

IL-10

IL-10, originally described as a Th2-cell-derived factor that inhibited Th1 effector functions, is now also known to suppress Th2 responses (Grutz 2005). The main source of IL-10 is the macrophage but T cells, monocytes, dendritic cells, B cells, eosinophils, mast cells, and keratinocytes are other potential sources (Weiss *et al.* 2004).

Studies examining the magnitude of IL-10 expression in AD have had conflicting results, but a recent study that looked at IL-10 expression as a function of disease severity offers a possible explanation (Seneviratne *et al.* 2006). In this study, patients with severe AD had lower frequencies of IL-10-producing allergen-specific CD4 T cells than those with mild disease. This suggests that a relative deficiency of IL-10 from T-regulatory cells might play a permissive role in disease expression.

Transforming growth factor β

TGF-β, similar to IL-10, is produced by a multitude of cell types and has pleiotropic effects on hemopoietic cells. Its main role in the immune system is to maintain tolerance via regulation of lymphocyte proliferation, differentiation, and survival (Li *et al.* 2006). A polymorphism in the TGF-β1 gene, indicating a low-producer TGF-β1 genotype, has been associated with increased risk of AD, especially with severe disease (Lee *et al.* 2000). Moreover in peripheral blood mononuclear cells of AD patients, spontaneous messenger RNA expression of TGF-β was lower than in controls. Of particular note, treatment of AD lesions with topical tacrolimus increases production of TGF-β, and the combination of TGF-β and tacrolimus increases the number of LCs in the epidermis but decreases their capacity to stimulate T cells, which may explain part of the drug's immunomodulatory effect (Caproni *et al.* 2006, Kwiek *et al.* 2008).

On the other hand, increased expression of TGF-β1 has also been reported in AD lesions, especially in chronic lesions (Toda *et al.* 2003).

FoxP3+ T-regulatory cells

A third type of T-regulatory cell, first identified in mice, has been described based on expression of the FoxP3 transcription factor. Deficiency of these cells in mice is associated with severe autoimmunity and an eczematous skin condition. The situation is not as simple in humans, however, where FoxP3 can be transiently expressed on activated T-effector cells in inflammatory diseases (Akdis *et al.* 1997). The finding of large numbers of CD25+ cells in lesional AD skin may indicate activated T cells rather than CD4+ CD25+ FoxP3+ T-regulatory cells.

There are conflicting data regarding circulating T-regulatory cells in AD. One study in patients with AD showed increased levels of circulating CD4+ CD25+ FoxP3+ T lymphocytes that expressed very low levels of CD69, an effector T-cell marker, suggesting that in the circulating pool true T-regulatory cells were present (Ou *et al.* 2004). These circulating T-regulatory cells lost their immunosuppressive activities when stimulated with staphylococcal enterotoxin B (SEB) at low concentration. This offers one explanation of how staphylococcal colonization could exacerbate dermatitis. Another recent study showed increased numbers of T cells with a 'regulatory phenotype' (CD25hi FoxP3+) linked to disease severity in AD (Reefer *et al.* 2008). Some of the regulatory T cells secreted Th2 cytokines that enhanced IL-5 production by effector T lymphocytes. SEB caused expansion and activation of these CD25hi Th2-like cells. On the other hand, Orihara *et al.* (2007) found that atopic patients with active disease had a lower Foxp3+ CD4+ ratio than asymptomatic control individuals having similar levels of serum IFN-γ, total IgE, and eosinophils.

With regard to cutaneous expression of T-regulatory cells, Verhagen *et al.* (2006) reported a deficiency of CD4+ CD25+ FoxP3+ T-regulatory cells in lesional AD skin and APT reactions.

Th17 cells in atopic dermatitis

The Th1–Th2 lymphocyte paradigm has proved to be an oversimplification with the recent description of lymphocytes (Th17 cells) that produce IL-17.

Development of Th17 cells from naïve T cells occurs under the influence of IL-23 from activated dendritic cells, monocytes, and macrophages (Langrish *et al.* 2005). Th17 cells are thought to play a role in defense against extracellular pathogens, autoimmune diseases, and diseases with chronic neutrophilic inflammation such as psoriasis (Lee *et al.* 2010). IL-17 has been identified in acute AD lesions much more so than in chronic lesions, and Th17 cells are present in the peripheral blood related to the severity of the eczema (Toda *et al.* 2003, Koga *et al.* 2008). Moreover IL-17 has been shown to potentiate IgE production (Milovanovic *et al.* 2010). As AD patients have staphylococcal colonization and infection and lack neutrophilic infiltration, the precise role of Th17 cells in this disease remains to be clarified.

IL-22

IL-22 was originally identified as a product of Th17 cells but is also produced by CD8+ T cells in AD skin and by unique Th22 cells that do not express IL-17 (Fujita *et al.* 2009, Nograles *et al.* 2009, Hijnen *et al.* 2013). IL-22 may be involved in the epidermal hyperplasia found in AD (Souwer *et al.* 2010). Using genomic, molecular, and cellular profiling Gitler *et al.* (2012) have demonstrated progressive activation of Th2 and Th22 immune axes from the acute to chronic phases of AD and stress the importance of IL-22 activation.

OTHER CYTOKINES INVOLVED IN THE PATHOGENESIS OF ATOPIC DERMATITIS

In addition to the Th1, Th2, and Th17 cytokines previously mentioned, a number of other cytokines play an intimate role in the pathogenesis of atopic dermatitis. Epidermal keratinocytes produce a variety of cytokines, among them IL-1, TNF-α, granulocyte–macrophage colony-stimulating factor (GM-CSF), IL-18, IL-25, IL-33, and TSLP (Carmi-Levy *et al.* 2011). Some of these, such as IL-1 and TNF-α, are proinflammatory and essential to innate immune responses. Others, such as IL-25, IL-33, and TSLP, have been shown to be important in driving Th2 immune polarization.

IL-1

IL-1 is a proinflammatory cytokine produced by keratinocytes and dendritic cells that plays an important role in inflammatory and hyperproliferative skin disease (Luger *et al.* 1997). It induces inflammation through activation and recruitment of immune cells as part of an innate immune response (Feldmeyer *et al.* 2010). The three forms are IL-1α, IL-1β, and IL-1 receptor antagonist (IL-1RA), which has no agonistic activity. Keratinocytes contain large amounts of preformed, biologically active IL-1α and inactive pro-IL-1β, which requires IL-1β-converting enzyme (caspase 1) for activation. The major source of IL-1β is dendritic cells. Barrier disruption and exposure to low humidity cause increased epidermal IL-1α as well as increased release of preformed IL-1α (Wood *et al.* 1996, Ashida *et al.* 2001). In addition topical application of house dust mite protein antigens induces upregulation of IL-1β and TNF-α in the epidermis of AD patients who are sensitized to these antigens, but not in the epidermis of normal individuals (Junghans *et al.* 1998).

IL-18, -25, AND -33

IL-18, -25, and -33 are keratinocyte-derived cytokines that are important in the pathogenesis of AD. IL-18 is also produced by dendritic cells and is thought to play a role in Th1 polarization. It is discussed in more detail later in the chapter. IL-25 is also produced by Th2 cells, allergen-activated mast cells, eosinophils, and basophils, and has been found to be coexpressed in the dermis in AD patients, likely on dendritic cells (Carmi-Levy *et al.* 2011). IL-25, along with thymic stromal lymphopoietin (TSLP), is intimately involved in the skewing and augmentation of Th2 responses by dendritic cells. IL-25 also decreases filaggrin production by keratinocytes and thus has more than one mechanism of action in promoting eczema (Hvid *et al.* 2011). IL-33, although a member of the proinflammatory IL-1 family, induces a Th2 response similar to IL-25 and TSLP.

IL-31 AND ITCH

A key cytokine intimately related to pruritus has been identified in a mouse model and in human AD (Takaoka *et al.* 2005). In a mouse model of AD, expression of IL-31 mRNA in NC/Nga mice was shown to be intimately associated with scratching behavior. In humans, IL-31 was also found to be expressed in pruritic dermatoses, especially prurigo nodularis, and was also induced by staphylococcal superantigen (Sonkoly *et al.* 2006). IL-31 expression has been shown to be associated with CLA+ T cells infiltrating AD skin lesions and its receptor, IL-31RA, is expressed by keratinocytes and infiltrating macrophages in skin biopsy specimens from patients with AD (Bilsborough *et al.* 2006). Expression of IL-31 is increased in AD lesional tissue at both the mRNA level and the protein level, and serum levels correlate with disease activity in adults and children regardless of the AD phenotype (Raap *et al.* 2008a, 2012, Nobbe *et al.* 2011). Moreover, in a mouse model of AD, intraperitoneal injection of IL-31 induced scratching behavior (Grimstad *et al.* 2009).

IL-31 expression is not only increased in AD but also in allergic contact dermatitis; in both types of dermatitis, its expression is associated with the expression of the Th2 cytokines IL-4 and IL-13 (Neis *et al.* 2006). One study suggests that IL-31-specific activation of dendritic cells may be part of a positive feedback loop driving the progression of inflammatory skin diseases (Horejs-Hoeck *et al.* 2012). Thus IL-31 represents an important cytokine produced by T cells associated with allergic inflammation and pruritus, and interventions against IL-31 might represent a potential treatment of AD pruritus. Indeed a preliminary study showed a decrease in IL-31 levels at 1 month in AD patients treated with cyclosporine (ciclosporin), a drug known to decrease AD pruritus (Otsuka *et al.* 2011).

LESION FORMATION IN ATOPIC DERMATITIS

At one end of the spectrum of AD lesions are acute, erythematous, crusted patches as seen on the cheeks of infants. A similar morphology occurs in acute lesions of allergic contact dermatitis. AD patients may also have drier, subacute, and chronic eczematous lesions, and thickened, lichenified plaques.

ACUTE LESION FORMATION

The histological hallmark of acute eczematous lesions is termed 'spongiosis.' It entails condensation of keratinocytes with widening of the intercellular spaces, intercellular edema, and distension of the remaining intercellular contacts which give the epidermis a 'sponge-like' appearance (Trautmann *et al.* 2001). Microvesiculation occurs and consolidation of microvesicles results in visible vesiculation on the skin surface which, with rupture, gives rise to a serous discharge. Intercellular adhesion is normally anchored by desmosomes and adherens junctions. The latter contain E-cadherin, a transmembrane glycoprotein essential in mediating keratinocyte adhesion. Trautmann *et al.* (2001) have demonstrated that T-cell-mediated keratinocyte apoptosis causes spongiosis in acute allergic contact dermatitis and AD (**Figs 6.7** and **6.8**). Keratinocytes normally express low levels of the death receptor Fas; the presence of IFN-γ

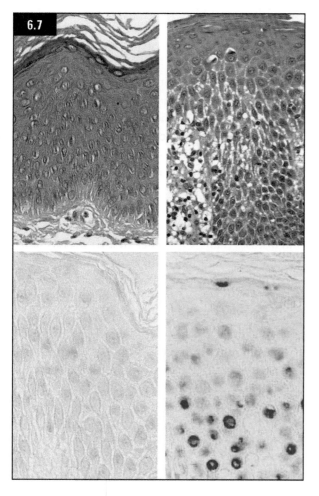

Fig 6.7 Demonstration of apoptosis in spongiotic eczema by the TUNEL method. Top left: normal skin H&E (hematoxylin and eosin staining). Top right: spongiotic eczema (H&E). Bottom left: no apoptotic cells. Bottom right: numerous apoptotic cells staining red. (Courtesy of Axel Trautmann, MD.)

increases Fas expression and renders it susceptible to apoptosis. Activated T cells infiltrating the epidermis have enhanced expression of Fas ligand (FasL) which delivers the *coup de grâce* to keratinocytes expressing high levels of Fas. Investigators have also demonstrated that cleavage of E-cadherin occurs with apoptosis of keratinocytes decreasing adhesion between cells, whereas desmosomal cadherins are left intact (Trautmann *et al.* 2001).

Spongiosis is limited to the suprabasal epidermis. This is because expression of the cell-intrinsic, caspase-8 inhibitor, cellular Flice-inhibitory protein (cFLIP), which modulates Fas–FasL signaling, is tightly restricted to the basal layer protecting basal

keratinocytes from apoptosis (Armbruster *et al.* 2009). It has recently been demonstrated that dysregulation of the metalloprotease, ADAM10, results in increased shedding of E-cadherin with subsequent loss of keratinocyte adhesion (Maretzky *et al.* 2008).

Finally, influx of serum into the malpighian layer occurs because of the osmotic pressure gradient resulting from increased hyaluronan in the epidermis (Ohtani *et al.* 2009). Ohtani *et al.* (2009) demonstrated, by immunohistochemical staining and *in situ* hybridization, intercellular accumulation of hyaluronan in the spongiotic epidermis and augmented hyaluronan synthase-3 (HAS3) expression by spongiotic keratinocytes. E-cadherin expression

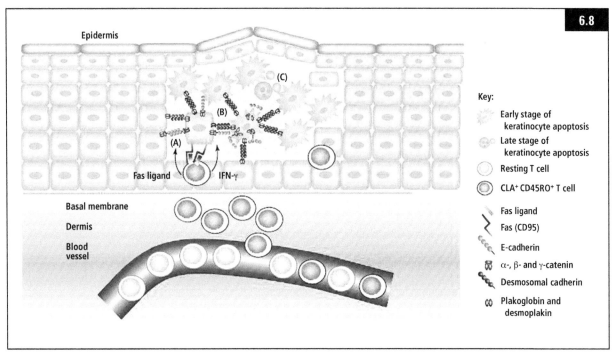

Fig 6.8 Apoptosis in eczematous dermatitis: T cells attack keratinocytes (KCs) in the elicitation phase of eczematous dermatitis. The infiltration of activated CD4+ and CD8+ T cells into the dermis and epidermis results in eczematous changes to the epidermis. Apoptosis of KCs is characterized by impairment of cohesion between KCs (spongiosis). The key pathogenic steps are: (A) Interferon-γ (IFN-γ) secreted by activated T cells (CLA+ CD45RO+) enhances the expression of Fas on KCs. Membrane-bound and soluble Fas ligand produced by activated T cells triggers Fas on the KCs. (B) During the early stages of the apoptosis of KCs, E-cadherin is cleaved by caspases that remove the β-catenin-binding domain from its cytoplasmic tail. Desmosomal cadherins (eg, desmogleins and desmocollins) remain intact. The intracellular domain of E-cadherin is linked to actin microfilaments through its association with α-catenin, β-catenin, and γ-catenin (plakoglobin). Desmosomal cadherins bind to the cytoplasmic proteins plakoglobin and desmoplakin, and are linked to keratin intermediate filaments. (C) Finally, DNA is fragmented and apoptotic bodies form. CLA, cutaneous lymphocyte-associated antigen. (Reprinted from Trautmann *et al.* 2001. © 2001 with permission from Elsevier.)

was reduced in intercellular spaces, which stained strongly for hyaluronan. Increased hyaluronan results from cytokine stimulation of keratinocytes. Among a number of cytokines tested, only IL-4, IL-13, and IFN-γ increased hyaluronan production, enhanced HAS3 mRNA expression, and decreased membrane E-cadherin expression by human keratinocytes. Thus IFN-γ with its proapoptotic role in the epidermis, along with IL-4 and IL-13, acts to decrease E-cadherin expression and contributes to the synthesis of hyaluronan. Increased hyaluronan in the intercellular space then can induce the movement of water into the epidermis by osmosis (**Box 6.3**).

CHRONIC LESION FORMATION

With chronic lesions it is difficult to dissect out the effects of continuous rubbing and scratching from those of ongoing inflammation unrelated to scratching. Clinically, in areas of rubbing, discrete lichenoid papules coalesce into lichenified plaques with thickening and exaggerated skin markings. Lichenification is not only seen in atopic dermatitis but can also be seen to some degree in other pruritic dermatoses. The term 'lichen simplex chronicus,' previously termed 'localized neurodermatitis,' refers to a localized, usually circumscribed area of lichenification that is extremely pruritic. It usually occurs on the nape of the neck, scrotum, vulva, and lower legs in patients who may or may not be atopic. It is the act of rubbing that causes these lesions and the original source of itching may no longer be apparent. Botulinum toxin relieved the itch of recalcitrant lichen simplex chronicus, notalgia paresthetica, and dyshidrotic eczema (Heckmann *et al.* 2002, Wollina and Karamfilov 2002). The mechanism by which botulinum toxin relieves itch is not known but may involve acetylcholine, calcitonin gene-related peptide (CGRP), or substance P (Wollina 2008), which could be involved in lichen simplex chronicus. On the other hand, very little work has been done on the actual mechanism by which chronic rubbing causes clinical lichenification.

Box 6.3   Mechanism for the induction of spongiosis

- Intracellular adhesion of keratinocytes is anchored by desmosomes and adherens junctions which contain E-cadherin
- Keratinocyte low-level Fas expression is increased by interferon-γ (IFN-γ) and renders them susceptible to apoptosis
- Enhanced FasL expression on infiltrating lymphocytes delivers the *coup de grâce*
- Cleavage of E-cadherin accompanies apoptosis decreasing adhesion between cells
- Dysregulated metalloproteinase ADAM10 causes ↑ shedding of E-cadherin
- Spongiotic keratinocytes have ↑ expression of hyaluronan (interleukin [IL]-4, IL-13, and IFN-γ increase hyaluronan production)
- ↑ hyaluronan in intercellular space induces water influx by osmosis

The histological changes of lichen simplex chronicus, caused by chronic rubbing, are psoriasiform epidermal hyperplasia, and thickened papillary dermis with laminated coarse collagen bundles parallel to the rete and perpendicular to the surface in 'vertical streaks' (Ackerman 1978).

In mice, scratching can switch the local skin immune response from Th2 milieu induced by epicutaneous antigen sensitization to Th1 with significant expression of IFN-γ but not IL-13 (Matsushima et al. 2003). This is analogous to the situation in chronic lesions of AD. Toda et al. (2003) demonstrated increased type I collagen deposition in chronic skin lesions of AD compared with acute lesions, particularly in the upper dermis. Type I collagen deposition in chronic lesions correlated with the presence of IL-11, a cytokine known to enhance collagen deposition. Expression of the fibrogenic cytokine TGF-β1 was increased in acute lesions and to a greater extent in chronic lesions. IL-17 released by Th17 CD4+ cells can induce proinflammatory mediators from macrophages and fibroblasts, and is present in acute AD lesional skin (Toda et al. 2003). Tissue fibrosis may be initiated by T-cell-secreted IL-17 with subsequent release of IL-11 from eosinophils and deposition of type I collagen.

Katoh et al. (2002) demonstrated that serum levels of *tissue inhibitor of metalloprotease-1* (TIMP-1) were elevated in patients with exacerbations of AD compared with normal individuals, especially in those with lichenification or prurigo lesions. Matrix metalloproteases and their inhibitors (TIMPs) play a role in inflammation-induced tissue destruction and remodeling (Katoh et al. 2002). Finally, aquaporin-3 (AQP3), a water-/glycerol-transporting protein expressed in keratinocytes and involved in keratinocyte migration and proliferation, is upregulated in the AD epidermis and may contribute to the epidermal hyperplasia (Nakahigashi et al. 2010).

DENDRITIC CELLS

Dendritic cells (DCs) are specialized antigen presenting cells (APC)s that serve a surveillance function and are intimately involved with the interface between innate immunity and the generation of specific adaptive immune responses. Studies of allergic contact dermatitis established the role of LCs in antigen presentation and opened the door to the study of dendritic cell biology. The two major subtypes of DCs are the myeloid DCs (mDCs), typified by LCs, and inflammatory dendritic epidermal cells (IDECs) and the plasmacytoid DCs or DC2 (Novak et al. 2008). LCs contain Birbeck granules, express CD1a and HLA-DR but are CD11b negative. As noted earlier, immunohistochemical studies of lesional skin in AD showed IgE in contact with LCs. In addition, enriched populations of AD LCs were shown to be highly stimulatory to autologous T cells (Taylor et al. 1991).

The most important IgE-binding receptor on LCs is the high-affinity IgE receptor FcεR1, which is also expressed on a type of mDC known as the inflammatory dendritic epidermal cell (Bieber et al. 1992). The high-affinity IgE receptor is also present in a different configuration on other immunocytes such as mast cells and basophils.

Whereas LCs are normally resident in the epidermis, IDECs migrate there anew during inflammatory reactions (Wollenberg et al. 1996). IDECs are not seen in normal appearing skin of patients with AD but appear in the epidermis approximately 24 h after the initiation of inflammation (Kerschenlohr et al. 2003). They also appear to be more proinflammatory than LCs and, although LCs favor a Th2 T-cell response, IDECs induce a Th1 polarization (Novak and Bieber 2005). Thus LCs are thought to be most important in initiating the allergic Th2 immune response, whereas IDECs predominate in chronic AD lesions and may provide the IL-12 necessary to cause the *Th1 switch* (Werfel 2009).

FcεR1 is not constitutively expressed on DCs as is its counterpart on mast cells and basophils, but its expression on LCs and IDECs correlates with serum IgE levels. In atopiform ('intrinsic atopic') dermatitis, a comparable percentage of CD1a+ cells express CD36, a marker of overall inflammatory activity as in truly atopic dermatitis, but there is significantly lower expression of FcεR1. This is easy to understand because increased IgE levels and allergen-specific IgE are absent in these patients (Oppel et al. 2000).

LCs and IDECs are thought to play a pivotal role in orchestrating the inflammatory response in

AD (Miraglia del Giudice *et al.* 2006). DCs in the periphery internalize antigens, undergo maturation, and migrate to draining lymph nodes where they present antigen to naïve CD4 lymphocytes.

Interactions between the epidermal barrier and resident DCs have a profound influence on the priming of T cells by DCs (Ziegler and Liu 2006), eg, in patients with AD, keratinocytes produce a key cytokine TSLP that induces maturation of LCs and their migration to draining lymph nodes. TSLP-activated DCs prime allergen-specific Th2 responses. Naïve allogeneic CD4 cells stimulated by allogeneic TSLP-activated DCs secrete IL-4, -5, and -13 but not IFN-γ.

TSLP CONTROLS ALLERGIC INFLAMMATION

The identification of TSLP, an IL-7 analog, elucidated aspects of innate and adaptive immunity, especially the way in which keratinocyte innate reactions contribute to the development of Th2 adaptive immunity. As mentioned previously, LCs are thought to be most prominent in the early phase of AD where they induce Th2 polarization in T cells. The immune polarization induced by DCs, Th1 or Th2, is dictated by stimuli that they receive early in their development (Liu 2007). In AD this stimulation is provided by keratinocyte-derived TSLP, which causes them to induce a Th2 response in lymphocytes. Although the major source of TSLP in humans is epithelial cells, it is also produced by fibroblasts, smooth muscle cells, and mast cells. TSLP facilitates the induction by DCs of a Th2 microenvironment; it does not induce production by DCs of the Th1-polarizing cytokine IL-12 or the proinflammatory cytokines, TNF-α, IL-1β, and IL-6 (Liu 2007).

INFLAMMATORY TH2 CELLS

Many sources define Th2 cells as those producing IL-4, -5, -13, and -10, and Th1 cells as those producing IFN-γ and TNF-α. Stimulation of naïve CD4 T-cells by TSLP–DCs produce a unique type of Th2 cell that expresses classic Th2 cytokines, IL-4, IL-5, and IL-13, as well as significant quantities of TNF-α but limited if any IL-10. Liu (2007) has defined these Th2 cells that produce TNF-α as *inflammatory Th2 cells* and consider them to be the pathogenic T cells involved in AD and asthma (**Fig 6.9**). Th2 cells that produce IL-10 in addition to IL-4, IL-5 and IL-13 are termed 'regulatory Th2 cells.'

The induction of inflammatory Th2 cells results from the production of OX40-ligand (OX40-L) by TSLP–DCs in the absence of IL-12. If IL-12 is present, the production of inflammatory Th2 cells is blocked. It has recently been demonstrated that TSLP also has a direct effect on activated CD4+ T lymphocytes (Rochman *et al.* 2007). Thus, TSLP that is released by epithelial cells in response to trauma, microbes, and inflammation links the innate immune response with a polarized adaptive immune response. In addition, TSLP induces mast cells to produce Th2

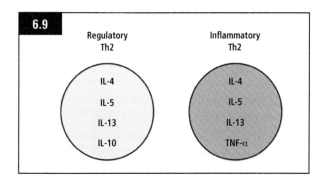

Fig 6.9 Inflammatory T-helper type 2 (Th2) cells: two types of Th2 cells defined by their interleukin (IL)-10 and tumor necrosis factor α (TNF-α) production. Regulatory Th2 cells produce IL-4, -5, -13, and -10. Inflammatory Th2 cells produce IL-4, -5, and -13, and TNF-α. It is proposed that only the inflammatory Th2 cells are associated with allergic diseases. (Reprinted from Liu 2007. © 2007 with permission from Elsevier.)

cytokines such as IL-13, further contributing to the Th2 microenvironment (Allakhverdi *et al.* 2007).

How does this relate to the pathogenesis of AD? We know that early-stage AD is characterized by a Th2 microenvironment and that Th2 cells specific for aeroallergens can be demonstrated in the infiltrate. It is hypothesized that aeroallergens such as products from house dust mites (HDM) and even food antigens can penetrate an impaired skin barrier and interact with epidermal LCs and promote an antigen-specific Th2 immune response. It is also considered that this epicutaneous sensitization can give rise to the development of asthma.

TSLP AND THE ATOPIC MARCH

The 'atopic march' is a term that was coined to describe the temporal progression of clinical signs of atopy, usually starting with AD and progressing to asthma and allergic rhinitis (Spergel 2005). At any given time one clinical sign is prominent whereas others subside. A great deal of literature has been published over the years since the time of Coca espousing the allergic nature of AD. The recent descriptions of filaggrin mutations associated with AD and asthma have fortified the contention by many investigators that barrier disruption favors epicutaneous penetration of aeroallergens, and that the skin becomes the earliest or primary site of sensitization, ultimately resulting in manifestations of allergy in the lungs (asthma) and nose (seasonal rhinitis). The concept that primary sensitization to allergens predominantly occurs through barrier-damaged skin has far-reaching implications, both clinical and financial, eg, Boussault *et al.* (2007) have suggested avoiding the use of topical preparations containing oat proteins in infants with AD because of the risk of epicutaneous sensitization, but this view has been questioned (Goujon-Henry *et al.* 2008). Are we putting children at risk for asthma and gastrointestinal allergies with certain widely used topical products, or could we prevent sensitization to food allergens by using certain brand emollients?

The concept of an atopic march progressing from eczema to other allergic diseases is not universally accepted because many patients develop asthma before or simultaneously with the development of AD (Illi *et al.* 2004, Barberio *et al.* 2008). Burgess *et al.* (2009) examined longitudinal population data and concluded that childhood eczema increased the likelihood of childhood asthma, new-onset asthma later in life, and asthma persisting into middle age. Another study found that eczema in the first 2 years of life was associated with an increased risk of childhood asthma only in boys (Lowe *et al.* 2008). One editorialist from a managed care pharmacy journal takes a more cynical view:

> The theory that AD progresses to AM *(atopic manifestations)* in an atopic march has been popularized by authors who are consultants to the manufacturers of drugs for AD and in BOGSAT (bunch of old guys sitting around talking) discussions (Curtiss 2007).

Some light has been shed on this debate by Bønnelykke *et al.* (2010) who followed infants at high risk for atopy prospectively for the development of eczema, asthma, and sensitization. Filaggrin loss-of-function variants were associated with early-onset eczema and asthma, but sensitization measured by RAST (radioallergosorbent test) occurred later. They concluded that *FLG*-associated asthma is 'mediated through a systemic, possibly immunological mechanism stimulated through the impaired skin barrier' but that the 'late effect on sensitization compared to the early increased risk of asthma … suggests that sensitization does not mediate the pathway from FLG deficiency to airway disease.'

In mice, epicutaneous sensitization with ovalbumin results in the induction of antigen-specific IgE and T cells that secrete Il-4 but not IFN-γ (Saloga *et al.* 1994, Wang *et al.* 1996). It induces a T-cell- and eosinophil-rich cellular infiltrate, IL-4, IL-5, and IFN-α mRNA, and interestingly can cause airway hyper-responsiveness to methacholine after a single inhalation challenge with ovalbumin (Spergel 2005). Thus it would seem that epicutaneous sensitization acting through TSLP–DCs and inflammatory Th2 cells could induce a sequential Th2 dermatitis and asthma, akin to the *atopic march*. On the other hand, epicutaneous sensitization may not be necessary: a chimeric mouse model with a barrier defect on a portion of their skin developed allergic-like dermatitis and susceptibility to asthma without epicutaneous sensitization (Demehri *et al.* 2009). TSLP was demonstrated to be the agent sensitizing the lung to allergens.

Direct production of TSLP by epidermal cells might also explain why patients with atopiform dermatitis without IgE involvement and infants before the development of IgE sensitization can develop eczematous lesions. It also helps explain the effect of scratching on the development of further lesions.

ATOPIFORM DERMATITIS (INTRINSIC AD, NONATOPIC DERMATITIS)

In various studies, approximately 20–30% of individuals with AD do not show elevated total IgE, allergen-specific IgE, or positive skin-prick tests to foods and aeroallergens. A prospective birth cohort study of 263 children followed for 5 years found that, among participants, 66.1% had eczema in the first 5 years of life, the majority in the first year (85.5%) (Kusel *et al.* 2005). A third of the cases were *nonatopic*. Those with *extrinsic* AD were more likely to be male, to have been breastfed longer, and to have food allergies, allergic rhinitis, and current wheeze. Those with atopiform (*intrinsic*) dermatitis were more likely to be female and to have experienced early day-care exposure. Another study found that 8% of AD patients studied had atopiform dermatitis (Brenninkmeijer *et al.* 2008). Patients with atopiform dermatitis were more likely to be female, had later onset of disease, and milder dermatitis than those with the extrinsic form. Despite acceptance of the concept of two types of AD by many investigators, others have urged a degree of skepticism with regard to this concept until 'it emerges from … studies that there is a consistent constellation of associations with different types of eczema in a way that increases our predictive ability' (Williams and Johansson 2005).

This is especially important because some patients with atopiform dermatitis eventually go on to develop specific IgE sensitization.

By definition, patients with atopiform dermatitis do not have elevated levels of IgE. On the other hand, a study examining sensitization to *Malassezia sympodialis* found elevated specific IgE in both AD (extrinsic) and atopiform dermatitis (intrinsic) (Casagrande *et al.* 2006). The authors posited that to a certain extent the term 'intrinsic atopic dermatitis' may be misleading and they also questioned the relevance of IgE in the pathogenesis of AD. Moreover, an APT study found positive responses to house dust mite in only 47.4% of adult males with extrinsic AD but surprisingly in 66.6% of patients with atopiform (intrinsic) dermatitis (Ingordo *et al.* 2002).

With regard to the two cytokines important for IgE production, IL-4 and IL-13, Akdis *et al.* (1999a) failed to detect IL-4 expression by immunohistochemistry in lesions of intrinsic AD or extrinsic AD. The expression of IL-13 was less in intrinsic AD than in the extrinsic form, and IL-5 was expressed by some but not all specimens from patients with both types of AD. IFN-γ was expressed only at relatively low levels in both.

Jeong *et al.* (2003), examining mRNA cytokine expression by reverse transcription polymerase chain reaction (RT-PCR), demonstrated increased expression of mRNA of IL-5, IL-13, and IL-1β in both extrinsic and intrinsic AD compared with normal control individuals. Expression of these mRNAs and eosinophilic infiltration were higher in extrinsic AD than in the intrinsic form. In infants, intrinsic AD is more common and there are lower eosinophil counts, lower eosinophil cationic protein (ECP) levels, and lower SCORAD indices than in extrinsic AD patients (Park *et al.* 2006). Clinical severity in intrinsic and extrinsic forms both correlated with eosinophil count and serum ECP levels. The clinical and immunological features of atopiform (intrinsic) dermatitis are summarized in *Table 6.2*.

Table 6.2 Features of atopiform (intrinsic) dermatitis

Clinical features	Incidence approximately 5–30% of those with eczema Later onset of disease Milder disease More common in females and associated with early day-care exposure Absence of asthma and allergic rhinitis
Immunological characteristics	Total IgE <150 (or 200) kU/L Absence of specific IgE to food allergens and aeroallergens (note exception of *Malassezia sympodialis*) Negative skin-prick tests to food allergens and aeroallergens Less Th2 *skewing* and relative overproduction of interferon-γ (Tokura 2010). Interleukins IL-5 and IL-13 are present in lesional skin but less than in 'extrinsic atopic dermatitis' Lower *Staphylococcus aureus* colonization

THE SKIN BARRIER IN ATOPIC DERMATITIS

The skin serves as a protective barrier, a sensory and immunological organ, and an organ of excretion and thermoregulation. It must adapt to diverse temperatures, humidity, ultraviolet light exposure, pathogens, allergens, and other physical insults. Not only does the skin provide a physical barrier against desiccation but its component cells also function as part of the innate immune system that acts as a first-line defense against infection.

INNATE IMMUNITY AND ANTIMICROBIAL PEPTIDES

The innate immune system includes all inborn, 'no need to learn' protective mechanisms that induce an immediate response against potentially harmful microorganisms (Wollenberg *et al.* 2010). The innate immune system comprises elements that not only recognize and help destroy pathogenic organisms but also play a role in directing specific adaptive immune responses. DCs, keratinocytes, and macrophages express receptors that recognize conserved pathogen-associated molecular patterns (PAMPs) (Baker 2006). Among these pattern recognition receptors (PRRs) are toll-like receptors (TLRs) and members of the NOD (nucleotide-binding oligomerization domain) family. Some single nucleotide polymorphisms (SNPs) have been described in TLR2, TLR4, and Nod1/CARD4 which are associated with AD.

ROLE OF PROTEASE-ACTIVATED RECEPTOR 2

Protease-activated receptors are a family of seven-transmembrane G-protein-coupled receptors that are stimulated by cleavage of their N-terminus by serine proteases rather than by direct occupancy of a receptor-binding site by a specific ligand (Macfarlane *et al.* 2001). Protease-activated receptor (PAR)-2 is one such receptor which, besides being involved in the pain pathway, has recently been shown to be associated with itchy skin diseases including AD (Kawagoe *et al.* 2002, Steinhoff *et al.* 2003).

Steinhoff *et al.* (2003) demonstrated staining for PAR-2 in lesional skin of patients with AD in keratinocytes, blood vessels, certain inflammatory cells, and nerve fiber-like structures (**Fig 6.10**). PAR-2 receptors provide an explanation for several phenomena occurring in AD. First, there is a pH-dependent increase in endogenous proteases in patients with barrier damage as in AD and, second, many allergens thought to be involved in AD as well as staphylococci have protease activity that can activate PAR-2 (Miedzobrodzki *et al.* 2002, Kato *et al.* 2009, Voegeli *et al.* 2009). Indeed, recent work suggests that the enhancement of protease activity through increased KLK7 expression by the Th2 cytokines IL-4 and IL-13 may be an important determinant of epidermal barrier dysfunction in patients with AD (Morizane *et al.* 2012). As PAR-2 activation by allergens with protease activity has been shown to delay barrier recovery and affect lamellar body secretion in barrier-disrupted skin in mice, it is not unreasonable to think that they might affect AD lesional skin similarly (Jeong *et al.* 2008). It is currently believed that upregulated proteases in AD stimulate PAR-2 and induce the production of cytokines and chemokines implicated in allergic inflammation, immune responses, pruritus, and ongoing barrier dysfunction, possibly allowing easier allergen penetration (Lee SE *et al.* 2010).

ANTIMICROBIAL PEPTIDES

Antimicrobial peptides (AMPs) are low-molecular-weight, primarily cationic proteins produced by keratinocytes that function as endogenous antibiotics active against bacteria, viruses, and fungi, and which directly modulate certain immune functions (Howell 2007). The two main classes of AMPs in skin are the β-defensins and canthelicidins. In human skin there are four known defensins, human β-defensins (HBDs) 1, 2, 3, and 4, and one canthelicidin LL-37. Dermicidin is an AMP present in sweat. Under normal circumstances, keratinocytes produce AMPs that inhibit the growth of pathogenic bacteria, fungi, and viruses on the skin surface.

As patients with AD are almost universally colonized with *Staphylococcus aureus*, are subject to eczema herpeticum, and may have an increased incidence of warts and molluscum contagiosum, investigators have looked at AMP expression in patients with AD compared with normal individuals and those with psoriasis. Ong *et al.* (2002) demonstrated decreased immunostaining for LL-37 and HBD-2 and their respective mRNAs in acute and chronic lesions of patients with AD compared with patients with psoriasis. They concluded that this downregulation may contribute to the development of infection and colonization of lesional and nonlesional AD skin with pathogenic staphylococci. The authors subsequently added that the multifunctional nature of AMPs suggested that distinctions between 'innate' and 'adaptive' immunity are arbitrary and should be looked at in the context of a coordinated immune response (Gallo and Leung 2003). Deficiency of other AMPs such as dermicidin, canthelicidin LL-37, and HBD-3 are also thought to contribute to the susceptibility of AD patients to skin infections (McGirt and Beck 2006, Werfel 2009).

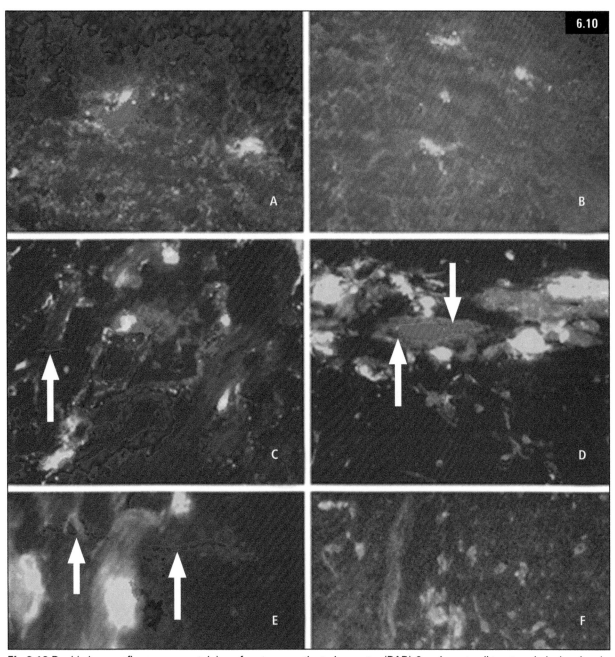

Fig 6.10 Double immunofluorescence staining of protease-activated receptor (PAR)-2 and mast cell tryptase in lesional and nonlesional human skin biopsies of patients with atopic dermatitis (AD). (A) In lesional skin of patients with AD, staining for PAR-2 (red) can be observed in keratinocytes, blood vessels, certain inflammatory cells, and nerve-fiber-like structures. Mast cells (green) associated with PAR-2-positive blood vessels (100 x). (B) Omission of antibodies against PAR-2 demonstrates only staining of mast cells by tryptase (100 x). (C) Higher magnification reveals staining of small nerve fibers (arrow) in the dermis associated with blood vessels (red) and mast cells (green) (400 x). (D) In lesional skin of patients with AD, increased staining for PAR-2 was observed in nerve fibers (arrows) closely associated with mast cells (green) (630 x) at higher magnification. (E) Staining for PAR-2 (arrows) was also observed in nerve fibers of nonlesional skin from patients with AD (630 x). (F) Control staining using the appropriate peptide for preabsorption did not result in any PAR-2-like or tryptase-like immunoreactivity in human skin tissue (630 x). (Reprinted from Steinhoff *et al.* 2003. © 2003 with permission of Society for Neuroscience.)

On the other hand, some investigators have found normal expression of AMPs in AD. Goo *et al.* (2010) found no difference in baseline expression of HBD-2 and LL-37 in foreskin biopsies from patients with AD and normal individuals. Moreover, Asano *et al.* (2008) found no decrease in levels of β-defensin-2 but rather increased levels compared with healthy controls, in the involved and uninvolved stratum corneum of patients with AD. *S. aureus* colonization was not inversely correlated with levels of β-defensin-2 in involved AD skin, suggesting that β-defensin-2 is induced in response to bacteria, injury, or inflammatory stimuli, and might not be associated with vulnerability to *S. aureus* colonization in patients with AD (Asano *et al.* 2008). Discordant results have been reported for the canthelicidin LL-37 as well, and it was suggested that upregulation of this AMP may be related to the process of re-epithelialization (Ballardini *et al.* 2009, Mallbris *et al.* 2010). In another study, Harder *et al.* (2010) showed increased expression of several AMPs including RNase 7, psoriasin, HBD-2, and HBD-3 in lesional AD skin compared with normal skin in AD patients and concluded that staphylococcal colonization and infection could not be fully explained by decreased AMPs in AD.

Human AMPs are also suspected to affect skin barrier integrity based on their effects on calcium mobilization and keratinocyte migration. As discussed below, there is ample evidence that *S. aureus* directly contributes to exacerbation of eczema.

THE EPIDERMAL BARRIER TO WATER LOSS

Crucial to the maintenance of internal hydration is the epidermal barrier to water loss, provided mostly by the outermost layer of the epidermis, the stratum corneum, and to some extent by tight junctions in the stratum granulosum (Harding 2004, Yuki *et al.* 2007, De Benedetto *et al.* 2010). Patients with AD frequently have extensive areas of itchy, dry-appearing skin that tends to worsen in the winter months and, in many patients, flares of the disease in winter are the rule. Exposure to low humidity and its effect on moisture content can increase keratinocyte proliferation, markers of inflammation, and the number of mast cells (Denda *et al.* 1998, Ashida and Denda 2003). Also, the observation of increased nerve growth in dry skin might explain the known association of xerosis with pruritus and be pertinent for AD (Tominaga *et al.* 2007). Numerous studies have pointed to a disruption of the cutaneous barrier to water loss and the decreased capacity of the stratum corneum to hold water in patients with AD.

An important question is whether innate inherited barrier abnormalities are primary to the disease process or whether underlying inflammation gives rise to these barrier defects. The recent association of loss-of-function mutations in the filaggrin gene with AD suggests that abnormalities of the stratum corneum may be constitutional for many patients with the disease. However, transepidermal water loss (TEWL) and water content of the stratum corneum appear to be normal in patients 'cured' of AD for several years, suggesting that barrier abnormalities, to a large extent, may be temporary and result from inflammation (Matsumoto *et al.* 2000).

Electron microscopic studies have shown the basic structure of the stratum corneum to be analogous to a brick wall in which terminally cornified, flattened keratinocytes, known as corneocytes, form the bricks, and lipid lamellae composed of ceramides, cholesterol, and free fatty acids constitute the mortar (Elias 1983, Candi *et al.* 2005). The plasma membrane of keratinocytes is replaced by an insoluble protein structure known as the cornified envelope (CE), which serves as a scaffold for lipid attachment and is essential for normal barrier function. The mostly proteinaceous CE is made up of filaggrin, loricrin, trichohyalin, involucrin, small proline-rich proteins, hornerin, and keratin intermediate filaments, which are crosslinked by transglutaminases (McGrath and Uitto 2008, Henry *et al.* 2011). Defects in the expression of multiple genes encoding the cornified envelope have been identified in AD, especially with regard to loricrin (expressed at 2% of the level of normal skin) (Guttman-Yassky *et al.* 2009) and also to hornerin. Attached covalently to the outer surface of this cornified envelope is a unique lipid layer referred to as the *corneocyte lipid envelope* (CLE) (Holleran *et al.* 2006).

The lipid lamellae and CLE of the stratum corneum are formed by an elegant mechanism in which preformed lipid precursors are released into the intercellular space, hydrolyzed and incorporated into these lipid structures. Lipid precursors in keratinocytes are bound in membrane-limited organelles known as lamellar bodies. Ceramides constitute more than 50% of intercellular lipids (Imokawa 2001). The ceramides are derived from sphingomyelin and glucosylceramide (GlcCer), the major constituents of lamellar granules. In the granular layer of the epidermis, lamellar bodies fuse with the apical plasma membrane of keratinocytes and extrude their protein and lipid contents into the intercellular space.

Hydrolysis of secreted lipid precursors to ceramides allows their incorporation into the intercellular lamellae and the CLEs, where they play an important role in barrier and water-holding function (Behne *et al.* 2000, Imokawa 2001). The formation of the CLE and lamellar membranes is illustrated in **Fig 6.11**.

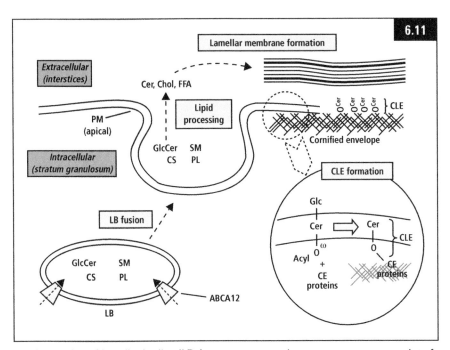

Fig 6.11 Formation and secretion of lamellar bodies (LBs) at stratum granulosum–stratum corneum interface. Precursor lipids, including glucosylceramide (GlcCer), sphingomyelin (SM), glycerophospholipids (PL), and cholesterol sulfate (CS), are packaged into LBs within the upper cell layers of the epidermis. Lipid packaging into the LB requires function of at least one ABC transporter protein, ABCA12, which appears to localize to limiting membranes of LBs. Fusion of LBs with the atypical plasma membrane (PM) in the uppermost nucleated cell layer of the epidermis (stratum granulosum) allows extrusion of lipid precursors into the extracellular domain(s). Subsequent enzymatic processing of precursor lipids generates the major lipid classes required for epidermal barrier function, ie, ceramides (Cer), cholesterol (Chol), and free fatty acids (FFAs). The corneocyte lipid envelope (CLE) consists of ω-hydroxy-ceramides that are covalently attached to the highly crosslinked proteins of the cornified envelope (CE), and is formed sequentially with the addition of ω-OH-GlcCer followed by deglucosylation. (Reprinted from Holleran *et al*. 2006. © 2006 with permission from Elsevier/FEBS.)

THE IMPORTANCE OF FILAGGRIN TO BARRIER FUNCTION AND EPIDERMAL HYDRATION

Filaggrin is a histidine-rich protein derived from a short-lived precursor protein, profilaggrin. The name derives from its ability to aggregate keratin filaments *in vitro* (Weidenthaler *et al.* 1993). Sybert *et al.* (1985) demonstrated absent or decreased levels of filaggrin in ichthyosis vulgaris, an autosomal disorder of keratinization commonly associated with AD. It is now known that homozygous or compound heterozygous mutations in the gene that encodes profilaggrin (*FLG*) cause icthyosis vulgaris and predispose to AD and possibly to nickel contact dermatitis (Palmer *et al.* 2006, Sandilands *et al.* 2006, 2009, Weidinger *et al.* 2006, Novak *et al.* 2007) (**Fig 6.12**). In **Fig 6.12**, immunohistochemical staining demonstrates the presence of filaggrin in normal skin and its absence in a patient who is homozygous for nonsense mutation *R501X* of the *FLG* gene. A clinical photo illustrates a patient with typical flexural atopic dermatitis. Loss-of-function mutations in *FLG* have been associated with a number of abnormalities summarized in **Fig 6.13**.

The importance of filaggrin relates to its crucial role in the formation of the cornified envelope and the role of its breakdown products in binding water in the stratum corneum. Caspase 14, which is downgraded by inflammatory cytokines, is required for the breakdown of filaggrin; it is decreased in AD skin, perhaps accounting in part for barrier abnormalities (Eckhart and Tschachler 2011, Hoste *et al.* 2011, Hvid *et al.* 2011).

These filaggrin breakdown products constitute an admixture of low-molecular-weight, water-soluble substances within corneocytes, mostly pyrrolidone carboxylic acid, urocanic acid, and free amino acids. They are referred to collectively as the 'natural moisturizing factor' (NMF). The water content of the stratum corneum of lesional and nonlesional atopic dry skin is decreased, probably as a result of a decrease in NMF and increased transepidermal water loss (Werner *et al.* 1982, Takehashi and Izekawa 2000). Indeed, lesional and nonlesional AD skin have been shown immunohistochemically to express reduced amounts of filaggrin and decreased free amino acids. The presence of parakeratotic cells in lesional skin, and to a lesser extent in nonlesional

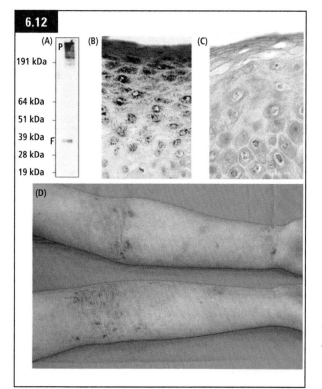

Fig 6.12 Filaggrin in human disease. (A) Post-translational processing of profilaggrin to filaggrin. Immunoblot of high-salt protein extract of human epidermis probed with monoclonal that recognizes an epitope within the filaggrin repeat domain and therefore detects both profilaggrin (P, upper band) and processed filaggrin (F, lower doublet, 37 kDa). (B) Immunohistochemical staining of human epidermis showing the great abundance of profilaggrin and/ or filaggrin in the upper granular layers of the epidermis. (C) Immunohistochemical staining of epidermis derived from an individual homozygous for nonsense mutation R501X in the first filaggrin repeat (compare with b). Filaggrin is completely absent in this individual, who has severe ichthyosis vulgaris, atopic eczema, and other allergies. (D) A patient with atopic eczema showing the flexural (referring to skinfolds, such as the inner surface of elbows) inflammation that is a classic clinical hallmark of this common, complex trait. Filaggrin-null mutations represent a major genetic risk factor for atopic eczema. (Reproduced with permission from Sandilands *et al.* 2009.)

skin, suggests that slight inflammation may induce epidermal hyperproliferation and decrease free amino acids as well.

Of note, it has been demonstrated that carriers of filaggrin mutations have decreased NMF in the stratum corneum compared with noncarriers (Kezic et al. 2008). Aside from AD, such carriers are also more susceptible to chronic irritant contact dermatitis (de Jongh et al. 2008).

In addition to there being a decrease in water-binding substances in patients with AD, there is a decreased barrier to water loss. Transepidermal water loss is increased in both lesional AD skin and to a lesser extent in nonlesional skin, but not in the normal skin of patients whose AD has totally resolved (Sakurai et al. 2002, Proksch et al. 2006). It is also worth noting that skin pH is significantly higher in patients with AD than in normal individuals and correlates with skin dryness (Eberlein-Konig et al. 2000).

LIPID AND CERAMIDE ABNORMALITIES

Much of the compromised barrier in AD skin results from abnormalities of lipid metabolism and decreased production of ceramides, especially ceramide-1. Moreover, lipid abnormalities are also thought to play a significant role in inflammation and itching responses. Interestingly, although TEWL is increased in all patients with AD compared with normal controls, TEWL is higher in nonfilaggrin-associated AD than in filaggrin-related AD on the extensor forearm and back but not on the flexor forearm (Nemoto-Hasebe et al. 2009). There is no clear relationship between filaggrin mutations and ceramide levels (Jungersted et al. 2010).

Stratum corneum ceramide levels are determined by the balance of enzymes that favor its production, ie, sphingomyelinase and β-glucocerebrocidase, and those that cause its degradation, eg, ceramidase.

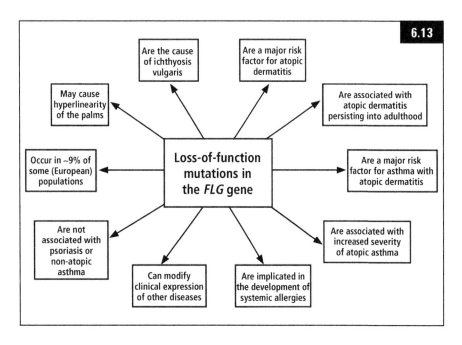

Fig 6.13 Clinical significance of loss-of-function mutations in the *FLG* gene. Mutations in *FLG* are directly associated with the cause, susceptibility to, or altered clinical expression of several dermatological and other disorders. (Reproduced from McGrath 2008 with permission from John Wiley & Sons.)

Reduced ceramide in AD may be caused by abnormally high expression of the enzyme, sphingomyelin (SM) deacylase, and decreased epidermal acid sphingomyelinase (SMase) activity (Hara et al. 2000, Jensen et al. 2004), eg, the stratum corneum from AD-lesional volar forearm skin expresses sphingomyelin deacylase at levels 5–17 times higher than normal skin and that of nonlesional skin of AD patients expresses levels 3–9 times higher. SM deacylase hydrolyzes sphingomyelin to produce sphingosophosphorylcholine (SPC) instead of ceramide normally formed by sphingomyelinase. In fact, levels of stratum corneum SPC have been shown to be upregulated in both involved and uninvolved AD skin (Okamoto et al. 2003). As SPC is a potent inducer of intercellular adhesion molecule-1 (ICAM-1) expression by keratinocytes, induces mast cell degranulaton and histamine release, and has a direct effect on nerves, it has been suggested that it may play an important role in AD epidermal inflammation and itching responses (Imokawa et al. 1999, Andoh et al. 2009, Kim et al. 2010). SPC also stimulates keratinocyte transglutaminase activity and cornified envelope formation, so it may alter the keratinization process in AD (Higuchi et al. 2001). Finally, SPC significantly decreases filaggrin gene transcription, implying that it plays a pivotal role in impairment of the epidermal permeability barrier in AD lesional skin (Choi et al. 2010).

Vulnerability to bacterial colonization may result in part from reduced expression of the natural antimicrobial agent, sphingosine. This results from decreased levels of ceramides, the substrate for sphingosine, and from diminished activities of its metabolic enzyme, acid ceramidase (Arikawa et al. 2002). Interestingly, bacteria colonizing patients with AD secrete ceramidase at higher levels than those colonizing normal individuals (Ohnishi et al. 1999).

TIGHT JUNCTIONS AND CLAUDIN

Although the stratum corneum accounts for most of the barrier to water loss from the skin, tight junctions (TJs), which occur in the stratum granulosum, also play a role (Yuki et al. 2007). Schlüter et al. (2004) have

demonstrated that cells of the stratum granulosum are connected by a continuous tight junction system that may act as a gate for the passage of water, solutes, and particles via the paracellular pathway; these may, it is speculated, regulate lipid targeting toward the stratum corneum (Schlüter et al. 2004, Niessen 2007). De Benedetto et al. (2010) have recently shown that there is a defect in the tight junctions in AD skin, with decreased levels of the TJ protein claudin associated with increased paracellular permeability. This is especially exciting in view of the recent study showing that activated LC dendrites elongate to penetrate keratinocyte tight junctions and thereby gain access to foreign antigens (Kubo et al. 2009) (see **Fig 6.1**). This presumably would be facilitated by defective tight junctions in AD and allow LC dendrites greater access to foreign antigens. On the other hand, as IgE is thought to be involved in antigen uptake in the context of AD and it is not clear that IgE is present at this level of the epidermis, other scenarios could be envisioned, eg, Sondell et al. (1997) showed staining of some but not all LCs by a monoclonal antibody reactive with stratum corneum chymotryptic enzyme (SCCE) (kallikrein 7) (Sondell et al. 1997). Igawa et al. (2011) have suggested that tight junctions can inhibit protease access to parts of the stratum corneum. Perhaps defects in tight junctions might allow direct access of stratum corneum proteases to LCs and induce some immunological effect.

THE ACID MANTLE – SKIN pH IN ATOPIC DERMATITIS

The term 'acid mantle' refers to the slightly acidic pH of normal skin that helps control the proliferation of pathogenic bacteria and is intimately involved in barrier homeostasis. A number of factors determine the skin pH such as age, anatomic site, ethnic differences, skin moisture, presence of sebum or sweat, and exogenous factors such as soaps and detergents (Rippke et al. 2002, Schmid-Wendtner and Korting 2006).

The normal acidic pH of the stratum corneum affects the barrier lipid formation and desquamation; raising the pH, as with alkaline soaps, has deleterious effects on barrier homeostasis, and stratum corneum integrity and cohesion (Hachem *et al.* 2005, 2010). At increased pH serine proteases (SPs) become activated, leading to deactivation and degradation of lipid-processing enzymes and corneodesmosomes (CDs) (Hachem *et al.* 2005).

One important factor that contributes to maintaining the acid mantle is the contribution of *trans*-urocanic acid (*trans*-UCA), which is one of the breakdown products of filaggrin and part of the NMF (Krien and Kermici 2000). Genetically determined decreased or absent filaggrin levels cause diminished production of UCA and contribute to a more alkaline skin surface pH, and adversely affect barrier homeostasis.

EPICUTANEOUS ANTIGEN PRESENTATION THROUGH AN IMPAIRED SKIN BARRIER

Impaired barrier function not only increases water loss from the epidermis but may also allow entry of foreign substances applied to the skin. The ability of haptens and small nonprotein molecules to penetrate the skin is well established, as exemplified by allergic contact dermatitis. It is the purported ability of protein molecules such as dust mite antigens to traverse the skin and reach APCs that is more controversial. There are certainly data to suggest that protein antigens or parts of them can penetrate the skin, such as in the occurrence of contact urticaria and protein-contact dermatitis after exposure to proteins (Berard *et al.* 2003). It is proposed that the enzymatic (proteolytic) activity of allergens such as dust mite allergens allows their penetration through the epidermis and direct access to APCs.

THE ATOPY PATCH TEST

Much of the support for epicutaneous sensitization has been based on an AD model, ie, aeroallergen patch testing also known as the atopy patch test. One of the difficulties encountered in trying to interpret studies that have used this procedure is the variability in methodology that has been used in various studies, including choice of antigen, size of the chamber used to present antigen, eg, 6 mm or 12 mm Finn chamber,

criteria for a positive test, time of patch test reading after application of antigen, and the use of 'tape stripping' before application of allergen in some studies. So, for example, one of the original studies suggesting a Th2 to Th1/Th0 switch in AD was based on APTs in which tape stripping with adhesive tape was performed before application of allergens (Thepen *et al.* 1996). Studies that used tape stripping before allergen application demonstrated the importance of IgE+ CD1a+ in the presentation of house dust mite antigen to T cells and in positive APT reactions (Mudde *et al.* 1990, Langeveld-Wildschut *et al.* 2000).

As mentioned previously, it has been suggested that epicutaneous sensitization to protein antigens is thought by some to be involved in the induction of asthma in patients with impaired skin barriers. In a mouse model using tape stripping and ovalbumin under an occlusive patch, skin changes similar to human positive APT reactions were seen, but more importantly bronchial hyper-responsiveness was also induced. This supports the premise that epicutaneous allergen processing might be involved in the 'atopic march.' So under certain conditions, such as tape stripping and occlusion, dust mite antigen and other allergens can penetrate the skin barrier and cause an eczematous dermatitis. Tape stripping is not entirely necessary for antigen penetration so dust mite antigen at higher concentrations in a petrolatum vehicle can also elicit a positive APT reaction (Oldhoff *et al.* 2004).

There are studies to suggest that house dust mite antigen can penetrate normal skin in patients with AD with scratching or with aeroallergen patch testing but there are few studies actually demonstrating the presence of aeroallergens in the skin of naturally occurring lesions of AD (Gondo *et al.* 1986, Tanaka *et al.* 1990). Maeda *et al.* (1992) detected house dust mite antigens by immunohistochemistry of lesional skin in 19 of 38 AD patients, all of whom had anti-HDM-specific IgE. Most of the HDM antigens were located near LCs or helper T cells.

On the other hand, other data suggest that the levels of dust mites found in beds and on human skin when getting up in the morning are unlikely to be an ongoing stimulus to symptoms in the great majority of mite-sensitive patients (Riley *et al.* 1998, Fitzharris and Riley 1999).

A recent study showed a high prevalence of positive APTs to indoor and outdoor aeroallergens in infants aged <1 year (Boralevi *et al.* 2008). Moreover the greater the TEWL, the higher the prevalence of sensitization to aeroallergens. It was suggested that this might result from facilitated epicutaneous sensitization. In considering these data it is important to consider studies in which APTs are used to establish the diagnosis of food allergy (Niggemann *et al.* 2000). It is now considered by some investigators that food allergens cause sensitization epicutaneously through an impaired skin barrier.

THE 500-DALTON RULE

There is good evidence that molecules >500 daltons (Da) in molecular weight do not cross the stratum corneum unless it has undergone significant disruption (Bos and Meinardi 2000). This is clinically relevant in AD because such molecules as cyclosporine with a molecular weight of 1202.63 Da are not absorbed adequately, even in damaged AD skin. Even tacrolimus, with a molecular weight of 822.04 Da, is formulated with propylene glycol to enhance absorption. It is argued that atopy-related allergens are themselves often proteases, allowing them to penetrate by degrading barrier proteins. But then one might ask what happens in the mucosal epithelia of the respiratory and gastrointestinal tracts. There is no corneal layer, no physical barrier, and atopy-related allergens would penetrate these surfaces in all individuals, sensitizing everyone, which of course is not happening. Clearly aeroallergens can penetrate the skin in the model of the APT but whether they induce ongoing dermatitis under real-life conditions remains to be proven.

SWEATING AND SWEAT ANTIGENS

What about Sulzberger's hypothesis of sweat duct obstruction and millions of minute injections of sweat and its solutes into the skin, provoking itching? It is known that sweating aggravates the itch in many patients with AD but the mechanism by which this occurs is unknown. A number of sweating abnormalities have been described in AD patients, including a depressed sweat loss rate despite increased borderline water loss, decreased cumulative sweat loss following thermal stimuli, and a retarded temporal sweating response (Parkkinen *et al.* 1991, 1992). The sweat of patients with AD has also been shown to contain specific IgE antibodies to inhalant allergens and it has been suggested that these may play a role in antigen trapping in the skin (Jung *et al.* 1996).

The presence of antigens in sweat relevant to AD has been suggested by some studies, eg, intracutaneous skin tests with autologous sweat were positive in 84.4% of AD patients but only in 11.1% of healthy volunteers (Hide *et al.* 2002). Experimental work also suggested that IgE antibody against antigen(s) in sweat may be present in the serum of patients with AD. Investigators have semi-purified a standardized sweat antigen consisting of a protein that induces degranulation of basophils and mast cells via antigen-specific IgE and FcεRI in patients with AD (Tanaka *et al.* 2006).

A more recent study gives some credence to Sulzberger's theory of sweat retention. The well-known phenomenon of miliaria has been attributed to blockage of sweat ducts by *extracellular polysaccharide substance* (EPS) produced by *Staphylococcus epidermidis* organisms on the skin (Mowad *et al.* 1995). Recently Freeny *et al.* (2011) and Allen and Mueller (2011) have identified biofilms of *S. epidermidis* on confocal and light microscopy in cultures from patients with flexural eczema. They suggest that eczema arises in areas of subclinical miliaria from insensible sweating, which results in scratching that then damages a predisposed epidermis.

STAPHYLOCOCCUS AUREUS AND OTHER MICROORGANISMS

The association of eczema with *S. aureus* has been known for over 100 years. At the turn of the twentieth century, Juan de Azúa Suárez (1901) reported a series of experiments affirming the role of *S. aureus* in the induction of eczematous lesions. The role of pruritus-induced traumatization of the skin was held to be an important factor in this regard. Hill, in his 1956 book *The Treatment of Eczema in Infants and Children,* noted that the concept of 'infectious eczematoid dermatitis,' ie, eczema caused by the 'irritating effects of a purulent discharge from such foci as chronic otitis media,' had been broadened to those eczemas that did not appear grossly infected but were 'kept active by low-grade infection and by allergic sensitivity to the infecting organism' (Hill 1956) (**Fig 6.14**).

Staphylococci frequently complicate AD lesions, particularly those with excoriation and fissures (Rajka 1989). One study found the carriage rate of *S. aureus* to be 93% in lesional skin, 76% in uninvolved skin, and 79% in the anterior nares (Aly *et al.* 1977). *S. aureus* constituted 91% of the total aerobic bacterial flora in lesional skin. Although staphylococcal colonization itself does not cause life-threatening sequelae, rare cases of septicemia, necrotizing fasciitis, and recurrent endocarditis of a prosthetic heart valve have occasionally been reported in AD patients (Hoeger *et al.* 2000, Brady and Levin 2007, Yamamoto *et al.* 2007).

As mentioned previously, reduced levels of stratum corneum-derived AMPs may favor colonization of AD skin by pathogenic staphylococci. Other factors that favor colonization include increased pH of AD lesional skin, decreased levels of sphingosine, and decreased secretion of dermcidin, an AMP derived from human sweat. In healthy individuals, sweating leads to a reduction of viable bacteria on the skin surface, but this does not occur in patients with AD, probably as a consequence of decreased dermcidin-derived peptides in their sweat (Rieg *et al.* 2005). The two major acidic breakdown products, urocanic acid and pyrrolidone carboxylic acid, which are markedly decreased in filaggrin null mutation carriers, profoundly affect staphylococcal proliferation, adhesion, and survival based on pH-dependent and possibly non-pH-dependent mechanisms (Miajlovic *et al.* 2010).

The mechanisms by which *S. aureus* affects AD are summarized in Chapter 9. Staphylococcal infection can cause direct damage to the epidermal barrier as well as provoke itching and excoriation, which may exacerbate dermatitis. Staphylococcal proteins may cause mast cell degranulation, formation of weals, and itching. Staphylococcal superantigens may penetrate

Fig 6.14 Infectious eczematoid dermatitis: drainage from an infectious focus such as chronic otitis causes sensitization and eczematous changes.

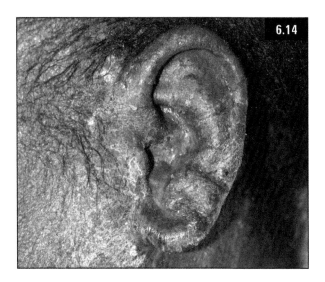
6.14

the skin barrier and contribute to the persistence and exacerbation of allergic skin inflammation in AD through several potential mechanisms:

- Massive stimulation of T cells
- Acting as allergens that induce relevant staphylococcal superantigen-specific IgE
- Direct stimulation of APCs including LCs, DCs, macrophages, and keratinocytes
- Expansion of the pool of skin-homing cutaneous lymphocyte-associated antigen (CLA)+ T cells
- Augmentation of allergen-induced skin inflammation
- Induction of corticosteroid resistance
- Induction of the pruritogenic cytokine IL-31 (Lin *et al.* 2007)
- Induction of IL-18.

Interestingly, staphylococcal epidermolytic toxin can bind to filaggrin and profilaggrin (Smith and Bailey 1986).

KERATINOCYTE-DERIVED FACTORS

Besides antimicrobial peptides, keratinocytes secrete a host of cytokines and chemical mediators that may play an important role in the development of AD lesions. Among these are IL-1α, IL-1β, TNF-α, GM-CSF, TGFβ, regulated upon activation normal T-cell expressed and secreted (RANTES), TSLP, thymus and activation-regulated chemokine (TARC), cutaneous T-cell-attracting cytokine (CTACK), macrophage-derived chemokine (MDC), and IL-18. Release or induction of some of these can result from scratching, eg, perturbations of the skin barrier induce keratinocyte expression and release of IL-1α, TNF-β, and GM-CSF, which can stimulate lipid synthesis and restoration of the epidermal barrier (Wood *et al.* 1996). These cytokines also have proinflammatory effects.

Unstimulated keratinocytes from AD patients tend to release higher levels of IL-1α, TNFα, and GM-CSF, then keratinocytes, than normal individuals (Pastore *et al.* 1998). Moreover, IFN-γ, a predominant cytokine in chronic AD lesions, significantly increases the release of each of these cytokines. GM-CSF is strongly expressed *in vivo* in AD lesional skin. It not only supports the survival of AD monocytes but also favors recruitment, proliferation, and activation of monocytes, basophils, and eosinophils. Most importantly, GM-CSF contributes to DC recruitment, survival, and maturation (Pastore *et al.* 1997).

As mentioned previously, TSLP is an important cytokine derived from keratinocytes that is highly expressed in acute and chronic lesions of AD (Ebner *et al.* 2007). TSLP-stimulated DCs prime naïve T-helper cells to produce the 'proallergic' cytokines IL-4, -5, and -13, and also TNF-α while downregulating IL-10 and IFN-γ (Soumelis *et al.* 2002). Moreover, TSLP expression is associated with LC migration and activation.

Ebner *et al.* (2007) propose the following sequence of events in the development of atopic dermatitis: keratinocytes produce TSLP that induces maturation and migration of LCs to draining lymph nodes; in the lymph node TSLP-'primed' LCs then cause the Th2 polarization of antigen-specific CD4 cells; and these *inflammatory Th2 cells*, when back in the skin, promote inflammation by their high production of TNF-α and low production of IL-10.

IL-18

IL-18 is a member of the IL-1 family of proinflammatory cytokines produced by keratinocytes and a variety of other cell types including IDECs; it is capable of enhancing both IL-12-driven Th1 responses and Th2 immune responses in the absence of IL-12 (Nakanishi *el al.* 2001). IL-18 can induce so-called *super-Th1* cells which produce IFN-γ and IL-13, and it is thought to be involved in the Th2–Th1 shift in AD lesional skin. IL-18, similar to IL-1, is stored as an inactive precursor in keratinocytes and is converted to its active form by caspase-1 after stimulation by danger signals. IL-18 is increased in the horn of patients with AD compared with normal individuals. Serum and stratum corneum levels of IL-18 correlate with severity of AD and, most interestingly, in patients with relatively low IgE levels (<1500 IU/m), horn IL-18 levels were significantly higher in patients in whom *S. aureus* was detected (Inoue *et al.* 2010).

EOSINOPHILS

It is not surprising that eosinophils are involved in the pathogenesis of AD. A number of extremely pruritic skin conditions manifest tissue eosinophilia such as bullous pemphigoid, insect bites, and eosinophilic folliculitis. Eosinophils are bone marrow-derived granulocytes that derive from CD34+ hemopoietic progenitor cells. As no cell surface protein specific for eosinophils has been identified, they are still delineated in tissue by their staining characteristics or by immunostaining of the eosinophil granule proteins, major basic protein (MBP), eosinophil-derived neurotoxin (EDN), and eosinophil cationic protein (ECP).

Increased total blood eosinophil counts are common in AD but the degree of eosinophilia varies greatly among individuals and over the course of the disease. Increased levels of circulating eosinophils expressing the activation molecule CD69 are common in infants with severe AD associated with elevated circulating IL-18 levels, a marker of eczema severity (Toma *et al.* 2005). Moreover, elevated blood levels of eosinophil MBP and other eosinophil granular proteins occur in more than half of AD patients, with or without peripheral blood eosinophilia (Wassom *et al.* 1981).

In skin lesions, the mixed perivascular infiltrate may contain some eosinophils but they are not consistently present (Mihm *et al.* 1976). On the other hand, eosinophil MBP is demonstrable in AD lesional skin on direct immunofluorescence (Leiferman *et al.* 1985). In most cases, there is fibrillar fluorescence in the upper dermis with few intact eosinophils and some patients show scattered MBP granules in the dermis. The presence of focal, patchy, upper dermal MBP localization in lesional skin and minimal deposition in uninvolved skin suggests that the MBP is not being deposited from the blood but occurs as a result of local eosinophil degranulation. This has been confirmed in an electron microscopic study of AD lesional skin which showed local eosinophil cytolysis and piecemeal degranulation (Cheng *et al.* 1997) (**Fig 6.15**). Thus intact eosinophils or their granule proteins are consistently found in AD lesional skin and likely play a role in pathogenesis.

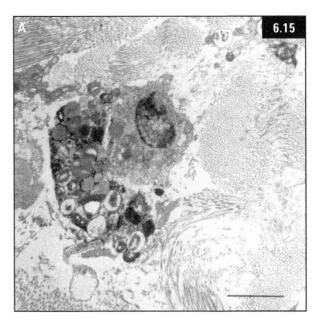

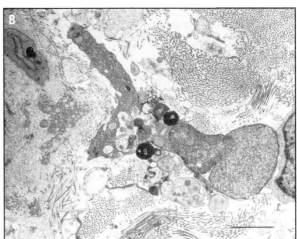

Fig 6.15 Electron photomicrographs of degenerating eosinophils with loss of cytoplasmic and/or nuclear membranes. (A) Eosinophil no longer contained by a cell membrane with markedly abnormal granules. (B) Degenerated eosinophil with loss of cytoplasmic membrane. Chromatolysis of the nucleus is also apparent. Abnormal eosinophil granules are in contact with the extracellular space. Scale bar = 2 μm. (Reprinted from Cheng *et al.* 1997. © 1997 with permission from Elsevier.)

Despite cytolysis of eosinophils in AD skin, circulating eosinophils appear to be resistant to apoptosis in the disease. Programmed cell death of circulating eosinophils is significantly delayed, not only in patients with truly atopic dermatitis but in atopiform ('intrinsic atopic') dermatitis resulting from the production by eosinophils of autocrine growth factors such as GM-CSF and IL-5 (Wedi et al. 1997). In support of this, expression of the activation molecule CD69 was noted on eosinophils, indicating possible 'preactivation.' Eosinophils from patients with AD have also been shown to resist Fas-induced apoptosis, possibly as a result of their expression of antiapoptotic BCL-2 protein family members (Dibbert et al. 1998, Wedi et al. 1999). They also have high expression of neurotrophin receptors, which may play a role in their resistance to apoptosis (Raap et al. 2008b).

A number of eosinophil-attracting cytokines are responsible for the trafficking of these cells to sites of cutaneous inflammation. These include IL-5, IL-8, RANTES, eotaxin, eotaxin-2, eotaxin-3, monocyte chemoattractant protein (MCP)-3, MCP-4 and TNF-α (Lampinen et al. 2004). Th2, mast, and epithelial cells are important sources of many of these mediators, and it is now recognized that eosinophils themselves produce many cytokines and play an important role in immunoregulation. Recently, the pluripotential cytokine macrophage migration inhibitory factor (MIF), which is expressed at higher levels in the skin and blood of patients with AD, has been proposed as a major factor causing eosinophil accumulation in the skin (Yoshihisa et al. 2010).

The exact role of eosinophils in atopic dermatitis is not known. Besides their ability to produce Th2 cytokines like IL-4 and IL-13, eosinophils also release toxic proteins such as MBP, ECP and EDN which can damage tissue and induce remodeling. Interestingly, a study of German patients with atopic dermatitis failed to find any polymorphisms in the genes encoding ECP, EDN, EPO and MBP (Parwez et al. 2008).

MAST CELLS

Mast cells were first described by Paul Ehrlich in his doctoral thesis (Vyas and Krishnaswamy 2006).

Although 'anaphylaxis' was described in 1902, and the physiological functions of histamine in 1910, it was not until 1952 that histamine was identified in mast cells. Although previously relegated primarily to a role in allergy, there has been renewed interest in mast cells both within and outside the field of immunology because of their involvement in a vast array of physiological processes, including innate immunity (Gregory and Brown 2006).

Mast cells derive from progenitor cells that are CD34+ and express the receptor for stem cell factor, c-kit, as well as CD13. Stem cell factor interactions with c-kit are crucial for the growth and development of mast cells. These *sentinels of innate immunity* produce and release a staggering array of vasoactive, proinflammatory, and nociceptive chemical mediators and cytokines with multiple effects (Galli et al. 1999). They can be triggered by a number of neuropeptides and electron microscopic studies have revealed their close apposition to unmyelinated nerve fibers (Wiesner-Menzel et al. 1981, Church et al. 1989).

Mast cells occur in normal-appearing and lesional AD skin and some show degranulation in close or direct proximity to nerve bundles (Toyoda and Morohashi 1998). Such changes are not seen in patients treated with cyclosporine (ciclosporin), a compound that rapidly reduces pruritus in AD patients. It is likely that mast cells play a role in AD pathogenesis both by secretion of granule proteins and by their expression of Th2 cytokines.

HISTAMINE

Mast cells are a major source of histamine, a powerful pleiotropic mediator with a controversial role in AD. Williams (1938) reported that intramuscular histamine produced a rise in skin temperature restricted to the face and neck in normal individuals, but in the sites of predilection for eczema such as the face, neck, upper chest, and flexures in AD patients. Johnson et al. (1960) described elevated histamine levels in the skin from the antecubital fossae of patients with AD. Other studies suggest an increased baseline histamine concentration in 20–30% of AD patients, especially those with severe disease and increased plasma levels in children after positive food challenges (Sampson and Jolie 1984, Ring and Thomas 1989). Enhanced releasability of histamine to immunological stimuli has also been indicated. Despite all these indications of a role for histamine in AD, H_1- and H_2-receptor antihistamines do not alleviate AD pruritus.

Recently a third histamine receptor (H_3) associated with scratching behavior in mice and a fourth histamine receptor (H_4) expressed on numerous immune and inflammatory cells have prompted a re-evaluation of the actions of histamine (Sugimoto et al. 2004, Thurmond et al. 2008).

The histamine H_4-receptor is expressed on Th2 lymphocytes and IDEC and H_4-receptor antagonism reduces hapten-induced scratching behavior, but not inflammation, in a mouse model (Dijkstra et al. 2008, Gutzmer et al. 2009, Rossbach et al. 2009). Certain polymorphisms in the H_4-receptor gene are also associated with AD (Yu et al. 2010). This raises the possibility that histamine may in fact be important in AD and that the lack of efficacy of H_1- and H_2-receptor antagonists in reducing pruritus is because they fail to block the appropriate receptor.

OTHER MAST CELL MEDIATORS

Mast cells also produce significant levels of IL-4, IL-5, IL-13, and mast cell chymase (Horsmanheimo et al. 1994, Obara et al. 2002).

Mast cell chymase expression is increased in chronic lesional AD skin and may affect inflammation and barrier function (Badertscher et al. 2005). It cleaves pro-IL-18 and generates a biologically active IL-18 fragment, which plays a significant role in the disease (Omoto et al. 2006). IL-18 is increased in the serum of patients with AD, and AD lesional tissue and serum levels correlate with disease activity (Park do and Youn 2007, Sohn et al. 2007). IL-18 may enhance eosinophil recruitment, induce increased IFN-γ, and affect IL-13 production (Shaker et al. 2009).

Another possible role for mast cells in AD is the promotion of angiogenesis. A recent study showed mast cells in the epidermis in 5 of 27 AD patients as well as in the papillary dermis (Groneberg et al. 2005). Epidermal mast cells were situated near the basal lamina, in the stratum spinosum, and in the granular layer. A large number were also in close proximity to endothelial cells. A 'tunnel' hypothesis was suggested through which epidermal mast cells propagate angiogenesis by secretion of proangiogenic factors, and facilitate growth by secreting matrix metalloproteases that induce a papillary 'tunnel' to make way for vessel growth. In fact a recent pilot study suggests that ablation of dermal vessels in chronic lesions of AD using a pulse dye laser can induce clinical improvement (Syed et al. 2008).

NERVES AND NEUROTROPHINS

Given that pruritus is the cardinal symptom of AD, peripheral nerves, free nerve endings and the factors that interact with them should take center stage in our attempts to understand the disease. Mechanisms and mediators of pruritus are reviewed in Chapter 5.

There is evidence that there may be alteration of peripheral nerve endings in AD. In a study of peripheral nerves in lesional skin, immunohistochemical staining with antibodies directed against protein gene product (PGP) and substance P showed significantly higher nerve fiber density in subacute, lichenified, and prurigo lesions than in uninvolved skin. However, another study, using electron microscopy, showed normal-appearing subepidermal and intraepidermal free nerve endings (Sugiura et al. 1997, Urashima and Mihara 1998). In a further study, nerve endings in normal skin showed branching at the dermoepidermal junction and multiple loops extending through the epidermis to just below the corneal layer (Bigliardi-Qi et al. 2005). In subacute and chronic AD lesions epidermal nerve endings appeared thin and barely visible, while running without curving through the epidermis. One hypothesis suggests that regular scratching results in epidermal hypertrophy, distortion of nerve fibers, and mechanical damage to nerve endings.

There appears to be a complex interaction of peripheral nerves, neurotrophic factors, lymphocytes, mast cells, eosinophils, and DCs in areas of allergic inflammation; eg, nerve growth factor (NGF), which is intimately involved in the development and survival of neurons, is prominent in allergic and inflammatory diseases and found in mast cells, eosinophils, Th2 cells, and keratinocytes (Leon et al. 1994, Aloe et al.

1997, Shaker *et al.* 2009). Levels of NGF are increased in the serum of patients with AD and increased levels of NGF mRNA occur in lesional AD tissue associated with an increased number of Schwann axon complexes on electron microscopic examination (Hodeib *et al.* 2010). NGF is not only produced and stored by eosinophils but can also activate them, suggesting a role in allergic inflammation. It can also induce T- and B-cell proliferation and cause mast cell degranulation.

Brain-derived neurotrophic factor (BDNF), a growth factor originally identified in the nervous system, is also produced, stored, and released by circulating eosinophils (Noga *et al.* 2003). In addition it inhibits eosinophil apoptosis (Raap *et al.* 2005). Levels of BDNF are significantly correlated with disease activity and nocturnal scratching in children with AD (Hon *et al.* 2007). Increased BDNF levels in AD have been suggested to derive not only from eosinophils but also from Th2 lymphocytes (Namura *et al.* 2007). Interestingly, BDNF is capable of enhancing the density of peripheral innervation and specific sensory receptors in mice, and has been suggested as a cause of heightened anxiety in patients with AD (LeMaster *et al.* 1999, Cremona *et al.* 2007).

Another aspect of the neurocutaneous connection is that nervous innervation of the skin can affect DCs, antigen presentation, and other epidermal processes. One study demonstrated CGRP-containing nerve fibers intimately associated with LCs in human epidermis, CGRP at the surface of some LCs, and CGRP-induced inhibition of LC antigen presentation (Hosoi *et al.* 1993). Another study showed neuropeptide-Y immunoreactivity in cutaneous LCs from patients with AD (Pincelli *et al.* 1990, Hosoi *et al.* 1993).

Nervous innervation may also affect epidermal proliferation, epidermal hydration, and susceptibility to eczema. In a mouse model, cutaneous denervation decreased keratinocyte proliferation and epidermal thickness (Huang *et al.* 1999). O'Riain (1973) reported the case of a child whose denervated finger failed to shrivel when immersed in water; after nerve repair, the finger shriveled normally like the other fingers. In addition, endogenous eczema has been reported in patients with cerebrovascular hemiplegia confined to the unaffected limb (Troilius and Moller 1989). Thus the nervous system is intimately related to immune responses, epidermal integrity, and eczema.

CONCLUSION

This chapter has presented a generalized overview of the pathophysiology of AD, looking at barrier defects, immune mechanisms, and the involvement of various cell types. Although AD appears to be an exceedingly complex disease, it is hoped that future research will clarify our understanding of its pathophysiology. It is further hoped that research will identify molecules, the modulation of which, perhaps by biological agents, will allow enhanced control of inflammation and pruritus, and clearance of AD similar to the gains that have been achieved with psoriasis.

ATOPIC DERMATITIS: THE ALLERGIST'S PERSPECTIVE

Mamta Reddy and Yudy K. Persaud

Recent epidemiological studies have demonstrated such a dramatic increase in atopic diseases that it is now widely recognized that we are in the midst of an allergy pandemic. Although attention has focused mostly on rising rates of asthma, rates of atopic dermatitis have risen similarly in the past 30 years (Wahn and von Mutius 2001, Schultz Larsen and Hanifin 2002). The definitive causes of this pandemic are still unknown. Although it is certain that genetic predisposition is a significant factor in the development of atopy, family history alone cannot explain the rapid increase in prevalence that has occurred over such a short time. Certain epidemiological observations suggest that a western lifestyle, urbanization, and development play significant roles in the increasing prevalence of atopic diseases (Diepgen 2001). Additional hypotheses suggest that specific features of a western lifestyle, including smaller family size, migration to urban areas, increased use of antibiotics, decreased incidence of early childhood infections, and high socioeconomic status, also contribute to this increased prevalence (von Mutius 2000). In light of the medical and economic burden of a growing allergy epidemic, future disease prevention and treatment strategies are increasingly desirable (Lewin Group I 2005).

THE HYGIENE HYPOTHESIS

Not only has increased exposure to allergens and air pollution been implicated in the current allergy pandemic (Diepgen 2001), but there is also a growing body of evidence from epidemiological studies to support what has been termed the 'hygiene hypothesis' to explain the development of allergic disease. As briefly stated by Strachan (1989):

> These observations ... could be explained if allergic diseases were prevented by infection in early childhood, transmitted by unhygienic contact with older siblings, or acquired prenatally. ... Over the past century declining family size, improved household amenities and higher standards of personal cleanliness have reduced opportunities for crossinfection in young families. This may have resulted in more widespread clinical expression of atopic disease.

A number of theories have been offered to explain the large geographic variations in the prevalence of asthma, allergic rhinoconjunctivitis, and atopic eczema. Environmental factors, in their broadest sense, may be critical for the development of these atopic conditions in childhood, and include air pollution, concentrations of indoor allergens, housing conditions, nutrition, and other lifestyle factors such as family size and early childhood infections (von Mutius *et al.* 1994, Bråbäck *et al.* 1995, Nowak *et al.* 1996, Early Treatment of the Atopic Child 1998).

The strongest arguments in favor of the hygiene hypothesis include the apparent protective effect of both early life infections and increased sibship size on the risk of atopy and asthma later in childhood. Early day-care attendance is considered an indicator of early life exposure to numerous infectious agents and is associated with a significantly reduced risk of atopy and asthma, particularly with day-care attendance in the first 6 months of life (Celedon *et al.* 1999, Ball *et al.* 2000, Illi *et al.* 2001). There is also increasing evidence that crowding and particularly sibship size affect the expression of atopy in families. Many authors have shown that the number of siblings is inversely related to the prevalence of self-reported inhalant allergy, atopic eczema, skin test reactivity, and the presence of specific IgE antibodies (Nowak *et al.* 1996, von Mutius 1998). Moreover, a number of studies suggest that exposure to an agricultural or farm environment is also associated with a lower prevalence of atopy (Naleway 2004).

The worldwide increase in the use of childhood vaccines and antibiotics has led to a reduction in exposure to various childhood infections and bacterial endotoxins. All of these components of a westernized, nonfarm environment, including decreased sibship size, use of vaccines and antibiotics, increased cleanliness, and so on, are thought to have altered the immune system development in many individuals, resulting in inappropriate allergic responses to common environmental allergens that would otherwise be innocuous (Patki 2007) (**Box 7.1**).

Box 7.1 Potential epidemiological factors in the recent allergy pandemic

- Western lifestyle, urbanization, and development
- Industrialization with a market economy
- Smaller family size
- Migration to urban areas
- Increased use of antibiotics and vaccines
- Decreased incidence of early childhood infections
- Higher socioeconomic status

A newer hypothesis, the *hapten-atopy hypothesis,* suggests that oral and skin exposure to chemicals in general, and to haptens in particular, may be an important factor contributing to the increased prevalence of atopic disease (McFadden *et al.* 2009, 2011). It is argued that initial innate immune responses, which normally favor a T-helper type 1 (Th1) cytokine milieu on exposure to chemical haptens, might, with prolonged low-level exposure to certain haptens, favor a Th2 immune response.

THE ATOPIC MARCH (THE CORRELATION OF ATOPIC DERMATITIS AND ASTHMA)

Atopic dermatitis is a cutaneous form of atopy that is associated with asthma, allergic rhinitis, and elevated levels of IgE. Up to 80% of children with atopic dermatitis will eventually develop allergic rhinitis or asthma later in childhood. The diseases in this classic 'atopic triad' have several pathophysiological elements in common, including cyclic nucleotide regulatory abnormalities, immune cell alterations, common inflammatory mediators, and allergic triggers (Eichenfield *et al.* 2003). In many cases atopic dermatitis predates the development of asthma and allergic rhinitis, suggesting that it is the first step in the development of subsequent allergic diseases. This procession is referred to as the *atopic march.*

Distinct types of atopic conditions are preferentially transmitted in families, suggesting that a parental background of atopy is likely to increase an offspring's risk for any atopic condition, not necessarily only for asthma (von Mutius and Nicolai 1996). It is known that multiple genes are responsible for the development of atopy and asthma via numerous pathways, including gene–gene interactions. Those with a genetic predisposition who are exposed to infections, allergens, pollutants, and other environmental exposures develop asthma during childhood and even later in adult life. The timing of exposure may play a critical role when considering potential adverse or beneficial effects of environmental stimuli in the development of atopic conditions (von Mutius 2001). Consequently, genes that encode proteins involved in the development and function of T-regulatory cells, such as toll-like receptor (TLR)-2, have been reported to associate with atopy and asthma phenotypes (Eder *et al.* 2004, Robinson *et al.* 2004).

Epicutaneous allergen sensitization may incite a systemic allergic response that crucially affects the development and course of asthma later in childhood (Beck and Leung 2000). Although the inflammatory process in atopic dermatitis is localized to the skin, IgE, eosinophils, and Th2 cells circulate throughout the body and can localize to sites of inflammation (Beck and Leung 2000). Evidence that allergic sensitization through the skin can directly affect Th2-mediated responses and airway reactivity has been demonstrated in animal models (Spergel *et al.* 1998). Such studies offer direct evidence that stimulation of inflammatory responses in the skin has systemic consequences. They provide a plausible explanation of how atopic dermatitis can lead to the development of asthma, and lend further support to the premise that atopic dermatitis is a risk factor for childhood asthma occurrence, severity, and persistence. The primary mechanisms by which atopic dermatitis influences the course of asthma are likely related to early IgE production and the consequent reactivity between allergens and IgE (von Mutius and Nicolai 1996).

Epidemiological investigations, such as the German multicenter atopy study that prospectively followed 1314 infants for more than 10 years, have shown a progression of atopic sensitization from food allergens to inhalant allergens over time. This study reported that approximately 10% of infants were sensitized to food allergens at 1 year of age but only 8% of children showed clinical food intolerance during the first 2 years. By age 6, only 3% of children were sensitized to food allergens. Conversely, 1.5% of infants were sensitized to inhalant allergens at 1 year but, by 5 years, 30% of children had become sensitized to inhalant allergens. Thus, the combination of atopic dermatitis, atopic family history, and food sensitivity is highly predictive of future respiratory allergy and asthma (Bergmann *et al.* 1994, 1998).

One study examining the relationship of atopic dermatitis in infancy, sensitization to aeroallergens, and presence of allergic airway disease reported that 69% of infants with atopic dermatitis in the first 3 months of life were sensitized against aeroallergens by age 5 years. The rate of aeroallergen sensitization increased to 77% of children if both parents had a positive history of atopic disease. By 5 years of age, 50% of children with early atopic dermatitis and a strong family history of allergy had allergic airway disease (Bardana 2004). Of these, 30–60% developed asthma and 35–66% allergic rhinitis (Lewin Group I 2005).

Atopic dermatitis is an intrinsic skin abnormality, perhaps analogous to the hyperirritable airway of asthma. Some evidence suggests a role for hyper-reactivity to cholinergic stimuli, which might relate to the reduced threshold of the itch response (Parslow *et al.* 2001). Atopic dermatitis and asthma can both be characterized as manifestations of an exaggerated inflammatory response to environmental triggers, including irritants and allergens. This response is accompanied by increased production of IgE and eosinophilia (Broide 2001, Leung *et al.* 2004a).

In recent years, new findings related to the filaggrin gene (*FLG*) have clarified the genetics of atopic dermatitis. Individuals with loss-of-function *FLG* mutations are known to be predisposed to ichthyosis vulgaris, a frequent concomitant of eczema. Studies of the filaggrin gene have demonstrated two major polymorphisms associated with atopic dermatitis in European populations (Irvine and McLean 2006). Additional studies have demonstrated a consistent association between *FLG* polymorphisms and atopic dermatitis in various populations (van den Oord and Sheikh 2009). Besides eczema, *FLG* mutations have been shown to be a risk factor for allergic sensitization and allergic rhinitis. Moreover, patients with filaggrin-related eczema are at increased risk of developing asthma (Weidinger *et al.* 2008). Observational studies, such as ISAAC II (Weidinger *et al.* 2008), showed a strong association with the complex asthma-plus-eczema phenotype with an odds ratio of 3.49 and, in the large longitudinal population-based Avon Longitudinal Study of Parents and Children, with an odds ratio of 3.42 (Henderson *et al.* 2008).

INTRINSIC VERSUS EXTRINSIC ATOPIC DERMATITIS

The controversial terminology of atopic dermatitis used in various countries has led the European Academy of Allergology and Clinical Immunology (EAACI) to propose a revised nomenclature that includes only IgE-associated forms of the disease as true atopic dermatitis. Some authors suggest that the term 'eczema' replace the current term 'atopic dermatitis' (Johansson *et al.* 2001, 2004, Lipozencić and Wolf 2007).

Researchers and clinicians have together classified two forms of atopic dermatitis: *intrinsic* (nonallergic) and *extrinsic* (allergic). Although the two forms are indistinguishable on physical examination, they vary in other aspects. Extrinsic atopic dermatitis, which comprises 70–85% of atopic dermatitis cases, is associated with high serum IgE levels, exhibits allergen-specific IgE to aeroallergens and foods, has positive skin-prick reactions, and has a cytokine profile characterized by high interleukin (IL)-4 and IL-13 levels. Patients with intrinsic atopic dermatitis (accounting for 15–30% of atopic dermatitis cases) by contrast have normal IgE levels, negative skin-prick reactions, and low IL-4 and IL-13 levels, and do not have allergen-specific IgE to aeroallergens and foods (Bardana 2004). The onset of extrinsic atopic dermatitis typically occurs during early childhood, whereas patients with intrinsic atopic dermatitis have a later onset of disease. Finally, patients with intrinsic atopic dermatitis are characterized by an absence of other atopic disease, asthma, and allergic rhinitis (Schmid-Grendelmeier *et al.* 2001). In addition, recent findings of susceptibility genes suggest that nonatopic dermatitis should be considered a distinct variety of childhood eczema. Affected children show eczematous skin changes with dry ichthyosiform lesions at an early age but an absence of sensitization to common allergens; 33% of them are without lesions by 5 years of age (Humbert *et al.* 1999).

ALLERGIC IMMUNOPATHOLOGY OF ATOPIC SKIN DISEASE

A key element of both asthma and atopic dermatitis is the development and activation of Th2 cells, a subset of T-helper cells that initiates and maintains local tissue inflammation (Romagnani 1992a, 1992b). As Th2-like cytokines are produced in the uterine environment to hamper rejection of the fetus, the immune response at birth is primarily directed toward Th2-like polarization. Repetitive infections promoting Th1 cytokine polarization, particularly early in childhood, allow T-cell immune responses to mature into a more balanced phenotype, which is less likely to favor allergen sensitization and atopic illness (Gern and Weiss 2000).

In allergic disease, IL-4 synthesis by Th2 cells stimulates production of IgE, and IL-5 synthesis by Th2 cells drives bone marrow differentiation of eosinophils (Spergel *et al.* 1998, Johansson *et al.* 2004). The characteristic skin lesions of atopic dermatitis result from this disturbed cellular immunity. Antigen uptake is thought to occur via epidermal Langerhans cells that express high- and low-affinity IgE receptors as well as via inflammatory dendritic epidermal cells (IDECs). There is increased production of IgE by B lymphocytes because of abnormal T-lymphocyte regulation. This results in upregulation of IgE receptors on dendritic cells, allowing further processing of allergens complexed to IgE. Much of the Th2 skewing of the immune response is now thought to result from barrier abnormalities and innate immune responses, eg, keratinocyte-derived thymic stromal lymphopoietin (TSLP) causes dendritic cells to evoke Th2 lymphocyte responses.

In addition, activated Th1 cells with increased production of interferon-γ in acute skin lesions bind to keratinocytes leading to apoptosis, spongiosis, and inflammatory skin changes. A relative imbalance between Th1 and Th2 subsets of CD4+ T-cell-producing cytokines is indicative of the prominent immune perturbations that occur in atopic dermatitis (Lugović *et al.* 2005). Antigen-presenting cells such as dendritic cells, Langerhans cells, and macrophages are involved in induction of allergic inflammation by presenting allergens to T lymphocytes. Owing to complex polygenic–environmental interactions, the atopic individual exhibits a dysregulation of T-cell-mediated immune mechanisms (von Bubnoff *et al.* 2001). IL-4, -5, and -13 cytokines play a role in the Th2 response, which is seen in the early stages of atopic dermatitis. Also, keratinocytes have been shown to intensify inflammatory reactions in the skin through release of cytokines and chemokines (Werfel 2009).

Chronic atopic dermatitis lesions principally, however, have a Th1 polarization with the cytokines IL-12 and interferon-γ playing a more dominant role (Hamid *et al.* 1994). The mechanisms responsible for the chronic inflammation in atopic dermatitis are likely linked to several interdependent factors. One of these is repeated exposure to allergens such as foods, aeroallergens, and microorganisms, leading to chronic allergic responses and Th2-like expansion (Adkinson and Middleton 2003). Lesions of chronic atopic dermatitis are related to type IV delayed-type hypersensitivity. Defective hypersensitivity skin test responses to recall antigens, deficient *in vitro* lymphocyte proliferation responses to mitogens and antigens, and reduced autologous mixed-lymphocyte reaction have all been reported in patients with atopic dermatitis. Many studies associate increased IgE production with the presence of predominant populations of T-helper cells with Th2 cytokine profiles. Other studies relate the excessive production of IgE by peripheral blood B lymphocytes to a deficiency of CD8 T lymphocytes (Broide 2001, Johansson *et al.* 2001).

Thus, according to the hygiene hypothesis, predominant activation of Th1-like T cells from recurrent viral or bacterial infections may prevent proliferation of Th2 clones and development of allergic disease (Romagnani 1992a, 1992b). Although evidence for Th-cell polarization was initially developed in experimental mouse models, numerous clinical studies have also shown Th2 dominance with IL-4 and IL-5 overproduction in patients with hayfever, allergic bronchial asthma, and atopic dermatitis (Hamid et al. 1994, Herz *et al.* 1998, Humbert *et al.* 1999). In addition, animal and human studies suggest that Th17 cells, which are involved in psoriasis, may be involved in atopic dermatitis as well. Studies have shown that Th17 cells are present in acute lesions of atopic dermatitis. In the absence of IL-4 and IL-13, topical application of allergens induces a strong Th17 response which under normal circumstances would induce antimicrobial peptide upregulation. However, in patients with atopic dermatitis, the presence of IL-4 and IL-13 partially inhibits upregulation of these natural antibiotics, thus contributing to the inability of these patients to clear *Staphylococcus aureus* (Koga *et al.* 2008, Eyerich *et al.* 2009, Oyoshi *et al.* 2009).

IMMUNOGLOBULIN E AND IgE RECEPTORS

Although most forms of childhood eczema improve by puberty, up to 40% of cases do not, and recurrences in adulthood are common. Factors associated with a more persistent course include early onset, severe disease at an early age, being the oldest or only child, respiratory disease, positive family history, and high serum IgE levels (Wüthrich 1999, Williams 2005). About 80% of affected adults have elevated serum IgE levels and also show sensitization against airborne and food allergens and/or concomitant allergic respiratory allergy. Conversely, a normal IgE level does not rule out the diagnosis (Humbert *et al.* 1999). Immunoglobulin E-mediated autoreactivity contributes to the defective tolerance of atopic dermatitis patients and can appear very early (during the first year of life) to contribute to disease flares (Lugović *et al.* 2006).

There are two types of myeloid dendritic cells, Langerhans cells, and inflammatory dendritic epidermal cells that express the high-affinity IgE receptor FcεR1. Each displays a different pathophysiological function. Langerhans cells are important in initiating cutaneous allergic immune responses and priming naïve T cells into Th2 cells with high expression of IL-4. Stimulation by allergens of FcεR1 receptors on Langerhans cells induces chemotactic signals that recruit inflammatory dendritic epidermal cells and T cells to areas of dermatitis. Stimulation of FcεR1E receptors on inflammatory dendritic epidermal cells causes the release of proinflammatory signals, which contribute to an allergic immune response (Humbert *et al.* 1999). Expression of FcεRI is prominent in atopic dermatitis skin lesions and is considered the relevant IgE-binding molecule on dendritic cells in the pathogenesis of the disease.

IgE-BLOCKING ANTIBODY

Omalizumab is a commercially available recombinant human monoclonal IgE–blocking antibody that inhibits IgE binding to FcεRI on mast cells and basophils. It is intended for use in patients with asthma and high IgE levels in whom IgE is a causative factor. Its mechanism of action, reduction in surface-bound IgE on FcεRI-bearing cells, limits allergic response mediator release. Treatment with omalizumab also reduces FcεRI receptor expression on basophils in atopic patients (Scheinfeld 2005, Genentech 2008).

IDENTIFYING ALLERGEN TRIGGERS

The skin is a unique immunological organ that acts as an interface between the external environment and the immune system. Eczema flares in patients with extrinsic atopic dermatitis are exacerbated by aeroallergens and foods, as reflected by elevated levels of antigen-specific IgE to these substances. Patients with intrinsic atopic dermatitis are not affected by foods and aeroallergens. Allergens complexed to IgE are thought to both trigger atopic dermatitis and cause an ongoing immunological reaction. The most frequent aeroallergens are animal dander, cockroaches, dust mites, human dander, molds, and pollens (Darsow *et al.* 2005). Evaluation of patients with atopic dermatitis should include identification of triggering factors, both nonallergenic, such as alkaline soaps, wool clothing, and ambient humidity, and allergenic, such as foods and aeroallergen exposure. Specific skin testing (prick and patch tests), *in vitro* IgE assays, and antigen challenge tests may be performed depending on disease severity and suspected exacerbating factors (Nassif *et al.* 1994).

DIAGNOSTIC TESTING

Prick/puncture tests are the most rapid, convenient, and specific screening method for detecting allergen-specific IgE and for confirming hypersensitivity to various allergens. It is important to note that skin tests are not necessarily diagnostic. As a result of a high frequency of false-positive or clinically irrelevant results, skin tests and *in vitro* allergen testing should be interpreted cautiously. Antigens should be selected judiciously, and results should be correlated with patients' clinical and exposure history. Skin testing for immediate hypersensitivity is usually performed on the upper back and/or on the volar surface of the arm. Peak reaction occurs within 15–20 min, at which time the reaction should be measured and documented in comparison to the control reaction. The size of the skin test reaction is not necessarily related to the degree of clinical sensitivity.

Serum immunoassays have been used extensively for the evaluation of IgE-mediated food allergy. However, clinical reactivity can be seen 10–25% of the time even with undetectable levels (Sampson 2001, Roberts and Lack 2005). Thus, both a negative skin-prick test and negative oral challenge may be needed to rule out a specific food allergy.

Referral for comanagement with an allergy/immunology specialist is recommended for selecting antigens to be tested and interpreting the results. Skin testing should be performed only in a setting in which trained personnel are available and equipped to treat any adverse reactions, some of which can be potentially dangerous. Skin testing should not be done on acutely inflamed skin and, for the testing to be valid, antihistamines and certain other medications may need to be discontinued for up to 72 h before performing the test.

Although skin tests are the preferred means of identifying IgE-mediated hypersensitivity, specific *in vitro* IgE immunoassays may be preferable to skin testing for certain subgroups of patients who cannot tolerate the discomfort of the procedure (**Box 7.2**).

> **Box 7.2** Consider *in vitro* IgE immunoassays if a patient
>
> - Has severe dermatographism, ichthyosis, and generalized eczema
> - Uses long-acting antihistamines or tricyclic antidepressants
> - Is at undue risk if medications are discontinued
> - Refuses skin testing
> - Is at risk for anaphylaxis with skin testing to a particular antigen

Of more than 6 million chemicals in the environment, approximately 3000 are known contact allergens. Patch testing can reveal sensitization to contact allergens in patients with eczema and may identify a subgroup of atopic dermatitis patients (Akdis *et al.* 2006). Approximately 20–30 contact allergens used in the routine contact allergen series may identify the inciting agent in 50–70% of cases of contact eczematous dermatitis. Testing is usually done on the upper back or arm depending on the number of antigens desired for testing. The peak reaction is noted after 48 h, and additional readings may be done for up to 7 days. Contact sensitization to topical medications or ingredients of certain emollients frequently occurs in atopic dermatitis patients, especially in adults. The possibility of contact allergy may be ruled out by patch testing in these patients (Echechipia *et al.* 2003).

The atopy patch test is of high value in assessing sensitization to inhalant allergens, particularly to dust mite antigens where its routine use also may improve the diagnosis of a dust-mite-induced respiratory allergy (Fuiano and Incorvaia 2004). To assess the contribution of aeroallergen sensitization in atopic dermatitis, clinicians should consider doing atopy patch tests if the results of a skin-prick test or radioallergosorbent test (RAST) studies are positive for an aeroallergen (Darsow *et al.* 2005).

In evaluating bronchial asthma, an inhaled methacholine challenge can be diagnostic. Intradermal methacholine testing may be useful in patients with atopic dermatitis. Testing initially produces a weal-and-flare response, followed in 2 min by blanching. This delayed blanch response is characteristic but not diagnostic of atopic dermatitis (Johansson *et al.* 2001).

ORAL ALLERGEN TRIGGERS

Cutaneous reactions to foods include: noneczematous reactions with pruritus, hives, and nonspecific rashes; isolated eczematous reactions, which are usually delayed hours to days; and combined eczematous and noneczematous reactions (Werfel *et al.* 2007).

Up to 8% of children aged younger than 3 years and approximately 2% of adults in the general population experience food-induced allergic disorders (Sampson 1999). It is estimated that between 20% and 40% of young children and infants with atopic dermatitis have clinically relevant food allergies that contribute to disease worsening, most commonly noted in children with moderate-to-severe atopic dermatitis (Eigenmann *et al.* 1998, Leung and Bieber 2003). However, serum-specific IgE is often present without clear relevance to the disease process (Sampson and Albergo 1984). The patient's clinical history is paramount in selecting antigens for food allergy testing. Having the patient maintain a journal of foods eaten that appear to cause symptoms may help determine specific foods to test. There has been a recent expansion of knowledge concerning the importance of IgE sensitization of food allergens in the gut. When food comes in contact with IgE on mast cells in the gut, it can produce local as well as systemic reactions. The gut's permeability can be changed by mediator release, causing allergens to bind with antibodies and deposit distally in areas such as the skin.

In randomized studies of dietary exclusion, elimination of food allergens resulted in clinical improvement of atopic dermatitis in some patients. Thus, if a specific food allergy is suspected, such as to hen eggs, a limited trial excluding the suspected food might be considered under the supervision of a pediatric dietitian (Lever 2001). Elimination diets are therapeutic trials that should be supervised by an allergy/immunology specialist and implemented only for a limited time period (10–14 days); variables such as height and weight should be monitored carefully. Long-term extensive food elimination diets are not helpful in managing patients with atopic dermatitis and may lead to nutritional deficiencies such as kwashiorkor or pellagra (Carvalho et al. 2001, Nguyen et al. 2001, Ladoyanni et al. 2007). Therefore, overzealous restriction of nonimplicated foods is strongly discouraged (Sampson and Albergo 1984). A limited number of foods is responsible for approximately 90% of food-induced atopic dermatitis. In children, these foods include cows' milk, eggs, peanuts, fish, and tree nuts; in adults, they include peanuts, tree nuts, fish, and shellfish (Bernstein and Storms 1995).

Blood RAST measures antigen-specific IgE. A negative test result rules out a particular food or aeroallergen suspected as playing a role in the disease process. A positive test result does not, however, especially for a food allergen, always correlate well with a patient's symptoms. Similarly, negative skin-prick test results are extremely useful in ruling out suspected allergens as causing immediate food hypersensitivity. Positive skin test results, on the other hand, have a low positive predictive value and offer only a nominal indicator of clinical hypersensitivity. This is because of the high rate of clinically false-positive results in atopic dermatitis patients, particularly those with elevated total serum IgE levels which cause nonspecific binding. Specialized quantification of food-specific IgE using the ImmunoCAP (Pharmacia CAP system) can be used to diagnose a symptomatic allergy to eggs, milk, peanuts, and fish in children, and eliminate the need for many patients with atopic dermatitis to undergo a double-blind, placebo-controlled, food challenge (Sampson 2001).

The double-blind, placebo-controlled, food challenge is considered the gold standard for diagnosing food allergies but should be avoided in patients with life-threatening symptoms or a history of anaphylaxis. This type of testing lets one specifically identify food allergies so that these foods can be avoided in the future. It also helps to decide which foods do not play a role in the patient's disease process (Niggemann 2004). If a patient has three or more positive skin-prick test results to foods, it is recommended that a double-blind, placebo-controlled, food challenge be conducted in a controlled setting to verify the results (Burks et al. 1998). However, the exposure to allergens to which the patient reacts positively on skin test, the size of the prick skin test reaction, or the concentration of food-specific serum IgE does not predict the amount of food that will cause a reaction, or the severity of that reaction upon ingesting the food (Sicherer et al. 2000).

Patients undergoing food challenges should strictly avoid the suspected food and receive aggressive topical therapy for about 2 weeks to clear the skin before testing (Greenhawt 2010). Ultraviolet light therapy and antihistamines should be discontinued before the food challenge, however. Children are often admitted to the hospital for 48 h to permit close and frequent skin monitoring and to facilitate adverse reactions such as anaphylaxis (Greenhawt 2010).

AEROALLERGEN TRIGGERS

Epicutaneous exposure to antigen in atopic dermatitis may enhance the development of asthma (Spergel et al. 1998). Skin or in vitro allergy tests usually produce positive results which may reflect concomitant respiratory allergies or asymptomatic sensitivities instead of allergic causes of the skin disease. House dust mite and human dander are the most clinically relevant, specific aeroallergens, but other antigens such as cockroaches, molds, and pollens may also play a role (Johansson et al. 2001). In general, aeroallergens are more critical in exacerbating the disease process in adults and older children (Savilahti et al. 1983).

PREVENTION

Prevention strategies are considered the key to minimizing the allergic response. Over the past 70 years, however, clinical studies analyzing the effectiveness of measures to prevent the manifestations of atopy have generated much controversy. Prevention of atopic conditions can be directed at three stages of allergic sensitization: primary, secondary, and tertiary prevention (**Box 7.3**). Primary prevention focuses on blocking IgE sensitization in high-risk individuals, such as patients with a strong family history of atopy but who have not as yet been sensitized. Secondary prevention attempts to inhibit the expression of disease despite prior IgE sensitization, such as in a patient who has been previously sensitized but who has not yet developed the disease or expresses only one type of atopic condition (eg, atopic dermatitis but not asthma). Tertiary prevention targets the factors that trigger symptoms after disease expression, such as in a patient who displays active disease but wishes to limit symptoms. Primary, secondary, and tertiary prevention strategies may be similar but are used at different stages of sensitization and disease expression. Based on the more recent understanding of the immunological basis of atopy, more objectively designed scientific studies must be done to evaluate the effects of certain dietary and environmental exclusion measures that prevent allergic disease (Leung *et al.* 2004b, Akdis *et al.* 2006).

Box 7.3   Proposed strategies for preventing atopy

Primary prevention of atopy
- Maternal avoidance of allergenic foods during pregnancy and lactation
- Prolonged breastfeeding
- Hypoallergenic protein hydrolysate formula feeding
- Delayed introduction of solid foods
- Infant avoidance of allergenic foods
- Aeroallergen avoidance

Secondary prevention of atopy
- Early identification of sensitization
- Early diagnosis of atopic conditions
- Avoidance of aeroallergens, environmental tobacco smoke, and pollution
- Pharmacological modification
- Specific allergen immunotherapy

Tertiary prevention of atopy
- Similar to secondary prevention
- Early and accurate diagnosis and treatment
- Avoidance of aeroallergens and confirmed food allergens

PRIMARY PREVENTION

Allergen sensitization and responsiveness are determined early in life. Although primary prevention of atopy would be optimal, controversy remains regarding the degree of benefit attainable by certain interventions directed at high-risk infant populations. Most sources cite the difficulty in identifying the many routes of potential food exposure as the high-risk fetus may encounter allergens via the placenta, breast milk, formula, solid food, and even airborne droplets or floor dust. However, the relative importance of these exposures and their contribution toward developing sensitizations are unclear (Lugović *et al.* 2006). The following is a review of various methods of primary prevention.

More than 70 years ago, the debate began about the effect of breastfeeding on the development of allergic diseases. In 1936, Grulee and Sanford reported a sevenfold decrease in the development of eczema in a cohort of 20 000 infants who had been breastfed compared with those who had been fed cows' milk. Since then, numerous studies have demonstrated both favorable and unfavorable effects of this approach to atopy prevention, and more recent prolonged investigations have failed to confirm the initial optimistic findings (Kramer and Moroz 1981, Pesonen *et al.* 2006).

There are conflicting data as to whether secretory IgA found in breast milk is responsible for inhibiting intestinal absorption of food antigens (Savilahti *et al.* 1983, Kleinman and Walker 1984). In addition, although IgA antibodies have been noted to be higher in breast milk of mothers of nonatopic infants, other studies have failed to show that elevated levels of breast milk-specific antibodies necessarily protected infants from sensitization (Machtinger and Moss 1986, Balloch *et al.* 1996). Nevertheless, breast milk is comprehensively regarded as the ideal nutritional, immunological, physiological, and psychological feeding choice of the newborn and should be promoted in all neonates, including those with atopic risk, even though nanogram amounts of food allergens may be present.

Early exposure to certain foods may predispose infants to develop atopy. Parental atopy and infant solid feeding patterns during the first 4 postnatal months have been correlated with an increased prevalence of eczema but not asthma (Fergusson *et al.* 1990). Therefore, delayed introduction of solid foods may counteract a predisposition for eczema in high-risk infants or at least may postpone expression of the disease. Extensively hydrolyzed protein hydrolysates are hypoallergenic as defined by the American Academy of Pediatrics (as 95% confidence that 90% of infants with documented cows' milk allergy will not react with defined symptoms to the formula under double-blind, placebo-controlled conditions). However, they are not totally nonallergenic (Rosenthal *et al.* 1991).

Numerous distinct interventions have been conducted involving food allergen avoidance by the mother and infant in high-risk families, but the specific interventions that elicit the desired effects have been difficult to isolate because of the multifactorial nature of these interventions. Most showed that avoidance strategies for more than 6 months were necessary to reduce development of eczema and food allergy in infancy, but the benefits derived were limited to the first 1–2 years of life and did not affect allergic respiratory disorders in the same way (Zeiger *et al.*

1989, Zeiger and Heller 1995). Maternal dietary restrictions in the third trimester, previously thought to be helpful, have been discredited and prenatal sensitization to foods is decidedly uncommon (Lilja *et al.* 1991).

Evidence does support the idea that efforts to delay the onset of atopic dermatitis in infants and children can be attempted using probiotics, particularly *Lactobacillus* spp., during pregnancy or infancy; however, more studies are needed (Hanifin *et al.* 2004). In animal studies, colonization of the gut by normal commensals has been shown to be a prerequisite for the developing immune tolerance and, thus, a strong protective determinant against developing atopy and atopy-related conditions (Stein *et al.* 1999). Whether the early composition of the gut flora leads to an induction of tolerance against environmental allergens remains controversial in humans. Some indirect evidence may corroborate the notion that lactobacilli in the gut flora may play a protective role against the development of atopy (Majamaa and Isolauri 1997, Sepp *et al.* 1997, Björkstén *et al.* 1999). However, these preliminary studies are regarded as being of limited validity; follow-up studies with larger numbers of patients and conforming to more rigid scientific methods need to be performed.

Primary prevention of allergy through avoidance of aeroallergens was prospectively studied in a series of infants at high risk for atopy from birth to 18 months of age. Recommendations were made to parents about infant diets and avoidance of common food allergens (either breastfeeding and/or hypoallergenic formula combined with avoiding solid foods during the first 6 months of life), aeroallergens, and tobacco smoke. At 18 months of age, compared with a control group of high-risk infants, the prevention group had significantly lower cumulative prevalence of atopic symptoms. Therefore, in at least a subset of patients with atopic dermatitis, avoiding food and inhalant allergens may improve clinical status (Halken *et al.* 1992).

Finally, a prospective long-term study of a nonsedating antihistamine (cetirizine) showed lower asthma prevalence in the subgroup of children with atopic dermatitis and IgE sensitization to pollens or house dust mites treated with cetirizine (International Study of Asthma and Allergies in Childhood [ISAAC] Steering Committee 1998). This was a study conducted by a pharmaceutical company and requires further study to show reproducibility.

SECONDARY PREVENTION

Until the efficacy of primary prevention is more widely validated, secondary prevention measures must be relied upon to minimize inflammation and hyper-reactivity.

CORRECTING SKIN BARRIER DYSFUNCTION

Patients with atopic dermatitis have an impaired cutaneous barrier. Changes in the pH of the stratum corneum impairs lipid metabolism, permitting penetration and susceptibility of irritants and allergens, triggering the inflammatory response, cutaneous hyper-reactivity, inflammation, and resulting skin damage (Irvine and McLean 2006).

A deficiency of filaggrin, the hereditary basis of ichthyosis vulgaris, affects a significant number of patients with atopic dermatitis. Impaired keratinocyte differentiation and barrier formation allow increased transepidermal water loss and entry of allergens, antigens, and chemicals from the environment (Irvine and McLean 2006).

ELIMINATING AND REDUCING TRIGGERS

In addition to a regimen of good skin care, secondary prevention of atopic dermatitis involves avoiding or at least reducing identifiable triggers. The specific prevention program must be tailored to each patient. Eliminating foods should be based on the results of a double-blind, placebo-controlled, food challenge (Rowlands et al. 2006).

Patients whose disease is exacerbated by dust mites should use several simple and inexpensive measures to reduce household dust mite burden including adequate household ventilation, mattress covers, pillow covers, avoiding wall-to-wall carpeting, frequent dust removal with a damp sponge, vacuuming floors and upholstery at least once a week, washing linens in hot water every 7–10 days, and decreasing indoor humidity levels with air conditioning (Tan et al. 1996, Friedmann and Tan 1998).

Secondary prevention of atopic dermatitis should include avoidance of skin irritants. If a patient's disease is worsened by sweating, progressive adaptation to exercise is advisable. Other options include water sports, such as swimming; however, patients must shower and apply emollients immediately after getting out of the swimming pool. Household temperature and humidity should be optimized to reduce sweating. In the winter, patients should be advised to increase emollient use.

Clothing containing synthetic fibers and wool should be avoided; loose-fitting cotton garments are less likely to cause skin irritation and are preferable.

Liquid laundry detergents should be substituted for powder detergents and a second rinse cycle added because residual laundry detergent in clothing can be irritating. Patients sensitive to enzyme-rich detergents should use nonenzymatic detergents. Mild soaps with a neutral pH and minimal defatting capabilities (eg, Dove, Cetaphil, Basis, Aveeno, and Neutrogena) should be used for bathing in all patients with atopic dermatitis. Patients should bathe in warm water once a day for 5–10 min, pat dry, and immediately apply emollients. Finally, nails should be trimmed to decrease excoriation of the skin. Education should include informing patients about the causes and triggers of atopic dermatitis.

TERTIARY PREVENTION

Preventing allergic symptoms is the arena with which clinicians are most familiar. Pediatricians and primary care providers are the first link in tertiary allergy prevention in that they are the first caregivers to recognize and diagnose allergic disease. A general practitioner should refer patients to an allergy specialist for early implementation of allergy-prevention measures and guidance, which should provide patients with specific advice about dietary and environmental control (**Box 7.4**). Methods of tertiary prevention to control the factors that trigger symptoms after disease expression are similar to methods for secondary prevention described above.

The use of immunotherapy to treat atopic dermatitis has been inconclusive. It is known that immunotherapy with aeroallergens is effective in the treatment of allergic rhinitis and asthma. However, there are selected individuals with atopic dermatitis who might benefit from immunotherapy (Kaufman and Roth 1974, Di Prisco et al. 1979, Zachariae *et al.* 1985, Glover and Atherton 1992). Expert opinion does recommend the use of immunotherapy for selected patients with atopic dermatitis (Leung *et al.* 2004b).

SUPERANTIGENS

Patients with later onset of disease (≥20 years of age) may have IgE sensitization against microbial antigens (*S. aureus* enterotoxins and *Candida albicans* or *Malassezia sympodialis*) with low total serum IgE levels. These cases develop into the extrinsic variant of atopic dermatitis, with increasing IgE serum levels and sensitization against airborne and food allergens later in life. It has been suggested that a defective CD4 helper T-lymphocyte population could explain the failure of CD8 T lymphocytes to function as suppressors of IgE production and to achieve sufficient cytotoxicity for effective immunity against secondary skin infections with such microbial antigens.

It is well known that *S. aureus*, which colonizes the skin of most patients with atopic dermatitis, plays a role in the pathogenesis, maintenance, and exacerbation of the disease. Although colonization is highest on lesional skin, *S. aureus* concentrations are increased on normal-appearing skin of patients with atopic dermatitis (Baker 2006, Boguniewicz and Leung 2006). *S. aureus* can secrete toxins that act as superantigens, which stimulate the proliferation of T cells and other immune cells and worsen atopic dermatitis. Moreover, IgE–specific antibodies against *S. aureus* superantigens have been found in the serum of patients with atopic dermatitis.

Box 7.4 Seeking consultation/comanagement with an allergy/immunology specialist

- Facilitate confirmation of the diagnosis and identification of causal factors
- Define IgE-mediated sensitivity in the differential diagnosis of skin diseases
- Perform and interpret diagnostic tests (skin test or *in vitro* assays)
- Identify the role of dust mite allergy and provide avoidance education
- Identify the role of food allergy, particularly in children
- Provide advice on the role of safe, targeted, elimination diets
- Conduct and supervise double-blind, placebo-controlled, oral food challenges in a controlled setting equipped to manage any adverse outcome such as anaphylaxis

ASSOCIATION WITH OTHER DISORDERS OF THE IMMUNE SYSTEM

Atopic dermatitis-like eruptions are a feature of the clinical constellations of several immunological deficiency disorders: Wiskott–Aldrich syndrome, ataxia–telangiectasia, X-linked hypogammaglobulinemia, hyper-IgE syndrome, immune deficiency polyendocrinopathy X-linked syndrome, Spink 5 deficiency/Netherton syndrome, and filaggrin deficiency; these are reviewed elsewhere in this book.

CONCLUSIONS

Although the contribution of allergic factors is controversial among many practitioners, there is good evidence that appropriate allergy testing, patient/parental education, and measures to reduce exposure to pertinent antigens are important in the overall management of many patients with atopic dermatitis. The role of allergen-specific immunotherapy is still not certain and awaits long-term prospective trials.

Clinical suggestions

1. Evaluation by an allergist is most helpful in diagnosing or excluding food and environmental aeroallergen sensitivity as exacerbating factors in atopic dermatitis. Such sensitivities can be identified in a percentage of patients in all age groups including infantile, childhood, and adolescent/adult forms, and in elderly patients.
2. Many parents are often convinced that something external, an allergen, is causing their child's eczema and are resistant to explanations to the contrary. If a baby or a young child with atopic dermatitis is not responding adequately to topical treatments, allergists are most qualified to identify pertinent allergens and perform objective testing such as RAST, skin-prick testing, and prospective double-blind food challenges. This satisfies the parents' desire to identify the culprit foods or aeroallergens if they exist and makes them more receptive to the idea that an external allergen is not causing the problem, when allergy testing is negative.
3. Based on allergy testing, allergists can recommend particular baby formulas that do not contain suspected antigens. Parents can be strongly advised to avoid self-initiated elimination diets such as those based on rice milk which can result in malnutrition.
4. Double-blind food challenges are best performed by allergists at a facility that can treat possible anaphylaxis and those with the expertise to differentiate urticarial food reactions from eczematous food reactions on challenge.
5. In the future specific immunotherapy and possibly anti-IgE may play a role in controlling selected cases of atopic dermatitis but evidence for these modalities is limited at present.

CHAPTER 8

SKIN BARRIER REPAIR IN ATOPIC DERMATITIS THERAPY

William Abramovits and Peter Elias

Human skin evolved from a simple chemical bilayer intended to encapsulate metabolic and reproductive processes into a complex anatomic and functional barrier. The skin protects deeper anatomic structures and their intrinsic biology from physical trauma, such as excessive pressure or friction, harmful chemicals, damaging radiation, and infectious agents. At the same time, the skin allows for health-promoting interchanges between the body that it covers and its surroundings. Thus, not surprisingly, disruptions in cutaneous functional integrity may result in systemic disease (Madison 2003).

CASE IN POINT: ATOPIC DERMATITIS (LEUNG *et al.* 2004, CORK *et al.* 2006, KIM *et al.* 2006)

Recent studies on the physiopathology of atopy suggest that the development of eczema is related less to dysregulation of the immune system and more to disruption of skin barrier function (*outside-inside hypothesis*) (Elias *et al.* 2008, Ong and Boguniewicz 2008). In all likelihood, defects in both mechanisms operate concomitantly, and result from faults at the genomic level.

EPIDERMAL BARRIER FUNCTION

To illustrate how the epidermis achieves its barrier function, a bricks-and-mortar model has been suggested (Elias 1983). Bricks represent keratinocytes whereas mortar represents intercellular space fillers (Harding 2004). A fundamental difference between the depiction of a static wall and the epidermis is that in the epidermis the 'bricks' are the source of the 'mortar' to a very large extent. The old concept was that keratinocytes passively underwent terminal differentiation into dead cells, flattening as their envelopes keratinized out of their plasma membranes. The dead, flat cells were thought to layer toward the epidermal surface because corneocytes comprising an insoluble amalgam of proteins were surrounded by a lipid envelope. They would thus be transformed into a physical and chemical cover. But this concept has been supplanted by the idea that keratinocytes very actively participate in the metabolic and immunological processes that lead to the development and maintenance of a functional barrier unit (Braff and Gallo 2006) (**Fig 8.1**).

During the transformation of basal layer keratinocytes to stratum corneum corneocytes, the intracellular structural protein profilaggrin is first converted to filaggrin by dephosphorylation and later to free amino acids through proteolysis (Rawlings and Matts 2005). These free amino acids, together with carboxylic, urocanic, and lactic acids, urea, sugars, and other intracellularly derived molecules, constitute the so-called *natural moisturizing factor* (NMF) (Rawlings and Harding 2004). Filaggrin is thought to aggregate keratin filaments, the main structural proteins in basal keratinocytes, into tight bundles. This causes progressive flattening of the cells as they transform into corneocytes (Candi *et al.* 2005). In addition, keratinocytes synthesize lipid bilayers in their Golgi apparatus from ceramides, cholesterol, and fatty acids, which are then extruded as lamellar bodies into the intercellular spaces of the stratum granulosum (**Fig 8.2**). This process is modulated by hyaluronic acid and water content gradients between the stratum granulosum and the cornified layer (Pasonen-Seppänen et al. 2003, Maytin *et al.* 2004).

Preservation of the physical, chemical, and biologic integrity of the skin and prevention of excessive water loss occur as a result of: the ability of NMF to retain water; the hygroscopic and hydrophilic properties of the lipid bilayers; and the effect of aquaporins, which are proteins expressed in decrescendo from the basal layer to the cornified layer that facilitate water transport across membranes (Warner *et al.* 2003, Cao *et al.* 2006, Hara-Chikuma and Verkman 2006, Olsson *et al.* 2006, Dumas *et al.* 2007).

Keratinocytes also form antimicrobial peptides, such as cathelcidins and defensins, which are active against staphylococcal colonization (Kisich *et al.* 2007). Moreover, keratinocytes express temperature sensor receptors which, when activated by heat, signal for the acceleration of barrier recovery mechanisms (Denda *et al.* 2007).

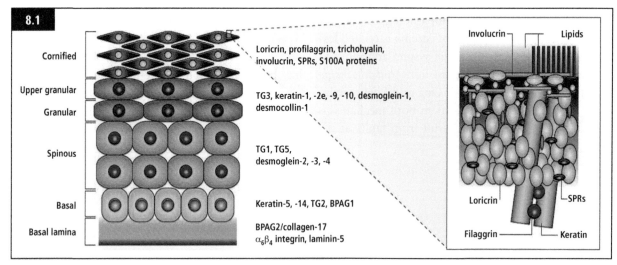

Fig 8.1 Terminal differentiation and apoptosis in the epidermis. The proteins that are expressed in particular locations in the epidermis during skin differentiation are shown. Apoptosis is restricted to the basal layer, whereas cornification occurs in the suprabasal layers, to form a cornified envelope (see inset). At the molecular level, the cornified envelope is formed by proteins that are highly crosslinked by transglutaminases, with specific lipids on the outside, to guarantee specific physical properties. BPAG, bullosus pemphigoid antigen; SPR, small proline-rich proteins; TG, transglutaminase. (Reprinted from Candi *et al.* 2005 by permission of Macmillan Publishers Ltd. © 2005.)

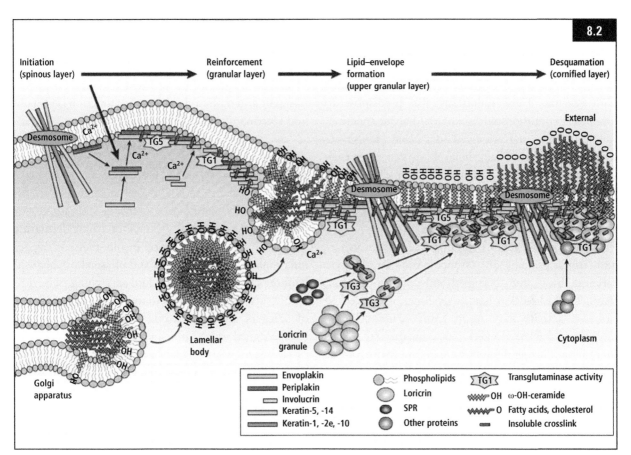

Fig 8.2 Progressive steps in the formation of the cornified envelope. The first step is the initiation stage, which takes place in the spinous layer, and involves the synthesis of the cornified envelope (CE) structural proteins and the synthesis and extrusion into the intercellular space of specific lipids. Transglutaminase (TG)-1 and TG-5 crosslink envoplakin and periplakin under the cell membrane, thereby anchoring them to the desmosome. The second step is the reinforcement phase, which takes place in the granular layer, and entails the covalent attachment of some lipids to the CE proteins, and the crosslinking of loricrin to small proline-rich proteins (SPRs) by TG-3 and TG-1. Heavy crosslinking occurs on the desmosome, where these proteins function as substrates for TGs. Next, during formation of the lipid envelope, also in the granular layer, lipids from the lamellar body, which are derived from the Golgi apparatus, are attached and crosslinked by TG-5 and TG-1 on the already crosslinked proteins (envoplakin, periplakin, involucrin) and are exposed on the outside of the membrane. The reinforcement and steps of lipid envelope formation take place concomitantly. Finally, the desquamation phase, which takes place in the cornified layer, involves further crosslinking of loricrin and other proteins by TG-1 on the protein scaffold, and the extrusion of ω-hydroxy-ceramides, fatty acids, and cholesterol. The physical properties of the cornified envelope depend on the nature of the substrates and on the crosslinks, as well as the lipid deposition. The location of the epidermal layers in which these progressive steps take place is indicated in **Fig 8.1**. (Reprinted from Candi *et al.* 2005 by permission of Macmillan Publishers Ltd. © 2005.)

Recently, loss-of-function mutations within genes that encode for profilaggrin have been found to predispose to atopic dermatitis with allergic sensitizations and to asthma when it is associated with eczema. These mutations also predispose to other skin conditions with impaired barrier function, ranging from self-perceived dry skin to severe ichthyosis vulgaris. Filaggrin levels are decreased even in nonlesional skin of patients with atopic dermatitis (Ginger *et al.* 2005, Irvine and McLean 2006, Palmer *et al.* 2006, Segre 2006, Weidinger *et al.* 2006, Sandilands *et al.* 2007).

Mutations in genes coding for certain proteases and transglutaminases, essential for keratinocyte differentiation and cornified envelope formation, may also lead to skin barrier dysfunction. Increased protease activity may result from serine protease inhibitor defects linked to genetic structural mutations. Phospholipases mediate the hydrolysis of phospholipids into free fatty acids which contribute to the acidification of the stratum corneum. This has the dual benefit of creating an *acid mantle* and preventing the premature dissolution of desmosomes between keratinocytes (Ishibashi *et al.* 2003, Bikle *et al.* 2004, Leyvraz *et al.* 2005).

The genetic makeup of atopic dermatitis thus appears to include a complex mixture of prevalent filaggrin gene mutations plus a large number of low-frequency mutations in genes that influence epidermal differentiation, such as those encoding the cornified envelope proteins loricrin and involucrin. These genetic effects, when combined, are thought to increase susceptibility to atopic dermatitis (Morar *et al.* 2007). Once the relevance of competent barrier function in atopic dermatitis is appreciated, one must address the possible therapeutic value of repairing and maintaining the barrier. The means of achieving this is discussed in this chapter.

A variety of methods is used to measure barrier function of the skin, from subjective physician visual scores or patient self-perception of dryness, moisture, or oiliness, to optical measurements of shine. Determinations of transepidermal water loss (TEWL), mechanical properties, skin capacitance, corneometry, permeability, histochemistry, and confocal microscopy both *in vitro* and *in vivo*, provide more objective, reproducible data. Although determination of water flux through the skin via TEWL measurement is indirect, imperfect, and limited, TEWL measurements are prevalent in the literature and are used to promote products purported to repair and maintain skin barrier function (Lebwohl and Herrmann 2005, Tagami *et al.* 2006).

THERAPEUTIC INTERVENTIONS

GENERAL MEASURES

The first step in the management of atopic dermatitis is to minimize environmental insults that can trigger inflammation. Both atopens and physical or chemical irritants can trigger itching and scratching, which in turn exacerbates or perpetuates eczema. Avoidance of triggers may be accomplished by education, psychological stress management, proper selection of cleansers, moisturizers, and humectants, artificial barriers, and pharmacological means (Choi *et al.* 2005, Draelos 2005).

Soaps and harsh surfactants in cleansers can damage skin proteins and lipids, and lead to tightness, dryness, itch, and irritation after washing (Gfatter *et al.* 1997, Abbas *et al.* 2004). They can also transiently increase surface pH and impair the antimicrobial acid mantle (Schmid and Korting 1995, Fluhr *et al.* 2001, Hanson *et al.* 2002, Schmid-Wendtner and Korting 2006). Newer surfactants containing synthetic detergents have been developed that react minimally with skin proteins and lipids (Ananthapadmanabhan *et al.* 2004). Neutral or slightly acidic cleansers may be less damaging to the cornified layer than those with an alkaline pH. In addition, mildness enhancers, moisturizers, lipidizers, and occlusives may be incorporated into cleanser formulations to minimize damage to the skin barrier. Cleansing atopic skin is important because it removes atopens such as house dust mites, bacteria, and dead cells; in addition it prepares the skin for topical therapy (Cardona *et al.* 2006). Bathing using antibacterial cleansers, dilute bleach in the bath water, antipruritics or emollients such as colloidal oatmeal can benefit patients with eczema. Colloidal oatmeal contains avenanthramides and anti-inflammatory polyphenolic antioxidants which reduce proinflammatory cytokines. Skin care regimens combining oatmeal-based body wash and a glycerin-containing cream were shown to decrease TEWL in atopic dermatitis patients (Eichenfield *et al.* 2007).

The ultimate moisturizer for dry skin is water (Levin and Maibach 2001). Some moisturizers deliver water to the skin and some help retain the water already contained in and below the cornified layer by coating the skin and inhibiting evaporation. Some deliver water-trapping molecules, and others provide ingredients that allow the skin to generate a physiological barrier (Harding 2004, Buraczewska *et al.* 2007).

Petrolatum or petroleum jelly, mineral and vegetable oils, paraffin, silicone derivatives dimethicone and cyclomethicone, squalene, waxes and their esters, including beeswax, lanolin and carnauba, propylene glycol, and others create an inert impermeable barrier that traps water in and under the cornified layer (Loden 2003, Rawlings *et al.* 2004). Moisturizers including glycerin, urea, hyaluronic acid, sodium and ammonium lactate, sodium pyrrolidone carboxylic acid, and gelatin are able to bind and retain water molecules up to 1000 times their own molecular weight.

Formulations with physiological lipids, or lipidizers, contain sterols such as cholesterol, ceramides, and free fatty acids, both essential such as linoleic and arachidonic acids, and nonessential such as palmitic and stearic acids. The lipids from these formulations are purported to serve as substrates for keratinocytes to synthesize new lipid bilayers. These, in turn, are thought to be extruded as lamellar bodies into the intercellular spaces of the granular layer. These ingredients must be delivered at critically precise ratios to work properly (Man *et al.* 1996, Zettersten *et al.* 1997). Some ceramide-dominant mixtures have been shown by TEWL measurements to repair skin barrier function and improve signs and symptoms of eczema in atopic dermatitis (Chamlin *et al.* 2002, Elias 2005, Simpson and Dutronc 2011).

Modern vehicle technologies facilitate the incorporation of these ingredients into barrier-repairing formulations. Newer formulations contain active ingredients in solution, or as suspensions or emulsions of nanoparticles, liposomes, microsponges, and microvesicles (Draelos 2000, Bergstrand 2003, Puig *et al.* 2004, Rosen 2005). Pharmacotherapeutic agents for atopic dermatitis, such as corticosteroids and calcineurin inhibitors, may now be compounded in complex formulations containing urea, salicylic acid, or retinoids intended to enhance delivery. At the same time, irritation usually associated with these agents can be minimized.

NEWER FORMULATIONS

Three creams have recently been introduced in the USA and other markets as medical devices for the treatment of signs and symptoms of atopic dermatitis. All three require a prescription in the USA. The first, Atopiclair, contains glycyrrhetinic acid, telmestine, and *Vitis vinifera* in a vehicle with hyaluronic acid and *Butyrospermum parkii* (shea butter), a botanical source of triglycerides, saturated fatty acids, and linoleic acid. This cream is intended to resemble the ceramide-dominant mixtures previously described.

The second cream introduced, Mimyx, contains the cannabinoid N-palmitoylethanolamine in a surfactant-free vehicle containing squalene, triglycerides, phospholipids, and phytosterol, to mimic the normal skin barrier.

In addition, two ceramide-dominant creams have been approved as medical devices in the USA, EpiCeram and Hylatopic Plus. These formulations reduce TEWL in atopic dermatitis patients. The anti-inflammatory properties of their key ingredients, on the one hand, the effect of their vehicles, on the other, or both, have been demonstrated to provide eczema relief (Chamlin *et al.* 2002, Abramovits *et al.* 2005, Abramovits and Perlmutter 2006a, 2006b, Sugarman and Parish 2009, Kircik and Del Rosso 2011). These medical devices are in general more expensive than petrolatum and are not usually covered by insurance. Also of note, a recent small study comparing the clinical efficacy and cost efficacy of a glycyrrhetinic acid-containing barrier repair cream (BRC-Gly, Atopiclair), a ceramide-dominant barrier repair cream (BRC-Cer, EpiCeram) and an OTC petroleum-based skin protectant moisturizer (OTC-Pet, Aquaphor Healing Ointment) as monotherapy for mild-to-moderate atopic dermatitis in children failed to show any clinical superiority of BRC-Gly or BRC-Cer over the petrolatum-based moisturizer (Miller *et al.* 2011). The petrolatum-based preparation was at least 47 times more cost-effective than the BRC-Gly and BRC-Cer preparations.

Several other products specifically intended to restore skin barrier function in pathological settings, such as atopic dermatitis, contain predominantly hyaluronic acid, hyaluronic acid sodium salt, trolamine, or are just hydrolipidic formulations. Hydrocortisone butyrate is now available in a hydrolipidic formulation and desonide is available as both a hydrogel and a foam. Both formulations have been shown to reduce TEWL. A clobetasone butyrate moisturizing emollient cream was also shown to reduce TEWL. Thus the iatrogenic barrier dysfunction associated with the atrophogenic effects of many corticosteroid formulations can be reduced with these vehicles (Sheu *et al.* 1997, Parneix-Spake *et al.* 2001, Faurschou *et al.* 2007, Kircik and Del Rosso 2007).

Pimecrolimus cream and tacrolimus ointment can also decrease TEWL, suggesting that correction of the inflammatory process underlying atopic dermatitis is another way to promote barrier function repair (Xhauflaire-Uhoda *et al.* 2007, Engel *et al.* 2008). In addition, despite their immunosuppressive effects, topical corticosteroids and calcineurin inhibitors actually reduce staphylococcal colonization of eczema lesions. The mechanism for this may involve the restoration of antimicrobial peptides as inflammation decreases (Park *et al.* 2005).

Although dietary deficiencies of zinc and essential fatty acids lead to syndromes reminiscent of eczema with increased TEWL, administration of lipid formulations such as linoleic acid have not shown sufficient or consistent efficacy in patients with atopic dermatitis to justify their routine use (Strobel *et al.* 1978, Borrek *et al.* 1997, Martens-Lobenhoffer and Meyer 1998, Takwale *et al.* 2003, Bettzuege-Pfaff and Melzer 2005, Umeda-Sawada *et al.* 2006).

CONCLUSION

In summary, the establishment and restoration of the barrier function of the skin in atopic dermatitis may be achieved: through proper selection of synthetic detergents with mild surfactants and mildness enhancers such as glycerin and lipids; by the use of moisturizers containing, in addition to water, an inert physical barrier to evaporation such as petrolatum; by humectants such as hyaluronic acid and urea; by physiological lipids that foster the production of a lipid bilayer and NMF by keratinocytes, such as ceramides and fatty acids; and by medicinal agents that address the dysregulated immune mechanisms which trigger and perpetuate the inflammation in eczema lesions.

CHAPTER 9

THE ROLE OF INFECTIOUS AGENTS IN ATOPIC DERMATITIS

Andrea L. Neimann, Jules Lipoff, Rachel Garner, Anat Lebow, and Steven R. Cohen

INTRODUCTION

Atopic dermatitis (AD) is a chronic inflammatory skin disease affecting 15–30% of children and 2–10% of adults (Bieber 2008). It is generally considered that patients with AD are prone to a variety of skin infections. This increased susceptibility is thought to be caused by an impaired skin barrier (making it easier for organisms to invade the skin and bind to cellular receptors), impaired innate and adaptive immunity, and defects in immunity resulting from treatment (eg, topical and systemic steroids and immunosuppressive agents) (Wollenberg *et al.* 2003a).

Recently an opposing perspective has received attention, one in which AD pathological alterations, such as impaired barrier function and cutaneous inflammation, are actually caused in part by infectious agents (Leung 2003, Lubbe 2003). Current evidence indicates that microorganisms, particularly *Staphylococcus aureus,* which colonizes the skin of most individuals with AD, play a significant role in its etiopathogenesis. Perturbations in innate and cell-mediated immunity also predispose AD patients to cutaneous viral infections such as eczema herpeticum. In this condition, widespread cutaneous dissemination of herpetic lesions occurs from what in normal hosts would merely be an innocuous cold sore. Warts and molluscum contagiosum are also held to be more prevalent in patients with AD, but there is little formal evidence to support this notion (Lever 1996, Lubbe 2003). Finally, an increased susceptibility to chronic dermatophytosis has also been suggested in patients with AD.

STAPHYLOCOCCUS AUREUS IN ATOPIC DERMATITIS

COLONIZATION

S. aureus is a common cause of cutaneous infections such as folliculitis, furunculosis, abscesses, cellulitis, and necrotizing soft tissue infections. Although it is widely stated that AD patients experience a much higher frequency of staphylococcal infections than people without AD, studies document only increased colonization and impetiginized eczema, uncommonly clinically severe infections (Hanifin and Rogge 1977). Rajka notes in his text, 'Interestingly, deep pyogenic infections such as furuncles, cellulitis, and erysipelas, despite frequent scratching, are less common than might be anticipated' (Rajka 1989).

On the other hand, several studies have demonstrated widespread colonization of lesional and nonlesional AD skin with *S. aureus.* In one study, lesional skin was colonized in 90% of patients with AD, whereas only 5% of individuals without AD showed colonization, usually intranasal or in intertriginous areas (Abeck and Mempel 1998).

Increased staphylococcal colonization of AD skin has been attributed to several factors. Decreased levels of naturally occurring antimicrobial peptides including β-defensins and canthelicidins are detected in patients with AD compared with those with psoriasis (Ong *et al.* 2002). Ong *et al.* (2002) demonstrated a deficiency of the antimicrobial peptides (AMPs) canthelicidin LL-37 and human β-defensin 2 (HBD-2) in acute and chronic lesional AD skin compared with psoriasis lesional skin, but in another study baseline levels of these AMPs did not differ between atopic and nonatopic foreskin (Goo *et al.* 2010). Reduced expression of HBD-3 has been reported at the mRNA and protein levels in AD patients (Nomura *et al.* 2003). Reduced expression or mobilization of AMPs such as HBD-2 and HBD-3 occurs as a result of increased expression of T-helper type 2 (Th2) cytokines, interleukin (IL)-4, -10, and -13 in AD skin (Howell *et al.* 2005, 2006, Kisich *et al.* 2008).

A deficiency of antistaphylococcal dermicidin-derived antimicrobial peptides in the sweat of patients with AD has also been established (Rieg *et al.* 2005). In contrast, a recent study showed that HBD-2 is induced in response to bacteria, injury, or inflammatory stimuli, suggesting that it is not associated with vulnerability to *S. aureus* baseline colonization in the skin of patients with AD (Asano *et al.* 2008).

Staphylococcal colonization is also favored by the more alkaline pH of AD skin and the presence in dermatitic skin of exposed fibrinogen and fibronectin, which facilitate binding of staphylococci (Wann *et al.* 2000, Cho *et al.* 2001). Reduced levels of filaggrin breakdown products urocanic acid and pyrrolidone carboxylic acid, caused by loss-of-function mutations in the filaggrin gene, may also favor staphylococcal colonization on the basis of pH-dependent and pH-independent mechanisms (Miajlovic *et al.* 2010). Other factors favoring staphylococcal colonization include decreased levels of sphingosine in AD stratum corneum, alterations in other bacteria that usually limit the growth of staphylococci, and possibly other AMPs. To reiterate, *S. aureus* is found in more than 90% of AD skin lesions. Compared with nonlesional atopic skin, moreover, inflamed AD lesions have a 1000-fold higher density of *S. aureus* (Williams *et al.* 1990, Gong *et al.* 2006). There is also a much higher frequency of *S. aureus* colonization in the anterior nares of AD patients, and bacterial counts correlate with levels of antistaphylococcal IgE in serum (Falanga *et al.* 1985).

PATHOGENIC ROLE OF STAPHYLOCOCCUS AUREUS IN ECZEMA

Although colonization by *S. aureus* is ubiquitous in atopic skin, the exact mechanism by which it contributes to the pathogenesis of AD has not been entirely elucidated. It is postulated that bacterial products directly damage the epidermis, inducing inflammation, provoking increased itching and excoriation, and altering cutaneous immune responses. There are several mechanisms implicated in the atopic inflammatory response to *S. aureus*. *S. aureus* cell protein A, when injected intradermally, evokes a biphasic weal-and-flare reaction (White and Noble 1985) and anti-*S. aureus*, IgE-mediated, mast cell degranulation has been postulated (Walsh *et al.* 1981). Circulating antistaphylococcal IgE antibodies have been detected in up to 30% of patients with AD (Schopfer *et al.* 1979, Walsh *et al.* 1981, Falanga *et al.* 1985, Friedman *et al.* 1985, Motala *et al.* 1986).

S. aureus superantigens are thought to promote Th2 skin inflammation, IgE production, T-regulatory cell subversion, expansion and migration of skin-homing T cells, and IgE antibody production (Cardona *et al.* 2006). *S. aureus*-producing superantigens, such as enterotoxins A, B, and toxic shock syndrome toxin 1 (TSST-1), can be cultured in more than 50% of AD patients (Leung *et al.* 1993, Bunikowski *et al.* 1999, Nomura *et al.* 1999). Specific IgE antibodies directed against these superantigens are correlated with the severity of disease. Staphylococcal colonization increases keratinocyte production of thymic stromal lymphopoietin production, which promotes Th2 immune polarization; it also augments keratinocyte production of IL-18, an important Th1 cytokine (Inoue *et al.* 2010, Vu *et al.* 2010). In addition, bacterial products from colonized skin cause dendritic cells to produce inflammatory cytokines such as IL-1β, IL-6, IL-10, and tumor necrosis factor β (TNF-β) (Voorhees *et al.* 2011). Finally, recent work suggests that specific allergic immune responses to a novel IgE-reactive protein, fibronectin-binding protein (FBP), from *S. aureus* may play a role in the development of AD (Reginald *et al.* 2011).

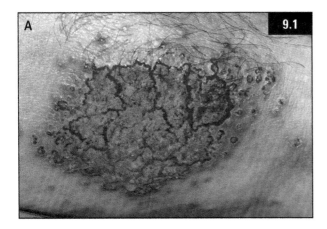

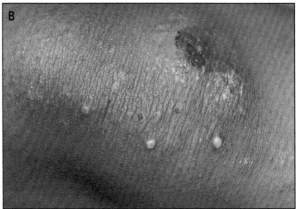

Fig 9.1 (A) Impetiginized eczema with fissuring and erosion surrounded by individual pustules, and (B) small area of impetiginized eczema with purulent folliculitis.

Fig 9.2 Flexural eczema with secondary impetiginization. It can be difficult to differentiate exuberant eczema colonized with *Staphylococcus aureus* from impetiginized eczema.

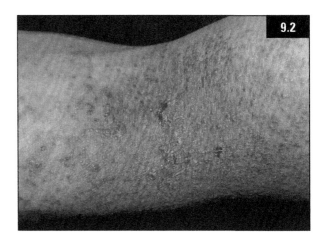

CLINICAL INFECTION

Although penetrating staphylococcal infections such as cellulitis, furunculosis and abscesses do not occur with increased frequency in patients with AD, impetiginized eczema is quite common and is associated with flares of disease (**Fig 9.1**). It may, in the clinical setting, be difficult to distinguish severe dermatitis colonized with staphylococci from frankly impetiginized skin (**Fig 9.2**). Hanifin and Rogge (1977) noted that superficial staphylococcal pustules in AD were associated with severe exacerbations of disease. These pustules typically appeared on unbroken skin, independent of hair follicles, were very itchy, and were rapidly effaced by scratching and rubbing. Other signs of impetiginization include weeping, crusting, and periauricular fissuring (David 1989).

There has been a recent surge in community-acquired methicillin (meticillin)-resistant *S. aureus* (MRSA) infections that might be expected to affect patients with AD. A 2004 study of German children with AD (mean age 2.7 years, age range 0.2–15 years) found all staphylococcal isolates to be sensitive to oxacillin, amoxicillin/clavulanic acid, cefadroxil, and cefuroxime (Hoeger 2004). Four years later a study in Germany of children, adolescents, and adults found a 3% incidence of MRSA (Niebuhr *et al.* 2008).

Low incidence rates of MRSA in AD have also been reported in studies from San Diego and New Zealand (Matiz *et al.* 2010, Hill *et al.* 2011). By contrast, a Philadelphia study reported that 16% of colonized patients were colonized with MRSA and a Korean study found that 75.4% of children with AD had *S. aureus* isolates, of which 18.3% were methicillin resistant (Chung *et al.* 2008, Suh *et al.* 2008). Five older children infected with MRSA manifested a characteristic 'fishy' odor during flares of disease (Hon *et al.* 2008).

In patients with acute exacerbation of eczema in whom secondary infection is thought to be the cause, bacterial culture of the skin should be performed and empiric therapy initiated with systemic antibiotics. Although *S. aureus* is the most common cause of bacterial infection in AD, other organisms, such as streptococci, may be found alone or in association with *S. aureus*. One prospective study of 190 atopic children found that 15% of patients with eczema exacerbations due to infection (presumed by response to anti-infective treatment) required hospitalization (David and Cambridge 1986). *S. aureus* was recovered in 97% of these patients, and β-*hemolytic streptococci* in combination with staphylococci were found in as many as 62%. Most other studies have not reported such a high frequency of streptococcal infection, but the possible presence of streptococci should be considered when planning systemic antibiotic coverage.

Treatment of bacterial skin infection in eczema is targeted at the most likely causative organism, *S. aureus*. Antibiotics of choice are the penicillinase-resistant penicillins, such as dicloxacillin, and first-generation oral cephalosporins (Williams *et al.* 1990, Ring *et al.* 1996). Patients colonized with MRSA should be treated with alternative antibiotic regimens such as sulfamethoxazole–trimethoprim, clindamycin, or doxycycline in older children who have their adult teeth. Patients with penicillin allergies may be treated with fusidic acid or clindamycin (Leclercq *et al.* 2000). Fusidic acid inhibits staphylococci at low concentrations, even in those with resistance to methicillin or oxacillin (Verbist 1990). Although not available in the USA, fusidic acid is widely available in Europe.

Another treatment strategy is to combine a topical glucocorticosteroid with a systemic or topical antibiotic such as mupirocin (Wachs and Maibach 1976, Leyden and Kligman 1977, Abeck and Mempel 1998). In one study, mupirocin significantly reduced bacterial counts and clinical severity in patients with AD (Lever *et al.* 1988). Improvement was maintained over 4 weeks, despite post-treatment recolonization with *new strains* not previously isolated. Other measures aimed at reducing staphylococcal colonization include dilute bleach baths (Metry *et al.* 2007) and garments made of silver-coated textiles or antibacterial silk fabric coated with alkoxysilane quaternary ammonium (Gauger *et al.* 2006, Ricci *et al.* 2006).

Dilute bleach baths, with or without intranasal mupirocin, seem to show promise in the treatment of infected AD. In a randomized, investigator-blinded, placebo-controlled study, 31 patients, aged 6 months to 17 years, with moderate-to-severe AD and evidence of secondary bacterial infection were randomized to receive intranasal mupirocin ointment treatment and sodium hypochlorite (bleach) baths (treatment arm) or intranasal petrolatum ointment treatment and plain water baths (placebo arm) for 3 months after an initial treatment course of oral cephalexin (Huang *et al.* 2009, 2011). The Eczema Area and Severity Index score showed significantly greater mean reductions from baseline in the bleach bath group at 1 month and 3 months compared with the control group but only in areas that were submerged (not on the face). Instructions for bleach baths are provided in **Box 9.1** (Krakowski *et al.* 2008). A video explaining the use of bleach baths can be found at www.eczemacenter.org/ecvc.htm#bleachbaths.

Ultraviolet (UV) phototherapy (UVB [broadband and narrowband] and psoralen plus UVA [PUVA]) has an antistaphylococcal effect in patients with AD (Jekler *et al.* 1992, Silva *et al.* 2006). Patients who did not respond to UV therapy were found to have higher *S. aureus* colonization rates than responders (Yoshimura *et al.* 1996, Schempp *et al.* 1997). Improvement in AD may be attributable, in part, to the reduction in staphylococcal superantigens by phototherapy (Yoshimura-Mishima *et al.* 1999, Silva *et al.* 2006). In general, UVB phototherapy is not

---

Box 9.1 A bleach bath primer

Explain to patients that their skin may benefit from 'swimming in pool water.' Then, give them these instructions for making a pool right in their very own bathroom:

- Add lukewarm water to fill the tub completely (about 40 gallons [150 liters] of water)
- Depending on the size of the tub/amount of water used, add ¼ to ½ cup of common bleach solution to the bath water. Any sodium hypochlorite 6% solution will do (eg, Clorox liquid bleach); the goal is to make a modified Dakin's solution with a final concentration of about 0.005%
- Stir the mixture to ensure that the bleach is completely diluted in the bath water
- Have patients soak in the chlorinated water for 5–10 min
- Thoroughly rinse skin clear with lukewarm, fresh water at the end of the bleach bath to prevent dryness and irritation
- As soon as the bath is over, pat the patient dry. Do not rub dry, as this is the same as scratching
- Immediately apply any prescribed medications/emollients
- Repeat bleach baths two to three times a week or as prescribed by the physician

The following restrictions apply:

- Do not use undiluted bleach directly on the skin. Even diluted bleach baths can potentially cause dryness and/or irritation
- Do not use bleach baths if there are many breaks or open areas in the skin (for fear of intense stinging and burning)
- Do not use bleach baths in patients with a known contact allergy to chlorine

(Reproduced with permission from Krakowski *et al.* 2008. © 2008 the American Academy of Pediatrics.)

---

used for acute exacerbations of AD whereas UVA1, PUVA, and extracorporeal phototherapy are effective for acute flares (Krutmann 2000). UVA1 therapy is available in only a few centers. Its long-term effects are unknown.

Although there is no doubt that frank skin infection needs to be treated, the use of systemic antibiotics routinely in the absence of manifest infection is not supported by the literature (Bath-Hextall *et al.* 2010, Schnopp *et al.* 2010). Although antibacterial and antiseptic regimens reduce staphylococcal colonization, their effect on eczema scores is less clear; however, the bleach bath approach shows promise (Bath-Hextall *et al.* 2010, Craig *et al.* 2010, Huang *et al.* 2011).

STREPTOCOCCAL INFECTIONS

As mentioned previously, some studies have reported an increased risk of streptococcal infections in patients with acute flares of AD (David and Cambridge 1986). Lancefield group A streptococcus (GAS) (β-hemolytic streptococci [*Streptococcus pyogenes*]) is the predominant type of streptococcus associated with AD (Brook *et al*. 1996). A study of streptococci associated with AD found that GAS accounted for 70.7%, group G streptococci for 19.5%, and group B streptococci for 9.8% (Adachi *et al*. 1998).

Patients with AD, in addition to impetiginized eczema, can have staphylococcal or streptococcal impetigo on normal-appearing skin. Streptococcal impetigo begins with vesicles and pustules, which subsequently rupture to form characteristic thick, honey-colored crusts (Akiyama *et al*. 1999). Patients with cultures positive for streptococci who were treated with oral penicillin had better clinical responses than those treated with topical antibiotics or disinfectants (Adachi *et al*. 1998).

Skin infection with GAS can predispose to acute glomerulonephritis, so affected children should be monitored carefully for hematuria or hypertension. Children who develop perianal erythema, soreness, and pain on defecation should be suspected of having perianal streptococcal dermatitis (cellulitis) and be treated with appropriate antibiotic therapy.

FUNGAL INFECTIONS

The role of yeasts and fungi in AD is controversial. Although not the cause of AD, *Malassezia* and *Candida* species may play a contributory role, ostensibly by evoking allergic reactions in a subgroup of patients, primarily adults resistant to treatment (Guého *et al*. 1998, Faergemann 1999, 2002, Savolainen *et al*. 2001). In patients with chronic tinea infections, dermatophyte fungi might also act as allergens (Klein *et al*. 1999, Faergemann 2002).

Several lines of evidence support a role for fungi and yeasts in atopic dermatitis, including presence of specific IgE to yeasts, prick test and atopy patch test data, and clinical improvement of eczema with antifungal therapy (Johansson *et al*. 2003). Several studies suggest improvement of AD with systemic antifungal therapy, especially with 'azoles' (Bäck *et al*. 1995, Bäck and Bartosik 2001, Ikezawa *et al*. 2004, Svejgaard *et al*. 2004, Takechi 2005).

The presence of specific IgE, positive prick tests, and response of eczema to antifungals do not necessarily prove a causal relationship of fungi and yeasts and AD. Children with AD frequently display specific IgE to multiple irrelevant food allergens, and antifungal drugs have anti-inflammatory effects apart from their antifungal action, eg, antimycotic azoles suppress IL-4 and IL-5 production in anti-CD3-/CD28-stimulated T cells from both AD patients and normal individuals (Kanda 2004).

MALASSEZIA SPP.

Malassezia spp. are normal skin commensals that vary in density between different body sites, in children compared with adults, and in normal compared with diseased skin (Faergemann *et al.* 1983). *Malassezia furfur* (*Pityrosporum ovale*) is commonly present in seborrheic areas such as the scalp, face, neck, and upper chest, and is cultured with the same frequency from patients with AD as in healthy age-matched controls (Broberg *et al.* 1992). IgE antibodies to *M. furfur* are, however, more common in AD patients than in nonatopic control individuals, suggesting that Th2 responses in AD may predispose to IgE production and hypersensitivity to *M. furfur* (Zargari *et al.* 2001, Johansson *et al.* 2002).

Specific serum IgE, positive skin-prick tests and positive atopy patch tests to *Malassezia* spp. have been demonstrated repeatedly in patients with AD (Faergemann 2002). Sensitization rates in European studies based on specific serum IgE levels have varied from 30% to 68% in adults. In an American study, adult AD patients with head, neck, and upper torso distribution showed high reaction rates to *Malassezia sympodialis* on atopy patch testing (Boguniewicz *et al.* 2006, Ramirez de Knott *et al.* 2006).

Sensitization to *M. sympodialis* occurs in AD patients with both intrinsic and extrinsic eczema, and should be considered in those with head and neck lesions, exacerbations during adolescence or young adulthood, and those with eczema recalcitrant to conventional therapy (Darabi *et al.* 2009). The relevance of malassezia sensitization is supported but not proven by reports of improvement of skin disease in patients with IgE antibodies to the yeast after antifungal therapy (Faergemann 2002, Leung 2003).

DERMATOPHYTES

The relationship between AD and chronic dermatophyte infections is controversial (Jones *et al.* 1974, Svejgaard *et al.* 1989). There is some evidence that patients with chronic tinea infections are more likely atopic and that atopic individuals may have a higher prevalence of chronic and possibly more severe dermatophyte infections than nonatopic individuals (Jones *et al.* 1973, Faergemann 2002). Conversely, patients with dermatophytosis may have more severe atopy. There are isolated case reports of improvement of recalcitrant AD in patients with culture-positive tinea infections and antitrichophyton IgE antibodies after successful treatment of the dermatophyte infection (Wilson *et al.* 1993, Klein *et al.* 1999). Nevertheless, the significance of raised IgE levels to dermatophytes in AD patients with chronic dermatophyte infections is not known (Jones *et al.* 1974). As mentioned, reports of a beneficial effect of antifungal treatment on AD must be interpreted with caution given the known anti-inflammatory activity of the azole drugs.

In summary, fungi are not causal, but may possibly *aggravate* AD via hypersensitivity mechanisms. The role of antifungal drugs in the treatment of AD awaits clarification.

VIRAL INFECTIONS

An increased frequency of viral infections occurs in AD patients as a result of altered innate immune mechanisms, defective cutaneous cell-mediated immunity, and possibly, in some cases, treatment with topical corticosteroids and calcineurin inhibitors.

MOLLUSCUM CONTAGIOSUM

Molluscum contagiosum is a poxvirus and the sole member of the molluscipox virus subfamily that presents as single or multiple pink- and flesh-colored umbilicated papules which contain a central molluscum body composed of white, cheesy material. According to some authors, patients with AD have an increased incidence of molluscum and tend to have more widespread disease, often with hundreds of lesions (Solomon and Telner 1966).

A recent retrospective review found that among children with molluscum contagiosum only 24% had a history of previous or active coexistent AD (Dohil et al. 2006). Children with AD were, however, more likely to have an increased number of lesions (**Fig 9.3**). Lesions are spread by autoinoculation and tend to be distributed in the flexures of the arms, axillae, and neck, and lateral aspects of the trunk, as well as the popliteal fossae. It is common for molluscum contagiosum to induce a perilesional eczematous reaction, which often resolves spontaneously (Binkley et al. 1956). Molluscum contagiosum lesions are particularly difficult to treat around the eyes, they may be huge, and may sometimes become infected (**Fig 9.4**).

Widespread dissemination of molluscum lesions in AD has been referred to as eczema molluscatum. This phenomenon is seen in untreated AD or as a result of treatment with topical calcineurin inhibitors (Wetzel and Wollenberg 2004, Fery-Blanco et al. 2007).

ECZEMA HERPETICUM

Eczema herpeticum (*Kaposi's varicelliform eruption*) is a disseminated cutaneous infection with herpes simplex virus characterized by a diffuse eruption of monomorphous, dome-shaped, umbilicated vesicles associated with fever, malaise, and lymphadenopathy (Bussmann et al. 2008) (**Fig 9.5**). Although fatal cases of eczema herpeticum have been reported, it may be more aptly described as 'an unpleasant disease that recovers on its own' (David and Longson 1985). Mortality rates approaching 75%, cited in the literature before the advent of effective antiviral therapy, were undoubtedly an overestimation (Wheeler and Abele 1966, Sanderson et al. 1987).

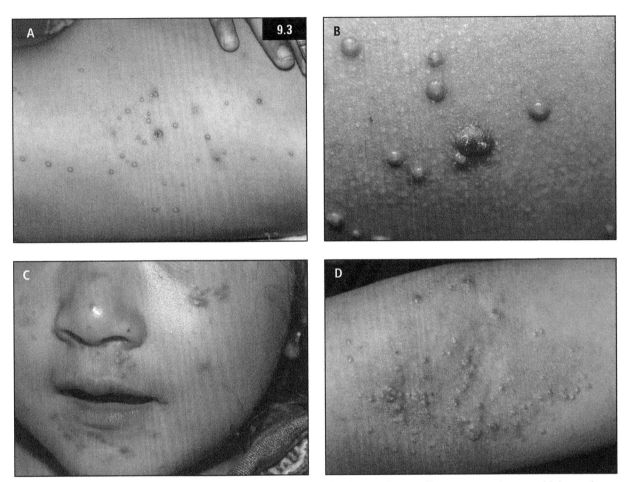

Fig 9.3 (A) Children with atopic dermatitis often develop viral infections such as molluscum contagiosum, which may be extensive. (B) Individual pink papules display a central dell and may become crusted, (C) frequently involve the face, and (D) may occur in areas of eczema or induce perilesional dermatitis.

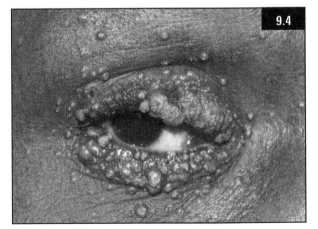

Fig 9.4 Molluscum contagiosum of the eyelid is a vexing therapeutic dilemma.

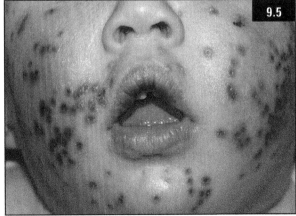

Fig 9.5 Eczema herpeticum: note discrete, punched-out erosions.

Eczema herpeticum is associated with both primary and secondary herpes simplex virus infection (Wollenberg *et al.* 2003b) and tends to affect the head, neck, and trunk, but more extensive involvement may occur (**Fig 9.6**). Within 2 weeks, blisters rupture, dry out, and form crusts that heal, leaving pitted scars. Although the time course of the cutaneous eruption is 2–3 weeks, uncommonly more severe complications (eg, keratoconjunctivitis and viremia) may occur, leading to multiple-organ involvement, meningitis, and encephalitis (Wollenberg *et al.* 2003b). Lesions in the periorbital region may rarely cause eye involvement, which should be managed by an ophthalmologist with topical and systemic antivirals (Sais *et al.* 1994) (**Figs 9.7** and **9.8**).

Evidence suggests that patients with early onset AD and a history of food allergy, concomitant asthma, and rhinitis (so-called atopic dermorespiratory syndrome), high IgE levels, filaggrin mutations, and reduced ability to produce the AMPs HBD-2, HBD-3, and canthelicidin are predisposed to eczema herpeticum (Bork and Brauninger 1988, Wollenberg *et al.* 2003b, Beck *et al.* 2009, Gao *et al.* 2009, Hata *et al.* 2010, Hinz *et al.* 2011). Topical corticosteroid therapy is not associated with eczema herpeticum and suggestions that topical calcineurin inhibitors might

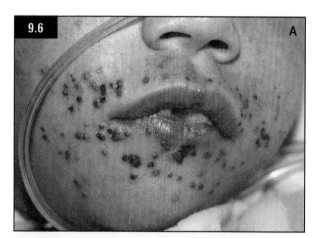

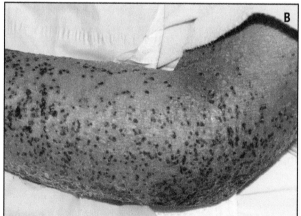

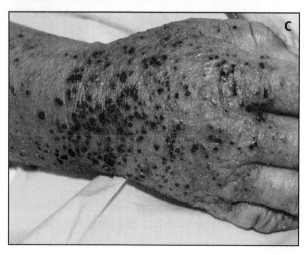

Fig 9.6 (A–C) Eczema herpeticum: child with extensive, painful vesicles, pustules, and erosions involving face and extremities. Discrete vesicles, pustules, and crusted erosions indicate the underlying herpetic nature of the eruption.

predispose to an increased frequency await more rigorous confirmation (Wahn *et al.* 2002). One group has reported an association of topical tacrolimus-induced eczema herpeticum in a subgroup of AD patients with genetic polymorphisms in the IL-18 gene promoter region (Osawa *et al.* 2007).

The diagnosis of eczema herpeticum is confirmed by positive Tzanck staining. Although viral cultures may be obtained, treatment should be instituted immediately when the diagnosis is suspected. Local disease may be treated on an outpatient basis; however, for children and immunocompromised individuals, it is prudent to start intravenous acyclovir (aciclovir) therapy in a hospital setting. This assures adequate blood levels of acyclovir, especially in patients who are toxic or who may reject or regurgitate oral therapy. Better absorption of oral valaciclovir and famciclovir make these agents preferable to acyclovir as an outpatient treatment in adults and older children. Topical antiseptic lotions may also help prevent bacterial superinfection and hasten drying of the vesicles. Adequate analgesia should be provided and bacterial superinfection treated aggressively with systemic and topical antibiotics.

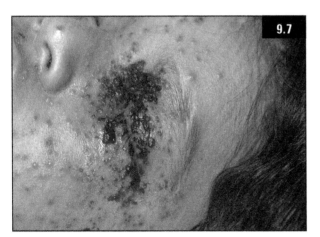

Fig 9.7 Severe eczema herpeticum of the eyelid: ophthalmological consultation is indicated to rule out involvement of the eye, which, although rare, may have serious consequences.

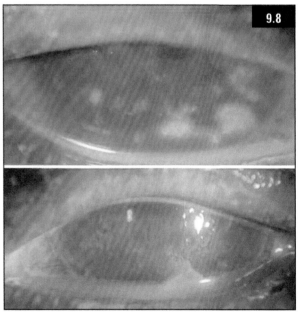

Fig 9.8 A rare case of bilateral dendritic herpetic keratitis manifesting as dendriform epithelial edema in a patient with eczema herpeticum. (Reprinted with kind permission from Springer Science and Business Media from Higaki *et al.* 2008.)

ECZEMA VACCINATUM

Routine immunization for smallpox was abandoned after worldwide eradication of variola in the 1970s. Today, immunization is restricted to military personnel, specialized laboratory workers, and, in some countries, hospital workers (Engler *et al.* 2002). Patients with AD may develop a disseminated eruption of firm, deep-seated blisters and pustules in the same stage of development with fever, malaise, and lymphadenopathy, known as eczema vaccinatum (Jen and Chang 2010) (**Fig 9.9**).

Although smallpox immunization is contraindicated in anyone with AD, eczema vaccinatum can still occur after accidental contact with immunized individuals such as in families of military personnel (Copeman and Wallace 1964, Lane and Millar 1971, Vora *et al.* 2008).

When immunization in the USA was recommended for the general population, the frequency of eczema vaccinatum was 123 per million primary vaccines, with a case fatality rate of 1–5% (Lane and Millar 1971). Recent data from a cohort of Israeli Defense Force recruits showed an overall complication rate of 4 per 100 000 immunizations, with a low rate of severe complications (Haim *et al.* 2000). Seemingly contradictory data indicate that two-thirds of those with eczema vaccinatum do not have active AD at the time of presumed vaccinia virus exposure (Copeman and Wallace 1964).

Federal law in the USA requires that public health authorities be informed if variola or eczema vaccinatum is suspected. Laboratory testing using polymerase chain reaction and electron microscopy is performed by health authorities in credible cases. Therapy involves rapid administration of vaccinia immunoglobulin, stored at the Centers for Disease Control in Atlanta, Georgia. This should be started as soon as possible, with a suggested initial dose of 0.6–1.0 ml/kg body weight (Kempe 1960). The antiviral agent cidofovir has activity against orthopox viruses and may be used in cases of severe eczema vaccinatum (Cono *et al.* 2003). Future treatments for eczema vaccinatum may include synthetic antimicrobial compounds called ceragenins and the use of monoclonal antibodies to vaccinia (Howell *et al.* 2009, Rico *et al.* 2009, Tomimori *et al.* 2011).

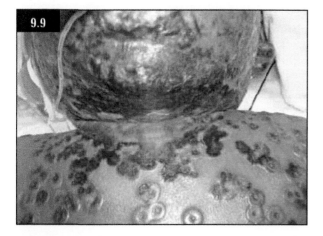

Fig 9.9 Severe eczema vaccinatum in a household contact of a smallpox vaccinee – day 7. (Reprinted from Vora *et al.* 2008 with permission of Oxford University Press.)

CONCLUSION

The increased prevalence of viruses, fungi, and especially bacteria in patients with AD is well described in the literature. These infections may precipitate atopic flares and contribute to disease activity. Although it has long been known that patients with AD have an impaired cutaneous immunity and susceptibility to infections, insights into mechanisms have only recently surfaced. These include decreased recruitment of plasmacytoid dendritic cells to the skin, as well as a potential role for defensins and canthelicidins (Ong *et al.* 2002, Wollenberg *et al.* 2002).

Regardless of the mechanisms, infections create challenging management problems for both patient and physician, warranting prompt evaluation and treatment.

Clinical suggestions

1. Although the ultimate efficacy of antibiotics for AD is controversial, *Staphylococcus aureus* is known to exacerbate the condition and many clinicians give a short course of antibiotics such as cephalexin together with topical corticosteroids to help control disease flares.
2. If antibiotic therapy is contemplated, it is well worth the effort to perform a bacterial culture to exclude MRSA and streptococcal involvement.
3. Dilute bleach baths (twice weekly for 5–10 min) together with intermittent intranasal mupirocin (twice daily for 5 days/month) help control AD and are a useful therapeutic adjunct in children aged >9 months (Huang *et al.* 2009). An instruction video for giving bleach baths is available at www.eczemacenter.org/ecvc.htm#bleachbaths. Care should be taken with children not to exceed the recommended concentration of bleach in bath water (final concentration: 0.005%). Dry skin, irritation, and itching occur rarely. The child should rinse off in the shower after the bath and emollients should be applied.
4. In patients with recalcitrant head and neck lesions that worsened during adolescence or young adulthood, suspect allergy to *Malassezia* spp. There is evidence in the literature suggesting that these patients may benefit from a 1- to 2-month course of oral antifungals. Ciclopirox cream may be useful in those in whom use of oral antifungals is not warranted or is contraindicated (Darabi *et al.* 2009).
5. Suspect eczema herpeticum in patients who present with sudden worsening of eczema, vesiculation, and the presence of tiny 'punched-out' erosions. Although localized disease can be treated in the outpatient setting, hospitalization and treatment with intravenous acyclovir (aciclovir) is warranted for children and immunocompromised patients.

CHAPTER 10

TOPICAL TREATMENT OF ATOPIC DERMATITIS

William Abramovits

Schemata (structured frameworks or plans) are frequently used in medicine to guide medical decision-making and put forward stepwise treatment plans. Although sometimes overly simplistic, they can provide a logical organizational basis for the topical treatment of diseases, such as atopic dermatitis. Such a schema is provided herein.

Systemic treatments and phototherapy of atopic dermatitis are discussed in Chapters 11 and 12 respectively. This chapter deals with topical therapy and is divided into two sections, one addressing barrier function repair, the other the use of medications intended to correct the immune dysfunction that characterizes the disease. **Fig 10.1** depicts a paradigm proposed for the treatment of atopic dermatitis.

For half a century, topical corticosteroids have been the uncontested gold standard of therapy for atopic dermatitis. At the turn of the millennium, the introduction of topical calcineurin inhibitors brought about a significant change in the approach to treatment of this condition (Abramovits *et al.* 2003, Abramovits 2005). More recently, this treatment paradigm has been changed by the marketing of topical agents as registered medical devices requiring prescription, which by definition do not contain active ingredients, but which are able to improve signs and symptoms of disease (Abramovits and Boguniewicz 2006, Abramovits and Perlmutter 2006). In addition, several over-the-counter remedies have been reported to relieve eczema based on purported 'controlled' studies.

The focus of this chapter is to provide treatment recommendations supported by rigorous studies conforming to principles of evidence-based medicine. When adequate studies are not available, an approach based on personal experience is proposed, clearly identifying inherent bias.

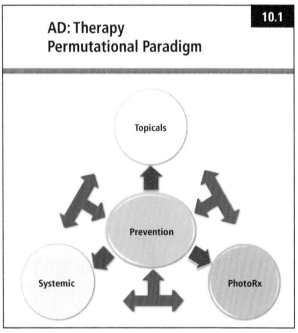

Fig 10.1 Permutational paradigm for the treatment of atopic dermatitis

GENERAL TREATMENT MEASURES

It is generally accepted that patient compliance often deviates substantially from treatment recommendations. The importance of educating patients and caregivers about possible triggers, moisturization, and proper use of medications cannot be overemphasized. Consider instruction about hydration, allergens and irritants, or agents that disrupt and repair barrier function (Chapter 8).

When recommending wet dressings, medicated or nonmedicated baths, and even when using seemingly simple applications, a demonstration in the medical office assures patient understanding and can make the difference between therapeutic success and failure. Certain vehicles such as foams, increasingly employed for their elegance, ease of application, and lack of sensitizers, are often expensive and typically require patient instruction to maximize the benefit–cost ratio.

Patients are sometimes confused as to how much cream or ointment to use in a particular area of involvement. Finlay *et al.* (1989) introduced the concept of the *fingertip unit* to simplify how much medication should be applied. One fingertip unit equals the amount of cream or ointment expressed from a tube with a 5-mm diameter nozzle, applied from the distal skin crease to the tip of an adult's index finger on the palmar aspect. Demonstrating the use of the fingertip unit helps patients understand how to dose creams and ointments without waste (**Fig 10.2**). Moreover, addressing issues such as steroid phobia or concerns about the risks of long-term toxicity

---

10.2

A parent's guide to the use of topical treatment

Use the adult fingertip unit (FTU) as your guide

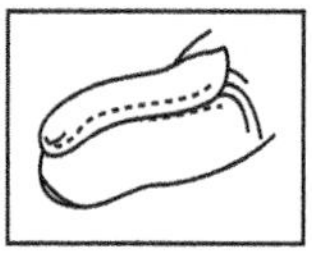

One adult FTU

The diagrams of the child (below) show how many FTUs of cream or ointment are required to cover each area of the child's body.

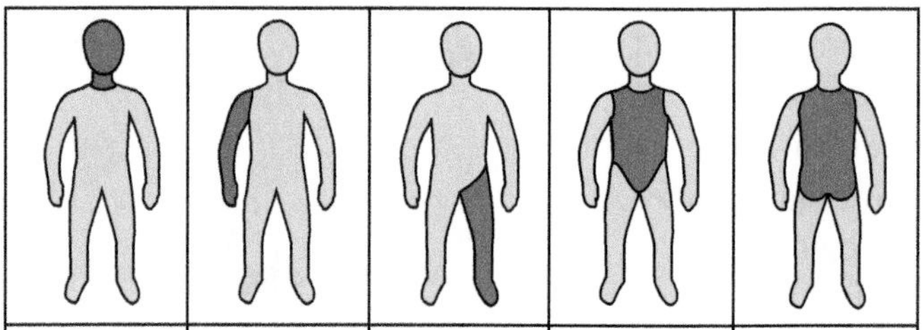

	Face & neck	Arm & hand	Leg & foot	Trunk (front)	Trunk (back) inc. buttocks
Age	Number of FTUs				
3–6 mth	1	1	1½	1	1½
1–2 y	1½	1½	2	2	3
3–5 y	1½	2	3	3	3½
6–10 y	2	2½	4½	3½	5

Fig 10.2 A patient/parent information sheet based on the 'fingertip unit' guidelines. (Reprinted from Long *et al.* 1998 with permission from John Wiley & Sons.)

at the start of treatment increases the likelihood of compliance. Finally, explaining that a topical agent can positively impact quality-of-life issues including sleep (through itch relief), odor, and beauty should also encourage compliance (Abramovits *et al.* 2005).

TOPICAL CORTICOSTEROIDS

Corticosteroid preparations remain the topical option most likely to succeed in the acute management of severe atopic dermatitis. Unfortunately pharmacologists have been unable to develop potent topical corticosteroid preparations devoid of local or systemic adverse effects, such as atrophy and hypothalamic–adrenal–axis suppression. On the one hand, superpotent preparations may be usable only for short periods of time to minimize toxicity, whereas, on the other, weaker agents may be used continuously but often lack efficacy for recalcitrant disease. Either way, the optimum choice may be unclear.

Prescribing a strong corticosteroid requires vigilance for early signs of toxicity. The clinician should monitor the patient for cutaneous atrophy, hypochromia, telangiectasias, bruising, and striae. Adrenal insufficiency, osteoporosis, hypertension, and hyperglycemia may occur but are less common. Frequent follow-up visits are the best way to monitor for harmful outcomes.

Starting with a potent preparation and bringing about rapid improvement may strengthen the physician–patient relationship. In addition, this approach brings opportunities for education, as well as the disclosure and review of personal, social, and economic issues. Lower-potency corticosteroids may be safer, but can require the gestalt of an experienced clinician to minimize failure. Many new corticosteroid preparations, mostly branded (and therefore more expensive), in novel vehicles or presentations are currently being marketed (*Box 10.1*). As potency may be determined by vehicle, it is emphasized that the same corticosteroid at the same concentration may be more potent in a cream than in a lotion, in a spray than in a cream, or in a hydroethanolic vehicle than in an emollient foam. Frequency of application may determine efficacy and safety as well.

Box 10.1   Generic Name

Class 1 – superpotent

Betamethasone dipropionate 0.05% augmented cream/ointment/gel

Clobetasol propionate 0.05% cream/ointment/lotion/solution

Diflorasone diacetate 0.05% cream/ointment

Halobetasol propionate 0.05% cream/ointment

Class 2 – potent

Amcinonide 0.1% cream/ointment

Betamethasone dipropionate 0.05% ointment

Desoximetasone 0.25% cream/ointment; 0.05% gel

Fluocinonide 0.05% cream/ointment

Halcinonide 0.1% cream/ointment

(continued)

Box 10.1   Generic Name

Class 3 upper mid-strength

Betamethasone dipropionate 0.05% cream

Betamethasone valerate 0.1% ointment

Fluticasone propionate 0.005% ointment

Mometasone furoate 0.1% ointment

Triamcinolone acetonide 0.5% cream

Class 4 mid-strength

Betamethasone valerate 0.12% foam

Clocortolone pivalate 0.1% cream

Desoximetasone 0.05% cream

Fluocinolone acetonide 0.025% ointment

Flurandrenolide 0.05% ointment

Triamcinolone 0.1% ointment

Class 5 lower mid-strength

Betamethasone dipropionate 0.05% lotion

Betamethasone valerate 0.1% cream/lotion

Fluocinolone acetonide 0.025% cream

Flurandrenolide 0.05% cream

Fluticasone propionate 0.05% cream

Hydrocortisone butyrate 0.1% cream

Hydrocortisone valerate 0.2% cream

Prednicarbate 0.1% cream

Triamcinolone 0.1% cream/lotion

Class 6 – mild strength

Aclometasone dipropionate 0.05% cream/ointment

Desonide 0.05% cream

Fluocinolone acetonide 0.01% cream/solution/oil

Class 7 – least potent

Topicals with hydrocortisone acetate, dexamethasone, flumethasone, methylprednisolone and prednisone

Before the introduction of effective alternatives to corticosteroids, options for ongoing therapy included preparations of lesser potency, 'pulse' dosing of higher potency topical steroids, or withdrawal of therapy; all fraught with the risk of losing control over the eczema (Thomas *et al.* 2002).

TOPICAL ANTIPRURITICS AND TAR

Topical antipruritics and antihistamines, including calamine plus diphenhydramine in shake lotions, and more recently in gels, plus promethazine creams, pramoxine, camphor, and menthol, among others, may provide transient itch reduction. Doxepin 5% cream is indicated in the USA for the short-term treatment of moderate pruritus associated with atopic dermatitis in adults, but carries the risk of sensitization and somnolence (Taylor *et al.* 1996, Sabroe *et al.* 1997). It should not be used in children aged under 12.

Tar derivatives have minor anti-inflammatory effects and relieve itch but they lack elegance and may cause irritation and folliculitis. For this reason they are rarely prescribed nowadays in the USA (Munkvad 1989, Langeveld-Wildschut *et al.* 2000).

TOPICAL CALCINEURIN INHIBITORS

A significant paradigm shift occurred in the treatment of atopic eczema with the introduction of topical calcineurin inhibitors (Abramovits *et al.* 2003). Unfortunately, a black box warning imposed by the US Food and Drug Administration (FDA) in late 2005 dampened initial enthusiasm for these agents by implying a theoretical risk of malignancy, including lymphomas. Understandably, many physicians, particularly nondermatologists, have become hesitant to prescribe this class of medications. Recent studies, however, involving large cohorts of patients with atopic dermatitis, support the safety of topical calcineurin inhibitors, and argue against any significant association with cancer (Koo *et al.* 2005, Fleischer 2006, Callen *et al.* 2007, Margolis *et al.* 2007). The potential risk of cancer was based on 20 case reports of lymphoma worldwide in postmarketing surveillance that did not verify

a causal relationship (Thaci and Salgo 2010). In studies of almost 10 000 patients treated in clinical trials with tacrolimus, no lymphomas occurred and only 2 cases of solid tumors were reported in 25 000 pimecrolimus-treated patients. This was less than in the control group (Thaci and Salgo 2010). Considering the large number of prescriptions that have been written for topical calcineurin inhibitors, the number of malignancies reported is less than that expected in the general population.

Pimecrolimus 1% cream and tacrolimus 0.03% and 0.1% ointment are marketed in most countries. Both reduce pruritus efficiently, and both decrease the severity of eczema signs and involved body surface area, thus minimizing the need for topical corticosteroids. Tacrolimus ointment-treated patients have significantly greater improvement in the validated Eczema Area Severity Index (EASI) score than those treated with pimecrolimus (Kaufmann *et al.* 2006, Fleischer *et al.* 2007). Transient burning may occur with both agents and is related to the severity of disease when treatment is initiated (Kempers *et al.* 2004, Paller *et al.* 2005).

The effectiveness of pimecrolimus in the treatment of eczema is similar to that of lower-potency corticosteroids, such as hydrocortisone, dexamethasone, and betamethasone valerate 0.1%. Tacrolimus potency matches or exceeds that of mid-potency products, hydrocortisone butyrate 0.1%, and betamethasone valerate 0.2% ointments (Rigopoulos *et al.* 2004, Ashcroft *et al.* 2005, Simpson and Noble 2005, Winiski *et al.* 2007). On the basis of large clinical trials, it is reasonable to use calcineurin inhibitors in patients with atopic dermatitis to prevent disease flares, reduce severity, lessen the need for topical corticosteroids, and sustain disease improvement.

Tacrolimus ointment may be used alone or in combination to treat all severities of atopic dermatitis, whereas pimecrolimus cream is indicated only for milder disease, mostly as a steroid-sparing agent (Alomar *et al.* 2004). Despite a theoretical risk that topical tacrolimus and pimecrolimus might increase skin infections, and the isolated reports of such occurrences, overall the rates of infection have not increased as a result of their use. Furthermore there is evidence suggesting a protective effect in eczema patients (Park *et al.* 2005).

MEDICAL DEVICES FOR THE TREATMENT OF ATOPIC DERMATITIS

The US FDA recently approved two products as medical devices for treating signs and symptoms of atopic dermatitis. The first, Mimyx, is a cream containing the cannabinoid palmitoylethanolamide, an endogenous bioactive fatty acid deficient in atopic skin; the other, Atopiclair, is a cream containing a mixture of ingredients including glycyrrhetinic acid, telmestine, *Vitis vinifera*, capryloyl glycine, shea butter, and hyaluronic acid. Palmitoylethanolamine binds to cannabinoid receptors on mast cells and other immune cells and modulates their response to antigens. Levels of histamine, and interleukin (IL)-4, IL-6, and IL-8 are reduced. Palmitoylethanolamine also binds to cannabinoid receptors in nerve fibers and decreases pruritus and burning messaging to the brain. Glycyrrhetinic acid (GA) inhibits 11β-hydroxysteroid dehydrogenase, an enzyme responsible for the conversion of cortisol into cortisone. GA also selectively inhibits the complement cascade. *Vitis vinifera* (grapevine) contains bioflavonoid antioxidants and telmestine. It has anti-inflammatory effects via inhibition of metalloproteases. The agents in both products are formulated to restore and maintain proper skin barrier function (Abramovits and Boguniewicz 2006, Abramovits and Perlmutter 2006).

The paucity of head-to-head studies makes it difficult to ascertain the relative efficacy of these *medical devices* compared with low-potency topical corticosteroids or pimecrolimus (Abramovits and Perlmutter 2007). In a study of patients with topical corticosteroid resistance, pimecrolimus was especially beneficial in the head and neck areas (Leung *et al.* 2009). Despite the lack of head-to-head comparison studies, insurance reimbursement issues and government restraints, and lack of consensus among various investigators, a paradigm is suggested for the topical treatment of atopic dermatitis (**Fig 10.3**).

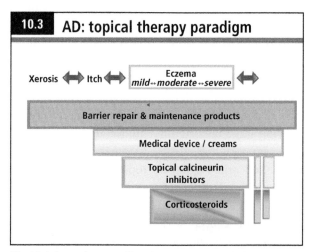

Fig 10.3 Stepwise paradigm for treating atopic dermatitis.

TOPICAL TREATMENT PARADIGM

Clinical suggestions

1. When eczema is mild it may be controlled with agents that preserve or repair barrier function; these should be tried first. The safety of these agents permits ongoing use until there is spontaneous resolution of the disease. Barrier repair and maintenance products have a steroid-sparing effect and thus lessen the need for topical corticosteroids and other agents.
2. When dermatitis is more severe, either of the two medical device creams – one containing palmitoylethanolamine and the other glycyrrhetinic acid – can be added. Alternatively, the clinician may opt for a topical calcineurin inhibitor. If the condition responds satisfactorily, the application frequency of topical calcineurin inhibitors may be stepped down with gradual discontinuation of these agents. (Note that maintenance may continue with barrier repairing agents or combinations of these drugs can be used uninterruptedly.)
3. If the condition is even more severe, combinations of high- and low-potency topical steroids will likely be required until the disorder is stable. Once in remission, a step-down approach should involve either intermittent applications and/or progressive reductions in corticosteroid potency. Corticosteroids may eventually be discontinued altogether or used sparingly together with topical calcineurin inhibitors, medical device creams, or barrier repair and maintenance products.
4. If this protocol fails, reconsideration of the permutational paradigm illustrated in **Fig 10.1**, inclusive of phototherapy, systemic therapy, and other supportive measures, must be pursued.

CHAPTER 11

SYSTEMIC AGENTS FOR THE TREATMENT OF ATOPIC DERMATITIS

Arash Akhavan and Donald Rudikoff

Atopic dermatitis (AD) is a chronic inflammatory skin condition with the potential for great social, economic, and psychological morbidity (Hong *et al.* 2008). A variety of treatment modalities are available for the management of AD, ranging from topical emollients to powerful systemic immunosuppressive agents with potentially serious side effects. Topical therapies include corticosteroid preparations, topical antibiotics, calcineurin inhibitors, and wet wraps followed by emollients or topical corticosteroids. In more severe cases refractory to topical treatment, phototherapy, systemic antibiotics, sedating antihistamines, leukotriene antagonists, systemic corticosteroids, and other immunomodulators may be of value. This chapter reviews the use of systemic immunomodulatory agents for the treatment of AD.

Systemic corticosteroids remain an effective and frequently utilized immunosuppressive treatment option for severe AD, but side effects limit their long-term use. Other immunomodulatory agents that have been used include the calcineurin inhibitor cyclosporine (ciclosporin; Neoral), azathioprine (Imuran), interferon (IFN)-γ therapy, methotrexate, mycophenolate mofetil (Cellcept), and to a limited extent a few of the newer biologic immunomodulators. Physicians and their patients must be aware that treatment with any of these agents is considered 'off-label' use. Patients receiving immunosuppressive drugs should undergo purified protein derivative (PPD) testing for tuberculosis and should not receive live vaccines. They should be used with extreme caution in patients from areas where strongyloidiasis is endemic (Ghosh and Ghosh 2007).

SYSTEMIC CORTICOSTEROIDS

Systemic corticosteroids are effective in treating acute flares of AD. With rare exceptions, they are not a good option for long-term treatment because of their known potential for severe adverse effects (Sonenthal *et al.* 1993). Ideally, therapy with systemic corticosteroids should be started only with a plan in place to transition to safer topical or systemic treatment as quickly as possible. A limited number of clinical trials, all in children, support the vast amount of anecdotal evidence for the use of systemic corticosteroids to treat AD flares (Heddle *et al.* 1984, La Rosaa *et al.* 1995).

Corticosteroids act via: inhibition of prostaglandin production and release; multiple actions on macrophages; apoptosis of eosinophils and activated lymphocytes; depletion of tissue mast cells; reduction of endothelial adhesion molecule expression, including intercellular adhesion molecule-1 (ICAM-1) and E-selectin; and limiting egress of leukocytes to areas of inflammation (Fauci *et al.* 1976, Vane and Botting 1987, Goldsmith *et al.* 1990, Nakano *et al.* 1990, Cronstein *et al.* 1992, Woolley *et al.* 1996, Finotto *et al.* 1997).

They also alter production of cytokines such as interleukin (IL)-4, IL-5, IL-10, and IFN-γ with differential effects depending on the stage of T-cell activation and, moreover, inactivate certain proinflammatory transcription factors (AP-1, NFκB, NF-AT) and upregulate cytokine inhibitory proteins (Brinkmann and Kristofic 1995, Almawi *et al.* 1999, Miyaura and Iwata 2002).

ADULTS

Treatment in adults is usually begun with prednisone at dosages of 1 mg/kg per day (usually 40–80 mg/day) in a single morning dose or in two divided doses for a period of about 1 week, and then rapidly tapered. Alternatively, triamcinolone acetonide can be administered by intramuscular injection at a dosage of 40–60 mg. Corticosteroid therapy can be accompanied by aggressive topical therapy and phototherapy to maintain remission.

CHILDREN

In children, a short course of oral corticosteroids at a dosage of 1 mg/kg body weight of prednisone or equivalent dose of prednisolone can be used in those whose disorder cannot be controlled by topical therapy, but long-term use should be avoided (Akdis et al. 2006). In cases in whom more prolonged courses of corticosteroids have been used, three critical clinical situations may occur: adrenal suppression, steroid withdrawal syndrome, and relapse/flare of the disease for which steroids were originally prescribed (Alves et al. 2008). Patients with adrenal insufficiency may display nonspecific symptoms such as anorexia, nausea, vomiting, weakness, malaise, myalgia, arthralgia, weight loss, postural hypotension, and depression, and may progress to adrenal crisis with cardiovascular collapse (Shulman et al. 2007). Steroid withdrawal syndrome manifests with physical or psychological symptoms, including many of the nonspecific symptoms previously mentioned and also emotional lability, mood swings, and sometimes delirium and psychotic states (Alves et al. 2008). A well-known pediatric dermatologist has written:

> There is no magic formula for corticosteroid use in children, except to say that it is safest to use the smallest possible dose for the shortest period of time (Lucky 1984).

ADVERSE EVENTS AND CAUTIONS

Risk of potential side effects increases with duration of use and includes growth retardation in children, Cushing syndrome, hypertension, glucose intolerance, osteoporosis, weight gain, changes in mood and sleep pattern, glaucoma, and cataracts. Should long-term therapy with systemic corticosteroids be required, alternate-day administration regimens can be used to decrease the risk of some, though not all, of these side effects. Adverse events not reduced with alternate-day dosing regimens include posterior subcapsular cataract formation, growth retardation, and osteoporosis (Truhan and Ahmed 1989).

It should be borne in mind, moreover, that withdrawal of steroids can sometimes result in a rebound phenomenon with worsening of skin lesions. Patients with rebound typically resemble those having an acute exacerbation of AD, both clinically and in their immunological profile, with a predominantly T-helper type 2 cell (Th2) pattern of immunity (Forte et al. 2005).

CYCLOSPORINE AND OTHER CALCINEURIN INHIBITORS

Cyclosporine is a macrolide inhibitor of calcineurin-dependent pathways that reduces levels of proinflammatory cytokines involved in AD skin inflammation. It forms a complex with cyclophilin, which blocks the translocation to the nucleus of cytosolic Nf-AT (Schreiber and Crabtree 1992). IL-2 is the most important cytokine so affected but cyclosporine may also have more subtle effects on Th1 and Th2 balance (Porter and Clipstone 2002), eg, studies of the effect of cyclosporine on T-regulatory cells have had conflicting results that might be explained by the different doses of the drug used in the studies (Brandt et al. 2009, Hijnen et al. 2009). Cyclosporine also affects keratinocyte differentiation and filaggrin production (Santini et al. 2001).

There are numerous studies proving the efficacy of cyclosporine in the treatment of AD, in both adults and children (Berth-Jones et al. 1996, 1997, Zonneveld et al. 1996, Harper et al. 2000). A reduction in pruritus can be seen within a week and marked improvement with alleviation of sleep disruption by 2 months.

Doses typically range from 2.5 mg/kg per day to 5 mg/kg per day. Cyclosporine can be started at the higher dosage range to obtain rapid control, and then be tapered to the lowest effective dose that provides adequate control of signs and symptoms of disease. Higher doses may be preferable in patients with extensive, severe disease for symptom relief, but are more likely to be complicated by an elevated creatinine level or hypertension. A recent study suggests that control of atopic dermatitis can be obtained in adults with low-dose cyclosporine (100 mg/day) if it is administered before meals (Nakamura *et al.* 2011). Cyclosporine has been reported to restore normal growth indices in children who have had growth retardation from extensive disease (Zaki *et al.* 1996). The drug is generally well tolerated in children although some have experienced headache and abdominal pain. Cyclosporine can also be given in 12-week intervals separated by a few months' rest with good results and less overall exposure to the drug (Harper *et al.* 2000).

Before starting cyclosporine it is customary to obtain two separate pretreatment creatinine levels and use the average of these two measurements as the *baseline creatinine level*. Should the creatinine level during treatment exceed this baseline by 25%, the cyclosporine level is reduced. Alternatively, cyclosporine can be started at the lower dosage range of 2.5–3.0 mg/kg per day and the daily dose can be increased if relief is not obtained. In children, nausea can be avoided by starting at the lower dose (Borchard and Orchard 2008). With its relatively rapid and dependable effect on AD, cyclosporine is a commonly used option for acute flares of severe AD.

Unfortunately relapse and, less commonly, flares of disease may occur with cessation of the drug, usually after 2–6 weeks (Berth-Jones *et al.* 1996). Approximately 10% of children treated with cyclosporine may experience a remission more than 6 months after discontinuation of treatment (Berth-Jones *et al.* 1996, Zaki *et al.* 1996).

Practitioners should be aware that there are two major preparations of cyclosporine: cyclosporine USP (Sandimmune) and cyclosporine USP modified (Neoral) with improved absorption. They are not biologically equivalent. The dosages quoted in the various studies in the treatment of AD refer to cyclosporine USP modified. If a patient's insurance plan requires generic substitution, it is best to stay with the same branded generic when refilling cyclosporine prescriptions to ensure stable blood levels of the drug.

ADVERSE EVENTS AND CAUTIONS

As a result of the potential for significant toxicity, continuous use of cyclosporine should be limited in duration, typically to periods of less than 1 year. The most significant adverse effects include nephrotoxicity, hypertension, and hyperlipidemia. Other side effects include hypertrichosis, gingival hyperplasia, liver toxicity, and paresthesias. There is also the potential for numerous drug interactions with cyclosporine via the cytochrome P450 pathway.

A baseline physical exam should be performed and certain laboratory work obtained before starting therapy with cyclosporine. As a result of the known potential for skin cancer and lymphoma in transplant recipients on cyclosporine therapy, physical examination should include assessment of the skin and examination of the lymph nodes, liver, and spleen. Careful monitoring for toxicity is imperative with ongoing use, including periodic complete blood cell counts, kidney and liver function tests, urinalysis, and serum magnesium level, and physical exam including blood pressure measurement (Sabbagh *et al.* 2008). To minimize the risk of permanent kidney damage, dosing protocols for cyclosporine have been established to respond to rising serum creatinine values (Griffiths *et al.* 2004).

Another strategy for minimizing long-term side effects of cyclosporine is using a dosage of 5 mg/kg per day as an acute management strategy for 6 weeks, followed by maintenance treatment with enteric-coated mycophenolate sodium (1440 mg/day) (Haeck *et al.* 2011). When compared with maintenance therapy with cyclosporine 3 mg/kg per day for 30 weeks, patients maintained on mycophenolate achieved greater disease control after discontinuation of treatment.

AZATHIOPRINE

Azathioprine is a purine analog that suppresses cell-mediated immunity and humoral immunity. Although azathioprine is cytotoxic to Langerhans cells (LCs) and inhibits their alloantigen-presenting capacity, its long-term immunosuppressant effect on LCs is probably based on depletion of these cells from the epidermis by bone marrow suppression (Liu and Wong 1997).

Results from several trials support the efficacy of azathioprine in the treatment of severe AD (Lear *et al.* 1996, Berth-Jones *et al.* 2002, Kuanprasert *et al.* 2002). Dosage of the medication ranges from 1 mg/kg per day to 3 mg/kg per day, but should be determined based on the patient's pretreatment level of thiopurine methyltransferase (TPMT), an enzyme that catalyzes the metabolism of the drug. Onset of action with azathioprine is typically slow, with benefits apparent 2–3 months after onset of treatment.

ADVERSE EVENTS AND CAUTIONS

Major concerns with azathioprine use include risk of bone marrow suppression and increased risk of malignancy, including non-Hodgkin lymphoma and squamous cell skin cancer (Meggitt and Reynolds 2001). In 2011, the US Food and Drug Administration (FDA) added a black box warning to azathioprine of the possibility of developing hepatosplenic T-cell lymphoma, which is highly aggressive and frequently lethal (Denby and Beck 2012). This type of lymphoma has not as yet been described in patients receiving azathioprine for AD.

Gastrointestinal side effects including severe nausea and epigastric pain can be quite common, including rates as high as 10% in at least one study. Drug hypersensitivity syndrome has been reported in some patients receiving azathioprine (Knowles *et al.* 1995). It presents with fever, hypotension and oliguria, and gastrointestinal symptoms but patients may also develop a maculopapular rash, urticaria, vasculitis, erythema multiforme, erythema nodosum, hepatotoxicity, and nephritis.

Patients with deficient activity of the enzyme thiopurine methyltransferase (TPMT) have an increased risk for myelosuppression from azathioprine use. TPMT catalyzes the *S*-methylation of azathioprine, and a deficiency of the enzyme can lead to toxic accumulation of the drug (Dicarlo and McCall 2001). Approximately one in 300 white individuals is homozygous for the autosomal recessive deficiency of TPMT, and one in 10 is heterozygous with intermediate levels (Krynetski and Evans 2000). The dose of the medication used for each individual can be tailored based on his or her level of TPMT activity, thereby decreasing risk of hematological toxicity. Both anecdotally and in published reports, AD patients with partial TPMT deficiency have been successfully and safely treated using reduced doses of azathioprine, with the benefit of decreased risk for other adverse events such as hepatotoxicity secondary to efficacy at lower doses of medication (Murphy and Atherton 2003). Patients with elevated levels of TPMT may require higher dosages of azathioprine. Recent work suggests that poor response to treatment with azathioprine may result from TPMT enzyme induction to levels higher than baseline, resulting in preferential metabolism of the drug to an inactive metabolite (el-Azhary *et al.* 2009, Wolverton 2009). A strategy, using measurement of levels of the active metabolite 6-thioguanine and the inactive metabolite 6-methylmercaptopurine, has been proposed to guide treatment with azathioprine (el-Azhary *et al.* 2009). It must also be kept in mind that myelotoxicity can occur even in the presence of normal TPMT levels, as pointed out by a recent case report; thus blood counts should be monitored carefully, especially at the initiation of treatment or for increases in dosage levels (Wee *et al.* 2011).

MYCOPHENOLATE MOFETIL

Mycophenolate mofetil is a new purine synthesis pathway inhibitor that blocks the activity of the enzyme inosine monophosphate dehydrogenase. It decreases guanine nucleotides needed for RNA-primed DNA synthesis in T and B lymphocytes which rely on the new purine biosynthesis pathway. Lymphocytes are selectively targeted; other body cells that use the *salvage pathway* for purine synthesis are for the most part not compromised.

Mycophenolate mofetil has been used widely in dermatology, most notably for bullous diseases. Doses of 1–2 g daily are typically used in the treatment of adult AD. It is best administered in divided doses two to four times daily to reduce gastrointestinal side effects. There are only a few, small, published uncontrolled studies supporting the use of mycophenolate mofetil in AD (Neuber *et al.* 2000, Grundmann-Kollmann *et al.* 2001, Murray and Cohen 2007). Most patients in these studies showed improvement in disease severity within 1–3 months of initiation of treatment. A recent retrospective study of eight patients with severe AD confirmed the efficacy of the drug (Ballester *et al.* 2009). Five patients improved by week 4 of treatment and experienced long-term improvement of their disease. Another retrospective analysis looked at the efficacy of mycophenolate as systemic monotherapy in children with severe recalcitrant AD (Heller *et al.* 2007). Of 14 patients with severe disease, 4 (29%) achieved complete clearance, 4 (29%) had >90% improvement, 5 (35%) had 60–90% improvement, and 1 (7%) failed to respond. Initial improvement was seen within 8 weeks (mean 4 weeks) and maximal effect after 8–12 weeks (mean 9 weeks). The dosage used in children was 40–50 mg/kg per day in younger children and 30–40 mg/kg per day in adolescents.

Although it works more slowly in AD compared with systemic corticosteroids and cyclosporine, and despite a comparatively limited number of published studies supporting its use for this disease, mycophenolate mofetil remains a valuable option for treating severe AD because of its relatively safe side-effect profile. As mentioned above, rapid improvement may be achieved with 6 weeks of cyclosporine 5 mg/kg per day followed by maintenance therapy with mycophenolate.

ADVERSE EVENTS AND CAUTIONS

The most commonly reported side effects with mycophenolate mofetil are gastrointestinal disturbances with nausea, diarrhea, and vomiting. As mentioned, the frequency of gastrointestinal complications can be reduced by dividing the daily dose into two to four equal doses per day. As with other systemic immunosuppressives, there is an increased risk of infection, but, unlike other medications in this class, long-term studies have not supported a strong carcinogenic role for the drug. It should be noted, however, that there are reports of central nervous system lymphomas in patients treated with the mycophenolate for lupus and myasthenia gravis (Dasgupta *et al.* 2005, Vernino *et al.* 2005, Tsang *et al.* 2010). A recent alert from the FDA highlighted a possible link between mycophenolate mofetil use and the development of progressive multifocal leukoencephalopathy (2008). Moreover, in one series, a patient developed herpes simplex retinitis while being treated for AD with mycophenolate mofetil (Grundmann-Kollmann *et al.* 2001).

Recently a new formulation of mycophenolate, Myfortic, has been introduced with enteric-coated mycophenolate sodium (EC-MPS), which may have fewer gastrointestinal side effects in some patients (Qureshi and Scheinfeld 2008). EC-MPS 720 mg twice daily is therapeutically equivalent to mycophenolate mofetil 1000 mg twice daily (Qureshi and Scheinfeld 2008). In a recent study, 10 patients aged 23–72 with severe, recalcitrant AD were treated with EC-MPS 720 mg twice daily for 6 months (van Velsen *et al.* 2009). In this small pilot study, treatment with EC-MPS resulted in a significant decrease in disease activity after 8 weeks of treatment.

METHOTREXATE

Methotrexate is a competitive inhibitor of dihydrofolate reductase that has immunosuppressive function through its inhibition of DNA synthesis in T lymphocytes. Although much more commonly used in dermatology in the treatment of psoriasis, there are several case reports and open-label prospective studies supporting the use of methotrexate in the treatment of AD (Egan *et al.* 1999, Shaffrali *et al.* 2003, Weatherhead *et al.* 2007, Lyakhovitsky *et al.* 2010). Goujon *et al.* (2006), in a retrospective study, reported on 20 patients (17–68 years old) who were treated for 3 months to 2.5 years with dosages of methotrexate varying from 7.5 mg to 25 mg once a week (Goujon *et al.* 2006). Of 20 patients, 15 (75%) improved after 3 months (beginning of improvement noted between weeks 4 and 8 of treatment) with

13/20 experiencing an improvement of greater than 70%. In another retrospective study, Lyakhovitsky *et al.* (2010) reported similar results. In their study, administration of methotrexate at weekly doses of 10–25 mg orally or by intramuscular injection for at least 8–12 weeks, with folic acid supplementation of 5 mg/week, resulted in an objective improvement in 16 of 20 patients. In both studies, some patients developed nausea and others elevation of liver function tests. Despite the retrospective nature of these studies, it would seem that methotrexate given once weekly may be an effective agent, especially in adults with severe disease. With regard to children, a retrospective study was conducted of 30 patients aged 2–16 years with severe AD treated with methotrexate (initial dose 0.5 mg/kg per week [maximum 15 mg]) and folic acid 1 mg per day on nontreatment days (Rouse and Siegfried 2008). Most patients experienced partial to complete response. Elevations in transaminases were unusual and transient and attributed to blood specimen collection within 1–2 days of drug administration.

ADVERSE EVENTS AND CAUTIONS

Methotrexate use is associated with serious potential side effects including liver toxicity, pulmonary fibrosis, and bone marrow suppression. The last is especially pertinent to elderly patients in whom serum creatinine may not accurately reflect true renal function. It is strongly recommended that practitioners using methotrexate review the 2009 guidelines for the use of methotrexate in psoriasis (Kalb *et al.* 2009). As with other systemic immunosuppressive medications, patients will need a baseline physical examination and laboratory work before initiating therapy. Patients on methotrexate must be closely monitored with complete blood cell counts, along with liver and kidney function tests. In the past, liver biopsy was recommended after psoriasis patients had been treated with a cumulative dose of 1–1.5 g to detect signs of progressive liver damage. Of interest, most rheumatologists rarely recommend liver biopsy

in patients being treated with methotrexate for rheumatoid arthritis. The 2009 National Psoriasis Foundation (NPF) Consensus Committee guidelines differentiate psoriasis patients into high- and low-risk groups based on the presence or absence of a history of or current alcohol consumption, persistently abnormal liver function tests, history of liver disease including hepatitis B or C, family history of inheritable liver disease, diabetes mellitus, obesity, history of hepatotoxic chemical or drug exposure, lack of folate supplementation, and hyperlipidemia. In high-risk patients, it is prudent to use an alternative systemic agent or to delay baseline liver biopsy to establish efficacy and tolerability first, before performing this invasive procedure. After baseline biopsy, the procedure is repeated after 1–1.5 g of cumulative therapy. Measurement of the serum procollagen III aminopeptide (P3NP) has been shown to be a valuable adjunct to the management of patients on long-term methotrexate therapy which may reduce the need for liver biopsy (Khan *et al.* 2006). This test is available in Europe but not in the USA.

There are a number of potentially dangerous drug interactions with methotrexate and a thorough medication history is needed before starting therapy. The concomitant use of trimethoprim–sulfamethoxazole with methotrexate is absolutely contraindicated because of the risk of profound neutropenia. Although trimethoprim–sulfamethoxazole has been advocated for the treatment of community-acquired methicillin (meticillin)-resistant *Staphylococcus aureus*, it should never be used in treating patients who are receiving methotrexate.

Nausea can be a common side effect of methotrexate therapy but can often be avoided by ongoing folate supplementation. Once clearance of disease has been attained, therapy should probably be limited to only a few months to a year with the hope that a prolonged remission may be maintained with topical treatment (Shaw *et al.* 2009).

INTERFERON-γ

IFN-γ is a Th1 cytokine, and an *in vitro* inhibitor of IL-4-induced IgE synthesis. Its mechanism of action in AD is, however, unclear, because studies have shown IFN-γ therapy to produce significant improvement in patients with AD without decreasing serum IgE levels (Musial *et al.* 1995). Several randomized, placebo-controlled trials have shown IFN-γ to be an effective and well-tolerated treatment for AD (Hanifin *et al.* 1993, Jang *et al.* 2000). IFN-γ is typically administered with oral analgesics to protect against the side effect of headaches and body aches. Despite initial enthusiasm with this agent, use of IFN-γ has not gained wide popularity among dermatologists, perhaps due to its high cost.

ADVERSE EVENTS AND CAUTIONS

Flu-like symptoms, with fever, muscle ache, headache, and chills, are common adverse events with INF-γ therapy. These adverse events can persist despite treatment with acetaminophen (paracetamol) and can limit acceptance of therapy.

IMMUNOBIOLOGICS

The great success of immunobiologics such as etanercept, adalimumab, and infliximab in the treatment of psoriasis has not been seen in the treatment of AD. Limited studies in patients with AD of infliximab, a chimeric monoclonal antibody to tumor necrosis factor (TNF)-α, have produced disappointing results (Jacobi *et al.* 2005).

Small studies with efalizumab, a humanized monoclonal antibody that binds to human CD11a, and rituximab, a chimeric monoclonal anti-CD20 antibody, have had somewhat more encouraging, albeit mixed, results (Chacko and Weinberg 2007, Forman and Garrett 2007, Sediva *et al.* 2008, Simon *et al.* 2008). Efalizumab has been removed from the US market because of concerns over reported cases of multifocal leukoencephalopathy with the drug.

Omalizumab, a humanized monoclonal antibody that specifically binds to the high-affinity FcεRI domain of free circulating IgE, and thus prevents binding of free serum IgE to mast cells and other effector cells, has shown some promise in treating patients with AD and elevated IgE (Caruso *et al.* 2010). In a pilot study, 21 patients aged 14–64 years with mild, moderate, and severe AD, and a mean pretreatment IgE level of 1521 IU/ml (range 18.2–8396 IU/ml), were treated with omalizumab over a period of 1–3 years (Sheinkopf *et al.* 2008). All patients showed clinical improvement with omalizumab therapy. In another small study, 11 patients with generalized AD and total serum IgE levels averaging >1000 IU/ml were treated with omalizumab 150 mg subcutaneously for 10 cycles in two 2-week intervals (Andres *et al.* 2008). Six patients showed clinical improvement, three were unchanged, and two had worsening of their eczema.

Another small study of omalizumab in three patients with AD and very high IgE levels (23 000, 5440, and 24 400 IU/ml) resulted in treatment failure, which was attributed to inadequate dosing of omalizumab relative to the levels of IgE (Krathen and Hsu 2005). It has been pointed out that patients with AD and IgE levels within the suggested dosing range (>700 IU/mL), for whom an expensive biologic agent might not be indicated, usually have milder disease (Beck and Saini 2006). A recent study showing lack of clinical efficacy of omalizumab for the treatment of AD, despite improvement in a number of IgE-related immune parameters, suggested that AD is not solely IgE-dependent and that the role of IgE in AD pathogenesis may be complex (Heil *et al.* 2010).

In summary, for now we must still rely on traditional systemic immunosuppressives for the treatment of severe and refractory AD.

Table 11.1   Drug mechanisms of action, adverse effects and drugs interactions

DRUG	MECHANISM OF ACTION	ADVERSE EFFECTS	DRUG INTERACTIONS
Systemic corticosteroids	Induce eosinopenia, monocytopenia, and lymphocytopenia Tissue mast cell depletion Inhibition of cytokines involved in inflammatory response	Fluid and electrolyte abnormalities: hypokalemic alkalosis Edema Hypertension Hyperglycemia Decreased immunity: infection, reactivation of dormant infections (tuberculosis, strongyloides infection) Peptic ulcer formation, when given with NSAIDs Myopathy Nervousness, insomnia, change in mood, psychosis Cataracts Osteoporosis and osteonecrosis Growth retardation in children Fetal abnormalities Cushingoid features: striae, fat redistribution, ecchymoses, acne, hirsuitism Effects resulting from withdrawal of therapy include: flare-up of AD, acute adrenal insufficiency, glucocorticoid withdrawal syndrome (fever, myalgias, arthalgias, malaise), pseudotumor cerebri	Erythromycin potentiates steroid effect (cytochrome P450 mediated) Diuretics (corticosteroids amplify diuretic-induced hypokalemia) Immunosuppressive agents: increased immunosuppression

Table 11.1   Drug mechanisms of action, adverse effects and drugs interactions *(continued)*

DRUG	MECHANISM OF ACTION	ADVERSE EFFECTS	DRUG INTERACTIONS
Cyclosporine (ciclosporin)	Binds to cyclophylin, inhibits calcineurin-dependent translocation of NFAT to nucleus, suppressing production of IL-2 and other cytokines Reduction of IL-2 receptor expression on T cells Decrease of eosinophil counts has been shown in patients with severe psoriasis	Nephrotoxicity Hypertension Tremor Hirsuitism Hyperlipidemia Gum hyperplasia	**Substances that inhibit CYP3A system microsomal enzymes can decrease cyclosporine metabolism and increase blood concentrations**: Calcium channel blockers (verapamil, nicardipine) Antifungal agents (itraconazole, fluconazole) Antibiotics (erythromycin) Glucocorticoids HIV-protease inhibitors (indinavir) Miscellaneous: allopurinol, metoclopramide, grapefruit juice **Substances that induce CYP3A activity decrease cyclosporine concentration**: Antibiotics (nafcillin, rifampin [rifampicin]) Anticonvulsants (phenobarbital, phenytoin) NSAIDs – additive Nephrotoxicity Elevated methotrexate levels when the drugs are coadministered Prednisolone, digoxin, and lovastatin are among the drugs that have reduced clearance when given with cyclosporine

(continued)

Table 11.1 Drug mechanisms of action, adverse effects and drugs interactions *(continued)*

DRUG	MECHANISM OF ACTION	ADVERSE EFFECTS	DRUG INTERACTIONS
Azathioprine	Affects purine nucleotide synthesis and metabolism, altering the synthesis of RNA and DNA, finally leading to the inhibition of T lymphocytes	Bone marrow suppression: leukopenia (common), thrombocytopenia (less common), anemia (uncommon) Infection: especially varicella and herpes simplex Hypersensitivity syndrome Miscellaneous: hepatotoxicity, alopecia, gastrointestinal toxicity, pancreatitis, and increased risk of neoplasia	Allopurinol blocks xanthine oxidase, an important enzyme in the catabolism of metabolites of azathioprine Coadministration with other myelosuppressive agents or angiotensin-converting enzyme inhibitors can lead to leukopenia, thrombocytopenia, and/or anemia, as a result of myelosuppression
Methotrexate	Inhibits dihydrofolate reductase, an enzyme that reduces folic acid to tetrahydrofolic acid, thus causing inhibition of DNA synthesis and decreased lymphocyte proliferation Promotes adenosine release Apoptosis of activated T cells	Toxicity against rapidly dividing cells of the bone marrow and gastrointestinal epithelium, reaching maximum 5–10 days after administration of the drug: mucositis, myelosuppression, thrombocytopenia Pneumonitis Hepatic fibrosis and cirrhosis Miscellaneous: alopecia, dermatitis, nephrotoxicity, defective oogenesis or spermatogenesis	Trimethroprim–sulfamethoxazole: profound myelosuppression Drugs that increase methotrexate levels: salicylates, NSAIDs, sulfonamides, phenothiazines, phenytoin, tetracyclines Agents that increase hepatotoxicity: isotretinoin, acitretin, alcohol
Mycophenolate mofetil	Inhibits inosine monophosphate dehydrogenase, an enzyme involved in the new pathway of purine synthesis This leads to inhibition of T and B lymphocytes	Gastrointestinal disturbances: vomiting and diarrhea Leukopenia Infections – herpes simplex and zoster, cytomegalovirus	Antacids containing aluminum or magnesium hydroxide decrease absorption Cholestyramine decreases mycophenolate levels Acyclovir (aciclovir) increases mycophenolate and acyclovir levels

Table 11.1   Drug mechanisms of action, adverse effects and drugs interactions *(continued)*

DRUG	MECHANISM OF ACTION	ADVERSE EFFECTS	DRUG INTERACTIONS
Recombinant interferon (rIFN)	Thought to inhibit Th2 cytokine milieu, important for initiating phase of AD	Flu-like symptoms: fever, chills, headache, myalgia, arthralgia, nausea, vomiting, diarrhea Rash Injection site reactions Less common: myelosuppression, neurotoxicity, and cardiovascular effects – only at higher doses	Not fully evaluated Use caution with other immunomodulatory agents rIFN-γ increases theophylline levels

AD, atopic dermatitis; CYP3A, cytochrome P450 variant; IL, interleukin; NSAID, nonsteroidal anti-inflammatory drug.
Reprinted from Akhavan and Rudikoff 2003. © 2003 with permission from Elsevier.

Table 11.2   Monitoring guidelines for the use of immunosuppressants

DRUG	MONITORING TESTS	FREQUENCY	GUIDELINES FOR DOSAGE MODIFICATION
Azathioprine	CBC with differential WBC and platelets	Weekly × 4, every 2 weeks × 2, then monthly	Decrease dose if WBC $<4 \times 10^9$/l, platelets $<10^{11}$/l; discontinue if WBC $<2.5 \times 10^9$/l
Methotrexate	CBC with differential WBC and platelets	Weekly × 2, every 2 weeks × 2, then monthly	Discontinue for 2–3 weeks if WBC $<3.5 \times 10^9$/l; discontinue if WBC $<2.5 \times 10^9$/l or platelets $<10^{11}$/l; increased MCV necessitates folate administration
	Renal function tests: BUN, creatinine	Every 3–4 months	
	Liver function tests	Every 1–2 months; ensure that it is at least 1 week after most recent dose	If persistently elevated, withhold for 1–2 weeks and repeat; if elevation persists for 2–3 months perform liver biopsy
	Liver biopsy	If no risk factors, at cumulative doses of 1.5 g, 3 g, and 4 g. If risk factors, first at 2–4 months of therapy, then at cumulative doses of 1–1.5g, 3g, and 4 g. After a cumulative dose of 4 g, biopsy every 1–1.5 g	

(continued)

Table 11.2 Monitoring guidelines for the use of immunosuppressants *(continued)*

DRUG	MONITORING TESTS	FREQUENCY	GUIDELINES FOR DOSAGE MODIFICATION
Cyclosporine (ciclosporin)	CBC with differential WBC and platelets	Every month, then every 2–3 months	
	Renal function tests: BUN and creatinine × 3	Biweekly × 6, then monthly	Decrease dose if creatinine increase is >30% over baseline; if persistent over two evaluations, discontinue
	Blood pressure	Biweekly × 6, then monthly	
	Urinalysis	Biweekly × 2, then monthly	
	Liver function tests	Biweekly × 2, then monthly	
	Potassium, uric acid, magnesium, cholesterol, triglycerides	Biweekly × 2, then monthly	
	Creatinine clearance	Not done routinely	
MMF	CBC with differential WBC and platelets	Weekly × 4, every 2 weeks × 4, then monthly	Decrease dose or discontinue if neutropenic

For all immunosuppressants, lymph node examination, complete physical examination, stool guaiac, skin cancer examination, and PAP smear every 6 months are recommended.

BUN, blood urea nitrogen; CBC, complete blood (cell) count; MCV, molluscum contagiosum virus; MMF, mycophenolate mofetil; WBC, white blood cell (count).

Adapted from Kazlow Stern *et al.* 2005. © 2005 with permission from Elsevier.

CONCLUSION

Treatment options for AD range from regular use of emollients to systemic immunosuppression (Buys 2007). Despite this broad array of therapies, many patients are left inadequately treated, refractory to traditional therapies, and unable to tolerate the adverse events associated with systemic immunosuppressives.

Still, as we wait for the development of newer treatment options with better side-effect profiles and heightened efficacy, the systemic immunosuppressives remain the clinician's best treatment option for severe and refractory AD. With careful monitoring of the patient some of these options can be used safely to control the disease in such patients.

Clinical suggestions

1. Consider using systemic therapy in patients who have not responded to topical agents and/or phototherapy, especially in those whose eczema is causing major problems functioning in school or at the workplace. None of these agents has FDA approval for the treatment of AD.
2. Short courses of corticosteroids or intramuscular triamcinolone may be used for flares but should be limited to no more than two courses or injections per year.
3. Azathioprine and mycophenolate have a much slower onset of action than cyclosporine (ciclosporin). Mycophenolate may play a role in maintaining the initial improvement attained with a 6-week course of cyclosporine.
4. Patients with decreased levels of thiopurine S-methyltransferase are at risk for myelosuppression with azathioprine, and those with high levels may have decreased efficacy. Obtain pretreatment levels of this enzyme and dose accordingly. Be aware that, besides non-Hodgkin lymphoma, highly aggressive hepatosplenic T-cell lymphoma can occur in patients being treated with azathioprine, although it has not as yet been described in patients being treated for AD (Denby and Beck 2012).
5. Methotrexate has shown efficacy in adult and childhood AD. It has multiple drug interactions and must never be coadministered with trimethoprim–sulfamethoxazole. Cyclosporine likewise has many drug interactions that clinicians should avoid.

PHOTO(CHEMO)THERAPY OF ATOPIC ECZEMA

Thilo Gambichler, Nordwig S. Tomi, and Stefanie Boms

The use of natural sunlight and more recently artificial ultraviolet (UV) phototherapy has been shown to be of benefit in the treatment of several skin disorders, among them psoriasis, eczema, and vitiligo. A well-known nineteenth-century American dermatologist wrote in his treatise on eczema: 'Ventilation and sunlight should not escape the careful physician's attention who seeks to cure an obstinate case of eczema' (Bulkley 1881). The first significant study of UV therapy for the treatment of atopic eczema (AE) was conducted by Nexmand (1948) on 57 patients, most of whom were children or young adults. The light source was a 'Universol' carbon arc lamp. Of the 57 patients, 10 (17.5.%) became symptom free (resolution of itching and physical changes) after an average of 20 irradiations, and 23 (40%) were improved (pruritus completely resolved or reduced but persistence of skin infiltration and lichenification). A number of subsequent studies have demonstrated a beneficial effect of sunlight exposure

(eg, heliotherapy, climatotherapy) and photo(chemo) therapy in AE (Harari *et al.* 2000, Autio *et al.* 2002). Photo(chemo)therapy is now considered one of the three fundamental modalities for treating AE, along with topical and systemic therapy. Several broadband UV spectra (UVA, UVB, UVA/UVB) and combined treatment modalities, such as salt-water baths plus UVB (balneophototherapy), and psoralen and UV light (PUVA), have demonstrated efficacy in the treatment of moderate-to-severe AE. Since 1993, however, with the advent of newer innovative phototherapeutic modalities such as UVA1, narrowband UVB (NB-UVB), and extracorporeal photopheresis, the paradigm for treating AE has changed (Larkö 1996, Horio 1998, Dawe 2003, Scheinfeld *et al.* 2003, Gambichler *et al.* 2005, Meduri *et al.* 2007). This chapter summarizes important study data regarding the treatment of AE and reviews current therapeutic options (*Table 12.1, Table 12.2*). It is important to realize that interpretation of these studies on the

Table 12.1 Recommendations* for the use of photo(chemo)therapeutic options in the management of atopic eczema

First line regimens	Second line regimens	Third line regimens
UVA1,	UVA/UVB,	Heliothalassotherapy,
NB UVB	Bath PUVA,	Balneophototherapy,
	BB UVA,	Oral PUVA,
	BB UVB	ECP

* the above suggested recommendations are based on treatment efficacy, safety, availability, practicability, and cost-effectiveness.

Table 12.2   Current therapeutic options for atopic eczema

MODALITY	INDICATIONS/ADVANTAGES	RISKS/DISADVANTAGES
NB-UVB	Nowadays widely available Useful for chronic AE in adults Can be used cautiously in children with AE Reduces epidermal hyperplasia in parallel with reduction of Th2 cytokines and IL-22	Less erythmogenic than BB-UVB (some AE studies used erythmogenic dose) Reactivation of herpes simplex infection
UVA-1	Acute flares of AE Similar result with high- and medium-dose UVA1. Low-dose UVA1 is less effective Duration of treatment usually 3–4 weeks	High-dose UVA1 should not be used in children Long-term adverse effects not established. Hyperpigmentation/tanning common Improvement duration only 4–8 weeks Considerable heat generated by metal halide lamps UVA1 equipment not widely available, expensive to maintain
BB-UVA/UVB and BB-UVB	BB-UVA/UVB somewhat superior to BB-UVB without UVA1	Widely available although NB-UVB has gained greater popularity BB-UVA/UVB and BB-UVB are useful in children who are intolerant of NB-UVB
PUVA	Effective for AE but has largely been replaced by NB-UVB and UVA	Not recommended in children because of known increase in cutaneous malignancies including melanoma May cause initial flare of AE that can be avoided by starting systemic corticosteroid before initiating PUVA Nausea, elevation of liver enzymes
Bath PUVA	Similar efficacy to NB-UVB Eliminates the need for protective lenses, reduces cumulative UVA doses, and facilitates uniform psoralen application	For adults; cooperation more complex in children Availability limited
Excimer laser	May be useful for localized AE in adults and children	For localized disease Combinations with NB-UVB promising but not well reported Availability limited
Extracorporeal photophoresis	May be of value in patients with severe and otherwise refractory AE	Not widely available
Heliothallasotherapy and balneotherapy	Efficacy suggested by several trials	Not widely available

AE, atopic eczema; BB, broadband; IL, interleukin; NB, narrow band; PUVA, psoralen + UVA; UV, ultraviolet.

efficacy of photo(chemo)therapy in the treatment of AE is hampered by several confounders such as publication bias, small sample sizes, high variability of treatment parameters used in different studies, and especially the lack of randomized controlled prospective trials comparing different photo(chemo) therapeutic modalities (Gambichler 2009).

ULTRAVIOLET A AND ULTRAVIOLET B

Combination therapy with UVA and broadband (BB) UVB (UVA/UVB) (wavelength region from 280 nm to 400 nm) was introduced to simulate the effects of natural sunlight. The efficacy of combined UVA/ UVB treatment of AE has been confirmed by several investigators (Hannuksela *et al.* 1985, Midelfart *et al.* 1985, Jekler and Larkö 1990a, 1991, Valkova and Velkova 2004). Hannuksela *et al.* (1985) conducted a retrospective study of 107 patients with AE who previously had received combined UVA/UVB or UVB only. Of those treated with UVB alone, 93% had a good response, with 50% of patients reporting a reduction in steroid use after cessation of phototherapy. In the UVA/UVB group, 94% achieved a good response with 85% reporting a reduction in steroid use after treatment. Similarly, Midelfart *et al.* (1985) compared the response to combined UVA/UVB versus UVB alone in a randomized study of 56 patients with AE (Midelfart *et al.* 1985). Of the patients treated with UVA/UVB, 96% achieved a good or even complete response with a mean of 18 treatments, whereas, among those treated with UVB alone, only 85% showed a good or complete response with a mean of 20 treatments.

Subsequently, Jekler and coworkers, in a randomized bilateral study, confirmed the superiority of combined UVA/UVB compared with UVB alone (Jekler and Larkö 1990a, 1990b, 1991). Outcome measures included reduction of lichenification, itching, scaling, and xerosis, and overall healing of their dermatitis. Significant differences in favor of UVA/UVB were observed for all variables analyzed, namely total score (p = 0.002), pruritus score (p = 0.04), and overall evaluation score (p = 0.03). There was no statistically significant difference in

healing rate, however. Twenty-five of 30 UVB-treated, and 26 of 30 UVA/UVB-treated body halves healed or improved considerably. Moreover, patients overwhelmingly preferred the combined treatment; 23 of 24 patients who completed a survey preferred UVA/UVB compared with only 1 of 24 who preferred UVB. The authors concluded that UVA/UVB is superior to UVB for treating AE and attributed this to the photoaugmentation and deeper depth of penetration provided by UVA and the lower level of skin irritation from UVA/UVB phototherapy (Jekler and Larkö 1991, Larkö 1996). Broadband UVB and broadband UVA/UVB remain useful treatment options in occasional patients who do not tolerate the newer modalities such as NB-UVB and NB-UVA1 (Pugashetti *et al.* 2010).

NARROWBAND ULTRAVIOLET B

'Narrowband UVB' is a term used for the UV radiation produced by a light source producing a narrow peak around 311 nm (TL01 bulbs). This modality was shown in 1988 to be equivalent to broadband UVB in the treatment of psoriasis but with less burning, and then in a small pilot study was found to be efficacious for the treatment of AE (Green *et al.* 1988, Grundmann-Kollmann *et al.* 1999). Subsequently, Reynolds *et al.* (2001) compared NB-UVB, broadband (BB) UVA, and visible light (placebo) phototherapy as adjunctive treatment in a randomized, controlled, double-blind trial in adults with moderate-to-severe AE (Reynolds *et al.* 2001). Phototherapy was administered twice weekly for 24 exposures (starting doses: 0.4 J/cm^2 NB-UVB, 5 J/cm^2 BB-UVA). After 24 treatments, mean reductions in total disease activity in patients who received NB-UVB (22 patients) and BB-UVA (19 patients) were, respectively, 9.4 points and 4.4 points more than the 19 patients who had received placebo light therapy. Mean reductions in the extent of disease with NB-UVB and BB-UVA were 6.7% and –1% respectively compared with placebo. At 3 months after the phototherapy phase, more patients in the NB-UVB group had lower disease activity than patients in the other two groups.

Although NB-UVB proved to be the most effective adjunctive treatment in this comparative study, it is difficult to draw any conclusions on the efficacy of NB-UVB alone because patients were permitted to use moderate-to-potent topical steroids throughout the treatment course.

In a randomized, investigator-blinded, half-side comparison study of severe, chronic AE comparing NB-UVB with bath PUVA, Der-Petrossian *et al.* (2000) determined the two modalities to be equally effective when given in erythemogenic doses. Half-side irradiation with threshold erythemogenic doses of NB-UVB and bath PUVA was administered to 12 patients three times weekly for 6 weeks. Mean baseline skin scores decreased by 65.7% with bath PUVA and by 64.1% with NB-UVB. In another randomized, half-side comparison study on nine patients with chronic AE treated with NB-UVB and medium-dose UVA1, NB-UVB was superior to medium-dose UVA1 (Legat *et al.* 2003). Physician relative score reduction for NB-UVB was 40% ($p = 0.004$) compared with 33% for UVA1 ($p = 0.055$); patient relative score reduction for NB-UVB was 71% ($p = 0.004$) compared with 40% for UVA1 ($p = 0.04$). A nonrandomized, half-side comparison study of 10 patients with AE failed to show a significant difference between NB-UVB and combined BB-UVA/BB-UVB treatment with regard to clinical score (Hjerppe *et al.* 2001). However, with regard to pruritus, NB-UVB was superior to UVA/UVB at 6 weeks ($p = 0.043$). Similar positive results have been reported in open prospective and retrospective trials on patients with moderate-to-severe adult or childhood AE, using NB-UVB as an adjunctive treatment combined with topical steroids (George *et al.* 1993, Collins and Ferguson 1995, Hudson-Peacock *et al.* 1996). In the aforementioned studies, NB-UVB not only decreased the total clinical score, but also substantially reduced the use of potent steroids.

A recent report confirms the efficacy of NB-UVB in the treatment of atopic dermatitis; it was shown to reduce epidermal hyperplasia in parallel with reduction of T-helper type 2 (Th2) cytokines and interleukin (IL)-22 (Tintle *et al.* 2011). NB-UVB is also reported to be effective in children with atopic dermatitis but, because of lack of information about the long-term safety of its use in children, it should be used cautiously and be followed up by yearly skin exams (Jury *et al.* 2006, Pavlovsky *et al.* 2011). Clearing or good remission is reported in about two-thirds of children treated for atopic dermatitis with NB-UVB, with remission duration of 5–6 months (Jury *et al.* 2006, Pavlovsky *et al.* 2011).

308-NM UVB LASER (EXCIMER LASER)

The success of NB-UVB in the treatment of atopic dermatitis has prompted investigation of the use of the 308-nm UVB laser, usually used in the spot treatment of psoriasis and vitiligo, on patients with localized atopic dermatitis. Baltás *et al.* (2006) treated 15 patients with limited atopic dermatitis (less than 20% body area involvement) with a xenon chloride excimer laser (XTRAC laser) twice weekly. Severity of atopic dermatitis in 14 evaluable patients, based on (1) a clinical score reflecting erythema intensity, infiltration, lichenification, and excoriation, (2) quality of life, determined by questionnaire, and (3) patient self-assessed severity of pruritus, was decreased by a mean of 58%. There was a mean decrease in Eczema Area Severity Index (EASI) score from 8.5 to 3.57. Nisticò *et al.* (2008) treated 12 adults and 6 children with a 308-nm monochromatic laser and reported complete remission in 12 of 18 patients (66.7%), partial remission in 3 of 18 (16.7%), and no remission in 3 of 18 (16.7%). In addition, Wollenschläger *et al.* (2009) reported efficacy in therapy-resistant localized atopic dermatitis using excimer laser. These preliminary results suggest that the 308 nm may be useful in the treatment of localized atopic dermatitis but controlled studies are necessary.

ULTRAVIOLET A1

A breakthrough in the field of photomedicine came in the early 1980s when Mutzhas *et al.* (1981) introduced an apparatus that could deliver high-dose radiation energy in the longer-wavelength region of the UVA spectrum (340–400 nm) referred to as UVA1. UVA1 is less erythemogenic than UVA2 (320–340 nm) and penetrates deeper into the skin (Krutmann 2000).

Ten years after the introduction of high-dose UVA1, Krutmann and associates (1992) showed that it was efficacious in the treatment of acute flares of AE. In these initial reports, UVA1 dosages of 130 J/cm^2 (high dose) were applied five times weekly for 2 or 3 weeks, with a cumulative exposure dose of 1300–1950 J/cm^2 and a reduction in the baseline clinical score by 54% and 74% respectively (Krutmann et al. 1992, 1998). In one study of 53 patients with AE (Krutmann et al. 1998), high-dose UVA1 monotherapy was superior to the combination of UVA/UVB and topical steroids (Krutmann et al. 1998).

Tzaneva et al. (2001) compared the efficacy of high- and medium-dose UVA1 (60 J/cm^2) in patients with severe AE. Patients, serving as their own experimental controls, received half-body radiation with high-dose UVA1 and contralateral half-body exposure to medium-dose UVA1. After 3 weeks of phototherapy there was no statistical difference in efficacy with regard to overall clinical response between the two dosage levels. High- and medium-dose regimens achieved similar responses with reductions in clinical scores of 34.7% and 28.2% respectively. Relapses appeared soon after therapy, however (median time 4 weeks), regardless of the dosing regimen used (Tzaneva et al. 2001). Whereas the previous study showed similar responses to high- and medium-dose UVA1, a study conducted by Kowalzick et al. (1995) comparing medium-dose UVA1 and low-dose UVA1 in 22 patients with acute AE found medium-dose UVA1 to be superior (Kowalzick et al. 1995). After 3 weeks of treatment, patients receiving medium-dose UVA1 had a 25.3% reduction in clinical scores compared with a 7.7% reduction in those who received the low-dose regimen.

One of the major problems with UVA1 therapy had been the heat generated by conventional UVA1 devices. Von Kobyletzki et al. (1999) investigated a new UVA1 apparatus designed to minimize this enormous heat load, the so-called UVA1 cold light, comparing it with conventional UVA1 and UVA/UVB therapy. In a study of 120 individuals with acute AE, the cold-light UVA1 regimen demonstrated superiority to both traditional UVA1 and UVA/UVB therapy in reducing disease severity after 3 weeks or 1 month of treatment.

Efficacy of medium-dose UVA1 in alleviating acute exacerbations of eczema was also demonstrated by Abeck et al. (2000). In this study there was a significant reduction of clinical score ratings ($p < 0.001$) at the end of the active UV treatment period and 1 month post-treatment ($p < 0.001$) (Abeck et al. 2000). However, at 3 months post-treatment the eczema had reverted to its pretreatment severity. Thus, medium-dose UVA1 also improves severe AE, is more effective than UVA/UVB, and is more effective than low-dose treatment, but remissions tend to be short according to this open study.

Polderman et al. (2005) compared the effects of 4 weeks of therapy of UVA1 with the usual 3 weeks of therapy in patients with AE ($n = 61$), using medium-dose UVA1 cold light (45 J/cm^2) 5 days a week. Although clinical score and quality of life improved in both groups, there were no significant differences in these outcomes between the 3- and 4-week treatments groups. Importantly, only patients treated for 4 weeks maintained their improvement 6 weeks after therapy. In both groups, 50% of the patients had intermittently used mild topical steroids during the follow-up. Hence, the extension of UVA1 therapy from 3 weeks to 4 weeks may result in more prolonged therapeutic effects (Polderman et al. 2005).

UVA1 phototherapy is thought to benefit AE based on the generation of singlet oxygen which induces apoptosis of skin infiltrating lymphocytes (Morita et al. 1997, Morita and Krutmann 2000). Medium-dose UVA1 phototherapy causes a decrease in the number of CD4+ cells, CD1a+ dendritic cells, and activated EG2+ eosinophils within the dermal infiltrate, but a significant increase in the percentage of dermal CD8+ cells (Breuckmann et al. 2002a, 2002b). UVA1 treatment also results in a significant decrease of IL-5, IL-13, and IL-31 mRNA expression and modulates the level of cathepsin G in the lesions of AE (Gambichler et al. 2008).

A recent report of two cases of Merkel cell carcinoma in immunocompromised patients receiving high-dose UVA1 therapy suggests caution in the use of this modality in immunosuppressed individuals (Calzavara-Pinton et al. 2010).

PSORALEN AND ULTRAVIOLET LIGHT AND EXTRACORPOREAL PHOTOPHERESIS

Psoralen and UV light (PUVA) was studied in the management of AE not long after its introduction for the treatment of psoriasis. The initial enthusiasm for PUVA therapy seems to have been dampened, however, by the greater complexities of administering psoralen and the potential risk of skin cancer with this treatment. Nevertheless, Yoshiike *et al.* (1993) attempted to formulate a guideline for the selection of AE patients to be treated with PUVA. According to this guideline, 114 patients were selected for PUVA treatment, 45% of whom had not responded adequately to other conventional forms of treatment (Yoshiike *et al.* 1993). Adverse effects from previous treatments, in particular steroids, occurred in almost 40% of the patients. After PUVA, the skin lesions significantly decreased in 81% of the inpatients and 67% of the outpatients. Some patients' lesions disappeared, despite the fact that, in many cases, other forms of treatment had been unsuccessful.

Atherton *et al.* (1988) reported 15 adolescent children with severe, chronic AE who had been treated with oral PUVA. Photochemotherapy resulted in initial clearance of eczema in 14 of the 15 children, 9 of whom achieved remission. Apart from its efficacy, notably a major benefit of this therapeutic approach was that it was associated with resumption of normal growth in children who had previously shown growth retardation, as a direct result of either severe eczema or its treatment. Nevertheless, the authors emphasized in their conclusion that, although there are considerable advantages to using PUVA in this group of patients, these advantages must be balanced with possible hazards, which include relatively high exposures that are required in some individuals, both initially to induce clearance and subsequently to maintain it. Over a 6-year period, oral PUVA was used to treat 53 children with refractory severe AE (Sheehan *et al.* 1993). Twice-weekly treatment resulted in clearance or near-clearance of disease in 39 patients (74%) after a mean of 9 weeks. Of these 39 children 32 (82%) subsequently achieved remission of disease after gradual withdrawal of treatment; the mean duration of treatment to remission was 37 weeks, the mean cumulative UVA dose was 1118 J/cm^2, and the mean number of treatments was 59.

Recently, Uetsu and Horio (2003) used oral PUVA to treat 113 patients with severe AE. At 4 and 8 weeks after PUVA therapy, the severity score of AE had decreased by 51% and 80% respectively. The amounts and strength of topical steroids were decreased during PUVA therapy and the quality of life of patients was greatly improved after treatment. The authors concluded that PUVA can be helpful in patients with refractory, severe, widespread AE.

Another recent, randomized, observer-blinded, crossover study compared UVA1 phototherapy with oral 5-methoxypsoralen (5-MOP) plus UVA (PUVA) in the treatment of 40 patients with severe generalized AE (Tzaneva *et al.* 2010). Patients received initial therapy of either 15 treatments with medium-dose UVA1 or 15 treatments with PUVA. In cases of relapse, those who had initial treatment with UVA1 received an additional 15 exposures to PUVA, and those who initially received PUVA were retreated with UVA1. Twenty-three patients completed the crossover treatment and, although both therapies were associated with clinical improvement, not only did PUVA reduce the baseline SCORAD score to a significantly greater extent than UVA1 (mean ± standard deviation [SD] 54.3 ± 25.7% vs 37.7 ± 22.8%; $p = 0.041$), it also resulted in a much greater length of remission of 12 weeks (interquartile range 4–26) after PUVA therapy ($p = 0.012$) compared with 4 weeks (interquartile range 4–12) after UVA1.

Use of psoralen in a dilute bath water solution (bath PUVA) may be used instead of standard systemic PUVA therapy. This technique avoids many adverse effects, reduces cumulative UVA doses, and facilitates uniform psoralen application. In a study of bath PUVA, 35 adults with severe AE were treated up to a maximum of 30 sessions (maximum single dose: 12 J/cm^2). A significant ($p <0.001$) reduction in symptoms was noted at the end of treatment in those who completed the study (de Kort and van Weelden 2000). As previously mentioned, bath PUVA and NB-UVB showed equal efficacy in treating AE in the study reported by Der-Petrossian *et al.* (2000).

Extracorporeal photopheresis is effective in a variety of diseases such as Sézary syndrome and graft-versus-host disease, but its use is limited to academic medical centers. The extracorporeal photopheresis procedure includes collection of peripheral mono-nuclear cells, extracorporeal radiation of these cells with UVA in the presence of 8-MOP, and reinfusion of treated cells back into the patient. In a study of patients with severe AE, Prinz et al. (1999) treated 14 patients with extracorporeal photopheresis at 2-week intervals in an open clinical trial. Disease activity was scored before each extracorporeal photopheresis cycle. Complete clinical remission was achieved in four patients (29%). Five patients (36%) experienced a substantial response with reduction of skin inflammation by at least 75%, whereas in one patient (7%), disease activity was reduced by more than 50%. However, four patients withdrew from the study because of failure to respond. The investigators concluded that extracorporeal photopheresis should be considered for patients with severe and otherwise refractory atopic skin disease. Other research groups have also reported encouraging results of extracorporeal photopheresis treatments in patients with AE in case series and small studies (Richter et al. 1998, Radenhausen et al. 2004, Sand et al. 2007).

MISCELLANEOUS

Change of climate and rest have often been advocated for skin disease in the older literature. More recently, improvement of AE was noted in children who went on holiday, especially to southerly locations such as the Mediterranean or further south compared with those who vacationed in northern Britain (Turner et al. 1991). In this telephone survey the authors were not able to identify the cause of improvement, be it rest, sunlight, or both. Other authors have supported the use of heliotherapy, climatotherapy, and spa for managing eczema but their studies must be interpreted with caution because of a lack of control groups (Horio 1998, Harari et al. 2000). Autio et al. (2002) studied 216 AE patients who participated in six different 2- or 3-week trips to the Canary Islands for heliotherapy. Eczema severity scores were assessed before heliotherapy, 2 weeks

after the start, and then 3 months after the conclusion of heliotherapy. Quality of life was assessed by means of a questionnaire mailed to all participants. The mean clinical eczema score was reduced by 70% after 2 weeks of heliotherapy and remained 45% lower than baseline 3 months after therapy ($p <0.0001$). Moreover, the use of topical steroids was still significantly reduced ($p <0.0001$) 3 months after the conclusion of treatment. The quality of life of patients improved, and their self-treatment and working capacity also increased. As the longer 3-week period provided no significant additional advantage over a 2-week period, 2 weeks of heliotherapy were considered optimal.

In a retrospective study of 1718 patients with AE, Harari et al. (2000) showed that treatments at the Dead Sea involving stays longer than 4 weeks caused a clearance of more than 95%. The length of sun exposure was no longer than 5 hours daily and the percentage of skin involvement had no impact on the clearance of patients staying more than 4 weeks. The authors concluded that climatotherapy of AE at the Dead Sea is a highly effective treatment modality. It is also a cost-effective method, because patients take no medications and experience no adverse effects.

As the aforementioned regimens are tied to special geographic settings, balneophototherapy was alternatively established in German rehabilitation centers, especially for treating psoriasis. Balneophototherapy represents a combined phototherapeutic regimen with salt-water baths and artificial UV radiation (Gambichler et al. 2000, Gambichler 2007). In a controlled prospective study by Dittmar et al. (1999), the efficacy of combined salt-water bath and UVA/UVB phototherapy was compared with UVA/UVB monophototherapy in patients with subacute AE. The patients in the balneophototherapy group ($n = 16$) were treated with baths containing 3–5% of a synthetic salt, followed immediately by UVA/UVB irradiation, whereas the other treatment group ($n = 12$) received UVA/UVB phototherapy only. After 20 treatments, the balneophototherapy group showed a statistically significant ($p <0.0015$) reduction in the clinical score from 69.5 before to 36.8 after therapy. No statistically significant reduction in the clinical score could be observed in the UVA/UVB phototherapy group (50.6 before to 44.3 after therapy). In another study, brine baths containing either 15% synthetic Dead Sea salt or 3% NaCl solution led to significantly better results in 80% of patients in the 15% salt-water group (Zimmermann *et al.* 1994).

Moreover, Schiffner *et al.* (2002) conducted an uncontrolled multicenter trial on combined treatment with NB-UVB and salt-water baths in outpatients with AE. The use of concomitant topical treatment such as steroids was not reported, however (Schiffner *et al.* 2002). Relative improvement of the skin score (percentage) was significant ($p < 0.05$) in 143 patients treated according to the protocol (55%) and in 615 patients in an intent-to-treat group (41%). The authors concluded that this treatment modality is especially recommended for patients with chronic types of AE, those who are highly motivated, and those with free time for therapy. Unfortunately, this large study did not include a NB-UVB monotherapy arm; therefore, the influence of bathing in salt water on the efficacy, tolerability, and practicability could not be assessed independently. In another study, Heinlin *et al.* (2011) prospectively compared treatment with synchronous balneophototherapy (sBPT), simulating treatment conditions at the Dead Sea with NB-UVB monotherapy in 180 patients with moderate-to-severe atopic dermatitis. They demonstrated a clinically relevant and statistically significant ($p < 0.001$) superiority of 26.2% in the sBPT group at the end of therapy, as well as superiority of sBPT after 6 months. Thus it would seem that balneophototherapy is a helpful treatment option although its availability is limited.

PHOTOTHERAPY IN CHILDREN

Given that most patients with AE are young, there have been a number of concerns regarding the widespread use of phototherapy and photochemotherapy, especially with regard to the possible risk of carcinogenicity and premature aging with long-term treatment (Dogra and De 2010). Studies on PUVA in children have been mentioned previously. Pavlovsky *et al.* (2011) conducted a retrospective review of children who had undergone NB-UVB phototherapy for psoriasis or AE. Outpatients were treated three times a week and inpatients six times a week; a face shield was used unless there was facial involvement and the genital area was protected with clothing in all children. Forty-one children with AE (18 males and 23 females; mean age 13 [±4.12]) received a mean duration of treatment of 3.3 (±2.43) months for a mean cumulative dose of 51.6 J/cm^2. Of the 36 children with AE available for final analysis 25% (9/36) achieved clearance, whereas another 44% (16/36) had a partial response. The median duration of remission was 5 months. Another retrospective study of childhood AE looked at 60 children aged 4–16 years (median 12) who were treated with NB-UVB (Clayton *et al.* 2007). Six of the children were aged <5 years. Of 50 children (83%) who received more than 10 exposures of NB-UVB, complete clearance or minimal residual activity was achieved in 20 children (40%). Improvement judged as 'good' was achieved in 10 children (23%), and moderate improvement obtained in 13 (26%). Interestingly, there was a statistically significant ($p = 0.02$) association between higher minimal erythema doses (MEDs >390 mJ/cm^2) and clinical clearing. The median duration of clearing was 3 months and treatment was well tolerated. According to current European Task Force on Atopic Dermatitis/European Academy of Dermatology and Venereology (ETFAD/EADV) guidelines, phototherapy of moderate-to-severe AE is recommended in children at the age of 12 and above (Darsow *et al.* 2010).

CONCLUSIONS

Interpreting the current literature with regard to the efficacy of photo(chemo)therapy in treating AE is limited by several factors, including publication bias, small sample sizes used in previous trials, high variability of parameters used in different studies, and, in particular, the lack of large randomized controlled trials comparing different photo(chemo)therapeutic modalities. Although photo(chemo) therapy is beneficial in most patients with AE, a small proportion of patients may have worsening of their eczema with UV light (photoaggravated AE). Moreover, the heat from some types of lamps (eg, UVA1) can trigger a vicious itch–scratch cycle in some patients.

On the basis of the current data, however, newer UV sources, such as medium-dose UVA1 and NB-UVB, with a high output and a narrow emission spectrum, may be considered the most effective regimens for treating acute and chronic AE, respectively (Meduri *et al.* 2007). Conventional broader-band UV regimens appear to have more drawbacks when compared with medium-UVA1 and NB-UVB. In general, phototherapy is not indicated in acute stage AE with the exception of UVA1, which is also useful in managing flares of disease (Darsow *et al.* 2010).

There are no prospective trials on AE patients comparing NB-UVB and UVA1 with more complex regimens, such as heliotherapy and balneophototherapy. Hence, the ultimate role of the latter treatment modalities in managing AE awaits further study. Support for the role of PUVA and extracorporeal photopheresis in AE is also generally weaker, and PUVA carries potential risk of squamous cell carcinoma and possibly melanoma, which may occur years after PUVA therapy has ceased (Stern 2001). By contrast, the evidence suggests that UVB phototherapy is a relatively safe treatment modality with regard to photocarcinogenicity (Weischer *et al.* 2004, Lee *et al.* 2005). NB-UVB is currently preferred over BB-UVB because it is less erythemogenic but BB-UVB may be used in occasional patients who do not tolerate NB-UVB (Darsow *et al.* 2010, Pugashetti *et al.* 2010). According to current ETFAD/EADV guidelines, topical steroids and emollients may be used at the beginning of phototherapy to reduce the chance of flare-up whereas topical immunomodulatory agents such as tacrolimus and pimecrolimus should be avoided (Darsow *et al.* 2010).

More common adverse effects associated with photo(chemo)therapy (eg, UVB, UVA) include skin burning and premature skin aging, which again tend to be worse with PUVA. Despite anxieties about possible long-term hazards, the authors believe that PUVA, in particular bath PUVA, may be justified in patients with severe AE who do not respond to other photo(chemo)therapeutic regimens (Tzaneva *et al.* 2010). When photo(chemo)therapy is used, its use is very much dictated by the availability and practicality of being able to attend the clinic several times a week. Careful planning and patient supervision are crucial to the successful delivery of photo(chemo)therapy.

CHAPTER 13

ECZEMA AND THE EYE

Kevin Stein and Frederick Perreira

The eye and ocular adnexae can be involved in a variety of eczematous conditions. This chapter discusses the ocular manifestations of atopic dermatitis, eczematous dermatitis of the eyelids, and corticosteroid-induced glaucoma and cataract.

A brief overview of ocular anatomy is pertinent to understanding eye disorders associated with eczematous dermatitis and complications related to treatment. The eye is arbitrarily divided into two segments. The anterior segment includes the lens and all structures anterior to it. The posterior segment includes vitreous humor, choroid, and retina. The anterior segment is further subdivided into anterior and posterior chambers. The anterior chamber includes the area behind the cornea and anterior to the iris. The posterior chamber lies behind the iris and anterior to the lens (**Fig 13.1**).

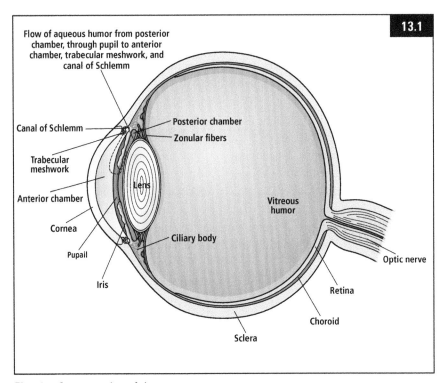

Fig 13.1 Cross-section of the eye.

The globe of the eye is encased in a fibrous membrane, the sclera. The cornea is a transparent, fibrous coat, continuous with the sclera. The cornea is moistened by tears, and it receives nourishment from the aqueous humor. Underneath the sclera is the vascular layer, the uveal tract, which includes the choroid, ciliary body, and iris. On top of the choroid lies the retina. The anterior surface of the eye and inner eyelid surfaces are covered by the conjunctiva, a vascular mucous membrane that is continuous with the lid margin skin.

The lens is a biconvex, transparent structure made up of multiple layers of epithelial cells enclosed in a capsule composed of collagen. These cells are densely packed with crystallins, a family of transparent proteins. Membrane-bound organelles are absent. The lens is attached to the ciliary body by very fine fibrous threads called zonular ligaments. Traction of these ligaments by muscles in the ciliary body changes the shape of the lens during accommodation (Lens *et al.* 1999, Kaufman and Alm 2003).

ATOPIC DERMATITIS

Eye disorders associated with atopic dermatitis include eyelid dermatitis, loss of eyelash or eyelid hair, tear abnormalities, blepharitis, conjunctivitis, keratitis, keratoconus, cataract, retinal detachment, and uveitis (Garrity and Liesegang 1984, Ohmachi *et al.* 1994, Carmi *et al.* 2006, Amer *et al.* 2007). Although they can occur in any race, these complications have a distinct predilection for Asian patients. Depending on the investigator, the population being studied, and the specific ocular abnormality being looked for, the incidence of associated eye disorders varies between 25% and 67% of patients with atopic dermatitis. All ocular manifestations of atopic dermatitis are exacerbated by eye rubbing.

KERATOCONJUNCTIVITIS

The most common ocular complication of atopic dermatitis is keratoconjunctivitis. In a series of 724 eyes of 362 patients with severe atopic dermatitis, biomicroscopic evidence of conjunctivitis coupled with superficial punctate keratopathy was observed in 67.5% of the patients (Dogru *et al.* 1999). Typical signs and symptoms of atopic keratoconjunctivitis include redness, pain, itch, photophobia, foreign body sensation, dry eye, and discharge.

Tear function abnormalities are a common feature of atopic keratoconjunctivitis (Dogru *et al.* 2005a, 2005b, 2006). The normal tear film consists of three layers: an outer lipid layer to prevent evaporation, an aqueous layer, and an inner mucin layer. Mucin enhances hydration, provides a barrier to prevent pathogens from contacting the eye surface, and ensures tear stability (Lens *et al.* 1999). The signs and symptoms of dry eye experienced by atopic keratoconjunctivitis patients result from abnormalities of mucin production. Squamous metaplasia of conjunctival mucin-secreting goblet cells causes reduction in secretion of normal mucin MUC5AC, as measured by MUC5AC mRNA expression (Dogru *et al.* 2005a). This leads to tear instability and rapid tear break-up. Aqueous tear production as measured by the Schirmer test is normal (Dogru *et al.* 2006).

Patients with atopic keratoconjunctivitis have impaired barrier function and corneal integrity, and the condition is associated with increased susceptibility to microbial infection (Yokoi *et al.* 1998, Nguyen 2007). Tears have antimicrobial properties (Lens *et al.* 1999). Atopic dermatitis is an important background disease in infectious keratitis, particularly in contact lens users. Gram-positive cocci are the most frequent infecting organisms (National Surveillance of Infectious Keratitis in Japan 2006).

The severity of corneal disease correlates with the presence of eosinophils from scrapings of the upper tarsal conjunctiva (Takano *et al.* 2004). Eosinophil cationic protein and eosinophil granule major basic protein have a cytotoxic effect on corneal epithelial cells *in vitro* (Takano *et al.* 2004, Yokoi *et al.* 1998). There is some evidence that the chronic inflammation associated with atopic keratoconjunctivitis may be a risk factor for conjunctival carcinoma (Kallen *et al.* 2003). Atopic keratoconjunctivitis is a potentially blinding disease because it can be associated with neovascularization (pannus formation), thinning, ulceration, and perforation (Tuft *et al.* 1991, Dogru *et al.* 1999). These complications can occur in the presence of minimal skin disease (Akova *et al.* 1993). Artificial tears devoid of preservatives help alleviate chronic dry-eye symptoms. Ophthalmic corticosteroids and topical cromolyns can be used in this condition and, in severe cases, topical tacrolimus ointment or topical and systemic cyclosporine (ciclosporin) is another treatment option (Hoang-Xuan *et al.* 1997, Cornish *et al.* 2010, Guglielmetti *et al.* 2010).

may complain of having to squint to see better, light sensitivity, and flares or halos around lights, especially when driving at night.

Treatment of keratoconus consists of corrective lenses; however, in severe cases, corneal transplantation surgery may be necessary (Ohmachi *et al.* 1994). Corneal transplantation in a patient with atopic keratoconjunctivitis is associated with a higher-than-average risk of infection and corneal clouding. Systemic cyclosporine has been shown to ameliorate this risk and improve graft prognosis (Reinhard and Sundmacher 1992, Reinhard *et al.* 1999).

KERATOCONUS

Keratoconus is an anterior bulging of the cornea due to thinning of the stroma (Bawazeer *et al.* 2000) (**Fig 13.2**). It is usually bilateral. An irregular corneal shape causes refractive changes and impairs vision. Although keratoconus is not common in atopic dermatitis, a significant percentage of patients with keratoconus have atopic dermatitis. In one study of 362 patients with severe atopic dermatitis, the incidence of keratoconus was 3.3% (Dogru *et al.* 1999). Another study of 240 atopic patients revealed an incidence of keratoconus of only 1.3% (Ohmachi *et al.* 1994). However, in a review of 125 keratoconus patients, 16% reported asthma and/or atopic dermatitis (Assiri *et al.* 2005). Rahi *et al.* (1977) reported a 35% incidence of atopy in keratoconus patients compared with an incidence of 12% in a control group.

In a case–control study of 49 patients with atopic dermatitis, trauma in the form of eye rubbing was identified as the major cause of keratoconus in a multivariate analysis; atopy itself was not a factor (Bawazeer *et al.* 2000). Ultraviolet light exposure and corneal inability to process reactive oxygen species have also been hypothesized to play roles in keratoconus development (Kenney and Brown 2003).

Keratoconus usually becomes symptomatic in the second decade of life or early 20s and can cause loss of visual acuity that cannot be compensated for with spectacles (Romero-Jiménez *et al.* 2010). Patients

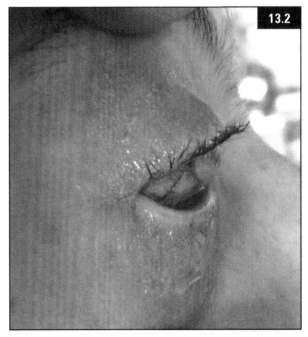

Fig 13.2 A 15-year-old female with severe atopic dermatitis. Exudation and lichenification are present in the periorbital region. There is severe keratoconjunctivitis and erythema of the palpebral and bulbar conjunctiva. Pronounced keratoconus is evident. (Courtesy of Dr Hara Schwartz.)

CATARACTS

An association between cataracts and atopic dermatitis has been known for decades. A cataract is an opacification of the lens resulting from denaturation of lens proteins. Cataracts form as a result of senescence, trauma, exposure to ultraviolet radiation, and a variety of metabolic insults. Oxygen byproducts such as hydroxyl radicals, superoxide, singlet oxygen, and hydrogen peroxide are particularly damaging to crystallins (Loewenstein and Lee 2004). Cataracts cause pathological dispersion of incoming light and refractive error. Symptoms include loss of contrast, increased light requirement for adequate vision, and progressive visual loss. Cataracts commonly occur with aging, but smoking, alcohol, and systemic disease such as diabetes, as well as corticosteroids and ultraviolet exposure, all increase the risk (Hutnik and Nichols 1999). The major indication for surgical removal is visual impairment that limits a person's functional capacity. Cataract extraction is usually accompanied by implanting a plastic or silicone lens. Potential surgical complications include infection, glaucoma, macular edema, and retinal detachment.

The incidence of cataract in atopic dermatitis patients is between 4.4% and 20% (Amemiya et al. 1980, Uehara et al. 1985, Ibarra-Duran et al. 1992). Atopic cataract formation correlates with severe disease, especially involving the face, elevated IgE, aqueous flare, and Asian ancestry (Matsuo et al. 1997, Sasabe et al. 1997, Uchio et al. 1998, Nagaki et al. 1999, Chen et al. 2000). 'Aqueous flare' refers to turbidity of the aqueous humor which may be elevated with increased protein content and inflammatory cells. Even in the absence of visual symptoms, ocular inflammation, eye rubbing, and subclinical cataractous changes are often observed in the lenses of atopic dermatitis patients (Sasaki et al. 1998). Cataract progression is accelerated by the use of corticosteroids and eye rubbing, but these factors are not considered causal (Sasaki et al. 1998, Uchio et al. 1998). The adverse effects of eye rubbing have been duplicated in animal models. Repeated vibratory stimulation of rabbit eyes causes opacification of the anterior and posterior subcapsular regions of the lens (Oshita et al. 2005). In a prospective study of 41 Japanese patients with atopic dermatitis, cataract progression correlated with facial skin lesions and eye rubbing (Nagaki et al. 1999). Atopic cataracts are often bilateral and frequently become clinically apparent in the second decade of life, sometimes earlier. Atopic cataracts are classically shield-like in morphology and anterior subcapsular in location (Brandonisio et al. 2001). However, they can occur anywhere in the lens and cannot be distinguished from corticosteroid-induced cataracts on the basis of clinical appearance and presentation (Amemiya et al. 1980, Castrow 1981).

Various pathogenic mechanisms for atopic cataract development have been proposed. These include the presence of autoantibodies to lens epithelium-derived growth factor, reduced capacity of atopic patients to counteract the effects of oxidative stressors, and trauma. The most intensely studied abnormality is the presence of autoantibodies to lens epithelium-derived growth factor (LEDGF). LEDGF is a protein present in the lens epithelial cells, epidermal cells, and various other cell types (Singh et al. 2000). It has been shown to be a prosurvival factor that confers resistance to apoptosis induced by stressors such as heat and oxidation (Singh et al. 1999). LEDGF has been detected in the nuclei of basal epidermal cells, but, as these cells differentiate, it moves into the cytoplasm (Sugiura et al. 2007). Likewise, in studies of rat lenticular epithelial cells, it has been shown that LEDGF translocates from the nucleus to the cytoplasm as cells differentiate (Kubo et al. 2003).

In the absence of LEDGF, lens epithelial cells become susceptible to stress; the presence of LEDGF is protective (Ayaki et al. 2002, Shinohara et al. 2002). Immunohistochemical studies of atopic cataracts suggest that apoptotic cell death plays a major role in the development of lens epithelial cell damage (Mihara et al. 2000). Autoantibodies directed against LEDGF may diminish its prosurvival functionality, thus leading to lenticular epithelial cell damage and cataract formation.

Approximately 30% of Japanese atopic dermatitis patients are found to have autoantibodies to LEDGF

(Ganapathy and Casiano 2004). However, there appears to be no statistically significant difference in the prevalence of autoantibodies to LEDGF in atopic dermatitis patients with cataracts compared with those without cataracts. It is believed that additional factors (eg, elevated histamine levels and eye rubbing) are necessary for cataract induction. These factors are thought to cause a breach of the blood–aqueous barrier, allowing entry of autoantibodies to LEDGF into the lens (Ayaki *et al.* 2002).

LEDGF also enhances survival of retinal pigment epithelial cells (Matsui *et al.* 2001). Autoantibodies to LEDGF have been identified in patients with atypical retinal degeneration and Vogt–Koyanagi–Harada syndrome, a disease associated with uveitis (Yamada *et al.* 2001, Chin *et al.* 2006). Although autoantibodies to LEDGF have been shown to be more prevalent in patients with atopic dermatitis, their presence is not common in patients with rheumatological disease (Ganapathy and Casiano 2004, Watanabe *et al.* 2004).

Hydrogen peroxide and other oxygen byproducts are an oxidative threat to the lens and play a role in cataract development. Aqueous humor contains significant amounts of hydrogen peroxide, the result of light-catalyzed reactions. Hydrogen peroxide is broken down in the aqueous humor by glutathione peroxidase. In animal models, deficiency of this enzyme leads to cataract formation. Decreased glutathione peroxidase occurs in people with atopic dermatitis and may contribute to cataract development (Namazi and Handjani 2006).

A gene abnormality, a $-56C/T$ single nucleotide polymorphism in the promoter region of the interferon-γ-1 receptor gene, has been identified in several atopic dermatitis patients with cataracts. The $-56T/T$ genotype increases promoter activity. Interferon-γ causes expression of inducible nitric oxide synthase (iNOS) in macrophages and lens epithelial cells (Matsuda *et al.* 2007). In animal models, nitric oxide plays a role in cataract development, and this may also apply to humans (Inomata *et al.* 2001, Ito *et al.* 2001, Nagai *et al.* 2006). The $-56C/T$ polymorphism was not detected in atopic dermatitis patients without cataracts.

RETINAL DETACHMENT

Retinal detachment is a separation of the sensory retina from the underlying pigment epithelium and choroid (**Fig 13.3**). It presents with floaters, light flashes (photopsia), and, most ominously, a descending curtain on the field of vision. Retinal detachment in atopic dermatitis usually involves a retinal tear (rhegmatogenous detachment), and this tearing can progress to involve the entire retina. Rhegmatogenous detachment also occurs in myopia, after cataract surgery, or after trauma.

Retinal detachment is treated with a variety of modalities including laser, cryotherapy, and electrosurgery. The basic purpose of these interventions is to create adhesions between the sensory retina and the pigment epithelium.

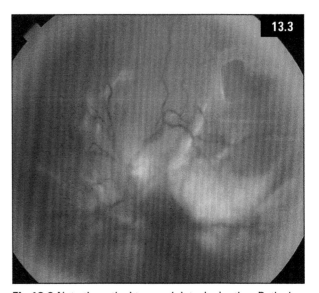

Fig 13.3 Note the retinal tear and detached retina. Retinal folding is present in one area. (Courtesy of Dr Allen Landers.)

The incidence of retinal detachment in Japanese atopic dermatitis patients with facial involvement is reported to be between 0.8% and 8%. It occurs predominantly between the ages of 10 and 30 years, and detachment is commonly associated with cataracts. Detachments are rhegmatogenous, with tears typically occurring at the extreme retinal periphery (Katsura and Hida 1984, Katsushima et al. 1994, Margolin et al. 2003). Atopic dermatitis was the underlying condition in 2.6% of 146 children with rhegmatogenous retinal detachment in a Taiwanese study (Chang et al. 2005).

Patients with facial dermatitis, especially those with eyelid eczema and blepharitis, frequently rub, scratch, or slap their eyes. Ocular trauma is a known risk factor for retinal detachment and worsening of cataracts (Wang et al. 2005, Chen et al. 2006). The fundoscopic findings of traumatic retinal detachment and atopic retinal detachment are similar: retinal breaks at the vitreous base border and the equatorial zone (Oka et al. 1994). A report analyzing 417 eyes of 348 Japanese patients with atopic dermatitis and rhegmatogenous retinal detachment concluded that self-induced trauma to the eyes was the most important causative factor, not atopic dermatitis itself (Hida et al. 2000).

Retinal detachment can complicate cataract surgery, but especially in atopic dermatitis patients (Katsura et al. 1994). Given the risk of retinal detachment in atopic patients, intraocular lens implantation has traditionally been avoided after cataract extraction. Without lens insertion, visual acuity remains poor. However, a recent study of patients with atopic cataracts showed increased visual acuity and decreased incidence of retinal detachment in patients receiving intraocular lens implantation compared with those who did not (Inoue et al. 2005).

UVEITIS

Uveitis is an inflammation of the uveal tract, which includes the iris, ciliary body, and choroid. Uveitis can be idiopathic, or be caused by infectious, autoimmune, or granulomatous disease. Symptoms vary and depend on site and severity of inflammation. Anterior disease involving the iris and ciliary body usually presents with pain, redness, and photophobia, whereas posterior disease involving the choroid produces floaters and decreased vision. Potential complications are cataract, ocular neovascularization, and visual loss. Uveitis in the setting of atopic dermatitis often represents a complication of some other ocular abnormality, particularly a retinal tear. It has been hypothesized that inflammation may result from release of antigen after such a tear (Lim and Chee 2004). Uveitis alone in atopic dermatitis usually takes the form of anterior uveitis (Singh and Mathur 1968, Amer et al. 2007).

BLEPHARITIS AND EYELID DERMATITIS

Blepharitis is characterized by erythema, scaling, and crusting around the eyelashes and eyelid margins. Although blepharitis is usually a manifestation of seborrheic dermatitis, it is also commonly seen in atopic dermatitis. A study of 280 patients with atopic dermatitis showed blepharitis in 52.5% of 560 eyes (Nakano et al. 1997). All forms of blepharitis are improved by cleaning the lid margins with water and baby shampoo.

Moistening the eye surface with artificial tears and moisturizing the skin around the eyes are additional therapeutic measures. Compared with healthy skin, the water retention capacity of eyelid skin in atopic dermatitis is reduced. This abnormality is present even in the absence of overt clinical findings of lichenification and erythema (Asano-Kato et al. 2001). Moisturizers containing ceramides appear to be particularly helpful in atopic blepharitis (Asano-Kato et al. 2003). In severe cases, topical corticosteroid ointments can be used. Ophthalmic preparations are preferred at the eyelid margin because the corticosteroid will contact the eye surface. Ophthalmic ointments are sterile and crystal size is fine.

Although the eyelids are commonly involved in atopic dermatitis, allergic contact dermatitis is the most common cause of eyelid dermatitis (**Fig 13.4**). Eyelid skin is thin (0.55 mm), and antigens can penetrate easily. Most patients with eyelid allergic contact dermatitis are women, and the most common allergens are cosmetic ingredients such as fragrances, surfactants, and preservatives (Amin and Belsito 2006). These chemicals are also found in topical dermatological medications and ophthalmological products (**Fig 13.5**). Airborne protein antigens such as ragweed, dust mites, pollens, and animal dander can also cause allergic contact dermatitis of the eyelids, as can allergens transferred from the hand such as nickel, nail products, and latex (Guin 2002) (**Fig 13.6**). Allergic contact dermatitis of the eyelids is usually associated with dermatitis elsewhere on the face or body. Isolated dermatitis localized to the eyelids alone is likely to be seborrheic dermatitis (Amin and Belsito 2006).

Assigning a precise cause involves careful history taking and patch testing. Patch testing involves applying specific, individual chemicals to skin to elicit a cell-mediated, type IV immunological reaction. 'Use testing' refers to applying the suspected whole product to a sensitive area of skin (such as the antecubital fossa) several times daily for 5 days to determine if the product causes dermatitis (Fisher 1986). False-positive irritant reactions are common, and patch testing is preferred.

Allergic contact dermatitis can be superimposed on atopic or seborrheic dermatitis; therefore, the presence of underlying dermatitis does not necessarily eliminate the need for patch testing. Any eyelid dermatitis can be perpetuated by chronic rubbing and scratching. Seborrheic dermatitis and allergic contact dermatitis of the eyelids are not associated with cataract; however, a case of a 34-year-old female with mild atopic dermatitis who abruptly developed cataracts after experiencing a sudden, severe, allergic contact dermatitis of the face has been reported (Uehara and Sato 1986).

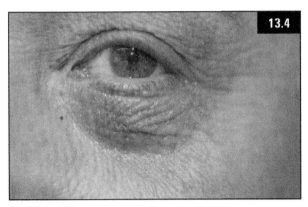

Fig 13.4 Eyelid atopic dermatitis: note the lower lid lichenification.

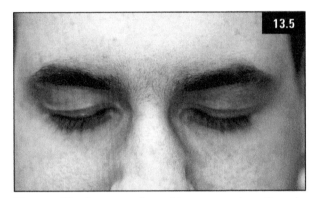

Fig 13.5 Allergic contact dermatitis to neomycin: unilateral left upper eyelid involvement suggests an exogenous cause.

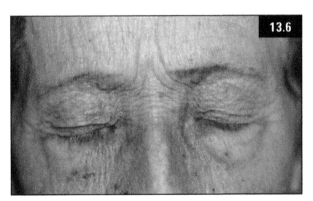

Fig 13.6 Airborne contact dermatitis: this is likely secondary to airborne ragweed. Note the lichenification of eyelid and facial skin.

Several other conditions uncommonly cause eyelid inflammation and should be considered in the differential diagnosis, particularly if the dermatitis does not respond to treatment. These conditions include psoriasis, dermatomyositis, rosacea, tinea, fixed drug eruption, cutaneous T-cell lymphoma, infections, infestations, and urticaria (Guin 2002). Also to be considered in the differential diagnosis of a recalcitrant dermatitis of the eyelids are *steroid rebound*, allergy to corticosteroids, and *perioral* dermatitis occurring in the periocular region (**Fig 13.7**).

Steroid rebound is a phenomenon characterized by redness, burning, edema, and apparent worsening of the original dermatosis on discontinuation of a topical corticosteroid, which may occur on eyelid skin. Prolonged use is necessary for this to occur, and the minimum duration of application is approximately 1 month. When steroid rebound occurs, the common (but erroneous) therapeutic intervention is applying more corticosteroid, often one of higher potency than the original. Repetitive cycles make the situation progressively worse and difficult to control. Eyelid skin appears to be particularly susceptible, and rebound can occur even after use of 'safe' corticosteroids such as over-the-counter hydrocortisone. The mechanism of steroid rebound is not known, but may be related to an accumulation of high levels of nitric oxide (an endogenous vasodilator) in vascular endothelium to counteract the vasoconstrictive effects of topical corticosteroids.

Appropriate treatment consists of discontinuation of topical corticosteroids around the eye coupled with cool compresses and bland emollients. Calcineurin inhibitors may be of value, but not during acute flares. It generally takes months for the skin to return to normal, and these patients require more than the usual amount of psychological reassurance (Rapaport and Rapaport 1999).

Allergic contact dermatitis to the steroid component of topical corticosteroids has been described and may be more common than realized (David *et al.* 2007). Allergy to a secondary chemical such as a preservative or surfactant is a well-recognized phenomenon. Ointments, in general, contain fewer secondary chemicals than creams or lotions, and their use is preferred for eyelid dermatitis. Atrophy, telangiectasia, and the fine papulopustular rash of perioral and periorbital dermatitis can also complicate the use of topical corticosteroids on eyelid skin.

CORTICOSTEROID-INDUCED CATARACT AND GLAUCOMA

The adverse cutaneous effects of long-term corticosteroid application around the eyes are bothersome and difficult to treat. However, prolonged use of topical corticosteroids on eyelid skin can also affect the eye itself and cause the sight-threatening complications of glaucoma and cataract.

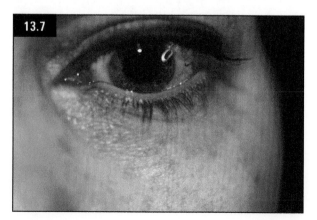

Fig 13.7 Eyelid periorbital dermatitis: fine papulopustules are present on the lower eyelid in a patient who has been using over-the-counter hydrocortisone cream on the area for several months.

In an ophthalmological context, the phrase 'topical steroids' means direct application of a corticosteroid to the surface of the eye. Topical corticosteroids are prescribed by ophthalmologists for many indications including allergic conjunctivitis, scleritis, episcleritis, interstitial keratitis, and uveitis. Topical corticosteroids applied to the periorbital region for dermatological indications can also inadvertently reach the surface of the eye. In all likelihood, topical corticosteroids applied to the skin reach the eye surface through the palpebral fissure, not directly through the eyelid skin.

An *in vitro* study showed that only extremely small amounts of a medium-potency corticosteroid – fluticasone – penetrated the thin eyelid skin (Tan *et al.* 2001). Ophthalmologists often observe flecks of cosmetics in tear films in females (Eisenlohr 1983). Also, the common experience of burning and stinging after applying sunscreens to the face supports the theory that chemicals reach the eye through the palpebral fissure, not through the skin. Transfer of medication from periorbital skin to the surface of the eye is especially likely to occur under conditions of sweating or eye rubbing.

Cataract formation is a known complication of systemic administration of corticosteroids, but topical corticosteroids used for ophthalmological and dermatological indications can also induce cataracts (Williamson and Jasani 1967, Donshik *et al.* 1981, Marsh and Pflugfelder 1999, Sim *et al.*

2009). Corticosteroid-induced cataracts are typically located posteriorly and subcapsularly (**Fig 13.8**). In an observational study, Yablonski treated 11 diabetic patients in one eye with topical dexamethasone for 14–36 months. In nine of these patients, cataract developed in the treated eye only (Yablonski *et al.* 1978). Munjal reported development of cataracts in 23 patients treated for inflamed eyes with topical corticosteroids for periods ranging from 9 months to 10 years. There appeared to be a correlation between duration of use and severity of cataract (Munjal *et al.* 1984). In a recent study from the Netherlands, long-term application of topical corticosteroids to the eye or periorbital skin did not correlate with the development of cataracts (Haeck *et al.* 2011). Other than surgical removal, there is no current medical treatment for any form of cataract.

The precise pathogenesis of steroid-induced cataract formation is not certain. Corticosteroids may covalently bind to lens proteins, leading to destabilization of the protein structure and subsequent oxidation (McGhee *et al.* 2002). Alternatively, it has been observed that only steroids with glucocorticoid activity have the capacity to induce cataracts. Cataract formation may therefore be the result of glucocorticoid receptor activation, and gene transcription within lens epithelial cells. This in turn would alter the balance of ocular cytokines and growth factors (Jobling and Augusteyn 2002).

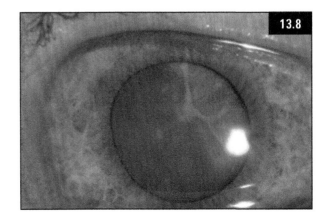

Fig 13.8 This patient who used topical hydrocortisone cream on the face for 20 years developed bilateral cortical cataracts. (Reprinted from Sim *et al.* 2009 with permission from Macmillan Publishers Ltd. © 2008.)

Lens tissue has higher levels of potassium (K$^+$) ions and lower levels of sodium (Na$^+$) and chloride (Cl$^-$) ions and water than the surrounding aqueous and vitreous humor. Chemical energy is needed to maintain the water and electrolyte composition of the lens. Water and Na$^+$ are extruded from the lens by Na$^+$/K$^+$ ATPase (the 'sodium pump'). Corticosteroids are known to inhibit Na$^+$/K$^+$ ATPase activity in lens epithelial cells. Decreased pump activity is associated with increased Na$^+$ and water content, which in turn damages lens epithelial cells, causes the formation of microscopic vacuoles, and promotes lens opacification (Mayman et al. 1979, Tao et al. 1999). For the lens to maintain transparency, it must remain dehydrated in relation to the surrounding environment. Studies comparing human cataractous lenses with those of normal age-matched controls show significant reduction in Na$^+$/K$^+$ ATPase activity (Kobatashi et al. 1982).

Glaucoma occurs as a complication of elevated intraocular pressure. Normal intraocular pressure depends on a balance between the production and outflow of the aqueous humor in the anterior segment of the eye. The function of aqueous humor is to maintain the shape of the eye and to provide nourishment to the lens and cornea. Aqueous humor is formed by the ciliary body in the posterior chamber. From there, it flows through the pupil to the anterior chamber. It leaves the anterior chamber through a sponge-like system of pores called the trabecular meshwork, located at the junction of the cornea and the root of the iris. The trabecular meshwork causes a resistance to flow and elevation of pressure. From the trabecular meshwork, fluid moves into the canal of Schlemm and then to the venous system. Under physiological conditions, a balance exists between fluid production and fluid outflow such that enough internal pressure is present to maintain the overall round shape of the eye. The normal intraocular pressure is 15 mmHg (Lens et al. 1999, Kaufman and Alm 2003). An elevation of intraocular pressure with no other abnormalities is known as *ocular hypertension*. Ocular hypertension associated with visual field defects or observable damage to the optic nerve is considered glaucoma.

Corticosteroids cause ocular hypertension and glaucoma. Topical application of corticosteroids is a much more potent inducer of elevated intraocular pressure than systemic administration, but at least several weeks of application are needed before elevation of intraocular pressure becomes detectable. Months or years may elapse before elevated intraocular pressure becomes evident from systemic corticosteroids (Carnahan and Goldstein 2000, Jones and Rhee 2006, Kersey and Broadway 2006). Corticosteroid-induced elevation of intraocular pressure is generally reversible when the medication is discontinued. If visual field defects are present, however, they usually persist even if the intraocular pressure returns to normal (Munjal et al. 1982, Mohan and Muralidharan 1989). On occasion, usually after long-term use of topical corticosteroids, intraocular pressure will remain permanently elevated and resistant to medical therapy even after discontinuation of medication (Kersey and Broadway 2006).

Visual loss brought about by steroid-induced glaucoma is insidious. Visual field defects often begin peripherally and are not noticed. By the time visual loss becomes apparent to the patient, that loss is significant and often irreversible (Kersey and Broadway 2006). Common complaints of patients with steroid-induced glaucoma include halos around bright objects and blurred vision.

Corticosteroids induce elevated intraocular pressure by interfering with the outflow of aqueous humor through the trabecular meshwork (Kersey and Broadway 2006). Several mechanisms have been proposed. Corticosteroids inhibit the activity of lysosomal hyaluronidase, leading to an accumulation of mucopolysaccharides within the extracellular matrix of the trabecular meshwork and resultant obstruction of flow (Spaeth et al. 1977, Francois 1984, Jones and Rhee 2006).

In vitro studies suggest that deposition of other materials, specifically laminin and collagen, in the outflow pathway of the trabecular meshwork may also play a role in corticosteroid-induced glaucoma (Tane et al. 2007). Corticosteroids interfere with the phagocytic abilities of trabecular meshwork cells. This may lead to accumulation of pigment and other debris within the trabecular meshwork which also could obstruct outflow (Zhang et al. 2007). Finally, it has been shown that dexamethasone causes development of crosslinked actin and actin-associated protein networks. These changes may lead to obstructed outflow (Clark *et al.* 2005, Rozsa *et al.* 2006).

People who experience elevated intraocular pressure after exposure to corticosteroids by any route are called *corticosteroid responders*. Approximately two-thirds of clinically healthy eyes are nonresponsive. One-third of clinically healthy eyes will show some elevation of intraocular pressure after topical application of corticosteroids to the eyes for 4–6 weeks. Approximately 5% of healthy eyes will show a high elevation of intraocular pressure after topical corticosteroid exposure (Armaly 1965). Risk factors for steroid responsiveness include a personal history of open-angle glaucoma, open-angle glaucoma in a first-degree relative, a prior episode of elevated intraocular pressure after steroid use, diabetes, high myopia, connective tissue disease (especially rheumatoid arthritis), long-term use of corticosteroids, use of potent steroids around the eyes, and a history of trauma to the anterior portion of the eye (Carnahan and Goldstein 2000, Garrott and Walland 2004, Kersey and Broadway 2006). Approximately 50% of patients with a history of open-angle glaucoma are steroid responders and, in glaucoma patients undergoing treatment, topical corticosteroids can result in loss of control of intraocular pressure (Garrott and Walland 2004). Elderly people and very young children are at particularly high risk for steroid responsiveness (Jones and Rhee 2006).

There have been several case reports describing glaucoma in patients using topical corticosteroids around the eyes for various dermatological conditions. (Cubey 1976, Zugerman *et al.* 1976, Vie 1980, Eisenlohr 1983, Aggarwal *et al.* 1993, Garrott and Walland 2004, Ross *et al.* 2004, Sahni *et al.* 2004, Van Boxtel *et al.* 2005). In most of these cases, the duration of treatment was long, sometimes years, and, in general, high-potency products were applied. The resultant glaucoma was often resistant to medical therapies and surgical intervention was needed. Significant visual loss was a consistent feature. In all cases, the patients were unaware of the risks associated with chronic topical corticosteroid use around the eyes.

Elevated intraocular pressure has not been reported as a complication of topical tacrolimus or pimecrolimus applied to eyelid skin. Tacrolimus ointment has been used safely in a patient with known glaucoma (Kymionis *et al.* 2004). It has also been shown to be effective in treating atopic eyelid dermatitis and atopic keratoconjunctivitis (Mayer *et al.* 2001, Rikkers *et al.* 2003, Freeman *et al.* 2004, Virganen *et al.* 2006, Nivenius *et al.* 2007). If eyelid dermatitis does not respond to bland emollients, a calcineurin inhibitor should be tried. These medications are apparently safe around the eyes, because they do not induce cataract or elevated intraocular pressure even after long-term use.

Calcineurin inhibitors, particularly tacrolimus, may sting on application. Stinging can be reduced somewhat if the medication is kept refrigerated and applied cold. Contact dermatitis to calcineurin inhibitors is rare, and rebound has not been reported with this class of medications (Shaw *et al.* 2004, Anderson and Broesby-Olsen 2006). In approximately 1% of patients who apply calcineurin inhibitors, however, flushing at the site of application can occur after oral ingestion of alcohol (Ehst and Warshaw 2004, Knight *et al.* 2005, Anonymous 2007). A case of eczema herpeticum was reported in a patient using 0.1% tacrolimus ointment around the eyes. Local immunosuppression from the medication, not eczema, was thought to be responsible. The authors cite a 4.2% incidence of eczema herpeticum in a 1998 multicenter study of tacrolimus ointment conducted in Japan (Miyake-Kashima *et al.* 2004).

If low- or medium-potency corticosteroids such as hydrocortisone or desonide are used for eyelid eczema, they are best applied for short periods, after which the patient should be transitioned to a calcineurin inhibitor. High-potency topical corticosteroids such as clobetasol or fluocinonide should be applied around the eyes with extreme caution, if at all.

Clinical suggestions

1. Patients with eyelid dermatitis, particularly atopic dermatitis, should be warned not to rub, scratch, or slap the eyes. This practice traumatizes the internal structures of the eye. It accelerates cataract progression, and is a known cause of rhegmatogenous retinal detachment. Rubbing the eyes worsens lichenification and increases the likelihood of transfer of medication to the eye surface. Periorbital itch is best treated by cold, wet compresses. If these are not available, gentle pressure on the eyelid skin will help. Frictional or slapping trauma must be avoided.

2. Inquire about personal or family history of glaucoma. People with a personal or family history are at particularly high risk of elevated intraocular pressure after topical corticosteroid use, and topical calcineurin inhibitors are the treatment of choice.

3. In cases of nonresponsive or worsening dermatitis around the eyes despite treatment with corticosteroids, re-evaluate the diagnosis and consider an uncommon cause such as dermatomyositis or tinea faciale. Consider also corticosteroid rebound or a superimposed contact dermatitis to the medication. Bear in mind that ointments generally contain fewer secondary chemicals than creams, gels, or lotions.

4. When writing a prescription for corticosteroids around the eyes, explicitly indicate the duration of treatment, make the prescription nonrefillable, and warn the patient of potential risks.

5. In patients with severe atopic dermatitis, particularly Asian patients, consider obtaining a baseline ophthalmological evaluation followed by periodic eye examinations. The skin, lens, and retina share a common neuroectodermal origin, and the eye can be a major target organ. Cooperation of dermatologists and ophthalmologists is essential.

CHAPTER 14

HAND DERMATITIS

Nina C. Botto and Erin M. Warshaw

The human hand is a versatile tool, useful in innumerable tasks, from activities vital to living and self-defense, to leisure pursuits such as knitting and cooking. As such, our hands come into contact with a wider range of chemicals and foreign substances than any other part of the body. As Sutton and Ayres noted in their 1953 treatise on hand dermatitis with regard to these remarkable instruments: 'they pick … pry … and investigate.' Hand dermatitis is, therefore, not surprisingly, a common, and often chronic, skin condition that can wreak havoc on the lives and livelihoods of affected individuals and on those who depend on, treat, employ, and insure them.

This chapter reviews the epidemiology, clinical features, occupational aspects, and long-term outcomes of hand dermatitis and supplements previous reviews by the senior author (Warshaw *et al.* 2003, Warshaw 2004). Therapeutic options are discussed in detail, with special focus on managing recalcitrant cases.

PREVALENCE

Current prevalence rates of hand dermatitis ranges from 2% to 9.5%; moreover, approximately 20–35% of all dermatoses affect the hands (Menné

et al. 1982, Elston *et al.* 2002). In addition it is estimated that approximately 80% of all *occupational* dermatoses involve the hands (Vestey *et al.* 1986). Thus, in a review of 958 cases of work-related skin diseases during a 1-year period, hand dermatitis comprised 88% of the total cases (Keil and Shmunes 1983). Another study found the overall prevalence of hand dermatitis among 167 inpatient nurses to be 55% (Lampel *et al.* 2007). Although it has been claimed that hand dermatitis has decreased in prevalence, it is arguably still the most common work-related dermatitis. Heightened awareness, legislation, and increased patient and employer education aimed at preventing occupational hand dermatitis may account, in part, for the recent purported decline in its prevalence.

A surveillance program implemented at a large food company alleged that the average incidence of work-related skin problems was declining (Smith 2004). However, such surveys tend to under-report cases so actual prevalence rates may be much higher (Mathias 1985). Individuals affected by hand dermatitis may not seek medical attention, despite persistent symptoms, as exemplified by a study which found that, although 63% of kitchen workers were affected by hand eczema, only 35% had consulted a physician about it (Nilsson 1994).

CLINICAL VARIANTS

In 1953, the prototypical hand dermatitis patient was portrayed as 'a young matron, who must keep house, cook, wash dishes, do the laundry, raise her children, and hold her husband' (Sutton and Ayres 1953). Today, neither gender roles nor individuals with hand dermatitis are so easily compartmentalized, but some original conceptions of eczematous hand dermatitis variants remain constant. These entities include contact (allergic and irritant), hyperkeratotic (psoriasiform, tylotic, frictional), nummular, atopic, and vesicular (pompholyx, dyshidrotic eczema, and chronic vesicular hand dermatitis). In clinical practice, however, arbitrary classification systems may be an oversimplification. Patients often exhibit their own unique amalgam of clinical variants and do not simply fit into a single pattern.

Some clinicians categorize hand dermatitis as either *endogenous/intrinsic* or *exogenous/extrinsic*, whereas others focus on reaction patterns. Clinical criteria in many publications are often not clearly defined; as such, the authors report the terms used in the original publications, although they may differ from the schema offered in this chapter. Importantly, the accurate diagnosis of hand dermatitis depends on a sound history and physical examination. In addition, patch testing, potassium hydroxide examination, and skin biopsy may be necessary if the diagnosis is in doubt. Key components of the history, physical examination, and useful diagnostic tests are listed in **Box 14.1.**

CONTACT DERMATITIS

The designation *contact dermatitis* comprises both irritant reactions and allergic contact dermatitis. Irritant contact dermatitis, by far the more common, is caused by direct cell damage from cutaneous exposure to an offending exogenous contactant; irritant contact dermatoses encompass about 80% of all cases of contact dermatitis (Centers for Disease Control 1986, Goh 1989). Allergic contact dermatitis, on the other hand, is a cell-mediated allergic reaction, caused by direct epidermal exposure to a contact allergen to which an individual has been previously sensitized. Other reactions such as contact urticaria and photosensitivity also cause hand dermatitis, and more than one cause or clinical pattern can be present concurrently in the same patient; eg, an irritant, by damaging the epidermal barrier and facilitating exposure and sensitization to contact allergens, might predispose one to an allergic contact dermatitis.

The pathogenic mechanism of irritant contact dermatitis involves direct chemical damage and innate immune responses. The combined exposure to several irritant substances, eg, water and soap, with repetitive activities such as hand washing that cause friction and trauma, ultimately leads to skin breakdown and dermatitis (Malten 1981). Regular or repetitive exposure to irritants also hinders intrinsic mechanisms that repair the damaged epidermis. Patients with atopic dermatitis, a condition that is known to have a dysfunctional skin barrier, are at particular risk of developing irritant hand dermatitis, especially those with loss-of-function mutations of the filaggrin gene (Nassif *et al.* 1994, de Jongh 2008). In addition, elderly individuals are more susceptible to asteatotic dermatitis, a subtype of irritant contact dermatitis, as a result of delayed barrier repair mechanisms (Seyfarth *et al.* 2011).

Whereas irritant contact dermatitis results from direct cell injury, allergic contact dermatitis is a cell-mediated, type IV, delayed-type hypersensitivity reaction elicited by exposure to a contact antigen.

Box 14.1   Key components in hand dermatitis evaluation

History
- Time of onset
- Occupation
- Hobbies
- Household activities
- Animal exposure
- Personal hygiene
- Temporal relationship to work, travel, and/or time off
- Change in dermatitis pattern or behavior
- Current and previous topical therapies
- Exposures at work, at home, or through hobbies to chemicals, detergents, medications, lubricants, cleansers, frictional forces, or gloves
- Hand-washing frequency
- Dermatitis at sites other than the hands
- Previous episodes or history of dermatitis
- Family history of dermatitis
- History of atopy

Physical examination
Hands:
- Dorsal versus palmar involvement
- Vesicles or pustules
- Nail pitting
- Fingertip and finger web involvement
- Wrist involvement

General:
- Full-body skin assessment
- Attention to the feet

Diagnostic testing
- Patch tests: standard antigens, corticosteroids, and exposure-specific antigens
- Potassium hydroxide (KOH) examination and fungal culture
- Biopsy to rule out other noneczematous skin diseases such as psoriasis, keratoderma, dermatomyositis, vesicular bullous pemphigoid, and cutaneous T-cell lymphoma
- Radioallergosorbent testing (RAST) or prick testing for contact urticaria to foods, latex, and other allergens in selected patients

Modified from Epstein (1984) and Warshaw *et al.* (2003)

This may be an oversimplification because many contact allergens act as irritants and induce an innate immune response with release of proinflammatory cytokines (Rustemeyer *et al.* 2011), eg, nickel, an extremely common contact sensitizer, has been shown to directly activate toll-like receptor 4 (TLR)-4, inducing a proinflammatory response (Schmidt *et al.* 2010).

Patch testing is an essential means of determining whether a given hand dermatitis is allergic in nature and, if so, identifying the responsible antigens. In various series, allergic contact dermatitis accounts for anywhere from 14% to 54% of cases of hand dermatitis; eg, in a study of 6953 hand dermatitis patients patch tested from 1994 to 2004 by the North American Contact Dermatitis Group, only 959 (14%) turned out to have allergic contact dermatitis alone, and, in another patch test series of 220 hand dermatitis patients, only 17% had allergic contact dermatitis (Jordan 1974, Warshaw *et al.* 2007). Other large studies have found allergic contact dermatitis to be the cause of hand dermatitis in 32–54% of cases (Meding 1994, Sun *et al.* 1995, Templet *et al.* 2004).

Also of note is that, in some studies, a correlation has been found between the pattern of hand dermatitis and the causative allergen. Of 5700 suspected allergic contact dermatitis patients, whole-hand dermatitis correlated with reactions to thiuram mix, *p*-phenylenediamine, chromate, and *Myroxylon pereirae* (balsam of Peru), whereas involvement of the interdigital spaces and fingers was associated with allergy to nickel, cobalt, and methylchloroisothiazolinone/methylisothiazolinone (MCI/MI). Palmar involvement corresponded to an allergy to nickel, cobalt, MCI/MI, and primin (Edman 2000). Common allergens identified in two large North American studies included quaternium-15, formaldehyde, nickel sulfate, fragrance mix, thiuram mix, balsam of Peru, and carba mix (Sun *et al.* 1995, Warshaw *et al.* 2007).

In summary, accurate diagnosis and management of hand dermatitis often rely heavily on patch testing. Patch testing identifies the responsible antigen(s), helps exclude irrelevant allergens, and forms a basis for patient education on avoidance of possible causative substances in the home and workplace.

CLINICAL FEATURES

Irritant and allergic contact dermatitis cannot be reliably distinguished based on clinical features alone. Many patients describe stinging, itching, and/or tenderness at the exposure site of both irritants and allergens. Visible signs of acute dermatitis include papules, vesicles, bullae, and edema, as well as weeping and crusting. With chronicity, both allergic and irritant contact dermatitis can manifest eczematous plaques with fissuring, hyperpigmentation, and lichenification (Sherertz 1999). Infrequently, lichenoid eruptions, contact leukoderma, and erythema multiforme-like reactions can be seen associated with tropical woods and photographic chemicals (Belsito 2000).

Finger web-space involvement with extension to the dorsal or ventral surfaces of the hand (the so-called 'apron' pattern), involvement of the dorsal aspects of the hands or fingers, and localization on the palms and ball of the thumb (in a nonvesicular pattern) have all been associated with *irritant* contact dermatitis (**Figs 14.1** and **14.2**) (Sun *et al.* 1995, Duarte *et al.* 1998). *Allergic* contact dermatitis is often associated with fingertip, nailfold, and dorsal hand involvement and frequently displays vesiculation (**Figs 14.3** and **14.4**). The palm is rarely primarily affected in allergic contact dermatitis, unless allergen exposure is limited to the palm, as might occur with gripping such objects as nickel-plated doorknobs or implements with rubber handles. Importantly, irritant contact dermatitis often precedes allergic contact dermatitis, so patterns of dermatitis may evolve; an irritant contact dermatitis may start in the web spaces and then move to the fingertips with the onset of sensitization. Similarly, palmar involvement may extend to include the dorsal surface of the hand, providing a clue to the clinician to consider patch testing.

The time course of irritant and allergic contact dermatitis may sometimes suggest a particular diagnosis. Irritant contact dermatitis often begins around 3 months after exposure, usually through 'wet work' (via repeated or extended exposure to water, irritants, and/or trauma). Upon re-exposure to irritants, the dermatitis quickly recurs, often much more rapidly than during the initial presentation. Upon removal of the responsible irritant(s), the reaction improves

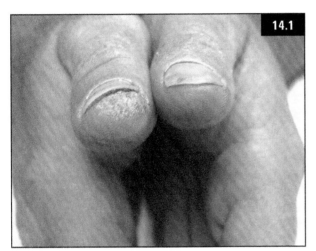

Fig 14.1 Irritant contact hand dermatitis. Note also onycholysis and fissuring.

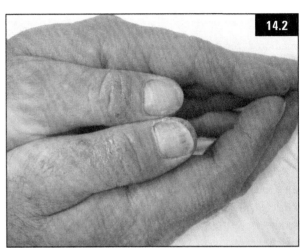

Fig 14.2 Irritant contact hand dermatitis.

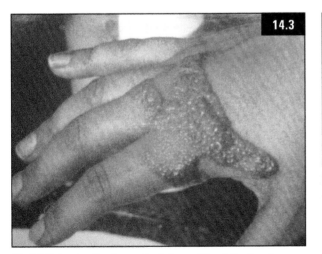

Fig 14.3 Acute allergic contact dermatitis of the hand caused by colophony resin in a bandage.

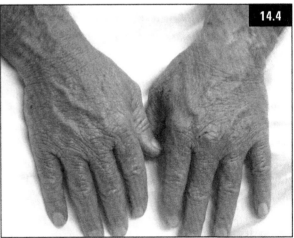

Fig 14.4 Allergic contact dermatitis of the hand due to formaldehyde-releasing preservative.

over time in a 'decrescendo' pattern. Allergic contact dermatitis, similar to irritant contact dermatitis, may be aggravated by exposure to water, humidity, gloves, occlusion, and other irritants. In addition, allergic contact dermatitis related to the workplace often abates on weekends or vacations and worsens 48–72 h after allergen re-exposure (Van der Walle 2000). As allergic contact dermatitis is a delayed-type cell-mediated reaction, reactions often 'crescendo' over 1–3 weeks before improving. Both irritant and allergic contact dermatitis can become chronic.

OCCUPATIONAL CONCERNS

The strong relationship between hand dermatitis and occupation is not surprising considering the critical role that hands play in most jobs; eg, in a study of 329 individuals with hand dermatitis, 56% of the cases were related to the occupation (both allergic and irritant contact dermatitis) and, of these, healthcare workers were most frequently affected (Templet et al. 2004). The preponderance of hand dermatitis among healthcare workers was confirmed by a Danish study which found that 21.4% of cases of occupationally induced hand eczema occurred in healthcare workers, followed by food service workers (11.3%). Occupations that involve wet work are more likely to cause both irritant and/or allergic contact dermatitis (Lushniak 1995). Healthcare workers, beauticians, food service workers, construction workers, homemakers, machinists, and warehouse workers are all at increased risk for hand dermatitis (Smit et al. 1993, Stingeni et al. 1995, Wigger-Alberti et al. 1999).

In most occupational studies, irritant contact dermatitis is more prevalent than allergic contact dermatitis, but this varies with the particular occupations studied. A Portuguese study of occupational hand dermatitis in 714 patients found that irritant dermatitis was more prevalent in healthcare workers, homemakers, and mechanics whereas contact allergy was more prevalent in hairdressers and bricklayers (Magina et al. 2003). Another study cited greater rates of irritant contact dermatitis in hairdressers, construction and steel workers, food handlers, and those who perform cleaning work (Diepgen and Fartasch 1994). In a study of hand dermatitis in North America, 7–11% of patients with allergic contact dermatitis had an associated occupational exposure (Warshaw et al. 2007).

CONTACT URTICARIA AND EVOLUTION TO ECZEMATOUS HAND DERMATITIS

Contact urticaria is a type I, IgE-mediated urticarial reaction, usually caused by exposure to protein antigens and much less commonly to low-molecular-weight compounds such as 2-ethylhexyl acrylate and acid anhydrides (Nicholson et al. 2010). Unfortunately, the literature regarding its prevalence is limited. An Australian study found that occupational contact urticaria (mostly on the hands but also on the face and arms) constituted 8.3% (143 of 1720) of the total number of patients with occupational skin disease (Williams et al. 2008). It was most commonly caused by natural rubber latex, foodstuffs, and ammonium persulfate in hairdressing bleach in healthcare workers, food handlers, and hairdressers respectively. A British study of work-related skin diseases from 1996 to 2001 found an incidence of contact urticaria (not limited to the hands) of about 4.2%; in comparison, contact dermatitis (allergic and irritant contact dermatitis) made up 78.6% of the cases (McDonald et al. 2006). In a 1999 Bureau of Labor Statistics report, 1% of the cases of occupational skin disease leading to time missed from work resulted from contact urticaria. The most frequent causes of occupational contact urticaria include cow dander, food and animal products, flour and grains, and natural rubber latex; the occupations most at risk include bakers, farmers, food preparers, and health workers (Nicholson et al. 2010).

One of the most important causes of contact urticaria of the hands is arguably latex in natural latex rubber gloves. Latex allergy occurs commonly in healthcare workers, food handlers, and rubber industry workers. Proteins found in the sap of the Hevea brasiliensis tree, from which rubber is derived, are the main allergens (Turjanmaa 1987). An epidemic of latex allergy in healthcare workers, likely due to low-quality, allergen-rich, natural rubber latex gloves, occurred in the 1980s and 1990s when universal precautions were first instituted. In the last decade, however, sensitization to latex appears to have decreased with the use of low-allergen and nonlatex gloves (Warshaw 1998). However, a 2011 study from the Duke University surveyed 4584 employees and found that 6% of these reported symptoms consistent with latex allergy (Epling *et al.* 2011). Nurses, medical or lab technicians, physicians' assistants, other clinical professionals, and housekeepers were the most frequently affected.

Contact urticaria may present with hives and itching (especially after donning rubber gloves), conjunctivitis, rhinitis, asthma (due to respiratory mucosal exposure to allergens absorbed onto glove powder), and rarely systemic symptoms. Anaphylaxis may occur after mucosal exposure of the rectum, vagina, or mouth during a gloved examination or surgery, or after sexual relations with a latex condom (Warshaw 1998). As allergic contact urticaria is a type I allergy, diagnosis can be confirmed by IgE radioallergoabsorbent testing (RAST), prick tests, or usage tests (Kelly *et al.* 1993); skin-prick testing has the greatest diagnostic efficiency with higher sensitivity and specificity than specific IgE determination or usage testing (Suli *et al.* 2006).

The number of years of latex glove use is a significant risk factor for latex allergy symptoms independent of the effects of atopy, gender, age, race, fruit, and other allergies (Epling *et al.* 2011). Moreover, chronic exposure to contact urticants in type I allergic patients may result in an eczematous dermatitis secondary to chronic inflammation and excoriation. As types I and IV hypersensitivities can coexist, it may be necessary to test for both immediate, type I allergic sensitivity (with the methods discussed above) and type IV, delayed hypersensitivity, with patch testing. Besides rubber chemicals, raw vegetables, fruit, and meats have all been well documented as causing type I allergy (Maibach 1976). Common agents that may cause contact urticaria of the hands are listed in Box 14.2.

Box 14.2 Potential causes of contact urticaria of the hands

Food:
- Seafood: fish, shrimp, oyster, calamari
- Meat: lamb, turkey, beef, pork, chicken, liver, animal blood
- Dairy products: milk, butter, cheese, eggs
- Fruit: apple, orange, pear, lemon, peach, plums, strawberries, tomato, banana, mango, kiwi
- Vegetables: onion, mushroom, cucumber, lettuce, beans, potato, carrot, celery
- Grains: rice, wheat, barley, rye, oats, buckwheat, maize

Metals:
- Aluminum
- Nickel
- Rhodium
- Platinum

Other:
- Natural rubber latex
- Wool
- Topical antibiotics

Modified from Warshaw *et al.* (2003).

HYPERKERATOTIC HAND DERMATITIS

Hyperkeratotic hand dermatitis (tylotic, psoriasiform, frictional), originally described by Sutton and Ayres (1953), is an uncommon clinical variant. Two separate studies found that hyperkeratotic hand dermatitis comprised only about 2% of all hand dermatoses and occurred most commonly in men between the ages of 40 and 60 years (Meding and Swanbeck 1989). Typically, hyperkeratotic hand dermatitis presents as symmetric plaques on the proximal or middle aspects of the palmar surfaces, accompanied by similar lesions on the feet (**Fig 14.5**). Hyperkeratotic hand dermatitis is often chronic and stable but painful fissures may complicate the condition.

The clinical differential diagnosis of hyperkeratotic hand dermatitis includes palmoplantar psoriasis, tinea manus, palmoplantar keratoderma, and allergic and/or irritant contact dermatitis, as well as frictional dermatitis from mechanical trauma. Skin biopsy, if performed, usually shows nonspecific changes of hyperkeratosis, focal parakeratosis, acanthosis, and/or spongiosis. These findings, often referred to as *psoriasiform changes*, do not necessarily imply palmoplantar psoriasis.

Although the cause of hyperkeratotic hand dermatitis is unclear, a history of manual labor (construction workers, forest workers, machinists, mechanics, and paper handlers) may be present

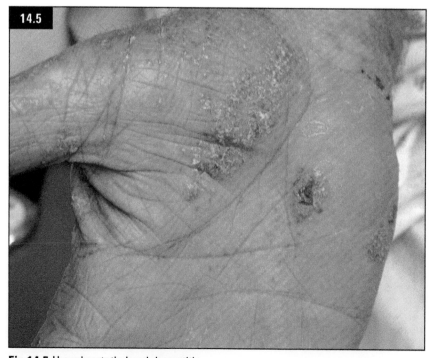

Fig 14.5 Hyperkeratotic hand dermatitis.

(Hersle and Mobacken 1982). Although some experts have postulated a link between hyperkeratotic hand dermatitis and psoriasis, a 10-year prospective cohort study of patients with hyperkeratotic palmar dermatitis failed to show an increased risk of psoriasis or, for that matter, fungal infection, increased serum IgE, or positive patch-test reactions.

When associated with frictional exposure, this variant is generally referred to as *frictional hand dermatitis*. A variety of mechanical forces may induce typical frictional dermatitis including shear forces, trauma, pressure, and vibration. Importantly, skin manifestations may take years to occur even with long-standing occupational exposures, and so may go unrecognized by practitioners. The clinical presentation of frictional hand dermatitis depends on the intensity and chronicity of the inciting force(s) involved (McMullen and Gawkrodger 2006). Forces of lower magnitude may induce hyperkeratotic plaques, whereas more intense forces may induce bullae (Pigatto *et al.* 1992). Acute frictional hand

dermatitis may develop into chronic frictional hand dermatitis, especially with continuous ongoing exposure. Sources of frictional dermatitis include fabric, paper, cardboard, steering wheels, tools, artificial fur, carpet, carbonless paper, bus tickets, tissue paper, and even pantyhose (Wahlberg 1985, Menné 1985, Gould 1991, Paulsen and Andersen 1991, Inui *et al.* 2004).

NUMMULAR HAND DERMATITIS

Nummular hand dermatitis typically presents with recurrent, asymmetric, tiny papules, papulovesicles, or coin-shaped eczematous plaques. Most often, the dorsal surfaces of the hands and distal fingers are affected (**Fig 14.6**). There are no known sex or age associations. It is important to rule out other causes of nummular and/or annular dermatoses, such as tinea manus (**Fig 14.7**). Contact urticaria and allergic contact dermatitis also can manifest in a nummular pattern.

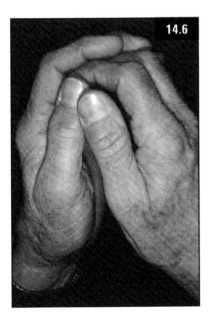

Fig 14.6 Nummular hand dermatitis.

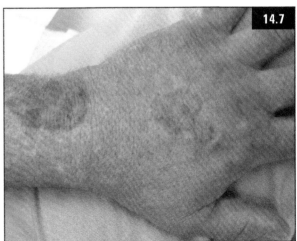

Fig 14.7 Tinea manus.

ATOPIC HAND DERMATITIS

There is a well-known association between adult hand dermatitis and a history of childhood atopic eczema (Kissling and Wüthrich 1994). The clinical picture of atopic hand dermatitis is heterogeneous, but a few specific morphological patterns have been delineated. Dorsal hand and finger involvement with thin, light-pink, xerotic, lichenified, poorly defined plaques has been reported as the most common presentation (Moller 2000). Dorsal hand, fingertip, and wrist involvement, along with nail changes, were similarly noted by Rajka (1989). Pruritus, thickening, and painful fissuring may be present and, when chronic, causes reduced finger mobility. Atopic dermatitis is unique from other types of hand dermatitis in that it often involves the wrists. In a study of 777 atopic dermatitis patients, 458 of whom (58.9%) had hand involvement, localization on the dorsal surface of the hand and involvement of the volar aspect of the wrist were most characteristic of atopic hand dermatitis (Simpson *et al.* 2006).

VESICULAR HAND DERMATOSES

Vesicular hand dermatoses include chronic vesicular hand dermatitis, pompholyx, and dyshidrotic eczema. The term 'chronic vesicular hand dermatitis' is used to describe hand eczema that is longstanding, pruritic, vesicular, and primarily involves the palmar surface of the hand. Frequently, vesicles surmount an erythematous base, distinguishing this entity from pompholyx or dyshidrotic eczema. Chronic vesicular hand dermatitis does not involve the wrist and either spares the dorsal surfaces of the hands completely or is limited to the dorsal fingertips. Sometimes, the soles of the feet may be affected. Chronic vesicular hand dermatitis is often more resistant to treatment than pompholyx and dyshidrotic eczema.

The term 'pompholyx' has long been considered synonymous with *dyshidrotic eczema*, although many experts maintain that it represents a unique clinical variant. Pompholyx is characterized by the sudden onset of large bullae on the palms, whereas dyshidrotic eczema is the chronic eruption of small noninflammatory papulovesicles on the lateral fingers and palms (**Fig 14.8**). Both usually resolve after 2 or 3 weeks but may recur at varying intervals. As sweat gland function is not altered in these patients, some have advocated eliminating the term 'dyshidrotic eczema' altogether because it implies eccrine gland dysfunction.

The term 'pompholyx' is derived from the Greek for *bubble*. Blisters often become quite large before rupturing, owing to the thick epidermis of the palms and soles, and may become secondarily infected. Papulovesicles are usually symmetrically distributed and heal with desquamation. In a prospective case–control study of 100 patients with pompholyx (matched with two controls for age and sex), both atopy and tinea pedis were shown to be statistically associated with pompholyx, although another study of 389 patients, evaluating the relationship of tinea pedis, atopy, nickel, and pompholyx, found that only tinea pedis was statistically associated with pompholyx (Bryld *et al.* 2003, Pitché *et al.* 2006). As dermatophytid reactions may stimulate pompholyx, examination of the feet for evidence of tinea pedis is important.

The role of allergy to nickel in the pathophysiology of vesicular hand dermatitis is controversial. Oral ingestion of 0.5–5.6 mg nickel has been reported to reactivate vesicular hand or finger dermatitis in nickel-sensitive patients (Veien and Menné 1990). However, many oral nickel-challenge studies have

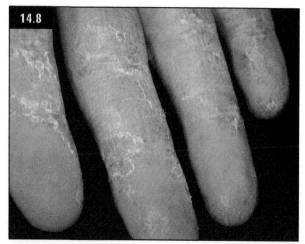

Fig 14.8 Dyshidrotic eczema (note: small, noninflammatory vesicles can be seen on fingertips).

been criticized because the daily dosages used in the challenges were much higher than amounts typically ingested in a standard diet (0.3–0.6 mg/day) (Jordan and King 1979). Some studies have reported improvement in patients with vesicular dermatitis who followed low-nickel diets but a randomized, double-blind, controlled study of 10 nickel-sensitive patients with hand dermatitis, each of whom had ingested 0.5 mg nickel daily, reported an exacerbation in only one patient (Kaaber et al. 1978, Veien et al. 1983). Disulfiram and other nickel chelators have been reported to improve dyshidrosiform dermatitis linked to nickel allergy; however, some patients experience an exacerbation on initiation of treatment (Menné and Kaaber 1978, Kaaber et al. 1983, Menné and Hjorth 1985, Klein and Fowler 1992). Such flares are thought to be due to the liberation of nickel from nickel–albumin or nickel–histidine complexes in the serum (Kaaber et al. 1979). Oral nickel does not appear to aggravate patients with other types of nonvesicular hand dermatitis (Veien et al. 1983).

Nickel may be the best-known allergen in vesicular hand dermatitis, but other contact allergens have also been implicated. In a patch-test study of 50 patients with clinical suspicion of pompholyx, 20 patients (40%) were positive to one or more allergens; the most common were nickel, potassium dichromate, p-phenylenediamine, nitrofurazone, fragrance mix, and cobalt chloride (Jain et al. 2004). Adachi and Horikawa (2007) reported an infant who was patch-test positive to chromium and developed recalcitrant pompholyx as a result of systemic metal allergy to chromium. The authors suggested that his mother's daily ingestion of large amounts of chocolate and cocoa, both of which contain substantial amounts of chromium, caused increased levels of chromium in her breast milk.

Other factors that have been reported to be associated with the development of pompholyx include intravenous immunoglobulin therapy, photoinduction by sunlight, and HIV infection (Man et al. 2004, Llombart et al. 2007, MacConnachie and Smith 2007). Severe dyshidrosis has been reported as a manifestation of immune reconstitution inflammatory syndrome in two patients undergoing treatment for HIV infection with highly active antiretroviral therapy (HAART) (Colebunders et al. 2005). Severe

pompholyx also has been reported after endoscopic thoracic sympathectomy for palmar hyperhidrosis (Niinai et al. 2004). Recently, a gene locus for a rare dominant form of pompholyx was identified in a large Chinese family. This may herald future gene-mapping studies and elucidation of pathogenic mechanisms (Chen et al. 2006).

HAND DERMATITIS RISK FACTORS

Hand dermatitis has been associated with both extrinsic and intrinsic factors, with *wet work* being the most common extrinsic factor and *atopy* the primary intrinsic factor.

EXTRINSIC FACTORS

Wet work is the most common extrinsic risk factor for developing hand dermatitis in adults. It comprises activities with ongoing exposure to liquids, typically for a few hours each day, frequent hand washing, and/or occlusion as with gloves. This is not a standard definition, and the need for such a standardized, international definition has been emphasized at a conference on occupational and environmental exposures of skin to chemicals (Flyvholm et al. 2006).

Several studies have highlighted the important etiologic role of wet work in hand dermatitis. A Danish study of workers with occupational hand dermatitis found that 59.6% of women with irritant contact dermatitis had been exposed to wet work, compared with 12.7% of men, supporting the premise that, despite changes in gender roles, women still have greater exposure to wet work and its sequelae than men (Skoet et al. 2004). Frequent hand washing, of the order of 35 times or more in a single shift, was also strongly associated with occupational hand dermatitis in a study of 126 intensive care unit workers (Forrester and Roth 1998).

The relationship between smoking and hand dermatitis is controversial. Whereas a twin study from Denmark found no association between smoking ± alcohol use and hand dermatitis, a Swedish study found smoking to slightly increase the 1-year prevalence of hand eczema (Montnémery et al. 2005, Lerbaek et al. 2007a).

INTRINSIC FACTORS

ATOPY

Atopy, especially a childhood history of eczema, is the principal endogenous factor associated with hand dermatitis in adulthood (Rystedt 1985). Meding and Swanbeck (1990a) reported childhood eczema to be the variable most predictive of future hand eczema, followed by gender, occupational exposure, asthma or hayfever, service occupations, and age. This was confirmed by Nyrén *et al.* (2005) who showed a 42% cumulative prevalence of hand eczema for those with a history of atopic dermatitis compared with a 13% prevalence in matched controls. The significant association between atopy and hand dermatitis was further confirmed in another study, but only in individuals younger than age 30 (Meding and Järvholm 2004). Other studies have shown atopy to be a more relevant risk factor than nickel sensitivity for hand eczema in females, an increased likelihood of atopic individuals to have allergic contact dermatitis of the hands, and an association of atopic dermatitis with a threefold risk of developing hand eczema with increased severity in both wet and dry work (Nilsson *et al.* 1985, Nilsson and Knutsson 1995, Heine *et al.* 2006).

Twin studies have shed some light on the importance of genetic factors in the development of hand eczema. A Danish twin study found that monozygotic twins were more than twice as likely as dizygotic twins to have hand eczema if their co-twin was affected (Lerbaek *et al.* 2007a). The same investigators looked at the importance of genetic and environmental risk factors independent of atopic dermatitis, which itself has a strong genetic component and is strongly associated with hand eczema, in relation to the occurrence and age of onset of hand dermatitis (Lerbaek *et al.* 2007b). In this large twin study, environmental factors accounted for 59% of the variance favoring the development of hand eczema. Similarly, early age of onset was favored by environmental factors. Analysis of this cohort with regard to filaggrin mutations confirmed an association with atopic dermatitis but not with hand eczema or contact allergy (Lerbaek *et al.* 2007c).

AGE

An association of age with the development of hand dermatitis has been reported, possibly related to age-related deterioration of barrier function (Patil and Maibach 1994, Ghadially *et al.* 1995). The skin of aged individuals is dryer and more sensitive to irritants. On the other hand, the prevalence of certain clinical variants of hand dermatitis is probably lower in individuals aged over 60 years. In a study of 1221 patients with hand dermatitis, the peak age for atopic, allergic, or irritant contact hand dermatitis was 21–25 years, whereas nummular and hyperkeratotic hand dermatitis showed no relationship to age (Diepgen and Fartasch 1994). In another report, age was found to be inversely related to the 1-year prevalence of hand dermatitis (Montnémery *et al.* 2005).

ETHNICITY

Ethnicity has not been shown to be an important risk factor for hand dermatitis. A study comparing 8610 white and 1014 African–American patients found no statistically significant difference between the two groups regarding rates of allergic or irritant contact dermatitis; this is in contradistinction to a previous investigation of transepidermal water loss (TEWL) and blood flow, in which African–American individuals were more sensitive to surfactants than white ones (Berardesca and Maibach 1988, Deleo *et al.* 2002). An additional investigation of irritant contact dermatitis failed to show differences in proliferation responses or variation in kinetics between white and African–American individuals, although better barrier function was noted in African–American individuals (Astner *et al.* 2006).

SEX

The relationship of sex to hand dermatitis appears to be linked more to gender-specific exposures than to any particular biological difference. Despite changes in sex roles in the last 50 years, females still remain more likely to perform wet work in the home and are also more likely to be exposed to irritants at work based on their particular occupations. Montnémery and colleagues (2005) found that the lifetime prevalence of hand dermatitis in females ranged from 5.7% to 16.7% compared with a lifetime prevalence of 5.2–9.5% in males. Not only is female sex an independent risk factor for the 1-year prevalence of hand eczema, but also in a Swedish study, females were found to have twice the rates of hand eczema compared with males (Meding 1994). Similarly, a study from the Netherlands of patients evaluated for skin disease reported a prevalence of hand dermatitis in females of 8% compared with 4.6% in males (Coenraads *et al.* 1983). Comparable results have been found in many other prevalence studies, although higher prevalence rates have also been reported in males (Smith *et al.* 2000).

With the current heightened interest in genetics and immunology, it is likely that the various risk factors for hand eczema will be elucidated by future studies involving its molecular mechanisms and immunological etiopathology.

PREVENTION AND LIFESTYLE MANAGEMENT

Although allergic contact dermatitis of the hands has been studied extensively, relatively little has been published on preventing hand dermatitis or treatment options for recalcitrant cases (Woolner and Soltani 1994). Behavioral changes including elimination of known irritants and allergens, creating physical barriers with gloves, and occasionally changing occupations are important considerations in the management of patients with hand dermatitis (Funke *et al.* 1996, Itschner *et al.* 1996, Uter *et al.* 1999, Mygind *et al.* 2006). Although occlusive gloves alone may actually worsen hand dermatitis, one study showed that adding a cotton glove liner inhibited the TEWL that occurred with vinyl glove use (Ramsing and Agner 1996). Cotton glove liners may be difficult for patients to obtain in local retail stores but are available at several internet locations. Liberal and frequent use of emollients is also an important intervention in rebuilding and maintaining the epidermal barrier.

Several studies have evaluated programs for primary, secondary, and tertiary prevention of occupational skin disease, especially involvement of the hands (Skudlik and Schwanitz 2004, Weisshaar *et al.* 2005, Löffler *et al.* 2006). A primary prevention study of nursing school trainees randomized subjects into two groups. The intervention group received regular education about prevention of occupational skin disease, and the control group received no such education. The 3-year prevalence of morphological skin changes was 66.7% in the intervention group and 89.3% in the control group. Another study evaluating a high-fat petrolatum-based moisturizer compared with gloves showed that the most striking improvements were not necessarily in those individuals practicing protective behavior, but, rather, in those participating in discussions on prevention. Educating atopic patients to avoid irritants and wet work in the home and at work is critical (Meding 1996). A sample patient handout on lifestyle management is listed in **Box 14.3** (overleaf).

Box 14.3   Sample patient handout on lifestyle management

Hand washing and moisturizing:
- Use lukewarm or cool water and mild cleansers without perfume, coloring, or antibacterial agents and with minimal preservatives. In general, bar soaps tend to have fewer preservatives than liquid soaps (Cetaphil or Aquanil liquid cleansers or generic equivalents are exceptions to this statement)
- Pat hands dry, especially between fingers
- Immediately after partial drying of hands (eg, within 3 min), apply a generous amount of a heavy cream or ointment (not lotion); petroleum jelly, a single-ingredient lubricant, is ideal
- It is helpful to have containers of creams or ointments next to every sink in your home (next to the bed, next to the TV, in the car, and at multiple places at work)
- Application of emollients should be repeated as often as feasible throughout the day, ideally 15 times per day
- Avoid using washcloths, rubbing, scrubbing, or overuse of soap or water

Occlusive therapy at night for intensive therapy:
- Apply a generous amount of your doctor's recommended emollient or prescribed medicine to your hands
- Then put on cotton gloves and wear overnight

When performing 'wet work':
- Wear cotton gloves under vinyl or other nonlatex gloves
- Try not to use hot water and decrease exposure to water to less than 15 min at a time, if possible
- Use running water rather than immersing hands, if possible
- Remove rings before wet or dry work

Protective, tight-fitting (leather, ideally) gloves should be worn in:
- Cold weather
- Work involving dust
- Frictional exposures

Avoid direct contact with the following, if possible:
- Fruit and vegetables, especially citrus fruit
- Shampoo
- Hair lotions, creams, and dyes
- Fragranced substances
- Detergents and strong cleansing agents
- Polishes of all kinds
- Solvents (eg white spirit, thinners, turpentine)
- 'Unknown' chemicals

Note
Heavy-duty vinyl gloves (available from Allerderm) are better than rubber, nitrile, or other synthetic gloves because vinyl is less likely to cause allergic reactions.

From Buxton (1987), Drake *et al.* (1995), and Warshaw *et al.* (2003).

THERAPY (TABLE 14.1)

TOPICAL AGENTS

TOPICAL CORTICOSTEROIDS

Topical corticosteroids are the first-line agents for treating hand dermatitis. Ointments are more effective than creams because they allow greater penetration of the active glucocorticoid, have a beneficial effect on barrier function, and require less potentially sensitizing preservatives than creams. Formulations free of propylene glycol are generally less irritating. It is important to be cognizant of the potential of corticosteroids to occasionally cause allergic contact dermatitis. One study found that 10.7% of patients with hand dermatitis were allergic to corticosteroids (Wilkinson *et al.* 1992). Preservatives such as formaldehyde releasers, parabens, and MCI/MI, in topical steroid creams, can also be responsible for allergic contact dermatitis (Rietschel *et al.* 1990). Generic triamcinolone ointment 0.1% in a petrolatum base is the authors' preferred topical corticosteroid preparation because of its effectiveness, its negligible potential for sensitization, its ease of use, and its low cost.

TOPICAL IMMUNOMODULATORS

Topical pimecrolimus and tacrolimus, ascomycin-derived agents that inhibit inflammatory cytokine production by T lymphocytes and mast cells, have been studied in the treatment of atopic dermatitis and allergic contact dermatitis (Grassberger *et al.* 1999). In a double-blind, vehicle-controlled study of patients with chronic hand dermatitis, twice-daily application of pimecrolimus 1% cream with overnight occlusion was superior to vehicle alone, especially in those without palmar involvement (Belsito *et al.* 2004). On the other hand, a questionnaire survey of patients with hand dermatitis failed to show any significant change in quality of life or work productivity with pimecrolimus treatment compared with vehicle (Reilly *et al.* 2003). A prospective, open, multicenter study of 29 patients with mild-to-moderate occupational hand dermatitis suggests that topical tacrolimus ointment 0.1% can also be an effective treatment option (Schliemann *et al.* 2008).

Transient skin burning and warmth are the most commonly reported adverse effects of topical tacrolimus and pimecrolimus. Systemic absorption is minimal with both; however, pimecrolimus may be a safer choice for widespread and long-term use owing to its lipophilicity and lower potential for systemic immunosuppression. Unlike corticosteroids, skin atrophy, telangiectasia, and tachyphylaxis do not occur with the topical use of tacrolimus or pimecrolimus (Reitamo *et al.* 1998, Queille-Roussel *et al.* 2001). Patients should be made aware of the *black box warning* regarding a possible increased chance of malignancy with these agents. Further research is needed to clarify whether these agents are as effective in treating hand dermatitis as they are in treating atopic dermatitis.

NONTRADITIONAL AGENTS

Successful treatment with nontraditional agents has been reported in small case studies. In one report of five patients with hyperkeratotic palmoplantar eczema treated with vitamin D_3 derivatives (calcipotriol 50 µg/g and maxacalcitol 25 µg/g), all patients improved within 2–9 weeks, without any adverse effects (Egawa 2005).

Tazarotene is another topical agent that has been used anecdotally to treat hyperkeratotic hand dermatitis; both tazarotene and calcipotriene affect epidermal cell maturation. Other anecdotal nonapproved treatments such as cyanoacrylate products (superglue) for fissuring in hand dermatitis may be useful. Older traditional regimens include tar and salicylic acid preparations. Twenty percent crude tar oil in alcohol may be effective in patients with hyperkeratotic hand dermatitis when painted on the hands twice a day, followed by 5% salicylic acid solution and a petrolatum-based emollient.

There are indications that future treatment of recalcitrant hyperkeratotic hand dermatitis may rely on the use of biologics. A recent study found a similar upregulation of interleukin (IL)-23 in hyperkeratotic hand dermatitis as in palmoplantar psoriasis (Lillis *et al.* 2010). As the highly effective antipsoriatic agent ustekinumab targets the shared p40 subunit of IL-23 and IL-12, it is possible that this agent might play a role in treating this stubborn form of hand eczema.

IONIZING RADIATION

Ionizing radiation comprises conventional radiograph and Grenz rays. Although less commonly used today, superficial radiograph therapy was utilized by some dermatologists in the early and mid-twentieth century to treat chronic hand dermatitis. In a double-blind, left–right hand, comparison study of 24 patients with chronic hand eczema, the combination of topical therapy and superficial radiograph therapy (100 rad at 50 kV every 3 weeks for three sessions) versus topical therapy alone showed significant improvement (greatest at 6–9 weeks) in hands receiving combination therapy (Fairris et al. 1984). A similar, double-blind, left–right study of 15 patients (7 with pompholyx and 8 with hyperkeratotic eczema) treated with superficial radiograph therapy (100 rad at 45 kV every week for 3 weeks) showed a statistically significant improvement after 1 month of therapy but not after 6 months (King and Chalmers 1984).

Grenz rays (ultrasoft radiographs or Bucky rays) have also been used to treat focal areas of dermatitis such as on the hands. Almost all of the radiation emitted is absorbed completely in the upper 3 mm of

Table 14.1 Authors' recommended therapies for hand dermatitis

THERAPEUTIC AGENT	ALLERGIC CONTACT DERMATITIS	IRRITANT CONTACT DERMATITIS	ATOPIC	HYPERKERATOTIC	NUMMULAR	VESICULAR
Corticosteroids topical	✓	✓	✓		✓	✓
Corticosteroids oral	✓					✓ (acute flares)
Cyclosporine (ciclosporin)	✓		✓			✓
Methotrexate	✓		✓	✓		✓
MMF	✓		✓		✓	✓
Tacrolimus, pimecrolimus, topical	✓	✓	✓		✓	✓
Phototherapy (UVB, PUVA, Grenz)	✓	✓	✓	✓	✓	✓
Retinoids, topical, and/or oral				✓		
Calcipotriene topical				✓		

MMF, mycophenolate mofetil; PUVA, psoralen plus UVA irradiation; UVB, ultraviolet B radiation.
Modified from Warshaw et al. (2003).

the skin, rendering Grenz rays the least penetrating form of ionizing radiation used by dermatologists (Edwards and Edwards 1990). The effectiveness of Grenz ray therapy is thought to involve reduction of the number of Langerhans cells within the epidermis (Cipollaro 1991). The therapeutic dosages used in Grenz ray therapy (150–300 rad) are not known to produce adverse effects such as erythema, exudation, and ulceration. Walling *et al.* (2008) reported the use of Grenz ray treatment at a weekly dose of 400 rad (4 Gy) in a dermatological surgeon with recalcitrant frictional hyperkeratotic hand dermatitis. He had marked improvement after 3-weekly treatments and has remained clear for 4 years following a total course of six Grenz ray sessions.

Hand dermatitis treatment regimens usually require 200–400 rad (2–4 Gy) every 1–3 weeks for up to six treatment sessions, followed by a 6-month period of rest (Lindelof *et al.* 1987, Lindelof and Beitner 1990). Similar to other radiotherapy treatments, low voltages are used whenever possible (5–20 kV); the total lifetime absorbed dosage of conventional superficial radiotherapy should not exceed 5000–10 000 rad (50–100 Gy) (Rowell 1978).

Not all studies have found Grenz ray therapy to be efficacious. A double-blind, right–left comparison study of 30 chronic hand eczema patients treated with Grenz ray therapy (total dosage 900 rad given in three equal doses at 21-day intervals) found it to be no better than placebo at multiple evaluations up to 18 weeks after therapy initiation (Cartwright and Rowell 1987). Another double-blind study of 25 patients with chronic, bilateral hand dermatitis comparing Grenz rays (900 rad) to conventional radiograph therapy (300 rad), both given in three divided dosages at 21-day intervals, found conventional radiograph therapy to be more effective (Fairris *et al.* 1985).

Megavoltage radiation has also been used to successfully treat chronic vesicular hand dermatitis. Derived from energy produced by a linear accelerator, this modality is commonly used by radiation oncologists to treat deep tumors. In nine patients with chronic vesicular dermatitis of the hands and feet treated with megavoltage irradiation (<1200 cGy per session), complete resolution was seen in 47% of the affected sites, with varying degrees of improvement in the remainder. Long-term adverse effects of this type of radiation are unknown, although serious adverse effects are unlikely with the low dosage used in these cases (Duff *et al.* 2006).

NONIONIZING RADIATION
Psoralen plus UVA radiation

Treatment with psoralen plus UVA irradiation (PUVA), both oral and topical, has been investigated in the treatment of various types of hand dermatitis (Morison *et al.* 1978, Grattan *et al.* 1991, De Rie *et al.* 1995, Schempp *et al.* 1997, Gritiyarangsan *et al.* 1998, Grundmann-Kollmann *et al.* 1999). A study of 20 patients with treatment-resistant palmoplantar dermatoses examined the clinical effectiveness of PUVA gel therapy versus traditional PUVA bath therapy. The easier-to-administer PUVA gel therapy was equivalent to traditional PUVA bath therapy (Schiener *et al.* 2005). Another study compared topical PUVA therapy with conventional radiotherapy in 21 chronic hand eczema patients; one hand was treated with radiotherapy and the other with topical PUVA. Although hands treated with superficial radiotherapy cleared more rapidly, at 12 weeks there was no significant overall difference between the two treatment regimens (Sheehan-Dare *et al.* 1989).

Psoralen and its derivatives (8-methoxypsoralen [8-MOP], 5-MOP, trioxsalen) are available in a variety of topical vehicles (creams, gels, lotions, and solutions) and oral preparations (8-MOP and psoralen-ultra). For topical PUVA treatment, 1% psoralen is applied and UVA administered at an initial dosage of 0.25–0.5 J/cm^2 with incremental increases of 0.25 J/cm^2 per treatment, usually given three times weekly (Zemtsov 1998).

Ultraviolet B radiation

The effectiveness of UVB radiation has also been evaluated in treating chronic eczematous hand dermatitis. In one randomized study, broadband UVB alone was inferior to topical PUVA in treating chronic hand dermatitis patients (allergic, irritant contact dermatitis, hyperkeratotic, and idiopathic types) (Rosén *et al.* 1987). Another study found no difference at 6 weeks between patients treated with topical PUVA and broadband UVB (Simons *et al.* 1997). Sezer and Etikan (2007) have suggested that narrowband UVB (NB-UVB) may be as effective as paint PUVA treatment based on a pilot left–right comparison study in 15 patients.

ULTRAVIOLET A1 THERAPY

Ultraviolet A1 (UVA1) radiation (340–400 nm) without psoralen has been used to treat several different skin conditions, including hand dermatitis. In open-label and randomized trials, UVA1 (40 J/cm^2 daily, five times weekly for 3 weeks) was effective in treating chronic vesicular dyshidrotic hand eczema (Schmidt et al. 1998, Polderman et al. 2003). In a study of 27 patients, localized UVA1 was found to be equivalent to PUVA using a cream vehicle in treating chronic vesicular dyshidrotic eczema (Petering et al. 2004).

SYSTEMIC GLUCOCORTICOIDS

Systemic glucocorticoids have a role in severe and recurrent cases of pompholyx, especially when initiated during the prodromal stage, or at the onset of itching. Short bursts of 60 mg prednisone as a single daily dose in the morning for 3–4 days are repeated every 2–4 months, as needed (Warshaw 2004). Despite the dramatic improvement obtained with these agents, the adverse effects, many of them long term, can outweigh the dramatic rapid relief. Side effects such as osteoporosis, glaucoma, cataracts, hypothalamic–pituitary–adrenal axis suppression, hyperglycemia, hypertension, and immunosuppression all limit the chronic use of systemic glucocorticoids (Nesbitt 1995). These complications can occur with intramuscular administration of glucocorticoids as well (Storrs 1979).

CYCLOSPORINE (CICLOSPORIN)

Cyclosporine works primarily by suppressing T-lymphocyte activation, making it useful for the treatment of many inflammatory skin conditions, such as atopic dermatitis and severe chronic hand dermatitis (Granlund et al. 1996, 1998, Schmitt et al. 2007). In a double-blind study of 41 hand dermatitis patients (21 of 41 participants diagnosed with irritant or allergic contact dermatitis and the remaining individuals unclassified), participants were randomized to receive either oral cyclosporine (3 mg/ kg per day) or a potent topical corticosteroid for

6 weeks (Granlund et al. 1996). There was a 50% decrease in disease activity in the cyclosporine group, compared with a 32% reduction in the corticosteroid group. However, 8 of the 20 patients receiving cyclosporine (40%) failed treatment, and both groups were noted to have a 50% relapse rate at the 2-week follow-up.

In a long-term follow-up study, the mean disease activity 1 year after cyclosporine treatment (3 mg/kg per day for 6 weeks) was decreased by more than 50% from both baseline and the treatment endpoint, in 21 of 27 chronic hand dermatitis patients (Granlund et al. 1998). Petersen and Menné (1992) reported a patient with chronic vesicular hand dermatitis and positive patch-test reactions to nickel, chrome, and formalin who responded to 2 weeks of oral cyclosporine at a slightly higher dose (5 mg/kg per day), but relapse occurred after discontinuation; it is noteworthy that previous treatments with azathioprine (both with and without prednisolone), methotrexate, and PUVA had all failed in this patient.

Oral cyclosporine treatment can be complicated by nephrotoxicity, hepatotoxicity, tremor, hypertension, and gingival hyperplasia. Topical cyclosporine is not effective, likely because of its large molecular size and low epidermal penetration (De Rie et al. 1991).

MYCOPHENOLATE MOFETIL

Mycophenolic acid, to which mycophenolate mofetil (MMF) is converted after digestion, is derived from the fungus Penicillium brevicompactum (Hartmann and Enk 2005). First approved to prevent renal allograft rejection, MMF inhibits the new synthesis of guanosine nucleotides, which are required for lymphocyte proliferation. Skin diseases treated with MMF include psoriasis, dyshidrotic eczema, bullous pemphigoid, chronic actinic dermatitis, and atopic dermatitis (Pickenäcker et al. 1998, Beissert and Luger 1999, Nousari et al. 1999a, 199b, Heller et al. 2007). Dosages of MMF used to treat adults with skin diseases are typically 2–3 g/day.

In a case report of a male with a 4-year history of recurrent and recalcitrant dyshidrotic eczema resistant to corticosteroids, iontophoresis, and phototherapy, treatment with MMF (1.5 g twice daily) resulted in complete clearing at 4 weeks (Pickenäcker et al. 1998). However, biopsy-proven MMF-induced dyshidrotic eczema, which cleared on discontinuation of the drug and flared on rechallenge, has also been reported (Semhoun-Ducloux *et al.* 2000).

The best-known adverse effects of MMF include nausea, loose stools, diarrhea, abdominal cramping, leukopenia, anemia, and an increased incidence of herpes zoster (Sollinger 1995). Hepatic toxicity is uncommon (Hantash and Fiorentino 2006).

ANTIMETABOLITES

Methotrexate is an inhibitor of dihydrofolate reductase, an enzyme necessary for DNA synthesis (Boffa and Chalmers 1996). At doses of 12.5–22.5 mg/week methotrexate partially or completely cleared pompholyx in a study of five patients; it has also shown effectiveness in treating moderate, severe, and refractory atopic dermatitis (Egan *et al.* 1999, Goujon *et al.* 2006, Weatherhead *et al.* 2007). Adverse effects are dose-dependent and include nausea, vomiting, diarrhea, hepatitis, liver cirrhosis, pancytopenia, and pulmonary fibrosis (Jolivet *et al.* 1983).

Azathioprine, another immunosuppressive agent, is derived from 6-mercaptopurine and acts by inhibiting RNA and DNA synthesis and function (Ahmed and Moy 1981). It is effective in treating atopic dermatitis and has shown efficacy in treating pompholyx (Scerri 1999, Berth-Jones *et al.* 2002). Thiopurine methyltransferase is a key enzyme in the metabolism of azathioprine. Variable levels of this enzyme can cause severe myelotoxicity, on the one hand, and treatment failure, on the other, in individuals receiving the drug. It is therefore recommended that starting dosages of azathioprine be based on an individual's thiopurine methyltransferase enzyme activity (Meggitt *et al.* 2006). Azathioprine at dosages of 50–150 mg/day may be effective in cases of recalcitrant allergic hand dermatitis. One disadvantage is its slow onset of action, typically 4–6 weeks. Adverse reactions include liver enzyme elevation, dyspepsia, leukopenia, red cell macrocytosis, and bone marrow suppression. Adverse effects involving the skin such as skin cancer may occur in transplant recipients (Zimmerman and Esch 1978).

RETINOIDS

Considered an experimental treatment in the USA, 9-*cis*-retinoic acid (9-*cis*-RA or alitretinoin) has been successfully used in Europe to treat patients with chronic hand eczema. In a multicenter, double-blind, randomized, controlled, prospective trial of 319 patients with moderate/severe and refractory chronic hand dermatitis, treatment with alitretinoin (10, 20, or 40 mg/day) was compared with placebo (Ruzicka *et al.* 2004). The treatment group had significant dose-dependent improvement defined as complete or nearly complete disappearance of disease signs and symptoms. Overall, 53% of alitretinoin-treated patients had complete or near-complete clearance. Adverse effects of headache, flushing, lipid level elevations, slight decreases in hemoglobin concentration, and decreased free thyroxine levels were seen at the highest dose (40 mg/day) only. At lower dosages, adverse effects were not significantly different from placebo. Headache, flushing, and cheilitis occurred commonly. In a similar study of 38 patients with treatment-resistant chronic hand eczema, 89% of those treated with 40 mg/day of alitretinoin, for an average of 2.3 months, had a 'good' or 'very good' response to the agent. These responses were more favorable than historical reports of response to oral etretinate (0%, $n = 11$), acitretin (6%, $n = 17$), or isotretinoin (0%, $n = 7$) (Bollag and Ott 1999).

More recently, the BACH (Benefit of Alitretinoin in Chronic Hand dermatitis) study of 1032 patients examined the effect on chronic severe hand eczema of 10 or 30 mg oral alitretinoin once daily for up to 24 weeks (Ruzicka *et al.* 2008). Up to 48% of patients treated with alitretinoin achieved clear or almost clear hands. In a follow-up study, patients originally treated with alitretinoin in the BACH study were randomized to receive either their previous alitretinoin dose or placebo for 12 or 24 weeks (Coenraads *et al.* 2008). Retreatment with alitretinoin was effective in most cases and was well tolerated; the best response rates were seen with the 30 mg dosage. In a commentary on the BACH study, Ingram *et al.* (2009) suggested that the authors' claim of remission in a high proportion of patients was *rather inflated* insofar as 'only slightly less than half of participants responded to the 30 mg dose; only 28% responded to the 10 mg dose; and the corresponding percentage responses for patient-reported outcomes were even less (40% and 24% respectively).'

OTHER THERAPIES

Iontophoresis (use of a direct current on the skin to induce the transfer of ions through the skin) was reported to be effective in an open-label study of 20 pompholyx patients (Odia *et al.* 1996). Botulinum toxin A also was efficacious in one small, open-label study of 10 patients with recurrent vesicular hand dermatitis; intradermal injections were performed on one hand, with the other hand serving as a control (Swartling *et al.* 2002). At 6 weeks, 7 of 10 patients, all of whom had pretreatment hyperhidrosis in addition to pompholyx, had improvement of their disease. Another study that evaluated six patients with pompholyx treated with topical corticosteroids plus intradermal botulinum toxin A, compared with topical steroids alone, found greater improvement in the botulinum toxin A group (Wollina and Karamfilov 2002). Both iontophoresis and intradermal botulinum toxin A are known to be effective therapies for hyperhidrosis. However, as pompholyx is not, as previously thought, related to hyperhidrosis and sweat gland obstruction, the improvement noted in these few small case series could be due to a placebo effect or to decreased sweat-induced irritation that occurs in atopic individuals (Morren *et al.* 1994). Other potential physiological mechanisms include inhibition of neurotransmitters or a direct inhibitory effect on the sensory system via afferent nerve fibers (Klein 2004).

Recently, etanercept, an antitumor necrosis factor (anti-TNF-α) agent, was reported to be effective in a patient with recalcitrant pompholyx (Ogden *et al.* 2006). Complete clearance of pompholyx was seen after 6 weeks of treatment, with remission lasting 4 months.

OUTCOME STUDIES

Patients and physicians may rate disease differently. A comparison study of 602 hand eczema patients found 18% of cases were deemed severe by a physician whereas almost twice as many patients (40%) rated their disease as severe (Cvetkovski *et al.* 2005).

QUALITY OF LIFE

Hand dermatitis can be chronic, aggravating, pervasive, and, in some individuals, a devastating condition. Investigations into quality of life related to hand dermatitis are revealing: in one evaluation of 1238 Swedish patients with hand dermatitis, 80% reported experiencing some kind of social or emotional disturbance owing to their condition, and 8% reported changing jobs. The most common occupations affected were hairdressing (18%), baking (11%), cleaning (8%), and nursing (7%) (Meding and Swanbeck 1990b). Of note, dermatitis of the hands has been significantly associated with worse quality-of-life outcomes than dermatitis in other body areas. In a study of 339 patients who completed a dermatology-specific quality-of-life instrument at the time of patch testing, hand dermatitis had a statistically significant impact on several parameters including itch/pain, embarrassment/self-consciousness, ability to clean house, shop, or garden, participation in social, leisure and sports activities, interference with work, social problems with partners or friends, and sleep. Moreover, treatments for dermatitis were deemed messy and/or time-consuming (Holness 2001). In a Danish occupational hand dermatitis study of 758 individuals, strong associations were found between a low quality of life and severity of hand eczema; lower socioeconomic status was also a substantial factor influencing reports of lower quality of life (Cvetkovski *et al.* 2006a).

More research is being devoted to the instruments used to evaluate quality of life. In a comparison of two different tools used to evaluate health-related quality of life and hand eczema, a generic questionnaire or the Short Form-36 (SF-36) provided a better assessment of emotional impact than the more specific Dermatology Life Quality Index, especially for women (Wallenhammar *et al.* 2004). Recently, the Dermatology Life Quality Index and the Work Productivity and Activity Impairment – Chronic Hand Dermatitis Questionnaires were validated for use in chronic hand dermatitis (Reilly *et al.* 2003).

OCCUPATIONAL CONCERNS

Patients with occupational hand dermatitis may experience financial stress related to their condition. Of 181 hospital workers with self-reported hand dermatitis, 48.1% of the participants reported psychological distress related to their disease. Psychological distress was a statistically significant predictor of those more likely to work longer hours and have more severe symptoms (Szepietowski and Salomon 2005). Interestingly, change of occupation in response to, and with the hope of improving, hand dermatitis does not necessarily improve prognosis. In a study of irritant contact dermatitis associated with cutting oils, chronicity was noted more than 70% of the time, regardless of occupation change, and, if irritant contact dermatitis did clear, it took up to 3 months to do so (Pryce *et al.* 1989). At the 6-month follow-up of 100 participants with occupational hand dermatitis, 33% were not working (92% of those due to skin disease), and 24% had changed jobs (92% of those due to their skin condition) (Holness 2004). In a survey of 149 allergic contact dermatitis patients (32% with hand dermatitis), 13% of the patients who changed jobs because of their condition reported a statistically significant poorer quality of life than those who did not change jobs (Kadyk *et al.* 2003). Furthermore, those with hand involvement and occupational allergic contact dermatitis had poorer quality-of-life scores. In a small study of 29 hairdressers with hand dermatitis and positive patch-test results, of 21 who were contacted, 14 (66%) changed jobs, but 3 of 14 still reported persistent hand dermatitis, despite change of occupation (Laing *et al.* 2006).

CHRONICITY, PROGNOSIS, AND PREDICTIVE FACTORS

Hand dermatitis often becomes chronic despite accurate diagnosis and appropriate therapy. In a 10-year follow-up of 83 hand eczema patients with contact allergy to colophony, 30% had ongoing symptoms for most of the 10 years, 30% cleared completely, and 40% were almost clear (Färm 1996). In a large, 12-year Swedish study of occupational hand dermatitis, 86% of patients reported 'symptoms on occasion,' and, of those with hand eczema at the time of follow-up, 88% reported enduring psychosocial effects owing to hand eczema (Meding *et al.* 2005a, 2005b). Another Swedish cross-sectional study reported a mean duration of hand eczema of approximately 12 years from time of diagnosis (Templet *et al.* 2004).

Early diagnosis may predict chronicity of disease. In one study of patients with occupational hand dermatitis, 53% with symptoms for less than 1 year had improvement within 6 months, whereas, of those with hand eczema for more than 1 year, only 23% improved in the same period (Holness 2001). Similarly, in a long-term follow-up study of 120 patients with occupational hand dermatitis from chromate exposure, delay of diagnosis for more than 1 year and ongoing exposure was significantly associated with chronicity (Halbert *et al.* 1992). Early evaluation in a specialty contact dermatitis clinic appears to be especially helpful with regard to diagnosis, prognosis, and intervention, as shown by studies of chronic eczema not limited to the hands (Paul *et al.* 1995, Soni and Sherertz 1997, Sherertz 2000).

PROGNOSTIC SIGNIFICANCE OF CHILDHOOD CONTACT ALLERGY OR ECZEMA

A 20-year follow-up study of Swedish women who were patch tested to nickel as children found that a childhood history of nickel sensitivity was not associated with an increased prevalence of hand dermatitis in adulthood. However, 31.4% of study participants with a history of atopic dermatitis reported hand eczema after age 15 years, as opposed to 10.6% of those women without a history of atopy (Josefson *et al.* 2006). Similarly, a follow-up study of 801 atopic dermatitis patients (not limited to the hands) reported that contact allergy did not worsen the prognosis of dermatitis in atopic patients (Mäkelä *et al.* 2007). In another study, a history of atopic dermatitis, age over 40 years, and low socioeconomic status were found to be reliable predictors of a poor prognosis in patients with occupational hand eczema; a history of contact dermatitis was not associated with poor prognosis (Cvetkovski *et al.* 2006b). Childhood atopic dermatitis was studied in relation to future work life by a review of 600 pediatric medical records and follow-up of those patients in adulthood. The self-reported cumulative prevalence of hand eczema was 42% for those with atopic dermatitis history and 13% for matched controls, with a rate of sick leave of 10% and 2% respectively, and a change in occupation of 9% of those with atopic dermatitis history compared with 2% of controls (Ramsing and Agner 1996).

Younger age at the onset of hand dermatitis also is associated with a poorer prognosis. In a 15-year follow-up of 868 individuals with hand eczema, the three most relevant predictive factors for poor prognosis were, in descending order: (1) the extent of eczema at the initial evaluation; (2) history of childhood eczema; and (3) age less than 20 years at the onset of hand eczema (Meding *et al.* 2005a, 2005b). A recent study further investigated the link between the extent of eczema and prognosis by including morphology and its relationship to prognosis (Meding *et al.* 2007). A correlation was found between morphology and the extent of eczema but only the latter was specifically associated with prognosis.

ECONOMICS

In 1993, 14% of workers affected with occupational skin diseases lost more than 10 days of work as a result of their condition (Burnett *et al.* 1998). This amounted to US$14 325 in direct costs per claimant in 1979, and a total of up to US$1bn of total direct and indirect costs in 1984 (Keil and Shmunes 1983, Mathias 1985). As hand dermatitis accounts for a considerable percentage of occupational dermatoses, its financial impact is likely similar to the figures described for overall occupational skin disease (Elston *et al.* 2002). In a Swedish study of 1238 patients with hand eczema, 69% of involved individuals sought medical attention with an overall average sick leave of 19 weeks (Meding and Swanbeck 1990b). In another study, occupational hand eczema contributed to almost 20% of episodes of prolonged sick leave, the highest proportion being in food service workers (27.2%), and wet work occupations (20.1%) (Cvetkovski *et al.* 2005). A study of 507 people, of whom 140 (27.61%) had chronic hand dermatitis, showed 25% higher medical costs among those affected (an incremental cost of US$70/month/patient) than among those without chronic hand dermatitis (Fowler *et al.* 2006). Prescription drugs comprised the biggest proportion of the cost.

CONCLUSIONS

Hand dermatitis is common, especially in certain occupations. It includes several clinical variants that can be classified based on cause, pathophysiology, host response, and/or site of predilection. Clarifying the causative or exacerbating factors in affected patients depends on a thorough and detailed history and a complete clinical examination.

Treatment of hand dermatitis can be frustrating both for the patient and for the practitioner, as many cases are chronic, relapsing, and recalcitrant. Of therapies reviewed, PUVA has been most extensively studied. More adequately powered, randomized, double-blind, controlled trials are necessary to further investigate the use of both topical and oral immunomodulators, antimetabolites, retinoids, and biologics. Moreover, basic science research is critical to further elucidate the pathophysiology involved in different types of hand dermatitis.

Clinical suggestions

1. In patients with hand dermatitis, it is important to establish the subtype: irritant or allergic contact dermatitis; contact urticaria evolving to eczematous hand dermatitis; hyperkeratotic hand dermatitis; nummular dermatitis; atopic dermatitis; or vesicular hand dermatitis (dyshidrosis/pompholyx). It is also important to exclude tinea infection and psoriasis.
2. A careful history including exposure to irritants and allergens on the job or in the home, wet work, possible improvement when the patient is away from work, results of previous treatment, or family history of atopy or skin disease should be obtained.
3. In cases of irritant or allergic contact dermatitis successful management will depend on avoidance, protection and substitution (Kedrowski and Warshaw 2008). Protective gloves (rubber or PVC with a cotton liner or worn over thin cotton gloves) are the mainstay of protection for irritant contact dermatitis. Choice of glove is dependent on the specific chemical exposure. (The website www.ansellpro.com/specware provides recommendations in this regard.) If it is impossible to avoid exposure at work, job change may be necessary.
4. Patch testing should be performed in patients with suspected allergic contact dermatitis. In addition to allergen avoidance, barrier creams may play a role.
5. In general, patients with hand dermatitis should avoid harsh soaps and use bland emollients after washing the hands and at bedtime.
6. Topical corticosteroids and in severe cases short courses of systemic corticosteroids or intramuscular corticosteroids are useful, especially for allergic contact dermatitis, nummular dermatitis, atopic dermatitis, and vesicular hand dermatitis.
7. Compresses or soaks play a role in the management of acute eczematous hand dermatitis and vesicular hand dermatitis. Suspected secondary infection should be treated with systemic antibiotics.
8. Patients with hyperkeratotic hand dermatitis are particularly difficult to treat because of chronicity, a propensity to relapse, exacerbations, and inconsistent response to therapy (Kedrowski and Warshaw 2008). Treatment includes measures used for irritant contact hand dermatitis, application of ointments under cotton glove occlusion at night, topical or systemic PUVA, and retinoids.

THE RELATIONSHIP BETWEEN ATOPIC DERMATITIS AND CONTACT DERMATITIS

Sharon Rose, Arash Akhavan, David H. Ciocon, and Steven R. Cohen

INTRODUCTION

Atopic dermatitis (AD) and contact dermatitis are common eczematous disorders with different inflammatory mechanisms. They are both characterized by a serous accumulation in the epidermis and a dermal inflammatory infiltrate, expressed clinically as erythema, with or without concomitant edema and/or blistering.

AD is a recurrent, hereditary, eczematous condition that typically begins in childhood, and affects patients with a personal or family history of hayfever, asthma, and/or eczema. Multiple genetic abnormalities render atopic individuals susceptible to flares of disease activity in the presence of environmental triggers including allergens, irritants, bacterial colonization, and variations in temperature and humidity. Moreover, exacerbation of AD may also be idiopathic and occur in the absence of any known environmental stimulus (Hanifin and Chan 1999).

Contact dermatitis is an inflammatory condition caused by exposure of the skin to an offending chemical and, in the case of photoallergic or phototoxic contact dermatitis, involves concomitant or subsequent exposure to ultraviolet light. Contact dermatitis reactions are classified as irritant contact dermatitis (ICD) or allergic contact dermatitis (ACD), but there may be overlap, eg, many contact allergens have a direct irritant effect and some irritants may function as allergens.

ICD is generally held to be an inflammatory reaction resulting from a chemical insult that causes direct cellular injury on skin contact. Most cases of ICD are associated with soaps, detergents, solvents, acids, and alkalis. Acute reactions occur minutes to hours after exposure to a very strong irritant chemical, whereas cumulative insult reactions follow repeated contact with milder irritants. As ICD is essentially an injury, most individuals will develop an eruption when certain parameters of chemical concentration and frequency of exposure are met.

On the other hand, ACD is an eczematous disorder mediated by acquired immunity requiring immunological memory. It occurs at sites of contact with small chemical haptens only in susceptible individuals who have been previously exposed and have become immunologically sensitized to a particular contact allergen. In contrast to ICD, only a small percentage of individuals are susceptible to ACD from a given contact allergen. The most common chemical allergens causing ACD in North

America are nickel neomycin sulfate, fragrances, and urushiol, the active moiety in plants of the Anacardiaceae family such as poison ivy, poison oak, and poison sumac (Cohen 1996, Mohammad *et al.* 2005, Mark and Slavin 2006). Patients with active ICD or AD have disturbed skin barrier function that may facilitate penetration of the skin by contact allergens, thereby increasing susceptibility to ACD.

Despite differing pathophysiological mechanisms, AD and contact dermatitis have been the focus of a number of studies examining their potential association or lack of association. Although early patch-test studies suggested that AD patients were less susceptible to contact allergic reactions as a result of altered immunity, more recent studies find that patients with AD develop ACD frequently (Schöpf and Baumgårtner 1989). AD patients are also known to be prone to ICD, especially of the hands (Schmunes 1986, Coenraads and Diepgen 1998). Understanding the potential links between AD and contact dermatitis, and the parallel aspects of their pathogenesis, diagnosis, and treatment, can be helpful to clinicians caring for patients with these disorders.

PATHOGENESIS

Genetic factors are very important in the pathogenesis of AD, but until recently have not been shown to play a major role in the development of ICD or ACD. Increased susceptibility to skin irritation has been demonstrated recently for individuals with the G to A transition at position −308 in the promoter region of the tumor necrosis factor (TNF)-α gene (de Jongh *et al.* 2008, Davis *et al.* 2010), and null mutations in the filaggrin gene may be associated with increased or altered tendency to nickel sensitization (Novak *et al.* 2008, Thyssen *et al.* 2010, Carlsen *et al.* 2010). Exposure to various environmental factors can exacerbate all three conditions. In contrast to ICD, which is caused by innate immune responses to direct cellular injury by an irritant chemical, ACD and AD are mediated through both innate and adaptive immunity mechanisms.

IMMUNOLOGY

ICD is caused by the release of proinflammatory cytokines from skin cells (mostly keratinocytes) in response to chemical and sometimes physical stimuli (Ale and Maibach 2010). On contact with the irritant, keratinocytes release preformed cytokines and inflammatory mediators (danger signals) such as interleukin (IL)-1α, TNF-α, and granulocyte–macrophage colony-stimulating factor (GM-CSF), which trigger the further release of IL-1α and other proinflammatory cytokines and chemokines (Rustemeyer *et al.* 2011). This causes an influx of immune cells and further release of inflammatory cytokines in a proinflammatory cascade. Unlike ACD, adaptive immunity and specific memory T cells are not a requirement. Yet ICD and ACD show similar histology and immunohistology, and share many common pathogenic pathways (Brasch *et al.* 1992). The percentages of T-cell subtypes, Langerhans cells (LCs), macrophages, and activation antigen HLA-DR are very similar. Whereas in ACD epidermal LCs migrate to draining lymph nodes to prime T-cells, in ICD LCs migrate out of the epidermis into the dermis and undergo a transformation to a macrophage-like phenotype in an IL-10-dependent manner (Ouwehand *et al.* 2010).

ACD has been considered a type-IV immune response (delayed-type hypersensitivity or DTH) but it is important to remember that, in addition to its antigen-specific aspects, ACD shares many of the innate immune system alarm signals and increased cytokine release seen in ICD (Rustemeyer *et al.* 2011). Nickel, one of the most common contact allergens in humans, directly activates the innate immune system sentinel, toll-like receptor (TLR)-4 leading to the production of type-I interferons and proinflammatory molecules independent of its antigenic effect (Schmidt *et al.* 2010, Rothenberg 2010). It is also known that many other contact allergens have irritant potential.

The mechanism of the classic cell-mediated pathogenic pathway is well described (Cohen 1996, Friedmann 1998). Briefly, the process is initiated when low-molecular-weight haptens bind to epidermal carrier molecules. This complex then binds to antigen-presenting LCs in the epidermis. The LCs have immune response-associated surface antigens (HLA-DR in humans) that bind to specific receptors on T lymphocytes, ultimately activating them. The activated T lymphocytes assume a variety of functions including cytotoxic properties, recruitment of other T lymphocytes, migration to regional lymph nodes, and formation of memory cells. In the lymph nodes, the T cells undergo further proliferation and then enter the circulation, from where they can access any skin surface. The immune system becomes sensitized to the hapten and, with re-exposure to the same chemical, a similar series of events will result in the eczematous rash of ACD. The T lymphocytes involved in ACD are believed to be mostly, but not totally, of the T-helper 1 (Th1) type, with cytokine production mostly consisting of interferon (IFN)-γ and IL-2 (Kapsenberg et al. 1992).

Although the mechanism of contact hypersensitivity (CHS) is closely related to DTH, certain data suggest that it is distinct in some ways, eg, the immunosuppressive cytokine IL-10 can suppress the induction of DTH but not CHS in mice (Schwarz et al. 1994). Moreover, murine CHS reactions demonstrate a prevalence of nickel-reactive Th0 and Th2 cells that produce high levels of IL-5 and variable amounts of IFN-γ and IL-4 on contact with nickel (Probst et al. 1995). Recent data suggest that ACD reactions entail two populations of reactive T cells: IFN-γ-producing CD8+ cells that mediate the CHS response, and CD4+ T cells producing IL-4 and IL-10 which modulate the magnitude and duration of the response (Dilulio et al. 1996). Other work suggests that both CD4+ Th1 and CD8+ type 1 cytotoxic T cells are important effector cells in certain murine CHS responses (Wang et al. 2000). In addition, the nature of the antigen can affect the make-up of the CHS response, eg, whereas most CHS responses are thought to be mediated by Th1 cells and regulated by Th2 cells, fluorescein isothiocyanate-induced murine CHS reactions are primarily the result of activation of Th2 cells (Dearman and Kimber 2000).

In recent years a CD4+ T-helper cell that produces IL-17 (Th17 cell) has been identified in mice and humans. This cell plays an important role in psoriasis,

AD, murine contact sensitivity, and human ACD. The effects in human ACD involve both innate and adaptive immunity (Larsen et al. 2009). In human ACD, IL17+ lymphocytes are enriched at sites of heavy spongiosis and vesiculation, and play a major role in linking and amplifying antigen-dependent and antigen-independent T-cell induction of keratinocyte apoptosis (Pennino et al. 2010).

LCs are dendritic cells in the classic paradigm of ACD, but recent work in murine contact sensitivity models with selective LC depletion suggests that other dendritic cell subsets may play a role in certain circumstances (Romani et al. 2010). Notably, langerin-positive dermal dendritic cells have been identified in mice but not as yet in humans (Bursch et al. 2007, Ginhoux et al. 2007, Poulin et al. 2007). Until this discovery, some rarely observed langerin-positive dendritic cells in the dermis were considered to be LCs in transit to lymph nodes. It is now thought, at least in the mouse, that there is redundancy in dendritic cell populations and that it may be the extent of hapten penetration into or past the epidermis that determines the relevant dendritic cell in contact sensitivity. LCs may even play a regulatory role in certain situations.

Although it is clear that AD is also an immune-mediated disease, the pathogenesis of the disorder is more difficult to understand due to the multiplicity and complexity of the immune system abnormalities present. In the past, the pathology of AD was thought to result from a positive feedback loop of humoral immunity, where LCs in the skin would interact with allergens through surface-bound immunoglobulin E (IgE) antibodies, ultimately activating T lymphocytes (Rudikoff and Lebwohl 1998). The T lymphocytes were believed to be almost exclusively of the Th2 type, producing mostly IL-4 and IL-5. IL-4 and IL-5 were known to cause eosinophilia and increase IgE levels, which would become bound to LCs, closing the positive feedback loop. The evidence supporting this mechanism of pathology is substantial. First, most patients with AD have elevated serum IgE levels, and the level rises in accordance with disease severity (Johnson et al. 1974). Also, the number of LCs is increased in the chronic lesions of AD patients, and they have increased amounts of IgE bound to them (Uno and Hanifin 1980, Bruynzeel-Koomen *et al.* 1986). Finally, eosinophilia in AD patients is common, which can be explained by IL-4 and IL-5 production found in a Th2 T lymphocyte immune response (Uehara *et al.* 1990).

Increasing evidence has supported an important role of Th1 cell immunity in AD. Th1-produced IFN-γ mRNA proteins have been shown to be highly expressed in approximately 80% of AD patients (Grewe *et al.* 1994). Moreover, it was found that the expression of IFN-γ and not that of IL-4 or IgE decreases to normal levels after therapy. *In situ* studies also have shown concomitant increases in Th2 and Th1 cytokines in diseased areas of skin in AD patients, suggesting that both a Th2 and a Th1 cell-type response are involved in AD pathology (Grewe *et al.* 1995). Thus, a two-phase mechanism of pathogenesis was proposed where a Th2 cell-driven initiation phase activates macrophages and eosinophils, which in turn release IL-12, an activator of Th1 cell-mediated immunity (Thepen *et al.* 1996). The activation of allergen-specific and -nonspecific IFN-γ-producing Th1 cells is responsible for the chronicity and severity of disease (Grewe *et al.* 1998).

We may conclude that a Th1 cell-type immune response is involved in the pathogenesis of both AD and ACD. A Th2 cell-type immune response is the primary type of immunity involved in the pathogenesis of AD, and may be involved in ACD to a certain extent (Szepietowski *et al.* 1997). This difference is illustrated in the way atopic individuals respond to an atopy patch test with an aeroallergen such as the house dust mite. Patients with AD undergoing a patch test typically have a positive reaction within 24 h (Young *et al.* 1985). This is in contrast to nonatopic individuals, including patients with ACD, who would be expected to have a reaction between 48 and 72 h, the typical timeframe for a type-IV immune response. It has been shown that the positive reaction in patients with AD within the first 24 h is a predominantly Th2-type cell response, switching to a mostly Th1 response at later time points (48–72 h) (Grewe *et al.* 1995, Thepen *et al.* 1996). In patients with ACD and in normal individuals, a skin response is seen after 48 h and is mediated almost exclusively by cells of the Th1 cell type.

Recently, other immune mediators have been implicated in both AD and ACD, ie, antimicrobial peptides (AMPs). AMPs are endogenous low-molecular-weight peptides that serve as a first-line defense system and are present constitutively in the epidermis, but may be increased with injury and inflammation. In humans, cathelicidins and defensins are the major groups of epidermal AMPs. AMPs exhibit potent killing of a broad range of microorganisms, including Gram-negative and Gram-positive bacteria, fungi, and viruses. AMPs are usually positively charged with a structure that separates charged, hydrophilic residues from hydrophobic residues. This amphipathic organization allows AMPs to associate with negatively charged microbial membranes and enter the lipid phase as a result of their hydrophobic amino acid cluster. Subsequently, microbial cell lysis occurs by various mechanisms such as pore formation or a detergent-like solubilization. In addition, AMPs have shown immunomodulatory effects as well as diverse roles in angiogenesis, wound healing, and chemotaxis in humans (Izadpanah and Gallo 2005).

AMPs appear to play an important role in AD because AD is complicated by recurrent skin infections. It has been found that patients with AD have a decreased ability to produce AMPs (specifically the cathelicidin LL-37 and human β-defensin HBD-2) compared with psoriasis patients, and AD lesions have a very low expression of cathelicidin and HBD-2. This inability to increase AMPs may be due to suppression by Th2 cytokines that are elevated in AD. The decreased level of AMPs in the skin of atopic patients increases their predisposition to infection with *Staphylococcus aureus*, herpes simplex virus, and vaccinia virus, further compromising their skin barrier function (Izadpanah and Gallo 2005).

Similarly, recent evidence suggests that low levels of cutaneous AMPs increase an individual's predisposition to developing ACD, because AMPs normally inhibit the immune inflammatory events required for the generation of ACD. Di Nardo *et al.* (2007) found that a deletion of the murine cathelicidin gene *Cnlp* enhanced an allergic contact response, whereas local administration of cathelicidin before sensitization inhibited the allergic response.

Cathelicidins inhibited TLR-4- but not TLR-2-mediated induction of dendritic cell maturation and cytokine release, and this inhibition was associated with an alteration of cell membrane function and structure, as well as receptor motility. Furthermore, the measurement of the cellular infiltrate in ears of sensitized mice showed that, despite an increase in swelling, $Cnlp^{-/-}$ mice had a fourfold decrease in cell infiltrate, suggesting that endogenous cathelicidin may act by influencing both allergic contact sensitization and cell recruitment (Di Nardo et al. 2007).

ASSOCIATION OF AD AND ACD

As mentioned previously, earlier studies indicated that patients with AD were less likely to develop ACD (Magnusson et al. 1969, Cronin et al. 1970, Marghescu 1985, de Groot 1990). Other studies suggested that contact sensitization in AD patients was inversely correlated with the clinical severity of the AD (Cronin 1993, Giordano-Labadie et al. 1999, Ingordo et al. 2001). In one sensitization trial in which the strong contact allergen dinitrochlorobenzene (DNCB) was applied to 150 patients with AD, 100% of patients with mild AD had a positive challenge test, compared with 33% of patients with severe AD (Uehara and Sawai 1989).

It is now generally accepted that the frequency of contact allergy in patients with AD is comparable to that of nonatopic individuals in both adults and children (Cohen et al. 1990, Lever and Forsyth 1992, Cronin 1993, Klas et al. 1996, Lugovic and Lipozencic 1997, Giordano-Labadie et al. 1999). In support of this observation, a study of nickel sensitization suggested similar cytokine profiles in atopic and nonatopic individuals who developed contact dermatitis (Szepietowski et al. 1997). Following nickel challenge, AD patients and nonatopic individuals had similar increases in IL-2, IL-4, and IFN-γ. The only difference in the immune response between the two groups was an increase just in IL-10 in nonatopic individuals.

Examining the prevalence of contact sensitization to preservatives in schoolchildren revealed that 44% of preservative-sensitive patients had AD (Jenkinson 1997). It is believed that this high prevalence resulted from the high frequency of preservative-containing topical products used by AD patients. In another study of 851 patients with AD, contact allergy to ingredients contained in topical medications was common; patients with severe and long-lasting dermatitis were most frequently sensitized (Lammintausta et al. 1992).

Mäkelä et al. (2007), in a study of 801 AD patients, found that contact allergy did not impair the prognosis of AD. On the contrary, it seemed to have a favorable influence on the course of AD; patients with contact sensitivities to common allergens most often became symptom-free during the 16-year follow-up period compared with those without contact allergy. The beneficial effect may have been a result of allergen avoidance or other immunological effects (Mäkelä et al. 2007).

In one very interesting study, patients with AD were compared with nonatopic individuals in their response to simultaneous exposure to an irritant, sodium lauryl sulfate (SLS), and a contact allergen, nickel sulfate (Seidenari 1994). The experimental design was intended to simulate the typical simultaneous exposure to both irritants and allergens that occurs in domestic and occupational environments. The study reported an increase in ACD after skin irritation in both atopic and nonatopic individuals. However, this effect was particularly enhanced in AD patients.

In conclusion, although there are studies that show that atopic individuals have a decreased prevalence of ACD, most recent studies indicate that there is an equal prevalence of ACD in AD patients and nonatopic individuals. The defective epidermal barrier and chronic exposure to the ingredients of skin-care medications in atopic individuals may offset any possible impairment of Th1 cell-type immunity in this patient population, making them no less susceptible to having ACD than other individuals. Systematic patch testing should be performed in the investigation of contact allergies among AD patients, and appropriate preventive measures taken to avoid contact with potential allergens.

ASSOCIATION OF AD AND ICD

The possible relationship of skin atopy and skin irritability has been investigated in numerous studies. Although some authors report no association between AD and ICD (Stolz et al. 1997, Basketter et al. 1998), most studies conducted show a definite enhancement of skin irritability in patients with AD (van der Valk et al. 1985, Tupker et al. 1990, Agner 1991a, 1991b, Seidenari 1994, Loffler and Effendy 1999). In a retrospective study of patients diagnosed with contact dermatitis, 9.6% of those with ICD were found to have a history of AD, and there was a statistically significant association between the two conditions (Nettis et al. 2002).

In another study, 95 volunteers were divided into 4 groups: (1) individuals with active AD; (2) individuals with a history of AD but without active skin lesions; (3) currently asymptomatic individuals with rhinoconjunctivitis or atopic asthma; and (4) healthy individuals (Loffler and Effendy 1999). Participants were patch tested on unaffected skin with aqueous SLS 0.5% for 48 h. Transepidermal water loss (TEWL) was used as an indicator of stratum corneum integrity and TEWL was measured before and after exposure to the SLS irritant. Only patients with active AD showed a significantly higher TEWL value after SLS, supporting an association between the condition and skin irritability.

DIAGNOSIS

Clinically differentiating between patients presenting with ACD, ICD, and AD can sometimes be difficult, eg, if a patient with atopy presents with a new or worsening rash, it is difficult to know whether the patient has an exacerbation of AD or a concomitant ACD or ICD. This is especially true given our recent understanding that both ACD and ICD can be quite common in AD. Still, there are ways in which the clinician can attempt to differentiate between the diagnoses.

A thorough history, including past or current history of personal or family atopy, as well as questions about environmental exposure in the patient's home, workplace, or during leisure activities is crucial. It is also important to examine the patient for a distinctive distribution of the rash that corresponds to areas of the body which have been selectively exposed to certain environmental stimuli. Causal symptoms and morphological features of eczematous conditions are typically quite similar to each other. They are less helpful in making a diagnosis. A skin biopsy has limited utility in diagnosing a cause of eczema, but it should be obtained in all cases of chronic dermatitis to exclude unexpected disorders, such as occult cutaneous T-cell lymphoma or subacute cutaneous lupus erythematosus. The diagnostic criteria of Hannifin and Rajka are a useful guide in the identification of AD (Hanifin and Rajka 1980).

Patch testing to identify a specific chemical or photochemical exposure(s) as a cause of ACD can be quite helpful. If the results of the patch test are positive and relevant to clinical circumstances, the diagnosis of ACD can be made with confidence. Patients with AD should undergo patch testing as needed if a diagnosis of concurrent ACD is suspected.

TREATMENT

Optimal treatment of ICD and ACD involves withdrawal or prevention of contact with the offending agent, including the use of protective barriers or complete avoidance of exposure. The treatment of ICD is relatively easy if the patient is compliant with instructions. Skin cleanliness and hydration are essential. Cleansing of the skin should rely mainly on tap water to remove dry particulate from the skin, and a slurry of cornmeal and water to remove soil or grease. The use of soap products should be limited. If necessary, neutral pH soap can be used to combat significant microbial contamination. Skin hydration is best achieved by soaking affected areas in tap water for 20–30 min followed by drying and application of a thin film of white petrolatum. The use of topical corticosteroids does not speed recovery from ICD, although it can help reduce symptoms during acute dermatitis.

The skin hydration measures used for ICD are not helpful for the treatment of ACD. The use of open wet dressings is a far more effective treatment for the blisters of ACD, because they are cooling, drying, and antipruritic. Burow solution may be used with open wet dressings for exudative dermatitis, adding some mild antimicrobial properties to the treatment, as well as more potent drying. However, as Burow solution may be irritating with repetitive applications, it should not be used for more than 3 days. If ACD is mild, the addition of potent topical steroids and oral antihistamines may be sufficient treatment. More extensive or severe disease may require the use of systemic corticosteroids.

Treatment goals for AD are similar to those for contact dermatitis: eliminate exposure to possible environmental triggers while also preserving and restoring the skin barrier and reducing inflammation. As with ACD, oral antihistamines reduce itch and tar ointments, alone or together with topical steroids, reduce inflammation. Emollients protect against drying and irritation. Phototherapy also has proven an effective treatment for AD. Patients with particularly severe AD recalcitrant to topical medications or phototherapy, or with AD affecting areas of the skin that significantly diminish quality of life, may benefit from systemic corticosteroids or other systemic immunosuppressive drugs (see Chapter 11).

Steroid-free topical calcineurin inhibitors (TCIs) have emerged in recent years as effective topical preparations to treat AD and ACD with a superior long-term safety profile over corticosteroid therapy. Structurally related macrolide lactones, TCIs specifically block T-cell activation and suppress the release of proinflammatory cytokines (ie, IL-2) by inhibiting the enzyme calcineurin. TCIs have a greater affinity for the skin than the bloodstream, leading to low systemic absorption. The two most common TCIs are tacrolimus ointment and pimecrolimus

cream. Tacrolimus is indicated for patients of all ages and AD severity, whereas pimecrolimus is approved by the US Food and Drug Administration (FDA) only for mild-to-moderate AD. As a result of a purported association with skin cancers and systemic lymphoma, both drugs are considered second-line agents. The most common adverse effects of TCIs are transient burning sensations and pruritus at the application site. Treatment can be started with topical corticosteroids to control the flare and then TCIs can be introduced. In this way the stinging associated with TCIs can be avoided to a large extent. Both TCIs prevent disease flares and cause improvement in AD symptoms over the long term (Stuetz et al. 2006, Alomar et al. 2007).

TCIs have also proven effective in the treatment of ACD, in both animal and human models, although they are not approved for this indication. In a porcine model of ACD, topical pimecrolimus 1% cream was as effective as high-potency topical corticosteroids. In this same model pimecrolimus 1% cream was also as effective as tacrolimus 0.1% ointment (Stuetz et al. 2006). In a recently described human model of ACD, patients with known contact hypersensitivity to nickel applied nickel patches to each arm for 4–8 h daily. Tacrolimus 0.1% ointment was applied to the patch site on one arm, whereas a control ointment vehicle was applied to the patch site on the other twice daily. After 8 weeks, contact dermatitis cleared or almost cleared in 45% of tacrolimus-treated patients on the basis of a physician's global assessment, compared with only 1% of patients using the ointment vehicle (Belsito et al. 2006).

Therapies for both AD and ACD still under investigation include genetically engineered vaccines that promise higher efficacy and fewer adverse effects compared with conventional topical therapy (Medi and Singh 2006). One approach for AD is administering modified hypoallergenic derivatives of recombinant allergens (ie, a few point mutations that leave the structural fold of the molecule unchanged), inducing tolerance with repeat challenge. Another method includes DNA vaccines with hypoallergenic forms of the allergen.

These vaccines have been shown to protect against sensitization and suppress Th2-mediated responses, while enhancing Th1-mediated immune responses. A third approach is immunotherapy with T-cell peptide epitopes by administration of short, allergen-derived synthetic peptides. T-cell peptide epitopes induce T-cell anergy and are unable to crosslink IgE. Furthermore, active immunization against IgE is an approach to inhibit the inflammatory cascade of AD. It has been shown to induce tolerance and reduce circulating IgE to a therapeutic level (Medi and Singh 2006). Unfortunately, studies of allergen-specific immunotherapy in AD have suffered from methodical shortcomings and no long-term studies have been performed to clarify their disease-modifying effect in the context of the 'allergic march' (Compalati *et al.* 2012).

In the case of ACD, T-cell receptor (TCR) 'mimic peptides' and DNA vaccines have also demonstrated some efficacy in mice but definitive human studies are lacking (Göllner *et al.* 2000, Medi and Singh 2006). In a murine model of ACD, Göllner *et al.* (2000) found that the topical application of a mimic peptide corresponding to the transmembrane region of the TCR can function as a local immunosuppressive agent by inhibiting T-cell signaling and function in the skin. Furthermore, injection of naked copy DNA encoding a sequence of the TCR chain suppressed the elicitation phase of ACD by inhibiting the development of an inflammatory infiltrate. In subsequent human case studies, TCR mimic peptides were able to suppress and prevent T-cell-mediated dermatoses, such as ACD, even more potently than in mice. The strongest effects were present when applied to newly arising skin lesions (Enk and Knop 2000, Göllner *et al.* 2000).

CONCLUSIONS

AD, ICD, and ACD are all eczematous disorders that represent similar pathological states. However, AD and ACD are both immune-mediated diseases, and AD most probably increases susceptibility to ICD. It is also known that AD is exacerbated in the presence of certain triggers, including other skin conditions such as contact dermatitis (Dahl 1990). These eczematous disorders have other, less well-defined similarities regarding pathogenesis, diagnosis, and treatment.

Although the relationship between AD and contact dermatitis is well investigated, large gaps in our understanding remain. There is a consensus that AD is a predisposing factor for ICD with all its ramifications for hand dermatitis in the occupational setting. The old dictum that ACD is decreased in patients with AD has been largely abandoned and most authors recommend patch testing in atopic individuals when clinically indicated.

NUMMULAR DERMATITIS

Noah Scheinfeld and Donald Rudikoff

BACKGROUND

Nummular dermatitis, or discoid eczema, is an idiopathic dermatosis, often resistant to treatment, characterized by coin-shaped eczematous plaques. According to one review, 'It is a survivor from the days of purely descriptive dermatology, when papules, vesicles, scales or crusts determined the status of an eczematous rash' (Gordon 1954).

Nummular dermatitis was first described by Rayer in 1845 but the term 'eczema nummulaire' was introduced by Devergie in 1854 (Pollitzer 1912, Shelley and Crissey 2003). Devergie described an eruption of small rounded plaques, each the size of a five-franc piece, occurring on the extremities and also on the trunk 'less remarkable for its nummular disposition than for its tenacity.'

Early French authors emphasized a connection with the nervous system; in fact, Bazin described an 'arthritic eczema' which corresponded to the picture of nummular eczema (Bazin 1862, Chipman 1934). Sulzberger and Garbe described an entity in 1937, mostly in middle-aged or older Jewish men, which has variously been called 'exudative discoid and lichenoid dermatitis of Sulzberger and Garbe' or 'oid-oid' disease (Sulzberger and Garbe 1937). Many authors consider that this entity was a variant of nummular dermatitis, though 40 years after its description Sulzberger maintained it was a unique dermatitis (Sulzberger 1979, Jansen *et al.* 1992). Notably, the entity was described as excruciatingly pruritic, with lichenoid lesions in addition to eczematoid lesions, and including facial and genital involvement which is not characteristic of nummular dermatitis.

EPIDEMIOLOGY

A public health service study (Johnson and Roberts 1978) found a prevalence for nummular dermatitis of 1.7 per 1000 population (males 1.0 and females 2.4). When stratified by age, the prevalence per 1000 individuals was 1.9 for children aged 1–5, 4.9 for those aged 18–24, 2.5 for those aged 25–34, and 3.2 in those aged 65–74. It occurs more frequently in the winter than in the summer. Nummular lesions are sometimes seen in children with otherwise typical atopic dermatitis but pure nummular dermatitis can occur in this population, albeit uncommonly (Hill 1956). The condition is rare in infancy.

In elderly individuals, there appears to be a connection with dry skin, and in younger people it may correlate with puberty.

CLINICAL MANIFESTATIONS

The eruption of nummular dermatitis consists of discrete, round, erythematous, edematous, and crusted plaques usually localized on the dorsal aspect of the hands, extensor surfaces of the arms, legs, thighs, and buttocks (Figs 16.1–16.3).

Plaques sometimes attain a large size and may be studded with papules or papulovesicles and weep serous fluid (Fig 16.4). They frequently begin as erythematous edematous papules and papulovesicles that coalesce into larger plaques. Lesions usually have a discrete border and, although not as well demarcated as psoriatic plaques, they are more sharply delineated than lesions of patch-stage mycosis fungoides, which have been described as having a *smudgy* border.

Individual plaques of stable nummular dermatitis are usually more than 1 cm in diameter but can range in size from 2 mm to 4 cm (Fig 16.5). The occurrence of nummular dermatitis around skin lesions such as seborrheic keratoses has been referred to as 'halo eczema,' 'perilesional nummular dermatitis,' or 'Meyerson phenomenon' (Rosen *et al.* 1990).

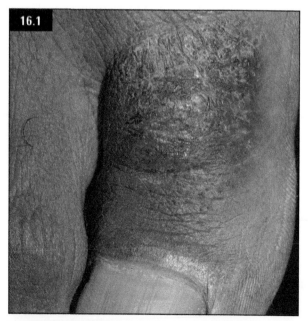

Fig 16.1 Nummular dermatitis is characterized by coin-shaped plaques most commonly located on the extremities.

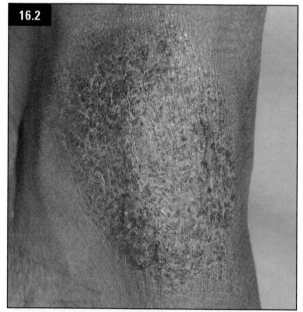

Fig 16.2 Oval, crusted, hyperpigmented plaque on the lower leg.

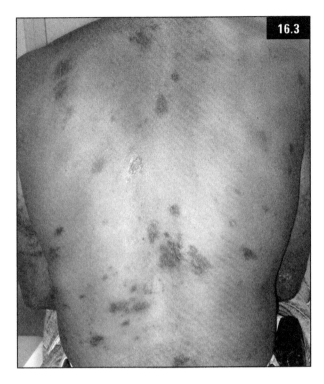

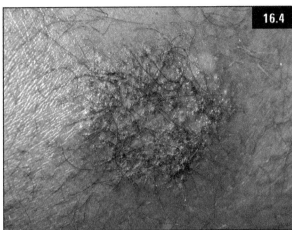

Fig 16.4 Lesions may be studded with papules and papulovesicles and weep serous fluid that forms crusts.

Fig 16.3 Lesions are usually acral but may occur on the trunk less commonly. (Courtesy of UCONN Department of Dermatology collection c/o Dr Justin Finch.)

Fig 16.5 Nummular dermatitis lesions vary in size from (A) 1 cm to (B) much larger plaques. They may be (A) single or (C) multiple.

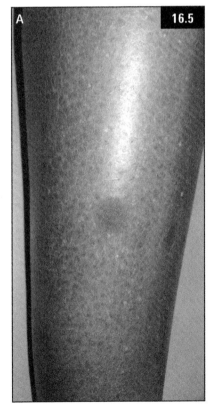

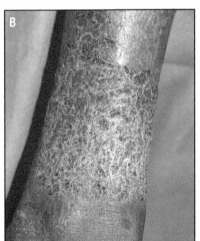

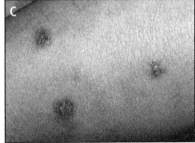

Nummular dermatitis lesions ordinarily appear pink or reddish in white people but are often brown, purple, or black in people of color. The surface may appear dry and scaly (**Fig 16.6**) or be studded with papules, papulovesicles, or blisters that give rise to erosions. Annular lesions may occur (**Fig 16.7**). Weeping and oozing lead to crust formation. The moist quality of the nummular lesions reflects epidermal spongiosis, the histopathological hallmark of the condition, and does not imply infection although lesions are frequently colonized with staphylococci. Recurrence after treatment displays papules and vesicles on the residual erythema of pre-existing lesions but may occur on previously uninvolved skin (Gordon 1954).

Nummular dermatitis lesions heal without scarring but often leave brown patches or hypopigmentation. This postinflammatory pigmentary alteration results from pigment incontinence, and may never completely fade, particularly when located below the knee. Pruritus is usually present to some degree and, when present, is usually worse at night. It can cause irritability and insomnia.

A so-called 'dry nummular dermatitis' has been described as a rare treatment-resistant variant of nummular dermatitis in which multiple, dry, scaly, round, or oval patches with occasional scattered microvesicles on an erythematous base appear on the palms and soles with minimal pruritus (Calnan and Meara 1956).

With regard to prognosis, a large review suggested that the disease either resolved within a year or, if not, tended to persist for many years (Cowan 1961).

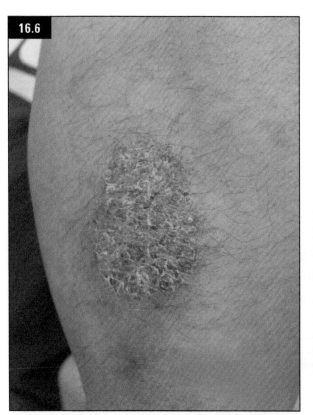

Fig 16.6 Nummular dermatitis lesion with dry surface.

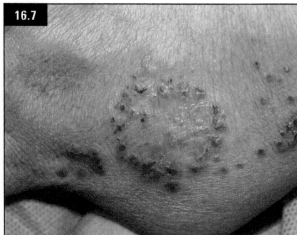

Fig 16.7 Annular lesions of nummular eczema.

CLINICAL ASSOCIATIONS

Nummular dermatitis appears to be associated with xerosis and asteatotic eczema, although this is not always the case. Patients also appear more susceptible to contact dermatitis, particularly from nickel, cobalt, or chromates. The presence of venous insufficiency, varicosities, stasis dermatitis, edema related to chronic heart failure, diabetes, hypertension, and elevated blood cholesterol correlates with an increased prevalence of nummular dermatitis, particularly on the lower legs.

Widespread plaques of nummular dermatitis may result from so-called 'autoeczematization,' ie, the development of eczema at a location distant from the initial site of involvement. Nummular dermatitis sometimes arises in the site of previous cutaneous injury, such as an insect bite, abrasion, or burn and, as mentioned previously, it can be a manifestation of atopic dermatitis (**Fig 16.8**).

LABORATORY AND HISTOLOGICAL FINDINGS

Bacterial cultures of nummular dermatitis lesions frequently grow *Staphylococcus aureus*, which usually represents bacterial colonization. That this is colonization and not infection is evident from the fact that corticosteroids without concomitant antibiotic therapy usually cause nummular dermatitis to resolve and antibiotics by themselves are ineffective. This would not be expected in truly infected skin.

Histological changes of nummular dermatitis vary with the stage of the lesions. In acute lesions, there are foci of spongiosis, papillary dermal edema, and a superficial perivascular infiltrate of lymphocytes, histiocytes, and sometimes eosinophils (Ackerman 1978). Subacute and chronic lesions may show psoriasiform epidermal hyperplasia and melanophages may be present in chronic lesions.

Increased numbers of mast cells have been observed in the plaques of nummular dermatitis as compared with normal skin, and this might relate to the sometimes intense pruritus (Järvikallio *et al.* 1997).

Fig 16.8 Nummular lesions may occur in patients with atopic dermatitis.

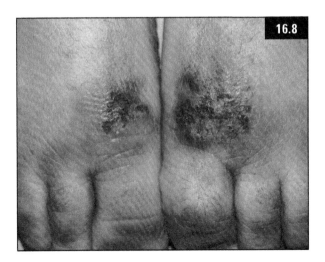

DIFFERENTIAL DIAGNOSIS

The differential diagnosis of nummular dermatitis includes atopic dermatitis, allergic contact dermatitis, psoriasis, lichen simplex chronicus, cutaneous drug eruption, mycosis fungoides, pityriasis rosea, impetigo, tinea, and syphilis (**Box 16.1**). Although patients with atopic dermatitis can have typical nummular dermatitis lesions, they will usually have symmetrical flexural eczema, lichenification, or other distinguishing clinical features. Nummular dermatitis might be confused with allergic contact dermatitis, especially if provoked by the base-metal back of a wristwatch, circular bandaids, or transdermal medicine patches. Although in most cases the diagnosis will be evident from the history and physical exam, patch testing can add a great deal of information.

A recent study of 50 patients with nummular dermatitis found significant positive patch-test reactions in 23 of the patients (Krupa Shankar and Shrestha 2005). The most frequent sensitizers were colophony, nitrofurazone, neomycin sulfate, and nickel sulfate (7.14% each). Antigens in topical medications, cosmetics, and toiletries accounted for almost two-thirds of the reactions.

Lichen simplex chronicus (LSC) can be differentiated from nummular dermatitis based on lesional morphology and typical sites of predilection (**Fig 16.9**). The surface of LSC lesions may be gray or brown and there is dry thickening of the skin accompanied by accentuation of skin markings. It is commonly localized on the ankles, neck, nuchal area, and scrotum.

Nummular dermatitis can occasionally be confused with psoriasis (**Fig 16.10**). Typical psoriasis presents with sharply demarcated plaques, often on the scalp, elbows, knees, and sacral area, covered with a micaceous scale. The plaques of nummular dermatitis are often studded with papules (**Fig 16.11**) and papulovesicles, and may appear moist. When lesions are dry, they lack the silvery psoriatic scale and do not display the Auspitz sign (dermal bleeding when a scale is removed).

Certain medications, particularly heavy metals (gold, bismuth, and arsenic) and interferon-α2b, can provoke a reaction resembling nummular dermatitis (*Table 16.1*). Calcium channel blockers have been

Box 16.1 Differential diagnosis of nummular dermatitis

Asteatotic eczema
Atopic dermatitis
Contact dermatitis, allergic
Contact dermatitis, irritant
Cutaneous drug eruption
Cutaneous T-cell lymphoma
Impetigo
Lichen simplex chronicus
Mycosis fungoides
Necrolytic acral erythema
Pityriasis rosea
Psoriasis, plaque
syphilis
Tinea corporis

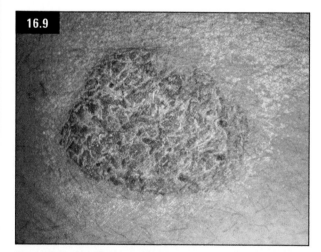

Fig 16.9 Lesion of nummular dermatitis with lichenification from rubbing. Note accentuation of skin markings.

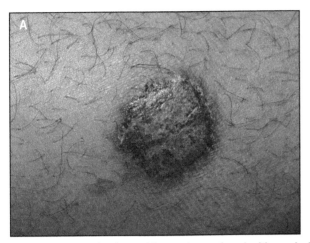
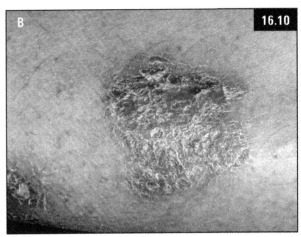

Fig 16.10 Nummular dermatitis may be confused with psoriasis. (A) This lesion in part appears to have typical psoriatic scale but is edematous and oozing. (B) Psoriatic lesions with silvery scale and sharp demarcation.

Fig 16.11 Confluent erythematous papules forming lesions of nummular dermatitis.

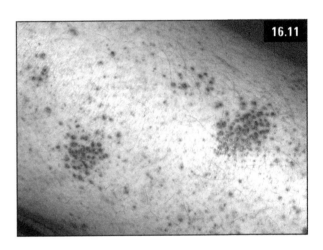

Table 16.1 Medications and contactants that can cause nummular dermatitis-like eruptions

Thimerosal	Patrizi *et al.* (1999)
Interferon-α2b plus ribavirin	Moore *et al.* (2004)
Ethylenediamine hydrochloride	Caraffini and Lisi (1987)
Isotretinoin	Bettoli *et al.* (1987)
Mercury	Adachi *et al.* (2000)
Gold	Wilkinson *et al.* (1992)
Tumor necrosis factor-α-blocking therapy	Flendrie *et al.* (2005)
Ethyl cyanoacrylate-containing glue	Belsito (1987)
Depilatory cream	Le Coz (2002)

reported to produce chronic eczematous reactions in elderly people (**Fig 16.12**). Additional clinical triggers of nummular dermatitis are listed in *Table 16.2*.

Nummular dermatitis should also be differentiated from mycosis fungoides. Patch-stage mycosis fungoides presents with brownish-red round or oval patches or a hypopigmented variant with an indistinct, 'smudgy' border (**Fig 16.13**). Lesions are frequently localized on the trunk, thighs, and buttocks, and may show slight atrophy and poikiloderma. Pityriasis rosea most commonly occurs on the trunk in a so-called 'Christmas tree' pattern. Individual lesions follow skin lines and often have a central collarette of scale with an inwardly pointing free edge. Occasionally a florid case of pityriasis rosea will have juicy, eczematoid patches that resemble nummular dermatitis. In rare cases, nummular dermatitis might be confused with sarcoid or secondary syphilis.

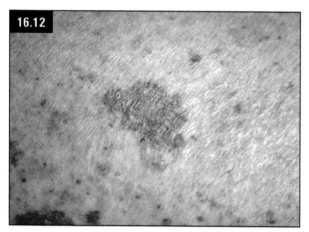

Fig 16.12 Eczematous lesions in an elderly female from a calcium channel blocker.

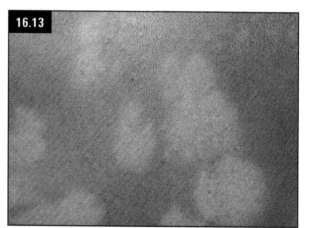

Fig 16.13 Nummular eczema may be confused with mycosis fungoides. This patient has multiple lesions of hypopigmented mycosis fungoides with *smudgy borders.*

Table 16.2   Miscellaneous triggers of nummular-like dermatitis

TRIGGER	REFERENCE
Scabies treatment	Kaminska and Mortenhumer (2003)
Odontogenic infection	Satoh *et al.* (2003)
Helicobacter pylori	Sakurane et al. (2002)
Leprosy	Pavithran (1990)
Giardiasis	Pietrzak *et al.* (2005)

PATHOGENESIS

There appears to be an as-yet undefined relationship between nummular dermatitis and epidermal barrier impairment. The exact relationship of nummular dermatitis with xerosis, asteatotic eczema (**Fig 16.14**), and irritant dermatitis, with which it may coexist, is not understood (Rollins 1968, Wilkinson 1979). It is significant that isotretinoin, a drug that causes dry skin, chapping, and likely affects epidermal integrity, has been reported to cause a nummular dermatitis-like eruption (Bettoli *et al.* 1987).

There is controversy as to whether nummular dermatitis is associated with atopy; an association has been found in some studies but not in others (Carr *et al.* 1964, Hellgren and Mobacken 1969). Moreover, IgE levels are usually normal. Some of the clinical studies of nummular dermatitis suggest a possible immune basis for the disease. An 8-year study of patients with nummular eruptions found a close association of nummular dermatitis with varicose veins and/or edema of the lower extremities. The study suggested that 'autoeczematization' was an important common denominator (Bendl 1979). A number of medications can also induce eruptions that resemble nummular dermatitis. The provocation of extensive nummular dermatitis by interferon-α2b plus ribavirin for hepatitis C suggests a possible immunological mechanism (Moore *et al.* 2004).

One report noted that elderly individuals with nummular dermatitis had increased sensitivity to environmental aeroallergens compared with age-matched controls (Aoyama *et al.* 1999). Another report noted a relationship with internal foci of infection including dental infection (Krogh 1960, Tanaka *et al.* 2009).

Fowle and Rice (1953) considered that staphylococci are important in nummular eczema both by invasion of the skin and by producing 'bacterial allergy.'

Nummular dermatitis such as seborrheic dermatitis can be related to neurological compromise. In patients with spinal cord injury, it may localize below the level of spinal injury (Reed *et al.* 1961).

To understand the immunological basis of nummular dermatitis, Bos *et al.* (1989) examined the epidermal and dermal lymphocytic infiltrate of several inflammatory skin diseases. The researchers found that nummular dermatitis lesional skin had more CD3+ epidermal lymphocytes than atopic dermatitis

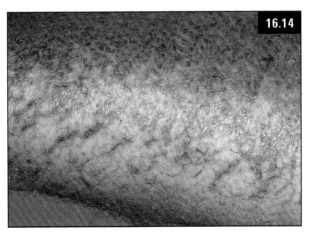

Fig 16.14 Nummular dermatitis is often associated with xerosis. This patient has a form of xerotic eczema referred to as eczema craquelé because of its resemblance to cracked china.

and normal skin but fewer than psoriatic skin. The epidermal CD4:CD8 ratio was 0.26, similar to normal skin. In the papillary dermis of nummular dermatitis lesions, there was a marked increase in CD3+ cells, most of which were CD4+ 'memory' (helper-inducer) cells (CD4:CD8 = 2.7).

The same group also reported a predominance of dendritic cells bearing the Langerhans cell marker (OKT6+) over interdigitating cell-expressing RFD1 in nummular dermatitis lesional skin (Bos *et al.* 1986).

Järvikallio *et al.* (2003), who previously demonstrated increased numbers of mast cells in nummular dermatitis skin, studied their association with sensory nerves and the distribution of the neuropeptides substance P (SP), vasoactive intestinal polypeptide (VIP), and calcitonin gene-related peptide (CGRP) in the skin of patients with atopic dermatitis and nummular dermatitis (Järvikallio *et al.* 1997, 2003). Nerve–mast cell contacts in the basement membrane zone were seen practically only in lesional nummular dermatitis. SP and CGRP fibers were prominently increased in lesional skin compared with nonlesional areas of nummular dermatitis in the epidermis and the papillary dermis. In both conditions, only small differences in VIP positivity were noted between lesional and nonlesional samples. The authors suggested that SP and mast cell tryptase play a prominent role in skin inflammation.

TREATMENT

General treatment methods for nummular dermatitis include the use of emollients such as bath oils, soap substitutes, and moisturizing creams to relieve itching, scaling, and dryness. Creams containing glycerin, cetomacrogol, white soft paraffin and liquid paraffin mixed, and wool-fat lotions have been advocated. Tar products have been suggested by earlier authors, but now the mainstay of treatment is topical corticosteroid preparations. A 2-week course of of high- or super-high-potency corticosteroid cream or ointment once or twice daily may be sufficient, followed by a less potent preparation. A course of oral antibiotics to treat staphylococci may be helpful in some cases. Oral antihistamines do not have any effect on the dermatitis but may be used for their soporific effect at bedtime.

For more severe and extensive cases, systemic corticosteroids and phototherapy have a major role. Intramuscular triamcinolone acetonide is usually beneficial especially if followed by broadband or narrowband ultraviolet (UV)B phototherapy. A recent retrospective study of nummular/discoid eczema in children advocates the use of methotrexate for moderate-to-severe pediatric discoid eczema that has failed to respond to conventional therapies (Roberts and Orchard 2010).

CONCLUSION

Nummular dermatitis remains notable among the eczemas for its striking morphology. The distinctive discoid lesions of this condition can sometimes be confused with other dermatoses that present with round lesions. As with all types of eczema, nummular dermatitis can be related to autoeczematization and can be related to medication use. In most cases, nummular dermatitis does not have a debilitating effect on patients' lives and it can usually be treated effectively. The association with xerosis is complex because, although it is more common in patients with xerosis, most patients with xerotic skin do not have nummular dermatitis. This striking condition still fascinates and interests dermatologists and it will likely continue to do so for years to come.

Clinical suggestions

1. Patients with nummular dermatitis should be evaluated for duration and extent of disease, severity of itching, previous treatment, bathing habits, and possible exacerbating factors such as contactants, medications, or occult infection.
2. If dermatitis is widespread, extremely itchy, and resistant to previous topical treatment, the authors recommend an aggressive approach. If there is no contraindication, the use of intramuscular triamcinolone acetonide 1 mg/kg often provides much needed relief, mitigates patient frustration, and promotes patient confidence in the practitioner. Alternatively if disease is limited, a high-potency corticosteroid ointment may be used.
3. Topical corticosteroids are applied using the soak-and-smear technique (Guttman *et al.* 2005). Basically, the patient is instructed to soak in a tapwater bath (not a shower) for 20 min at night and to apply a corticosteroid ointment immediately without drying the skin. Pajamas are worn over this. Moreover patients should apply emollients after bathing to maintain skin hydration.
4. As nummular dermatitis frequently relapses after anti-inflammatory treatment, it is useful to have a plan for maintenance therapy such as the use of UVB phototherapy or topical corticosteroids applied twice or three times weekly.
5. Antibiotics may be useful if an occult dental or other infection is suspected or if there is secondary infection of skin lesions. Systemic immunosuppressive agents may have a role for recalcitrant disease.

CHAPTER 17

STASIS DERMATITIS

Scott L. Flugman

BACKGROUND

Stasis dermatitis is a common inflammatory condition, typically affecting the lower legs of middle-aged and elderly patients (Farber and Barnes 1956). It presents as an eczematous dermatitis of the lower legs and ankles against a background of chronic venous insufficiency and lower extremity edema. The severity of stasis dermatitis varies widely from mild, asymptomatic, cutaneous pigmentary alteration to severe eczematous dermatitis with fibrosis and ulceration. The prevalence of stasis dermatitis is around 6–7% in patients aged over 50 years (Beauregard and Gilchrest 1987). This means that more than 15 million people in the USA may have this condition.

For patients older than 70 years, prevalence of stasis dermatitis is probably higher (around 20%) (Beauregard and Gilchrest 1987). In older patients, stasis dermatitis is more than twice as prevalent as psoriasis and only slightly less prevalent than seborrheic dermatitis (Droller 1955, Dooms-Goossens *et al.* 1979, Weismann *et al.* 1980, Beauregard and Gilchrest 1987). A slight female preponderance has been reported, resulting most likely from the stress that pregnancy places on the venous system, which makes venous insufficiency more common in women. Complications of stasis dermatitis (most significantly leg ulcerations and cellulitis) make this condition a significant cause of morbidity for patients in this age group. With a significant portion of the baby-boomer generation entering their 70s, stasis dermatitis is sure to become even more prevalent in the coming 10–20 years.

CLINICAL FEATURES

The typical patient affected with stasis dermatitis shows clinical signs of chronic venous insufficiency. Lower-leg edema is commonly present, as are varicosities affecting the veins of the affected leg(s) (**Fig 17.1**). Stasis dermatitis may be present in one or both legs; unilateral involvement is more common in patients with a history of extrinsic damage to the lower extremity venous system, such as by surgery or prior trauma. 'Stasis pigmentation' may precede the onset of clinically symptomatic stasis dermatitis by months or years. It consists of asymptomatic reddish-brown, nonblanching discoloration of the skin of the

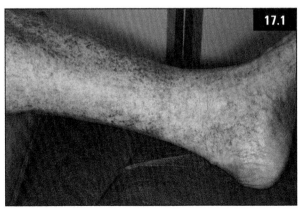

Fig 17.1 Stasis changes with varicose veins and hemosiderin deposition giving the skin a reddish-brown color. Note decreased involvement in areas where a sock provided compression.

lower leg. It results from deposition of hemosiderin in the dermis from extravasated red blood cells. Although asymptomatic, stasis pigmentation is permanent and may result in cosmetic distress for affected patients. Stasis dermatitis may rarely present on the arm as a result of vascular anomalies or surgery (Deguchi *et al.* 2010).

The most common early manifestation of stasis dermatitis is a pruritic, eczematous patch that starts on the medial aspect of the lower leg and ankle. The course may be insidious, occurring as mildly progressive symptoms over many years, or it may present as a severe and acute inflammatory eczematous exacerbation. It is hypothesized that this classic location of stasis dermatitis results from the medial lower leg being a 'watershed area' of venous blood flow, with relatively poor venous circulation compared with the rest of the leg. Therefore, this area is preferentially affected by venous hypertension (Browse and Burnand 1982).

The eczematous nature of stasis dermatitis is represented by erythema, scaling, and xerosis of the skin of the leg. If stasis dermatitis is not treated at an early stage, the condition may progress to involve larger areas of the leg. Frequently, the inflammation can completely encircle the lower leg; it also may move in a superior direction, affecting the calf and shin up to the knee. This more severe inflammatory manifestation is known as *stocking erythroderma* (Kirsner *et al.* 1993). In more advanced cases, dermatitis may affect the dorsal aspect of the foot.

Any change that can occur in other types of eczematous dermatitis may also occur in stasis dermatitis. Externally induced secondary changes are common. Skin changes from repeated excoriation are common, owing to the pruritic nature of the condition. These include superficial erosions as well as deeper traumatic ulcerations. Lichenification is also common as a result of constant rubbing and scratching; the patient may report repeatedly rubbing the affected area with the heel of the opposite foot while sitting (**Fig 17.2**). Purpura and ecchymoses may result from the trauma of scratching and from edema. Purpura and ecchymoses are especially prevalent in patients being treated with blood-thinning medications.

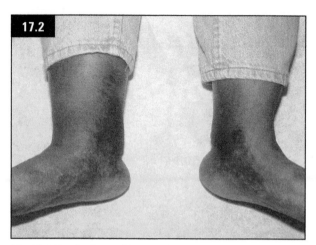

Fig 17.2 Stasis dermatitis with lichenification.

CLINICAL COMPLICATIONS OF STASIS DERMATITIS

As a result of the compromised nature of the skin barrier in affected patients, secondary infection is common in patients with stasis dermatitis. Bacterial superinfection is a significant cause of morbidity in those affected. This may be limited to superficial impetiginization with honey-colored crusting and a weeping or purulent discharge, or to bacterial folliculitis of lower-extremity hair follicles. Deeper bacterial infection affecting the dermis and subcutis manifests as cellulitis of the affected leg. As sepsis may result from virulent or neglected infection, patients with cellulitis are often hospitalized for intravenous antibiotics. Cellulitis presents as spreading erythema, induration, and pain of the affected leg, and initially may be difficult to distinguish from an exacerbation of the underlying stasis dermatitis (Kirsner *et al.* 1993). Patients may or may not show systemic signs of infection, such as fever, chills, and malaise.

Other less common forms of superinfection in stasis dermatitis patients include fungal infections, such as cutaneous candidiasis and dermatophyte infection. The diagnosis of candidiasis is suggested by worsening erythema with satellite pustules; it is more common in patients with immune dysfunction (such as individuals with malignancy, those who have undergone organ transplantation, and those with long-standing diabetes mellitus).

Dermatophyte infection is extremely common in the elderly population, especially recurrent tinea pedis and onychomycosis. Fungal involvement of the skin of the feet and toes may easily progress to involve the skin of the leg in patients whose cutaneous barrier is already compromised by stasis dermatitis. Susceptibility to tinea infection of the leg is further increased by frequent use of topical steroids, which can impair the capacity of the skin to contain cutaneous dermatophyte infections.

Stasis dermatitis is unique among forms of eczematous dermatitis in that it can be accompanied by deep dermal inflammation and scarring, known as *lipodermatosclerosis* and sometimes referred to as *hypodermitis sclerodermiformis*. This disorder consists of deep inflammation leading to fibrosis of the dermis and subcutis. It may occur as a complication in patients with long-standing stasis dermatitis, or it may present as an initial manifestation.

Clinically, lipodermatosclerosis presents as firm induration of the lower leg, with a taut, bound-down appearance of the overlying skin. In the acute inflammatory phase, lipodermatosclerosis is accompanied by exquisitely tender erythema, making simple palpation of the affected leg extremely painful for the patient. Chronic lipodermatosclerosis results in the classic 'inverted champagne bottle' appearance, with the scarred, bound-down, hyperpigmented lower leg giving way to the edematous, nonsclerotic, superior portion of the affected leg (Kirsner *et al.* 1993) (**Fig 17.3**). The painful, acute phase of lipodermatosclerosis is frequently misdiagnosed as cellulitis or erysipelas, and, even for the experienced dermatologist, it may be difficult to distinguish the two with certainty (Reich-Schupke *et al.* 2009). One clinical clue is that cellulitis is most often unilateral; only rarely are pathogenic bacteria able to breach the defenses of both legs at once. Therefore, many hospital consultations for 'bilateral cellulitis' are actually for exacerbations of lipodermatosclerosis.

Fig 17.3 (A, B) *Inverted champagne bottle* appearance of chronic lipodermatosclerosis.

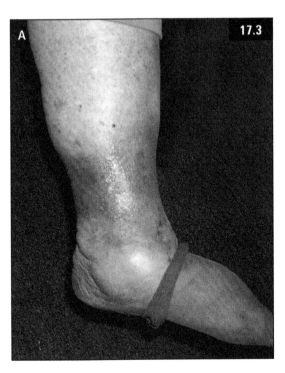
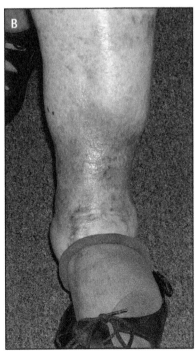

The clinical complication causing the greatest long-term morbidity in patents with stasis dermatitis is cutaneous venous ulceration. Lower extremity skin affected by chronic stasis dermatitis and/or lipodermatosclerosis may progress to clinical, nonhealing ulceration of the skin (Fig 17.4). The resulting venous stasis ulcers may persist for many years or even decades, necessitating prolonged treatment courses and multiple, painful, inflammatory recurrences. Venous stasis ulcers typically appear in the areas most commonly affected by stasis dermatitis, particularly the medial aspect of the ankle and lower leg. The ulcers may become large (>5 cm) and completely encircle the lower leg (Fig 17.5). Besides being painful and debilitating, chronic stasis ulcers are a portal of entry for infectious microorganisms. Moreover, they cause dermal scarring, which further impairs already compromised venous circulation (Kirsner *et al.* 1993, Pardes and Nemeth 1993). Although venous ulcers do not cause gangrene and amputation (as is the case with arterial insufficiency), they do cause major prolonged morbidity. The cost of caring for patients with chronic stasis ulcers also remains significant. The mean cost of caring for a venous ulcer in Germany is almost €10 000, most of it paid by statutory health insurance (Purwins *et al.* 2010).

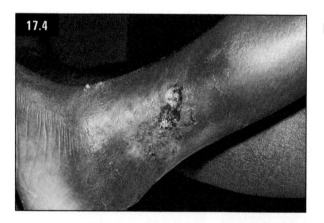

Fig 17.4 Chronic stasis dermatitis with *venous ulceration.*

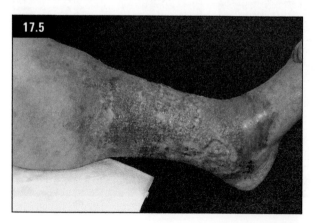

Fig 17.5 Chronic venous stasis ulcer encircling the leg.

PATHOPHYSIOLOGY OF STASIS DERMATITIS

Stasis dermatitis occurs as a direct consequence of venous insufficiency. Disturbed function of the one-way valvular system in the deep venous plexus of the legs results in backflow of blood from the deep venous system to the superficial venous system, with accompanying venous hypertension. This loss of valvular function can result from an age-related decrease in valve competency. Alternatively, specific events, such as deep venous thrombosis, traumatic injury, or surgery, can severely damage the function of the lower-extremity venous system (Lotti *et al.* 1987, Isoda *et al.* 2006) (**Fig 17.6**). Surgical causes include direct surgical manipulation of the venous system, such as vein stripping or harvesting of vein grafts for coronary bypass. Orthopedic procedures (eg, a knee arthroplasty or fracture repairs) may indirectly cause scarring, edema, or impairment of venous circulation. The mechanism by which venous hypertension causes the cutaneous inflammation of stasis dermatitis has been studied extensively for decades. Several theories have been proposed.

The earliest theories about the cause of cutaneous inflammation in venous insufficiency centered on oxygen perfusion of lower-extremity tissues (Dodd *et al.* 1985). Originally, an incompetent venous system was thought to lead to pooling or 'stasis' of blood in the superficial veins, with reduced flow and, therefore, reduced oxygen tension in the dermal capillaries (Browse and Burnand 1982, Dodd *et al.* 1985). This pooling hypothesis led to the term 'stasis dermatitis.' It was believed that the decreased oxygen content of pooled blood led to hypoxic damage to the overlying skin. Subsequent studies, however, failed to document this hypoxia. In fact, the venous blood in patients with venous insufficiency is actually characterized by increased flow and high oxygen tension (Coleridge Smith *et al.* 1988, Cheatle *et al.* 1990).

Additional research focused on the role of lower-extremity microcirculation in the pathogenesis of cutaneous inflammation caused by venous insufficiency. Studies done in the 1970s and 1980s showed that increased venous hydrostatic pressure is transmitted to the dermal microcirculation with a resulting increase in the permeability of dermal capillaries. This phenomenon enables macromolecules, such as fibrinogen, to leak out into the pericapillary tissue. Polymerization of fibrinogen to fibrin results in the formation of a fibrin cuff around dermal capillaries (Falanga *et al.* 1987, Coleridge Smith *et al.* 1988, Pascarella *et al.* 2005). Decreased cutaneous fibrinolytic activity has been proposed to contribute to the formation of fibrin cuffs. Fibrin cuffs are also found in ulcers caused by venous hypertension, and they are not found in ulcers resulting from other causes. It has been suggested that the fibrin cuff serves as a barrier to oxygen diffusion, with resulting tissue hypoxia and cell damage.

Fig 17.6 Stasis dermatitis associated with a combat scar.

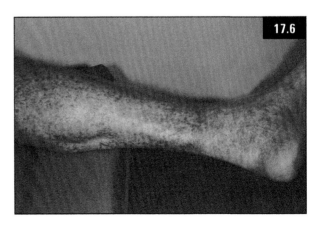

17.6

Formation of fibrin cuffs, coupled with decreased fibrinolysis, results in the dermal fibrosis that is the hallmark of advanced stasis dermatitis and lipodermatosclerosis. The pruritus and cutaneous inflammation likely result from the fact that fibrin cuffs serve as a depot for activated leukocytes. The leukocytes are attracted to and retained in the fibrin cuff by chemoattractants released in the fibrinogen-to-fibrin inflammatory cascade. These leukocytes, in turn, release inflammatory mediators into the surrounding dermis (Falanga *et al.* 1987, Pappas *et al.* 1999). Growth factors released by activated leukocytes and fibroblasts include transforming growth factor-$\beta 1$ (TGF-$\beta 1$), vascular intercellular adhesion molecule-1 (ICAM-1), and vascular cell adhesion molecule-1 (VCAM-1) (Peschen *et al.* 1999). These growth factors are important mediators that attract leukocytes while inducing inflammation and subsequent fibrosis. Other molecules released by activated leukocytes include proteolytic enzymes, matrix metalloproteases, leukotrienes, and free oxygen radicals (Cheatle *et al.* 1991a, Herouy *et al.* 2001). The finding of growth-factor-mediated cytokine production, aided by fibrin-cuff formation, provides a direct link between dysfunctional venous circulation and cutaneous inflammation with fibrosis (Pappas *et al.* 1999).

DIAGNOSIS OF STASIS DERMATITIS

Diagnosis of stasis dermatitis is typically based on its classic clinical appearance in a patient with signs of chronic venous insufficiency. Biopsy is not typically required; in fact, skin biopsy is frequently detrimental, owing to poor wound healing in affected patients. Biopsies are limited to those patients for whom histology is required to rule out other skin pathologies (eg, vasculitis, panniculitis, cutaneous T-cell lymphoma, or, in the case of nonhealing leg ulcers, basal or squamous cell carcinoma). Stasis dermatitis may occasionally present as a solitary lesion and be mistaken for a neoplasm, in which case a biopsy would be appropriate (Weaver and Billings 2009).

A skin biopsy of stasis dermatitis shows acute or subacute spongiotic dermatitis, which is frequently indistinguishable from other forms of eczematous dermatitis (except for the accompanying histological indications of venous insufficiency). Acute lesions may exhibit a superficial perivascular lymphocytic infiltrate, epidermal spongiosis, serous exudate, scaling, and crust. Chronic lesions may show signs of lichenification, such as epidermal acanthosis with hyperkeratosis. The dermis is characterized by deep dermal aggregates of siderophages due to uptake of hemosiderin from degraded erythrocytes that have leaked into the perivascular space. Dermal capillaries are frequently dilated and, along with dermal fibrosis, a biopsy may show intimal thickening of small arterioles and venules (Lever and Schaumburg-Lever 1990). In cases of long duration, there may be proliferation of small capillaries and venules along with fibrosis, which is known as *pseudo-Kaposi sarcoma* or *acroangiodermatitis*. Biopsy in patients with acroangiodermatitis is valuable in ruling out classic Kaposi sarcoma, which also occurs on the lower legs of elderly patients.

TREATMENT OF STASIS DERMATITIS

Initial therapy of stasis dermatitis is aimed at reducing epidermal inflammation and relieving symptoms (eg, pruritus). The most effective first-line treatment is topical steroid therapy. In affected patients, mid-potency steroids (eg, triamcinolone or fluticasone ointment) are usually highly effective (Cheatle et al. 1991b). As in other eczematous dermatoses, ointment vehicles are preferred owing to their ability to aid the repair of the epidermal water barrier. High-potency steroids are rarely required, except in the patient with significant lichenification and epidermal thickening. In fact, overuse of class 1 or 2 steroids may predispose the patient to epidermal ulceration, owing to the risk of atrophy of treated lower extremity skin.

Once the acute inflammation has been controlled with topical steroids, patients must be instructed about the regular use of emollient moisturizers to aid the epidermal water barrier and minimize risks of subsequent exacerbations. Regular over-the-counter emollients are typically effective and well tolerated. In patients with excessive xerosis of the lower extremities, keratolytic moisturizers containing ammonium lactate or salicylic acid may be indicated, although these preparations will cause discomfort on broken or inflamed skin. For patients with frequent flares of stasis dermatitis, overuse of topical steroids and induction of cutaneous atrophy are a concern. The topical calcineurin inhibitors, tacrolimus and pimecrolimus, are both effective at long-term suppression of inflammation without the risk of steroidal adverse effects (Dissemond et al. 2004).

The dyspigmentation of stasis dermatitis is usually permanent although a recent report suggests that the use of noncoherent intense pulsed light may be helpful in reducing pigmentation (Pimentel and Rodriguez-Salido 2008).

A special circumstance in the treatment of patients with stasis dermatitis arises when there is superimposed allergic contact dermatitis. Chronic inflammation of the skin, coupled with the use of multiple topical medications (both prescription and over the counter), frequently results in contact sensitization as a complication of stasis dermatitis. Two of the most frequent contact allergens that complicate stasis dermatitis are the topical antibiotics neomycin and bacitracin (Dooms-Goossens et al. 1979, Morris et al. 2002, Jappe et al. 2003). Preservatives and fragrances contained in over-the-counter moisturizers and antipruritics are also frequent causes of contact allergy. Affected patients may also become sensitized to rubber products found in some wraps and stockings (Gooptu and Powell 1999). Topical corticosteroid allergy from what is considered appropriate therapy, although uncommon, is a condition that can worsen stasis dermatitis and may elude diagnosis (Wilkinson and English 1992, Wilkinson 1994). In a patient with stasis dermatitis who appears not to be responding to standard topical treatments, patch testing should be done to rule out contact allergy. Expanded patch-test series – including fragrances, preservatives, and topical steroids – are strongly recommended.

The mainstay of treatment in stasis dermatitis patients (which typically has been compression therapy) is aimed at decreasing the clinical impact of the underlying venous insufficiency. Assessing the patient's peripheral arterial circulation (clinically or with a Doppler study) before recommending compression therapy is important; adding compression to a leg with compromised arterial circulation could put the patient at risk for ischemic damage. Frequently, peripheral pulses are difficult to assess in patients with venous stasis and leg edema. Vascular surgery consultation is prudent when there is any question of arterial insufficiency.

Compression is generally accomplished using specialized stockings that deliver a controlled gradient of pressure (measured in millimeters of mercury) to the affected leg. More aggressive compression can be achieved with elastic wraps such as Ace or Coban wraps. Medicated compression boots (the Unna boot) are frequently used in patients with ulcerations accompanying stasis dermatitis. More sophisticated devices (eg, end-diastolic compression boots) may be used in patients with severe edema (Dillon 1986). Frequently, leg elevation is a necessary adjunct to leg compression, with patients being counseled to keep the affected leg(s) elevated above the level of the heart, specifically while sleeping and sitting.

Counseling patients about the use of compression therapy is vital to successful management of stasis dermatitis. Patients frequently resist the idea of compression dressings and/or stockings because these modalities can cause considerable discomfort when first applied to edematous, inflamed, lower extremities; many patients consider these devices a major nuisance as well. In fact, almost two-thirds of patients with venous stasis fail to comply with regular use of support stockings (Raju *et al.* 2007). Compression stockings may be difficult to apply because of leg edema and discomfort (especially in patients with lipodermatosclerosis and ulceration). It is important, however, to reassure patients that this discomfort will lessen considerably as the leg edema reduces, and that the therapy must be maintained permanently to prevent recurrence of the dermatitis and leg ulcers. To facilitate their application, compression stockings should be applied early in the morning, before the patient has arisen from the bed, when leg edema is at its lowest. As leg edema improves, stockings with progressively higher compression ratings can be used.

Systemic therapy is not typically indicated in patients with stasis dermatitis. An exception to this is the case of autoeczematization (id reaction), in which severe, acute, localized stasis dermatitis induces a systemic reaction, possibly by upregulation of circulating activated T lymphocytes (Kasteler *et al.* 1992).

Autoeczematization consists clinically of widespread, pruritic, eczematous papules and plaques that can be widely distributed over the trunk and extremities. In these severely symptomatic patients, systemic steroid therapy is usually required to alleviate pruritus. Once the autoeczematization reaction has been controlled, the underlying stasis dermatitis can be managed with topical therapy as described previously. Recent new theories about the pathogenesis of cutaneous inflammation in venous insufficiency have led to the investigation of systemic maintenance therapies, which have been hypothesized as having beneficial effects on neutrophil function.

Other systemic therapies in stasis dermatitis patients are typically aimed at decreasing leg edema with diuretics. Also, because uncontrolled hypertension can lead to diastolic dysfunction (which increases pressures in the venous system), control of hypertension is essential. These treatments are typically managed by the patient's internist or cardiologist.

Pentoxifylline has been studied for the treatment of venous ulcers; it is hypothesized that this medication decreases cytokine-mediated neutrophil activation, leading to reduced inflammation (Pascarella *et al.* 2005). Although the effectiveness of pentoxifylline has not been proven conclusively, it is a well-tolerated and inexpensive therapy that shows benefit in a certain subset of patients with stasis dermatitis. One might speculate that it could be exerting a beneficial effect through its ability to reduce tumor necrosis factor (TNF)-α. This cytokine appears to be involved in the inflammation of chronic wounds such as venous leg ulcers, raising the question of whether anti-TNF-α biological agents might have a role in the treatment of ulcers associated with stasis dermatitis (Cowin *et al.* 2006, Charles *et al.* 2009).

CONCLUSION

Stasis dermatitis is a common source of morbidity in the dermatology patient population. Management of stasis dermatitis and its complications requires multiple short- and long-term treatment modalities as described previously. Patients must be counseled repeatedly about chronic management, especially regarding the use of compression stockings, elevating the lower extremities, and using emollients to prevent exacerbations. Although a cure for venous insufficiency is not possible, patients can remain free of morbidity resulting from stasis dermatitis if they follow a comprehensive treatment plan. This treatment plan includes frequent follow-ups and early application of topical therapy to extinguish inflammatory flare-ups before they have the opportunity to predispose the patient to ulceration and infection. Coordination with other specialists such as internal medicine and vascular surgery can complement dermatological management of patients with stasis dermatitis.

ACKNOWLEDGMENTS

Special thanks to Richard A.F. Clark, MD, for inspiring my clinical and academic interest in this topic.

CHAPTER 18

SEBORRHEIC DERMATITIS

Karen Chernoff, Richie Lin, and Steven R. Cohen

INTRODUCTION

Seborrheic dermatitis is a common inflammatory skin disorder characterized by erythema, scaling, and flaking. It exists in adult, adolescent, and infantile forms, each of which is defined by age of onset, distribution of lesions, degree of chronicity, and, possibly, etiology. The condition is often seen with increased frequency and/or severity in patients with immunodeficiency or neurological diseases (Krfstin 1927, Berger *et al.* 1988, Marino *et al.* 1991).

The cause of seborrheic dermatitis is controversial, especially in the infantile form, but most evidence strongly supports the role of the *Malassezia* species of yeast, sebaceous fatty acids/triglycerides, and individual susceptibility (DeAngelis *et al.* 2005). Infantile seborrheic dermatitis is unique in its lack of chronicity and more frequent generalized involvement, which differs from the adult form. In addition, it has a greater overlap with other skin disorders that affect infants, including atopic dermatitis. Some authors do not consider infantile seborrheic dermatitis a distinct unique disease entity, but, rather, a variant of atopic dermatitis (Vickers 1980, Ruiz-Maldonado *et al.* 1989a), or a distinct syndrome based on similar clinical findings (Moises-Alfaro *et al.* 2002).

The focus of this chapter is on the classification, causes, clinical manifestations, differential diagnosis, histology, treatment, and prognosis of seborrheic dermatitis in both its adult and infantile forms.

DEFINITION AND CLASSIFICATION

The term 'seborrheic dermatitis' implies an inflammatory disorder of the skin secondary to a disorder of the sebaceous glands. And, indeed, the disorder is found in areas of the skin with increased density of sebaceous glands, including the scalp, face, trunk, body folds, and genitalia. However, sebum production is not increased in patients with seborrheic dermatitis. So, a more accurate description of the disease might be *dermatitis of the seborrheic areas* (Eyre *et al.* 1984). In contrast, the term 'seborrhea,' which is often used interchangeably with *seborrheic dermatitis*, actually refers to excessive oiliness of the skin secondary to hyperfunctioning sebaceous glands. The scales that are seen in association with seborrhea are referred to as *scurf*.

Seborrheic dermatitis in adults comprises several subtypes. When the scalp is the only site of involvement, the term 'dandruff' is often treated as a synonym for seborrheic dermatitis (Gupta and Bluhm 2004), although other authors refer to dandruff as any form of scalp flaking regardless of cause (Kligman *et al.* 1976, Priestley and Savin 1976, Piérard-Franchimont *et al.* 2000). Alternatively, dandruff is viewed as a mild form of seborrheic dermatitis without erythema. When truncal involvement is evident, the disorder is subcategorized into the familiar petaloid type and the less common pityriasiform type (Janniger and Schwartz 1995).

Although infantile and adult seborrheic dermatitis are considered the same disease, early childhood and adult/adolescent forms differ in several ways. The course of infantile disease is nearly always self-limited, resolving within a few months. It typically has a more widespread distribution with greater involvement of the groin, and less involvement of the paranasal area. In addition, pruritus is less commonly encountered in infantile seborrheic dermatitis.

The classification of infantile seborrheic dermatitis is complicated by various symptoms and signs that may in fact define separate entities. 'Cradle cap,' for instance, is referred to as *seborrhea capitis*, but some authors consider it a distinct entity from infantile seborrheic dermatitis. Similarly, napkin dermatitis, which is a characteristic finding in infantile seborrheic dermatitis, also occurs independently, secondary to irritants, and frequently secondary to bacterial or candidal infection (Rook *et al.* 1998). Some authors consider napkin dermatitis to be a separate entity, more closely related to psoriasis than to seborrheic dermatitis (Andersen and Thomsen 1971, Neville and Finn 1975). Nevertheless, it is compelling to make the association because napkin dermatitis is so often preceded by infantile seborrheic dermatitis (Ilchyshyn *et al.* 1987).

Some authors have additionally subclassified infantile seborrheic dermatitis by clinical patterns, including psoriasiform, seborrheic, localized napkin dermatitis, and generalized napkin dermatitis. An alternative classification system divides infantile seborrheic dermatitis into true seborrheic dermatitis, psoriasiform seborrheic dermatitis, and erythrodermic seborrheic dermatitis (Menni *et al.* 1989, Janniger 1993). Such differences in subclassification make it difficult to compare the results of diverse studies, eg, one study by Yates *et al.* (1983) looking at the clinical differences between infantile seborrheic dermatitis and infantile atopic dermatitis did not distinguish *napkin psoriasis* from seborrheic dermatitis. In addition, some authors consider infantile seborrheic dermatitis to be a variant of atopic dermatitis (Podmore *et al.* 1986). A consensus on the classification of infantile seborrheic dermatitis is needed.

One final subclassification in infantile seborrheic dermatitis that warrants further examination is erythrodermic infantile seborrheic dermatitis, referred to as *Leiner disease*. True Leiner disease also includes failure to thrive, protracted diarrhea, and associated immune abnormalities, such as C5 deficiency. It has been suggested that severe, erythrodermic, infantile seborrheic dermatitis in the absence of C5 deficiency and diarrhea be classified as *Leiner-like seborrheic dermatitis* (Ruiz-Maldonado *et al.* 1989b).

CLINICAL FEATURES

Adult seborrheic dermatitis typically presents between the ages of 12 and 45 years, with peaks in adolescence and in those over 50 (DHEW 1978, Kligman 1979, Lynch 1982). The onset is usually manifested by flaking (scale) of the scalp (**Fig 18.1**) and/or erythema of the nasolabial folds (**Fig 18.2**). The course is gradual but low humidity and physiological and emotional stress are both recognized exacerbating factors.

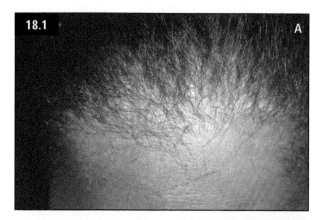

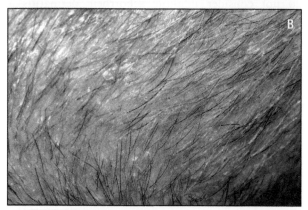

Fig 18.1 (A) Seborrheic dermatitis of the scalp with white scale. (B) Close-up of scalp seborrheic dermatitis showing granular scale.

The lesions of seborrheic dermatitis are orange–red or gray–white macules and papules covered with greasy white scales (**Fig 18.3**). As previously noted, the colloquial designation for scaling of the scalp is *dandruff*. Sites of predilection include hair-bearing skin of the head – namely, the scalp, eyebrows, eyelashes, and beard area (**Fig 18.4**). Equally common sites of predilection are the nasolabial folds, glabella,

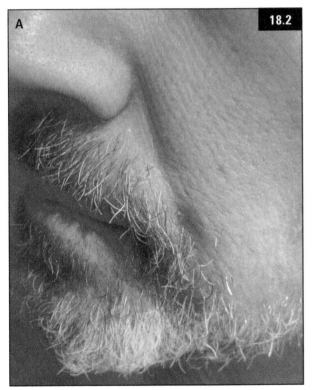

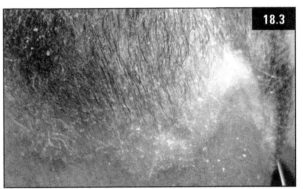

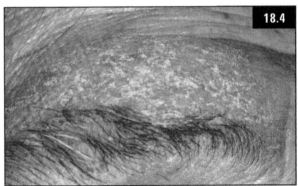

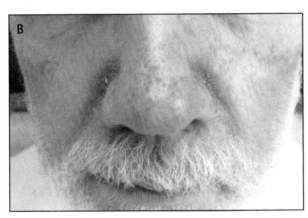

Fig 18.2 (A) Seborrheic dermatitis: subtle erythema and scaling in the nasolabial and melolabial folds. (B) Marked erythema and scaling of the nasolabial and melolabial folds. (Courtesy of Herbert Goodheart, MD.)

Fig 18.3 Seborrheic dermatitis: greasy scaling of the forehead, temples and scalp. (Courtesy of Herbert Goodheart, MD.)

Fig 18.4 Seborrheic dermatitis with scaling of the eyebrows.

forehead, conch of the ear, and pre- and postauricular areas (**Figs 18.5** and **18.6**). When the external ear is involved, crusts and fissures are common and secondary infection may occur (**Fig 18.7**). In individuals with darker complexions seborrheic dermatitis can cause areas of hypopigmentation (**Fig 18.8**). Annular lesions may occur on the face and suggest dermatophyte infection or secondary syphilis (**Fig 18.9**). Truncal disease may be either petaloid or pityriasiform, appearing as yellow–brown patches over the sternum with less frequent involvement of the axillae, groin, umbilicus, and inframammary skin (**Figs 18.10** and **18.11**). Diffuse, brightly erythematous, sharply marginated plaques can mimic psoriasis. Erosions and fissuring are common when the body folds are involved. Rarely, yellow crusts and psoriasiform lesions may occur on the external genitalia.

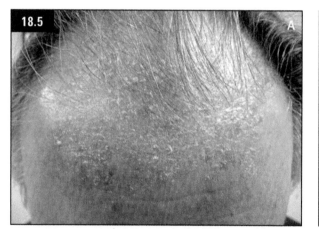
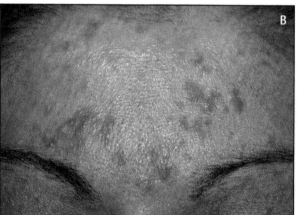

Fig 18.5 (A) Scaling of the forehead and scalp in a patient with seborrheic dermatitis. (Courtesy of Herbert Goodheart, MD.) (B) Petaloid erythematous scaly macules on the forehead.

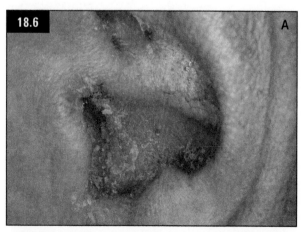
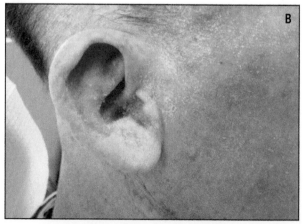

Fig 18.6 (A) Scaling of the conch of the ears. (B) Scaling of the external ear and preauricular area. (Courtesy of Herbert Goodheart, MD.)

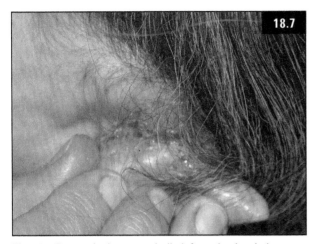

Fig 18.7 Postauricular secondarily infected seborrheic dermatitis with erosion.

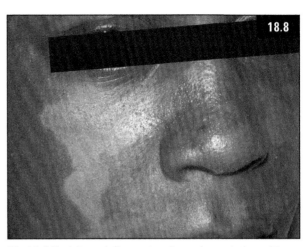

Fig 18.8 Facial postinflammatory hypopigmentation with seborrheic dermatitis in an African–American teenager.

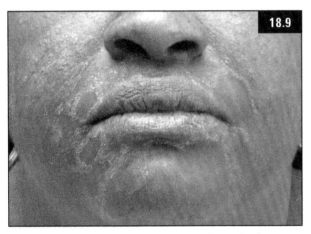

Fig 18.9 Seborrheic dermatitis with annular scaly plaques that might be confused with secondary syphilis or dermatophyte infection. (Courtesy of UConn Dermatology Residency Collection c/o Dr Justin Finch.)

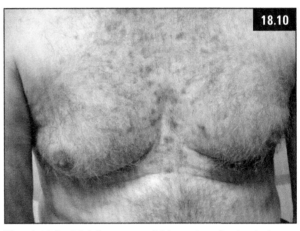

Fig 18.10 Reddish-brown *petaloid* papules of seborrheic dermatitis in the presternal area. (Courtesy of Herbert Goodheart, MD.)

Fig 18.11 Seborrheic dermatitis of the umbilicus. (Courtesy of Herbert Goodheart, MD.)

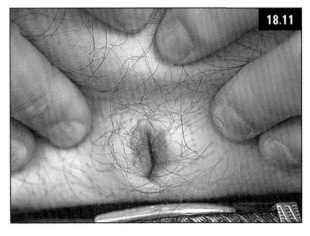

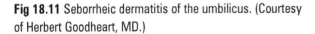

Infantile seborrheic dermatitis generally starts in the first few weeks of life and lasts 3–4 months if left untreated (Ruiz-Maldonado *et al.* 1989b). The mean age of onset in one study was 4.9 weeks with a range of 3–23 weeks (Yates *et al.* 1983). It usually appears first in the diaper area, although lesions may arise initially on the face and scalp. Simultaneous onset may occur in both the diaper area and the area of the face and scalp. In contrast to the adult disease, infantile seborrheic dermatitis is characteristically asymptomatic. As infants lack the ability to scratch until 6–8 weeks of life, a tranquil disposition in the setting of active dermatitis has led most observers to exclude pruritus as a clinical feature.

The eruption of infantile seborrheic dermatitis comprises thick greasy scales that vary in the scalp from white to yellow. 'Cradle cap' is defined by prominent scaling over the vertex, possibly resulting from the hesitancy of new parents to wash the fontanelle (Ruiz-Maldonado *et al.* 1989b). More diffuse fine scaling may be seen on the scalp, as well as the central face, forehead, and ears (see **Fig 3.46**). When scales are large and dry, the term 'psoriasiform seborrheic dermatitis' is sometimes used. The underlying skin may be mildly erythematous, but hair loss is unusual, minimal, and temporary, occurring after removal of scale when it does occur (Schachner and Hansen 1988, Caputo and Gelmetti 2002).

The distribution of infantile seborrheic dermatitis also includes the parietal scalp, central face, neck folds, and mid-chest. Axillary, inguinal, and intergluteal fold involvement may be discrete or coalescent with greasy, glazed, sharply circumscribed erythematous or salmon-colored plaques. When the diaper area is affected, the genitalia and anus are almost always involved, but it may spread peripherally to the inguinal flexures (Keipert 1990). Microvesicles may be present. Truncal involvement in the infant is initially patchy but may become confluent with time. In some instances seborrheic involvement simulates guttate psoriasis (Yates *et al.* 1983).

Seborrheic dermatitis in adults is often associated with other dermatological disorders such as rosacea, and ocular irritation may occur as a result of blepharitis from either seborrheic dermatitis or rosacea (McCulley and Dougherty 1985, Zug *et al.* 1996, Gupta 2001). Blepharitis may be accompanied by meibomian gland occlusion and abscess formation. An association of seborrheic dermatitis with acne vulgaris was previously considered evidence of the now disproven theory that seborrheic dermatitis resulted from increased sebaceous-gland secretions, as seen in acne. Finally, diseases associated with *Malassezia* spp. are commonly found in patients with seborrheic dermatitis, including pityriasis versicolor and pityrosporum folliculitis (Faergemann *et al.* 1986).

In infants, seborrheic dermatitis is sometimes associated with atopic dermatitis and psoriasis, although generally not concurrently. In a study of 191 children with infantile seborrheic dermatitis, 7 of 88 available for follow-up approximately 10 years later went on to develop adult/adolescent-type seborrheic dermatitis, 5 had atopic dermatitis, and 1 had psoriasis. In two other studies, 19% and 27.5% of the patients with infantile seborrheic dermatitis were found to have developed atopic dermatitis 12 and 13 years later, respectively. However, this may be due to misdiagnosis of the initial condition rather than infantile seborrheic dermatitis being an actual precursor to the development of atopic dermatitis (Neville and Finn 1975, Kligman 1979). In addition, 20 of 88 children with infantile seborrheic dermatitis were found to have a sibling who was later diagnosed with the condition (Mimouni *et al.* 1995).

Both infantile and adult seborrheic dermatitis can also be associated with non-dermatological disorders. In adults, seborrheic dermatitis is highly associated with HIV infection and AIDS. Although the prevalence of seborrheic dermatitis in the general population is close to 3%, in patients with HIV and AIDS, that figure rises to between 34% and 83%. In fact, seborrheic dermatitis, which is rarely seen in Mali, has been used as a predictor of HIV infection in that country (Mahé *et al.* 1994, 1996). Not only is seborrheic dermatitis more common in patients with HIV infection but it is also frequently more severe and extensive (Eisenstat and Wormser 1984, Mathes and Douglass 1985), with more frequent involvement of the extremities (Soeprono *et al.* 1986). The number of lesions, and severity and extent of involvement, increase with progression to advanced acquired immune deficiency syndrome (AIDS) (Matis et al. 1987, Alessi et al. 1988). At least one study found a relationship between CD4 T-cell counts and the severity of seborrheic dermatitis (Kaplan et al. 1987); however, some studies have shown no relationship between the severity of seborrheic dermatitis and that of HIV infection (Senaldi et al. 1987, Vidal et al. 1990).

Seborrheic dermatitis is also associated with neurological conditions, most notably Parkinson disease (Krfstin 1927). In such patients, involvement of seborrheic dermatitis is more often bilateral (Burton et al. 1973a), and patients often demonstrate increased sebum levels, thought to result from facial immobility (Burton et al. 1973a, Cowley et al. 1990). Interestingly, unilateral facial paralysis, due to facial nerve palsy or stroke, is associated with an increased rate of seborrheic dermatitis, usually on the paralyzed side (Burton et al. 1971, Faergemann 1999). An increased incidence of seborrheic dermatitis also occurs in some patients with psychiatric disorders. One study reported that 38 of 150 (25.3%) patients with psychiatric illness had seborrheic dermatitis compared with only 13 of 150 (9%) control patients without significant psychiatric disease (Maietta et al. 1990).

Other conditions linked to seborrheic dermatitis but studied less extensively include alcohol-induced chronic pancreatitis (Barba et al. 1982), hepatitis C infection (Cribier et al. 1998), malignancy (Clift et al. 1988), and genetic disorders such as Down syndrome (Ercis et al. 1996) and cardiofaciocutaneous syndrome (Gross-Tsur et al. 1990), among others. One study showed that 30.9% of children with Down syndrome had seborrheic dermatitis.

In the infant, seborrheic dermatitis has been associated with Leiner disease but this is extremely rare. Mortality in this rare condition is associated with bacterial superinfection. Evaluation for immunodeficiencies has been recommended in infants with generalized seborrheic dermatitis, diarrhea, and failure to thrive (Jacobs and Miller 1972, Sonea et al. 1987).

DIFFERENTIAL DIAGNOSIS

The differential diagnosis of seborrheic dermatitis in adults and infants centers on conditions that cause erythema and scaling. In adults, scalp psoriasis can be nearly indistinguishable from seborrheic dermatitis. However, psoriatic plaques are often more sharply demarcated, and in psoriasis other signs, such as nail pitting, onycholysis, or psoriatic lesions in other areas, are usually present (Janniger et al. 2005). An erythematous scaly dermatitis that may be confused with seborrheic dermatitis may occur on the scalp of patients with dermatomyositis (Kasteler and Callen 1994). Nonscarring alopecia may occur in 30–40% of these patients, a feature not characteristic of seborrheic dermatitis (Tilstra et al. 2009).

Seborrheic dermatitis may also be confused with dermatophytosis (tinea capitis, tinea facialis, and tinea corporis), pityriasis versicolor, and intertriginous candida infection. Potassium hydroxide examination will help distinguish these conditions. Clinicians should also maintain index of suspicion for streptococcal intertrigo characterized by intense, fiery-red erythema and maceration in the intertriginous folds of the neck, axillae, or inguinal spaces, often with a distinctive foul odor (Honig et al. 2003).

Facial seborrheic dermatitis may also be confused with the butterfly rash of lupus erythematosus, subacute lupus, and rosacea. It may coexist with the latter condition. These eruptions do not have the greasy scale of seborrheic dermatitis and may have nasolabial sparing. Rosacea usually has central facial erythema and telangiectasia and often erythematous papules. In some patients with rosacea, the forehead may be the only site of involvement (Schwartz et al. 2006). Other less common disorders that could be confused with seborrheic dermatitis include 'seborrheic' papules in secondary syphilis, cutaneous lymphoma, and glucagonoma syndrome.

Atopic dermatitis is unlikely to be confused with seborrheic dermatitis in the adult; however, these two conditions may be difficult to distinguish in infancy. Atopic dermatitis in the infant may appear on the scalp, face, diaper areas, or extensor surfaces, mimicking seborrheic dermatitis (Turner and Schwartz 2006).

As mentioned previously, some authors view infantile seborrheic dermatitis as a variant of atopic dermatitis (Vickers 1980). The two conditions have a striking difference in prognosis and an attempt should be made to differentiate them. Infantile seborrheic dermatitis usually resolves in a few months without treatment, whereas atopic dermatitis is often chronic and can be associated with the subsequent development of asthma in a significant number of children.

Skin lesions of infantile seborrheic dermatitis are usually not itchy and lack the oozing and weeping often seen in atopic dermatitis (Schwartz et al. 2006). However, a study by Yates et al. (1983) found that pruritus or its absence is not a reliable diagnostic feature. Although 90% of atopic infants experienced pruritus, approximately a third of infants with infantile seborrheic dermatitis also had pruritus (Yates et al. 1983). In terms of distribution, scalp and cheek involvement occur in both infantile seborrheic dermatitis and atopic dermatitis. By comparison, axillary involvement suggests infantile seborrheic dermatitis; eczema on the shins favors a diagnosis of atopic dermatitis. Owing to clinical similarities, it is often necessary to follow the natural course of the disease in order to make a definitive diagnosis.

Certain laboratory parameters may also be helpful in differentiating the two conditions. Radioallergosorbent testing (RAST) for specific IgE antibodies against egg white or cows' milk has been investigated. In one study, 80% of atopic infants had positive RAST results, whereas only 15% of infants with infantile seborrheic dermatitis had positive ones (Yates et al. 1983). Total IgE levels were also found to be elevated in infants with atopic dermatitis, compared with infantile seborrheic dermatitis. Total eosinophil count and specific IgE levels to antigens including dust mite, pollen, and cat dander showed no difference between infantile seborrheic dermatitis and atopic dermatitis. In a study by Podmore et al. (1986), T-cell counts could not be used to distinguish infantile seborrheic dermatitis from atopic dermatitis. Surprisingly, IgE antibodies to *Malassezia* spp., a purported causative factor of seborrheic dermatitis, were found in greater percentages among patients with atopic dermatitis than those with seborrheic dermatitis (35% vs 12%) (Mayser and Gross 2000). However, this study did not focus on infants and, as such, the implications for infantile seborrheic dermatitis are unclear.

A rare but serious disorder which presents with skin lesions that can be confused with those of infantile seborrheic dermatitis is Langerhans cell histiocytosis, previously called *histiocytosis X*. Infants present with erythematous scaly papules on the scalp, posterior auricular areas, axillae, groin, and perineal areas. Vesicles, crusted papules, and purpuric papules may be seen. Infants with Langerhans cell histiocytosis also present with systemic signs, including fever, anemia, thrombocytopenia, hepatosplenomegaly, and lymphadenopathy.

Wiskott–Aldrich syndrome and other congenital immune deficiency syndromes may also present with a generalized eczematous reaction mimicking severe infantile seborrheic dermatitis.

Finally, nutritional deficiencies can mimic infantile seborrheic dermatitis. Acrodermatitis enteropathica, a rare disorder of zinc deficiency, can cause skin lesions that may be confused with generalized infantile seborrheic dermatitis. It classically presents with periorificial blistering erythema and erosions with acral erythema and scaling (Caputo and Gelmetti 2002). If the disease is chronic, involvement of the body folds may also occur. Acrodermatitis enteropathica may result from a congenital defect in zinc absorption or insufficient intake in breastfed babies. In addition, riboflavin, biotin, and pyridoxine deficiencies have been associated with seborrheic dermatitis-like lesions in the infant (Brenner and Horwitz 1988).

HISTOPATHOLOGY

It is rarely necessary to biopsy patients with obvious seborrheic dermatitis, especially infants. In adults and infants who do not respond to treatment or where a more serious disorder is suspected, skin biopsy may be indicated. Histologically, seborrheic dermatitis may be difficult to differentiate from psoriasis and overlap of features is common (see below) (Barr and Young 1985). Histopathology demonstrates regular or irregular acanthosis, variable focal spongiosis with exocytosis of mononuclear cells, and occasional neutrophils. The last also may involve the follicular infundibula. Parakeratosis, the persistence of nuclei in the stratum corneum, and Munro microabscesses are predominantly at the margins of the follicular ostia (*shoulder parakeratosis*) and examination of scale crust reveals collections of plasma and neutrophils (Barr and Young 1985, Caputo and Gelmetti 2002). Parakeratosis is reported to be more prominent in seborrheic dermatitis associated with HIV infection or AIDS (Schwartz *et al.* 2006). There is a sparse perivascular lymphohistiocytic infiltrate with few neutrophils present in the dermis.

Direct immunofluorescence in infantile seborrheic dermatitis reveals no significant deposition of IgG, IgM, IgE, IgA, C1q, C3, properdin, or fibrinogen, either at the dermoepidermal junction or around blood vessels. However, helper T cells have been found in a perivascular location with a few scattered helper T cells in the epidermis.

Despite some overlap of features, biopsy can be useful for distinguishing seborrheic dermatitis from psoriasis. Psoriasis lesions demonstrate neutrophils in the horny layer (so-called *neuts in the horn*), thinning of the suprapapillary plates, and tortuous capillaries in the dermal papillae – findings not generally seen in seborrheic dermatitis. In contrast, spongiosis is more commonly seen in seborrheic dermatitis, which also has a lesser degree of psoriasiform hyperplasia (Caputo and Gelmetti 2002). Of note, however, chronic seborrheic dermatitis lesions become less spongiotic and closer in appearance to psoriasis with follicular plugs of orthokeratotic and parakeratotic cells and uneven rete ridges (Ackerman 1977). Nevertheless, a biopsy can be a useful adjunct in clinically indistinct cases of seborrheic dermatitis.

CAUSES

The cause of seborrheic dermatitis is unknown but probably involves malassezia yeasts, sebaceous triglycerides and fatty acids, and individual susceptibility. Much of the recent work has focused on the role of sebum and fatty acids in seborrheic dermatitis, as the distribution of lesions closely reflects the distribution of the sebaceous glands (Gupta and Bluhm 2004). Some studies have revealed the rate of sebum production in seborrheic dermatitis to be normal when compared with control individuals (Burton and Pye 1983). Current opinion favors seborrhea as a predisposing factor to seborrheic dermatitis but not a direct causal agent.

The chemical make-up of sebum with regard to triglycerides and fatty acids, rather than the rate of sebum production itself, is thought to play an important role in the development of seborrheic dermatitis. An altered pattern of fatty acids has been suggested as a cause of infantile seborrheic dermatitis and the adult/adolescent form. Serum fatty acid levels were found to be altered in children with infantile seborrheic dermatitis, consistent with a transient decrease in function of the δ6-desaturase enzyme (Tollesson *et al.* 1993). Infants with seborrheic dermatitis were found to have increased levels of fatty acid ($20{:}2\omega6$), an elongation product of linoleic acid ($18{:}2\omega6$,) and an absence of γ-linolenic acid ($18{:}3\omega6$), the normal product of linoleic acid desaturation.

Linoleic acid, γ-linolenic acid, and arachidonic acid ($20{:}4\omega6$) are considered essential for maintaining a normal epidermal barrier in the skin. A deficiency of the enzyme δ6-desaturase would explain the abnormalities found. The enzymes involved in fatty acid metabolism are thought to be immature in infants, and by 6–11 months of age, when the abnormalities of fatty acid metabolism normalize, clinical recovery occurs (Tollesson *et al.* 1993). Such normalization of fatty acid levels parallels clinical recovery of infantile seborrheic dermatitis at any age in which it occurs. This may explain why infantile seborrheic dermatitis will resolve spontaneously in time, even without treatment. In addition, clinical improvement was noted when topical borage oil, which is a natural source of γ-linolenic acid, was administered (Tollesson and Frithz 1993). The studies of fatty acid metabolism in adults have been less convincing although some reports do show abnormal composition of fatty acids and triglycerides in adult patients with seborrheic dermatitis (Passi *et al.* 1991, Ostlere *et al.* 1996).

Malassezia furfur, or its yeast form *Pityrosporum ovale*, has long been thought to be a causative factor in seborrheic dermatitis (Moore and Kile 1935). In 1996, the malassezia taxonomy was revised, and the species implicated in seborrheic dermatitis are still being defined. Species with the most evidence supporting a link to seborrheic dermatitis are *M. globosa* and *M. restricta* (Dawson 2007, Tajima *et al.* 2008, Prohic 2010). However, other species including *M. furfur, M. sympodialis, M. obtusa*, and *M. slooffiae* were found in one study to be increased in patients with seborrheic dermatitis (Nakabayashi *et al.* 2000). All species of malassezia yeasts implicated in seborrheic dermatitis require lipids for survival. These are most commonly found in sebum-rich areas and thus parallel the distribution of seborrheic dermatitis (Gupta *et al.* 2004a). A number of studies have shown improvement in seborrheic dermatitis with various antifungal agents, including azoles and zinc (Shuster 1984). The relationship between the level of malassezia yeasts and seborrheic dermatitis remains uncertain. Some studies report higher counts in patients with seborrheic dermatitis (Lynch 1982), whereas others find no difference (Gupta *et al.* 2004b).

There is also debate about levels of malassezia yeasts in lesional versus nonlesional skin. One study found increased numbers of yeast in patients with dandruff or seborrheic dermatitis (McGinley *et al.* 1975); other studies did not confirm this association (Bergbrant and Faergemann 1989). Although the role of malassezia levels remains unclear, clinical improvement is associated with a reduction of *Malassezia* spp. on the scalp in adults (Pierard *et al.* 1997). Infantile seborrheic dermatitis is not associated with a significant change in colonization rates after clearing or 1 year later (Tollesson *et al.* 1997). Infants in this study did have abnormal patterns of essential

fatty acids, suggesting that the cause of seborrheic dermatitis in infants might be more heavily dependent on fatty acid metabolism than *Malassezia* spp.

The manner in which malassezia yeasts are involved in initiating the erythema and scaling of seborrheic dermatitis has not yet been fully elucidated. However, the yeasts have been found to alter fatty acid metabolism in patients with seborrheic dermatitis. A study focusing on *M. restricta* and *M. globosa* demonstrated that these organisms degrade sebum, release free fatty acids from triglycerides, and consume specific saturated fatty acids, leaving behind the unsaturated compounds (Ro and Dawson 2005). The authors consider that altered composition of sebaceous secretions causes inflammation, irritation, and flaking of the scalp. In another study a gene *LIP1* which encodes lipase was identified in *M. globosa*; the isolated lipase is thought to break down sebaceous lipids and release irritating free fatty acids (DeAngelis *et al.* 2007). The effect of *Malassezia* spp. on fatty acid metabolism links the two leading causative factors in the development of seborrheic dermatitis.

Recently, *M. furfur* strains from patients with seborrheic dermatitis have been shown to selectively produce aryl hydrocarbon receptor (AhR) ligands, the indoles malassezin, and indolo[3,2-b]carbazole (ICZ) which may be involved in triggering seborrheic dermatitis (Gaitanis *et al.* 2008).

What has not been shown is why some individuals react to the presence of malassezia yeasts or altered fatty acid composition by developing seborrheic dermatitis, whereas others remain asymptomatic. One theory is that immune dysfunction or individual susceptibility plays a role. The dramatically elevated prevalence of seborrheic dermatitis in HIV-infected patients and patients with other immunodeficiencies, including congenital defects, supports this hypothesis. Some authors also cite the tendency of patients to relapse after treatment of seborrheic dermatitis to support an immune defect (Valia 2006). Specifically, it has been reported that patients with seborrheic dermatitis have depressed T-cell function and increased prevalence of natural killer cells (Bergbrant *et al.* 1991). It also has been proposed that impaired cell-mediated immunity may facilitate fungal survival in the skin (Guého *et al.* 1994). Prohic (2010) demonstrated low helper/suppressor ratios in 70% of patients, because of an increase in the suppressor T-cell population, suggesting impaired cellular immunity.

Increased levels of total serum IgA and IgG also have been associated with seborrheic dermatitis in some studies but others have shown that elevation in IgG is not related or specific to *Malassezia* spp., and that patients with seborrheic dermatitis do not have elevated IgG antibody titers against yeasts (Bergbrant *et al.* 1991). It is interesting that IgE antibodies against *Malassezia* spp. are found in greater percentages among patients with atopic dermatitis compared with patients with seborrheic dermatitis (35% vs 12%) (Mayser and Gross 2000). It has been postulated that seborrheic dermatitis is caused by an abnormal cutaneous reaction to yeasts, but not mediated directly by antibodies. The most plausible explanation involving the cause of seborrheic dermatitis is multifactorial, involving fatty acid metabolism, malassezia yeasts, and individual susceptibility mediated via the immune system. The role each factor plays likely differs between the infantile and adult forms of seborrheic dermatitis and even from individual to individual.

Of note, recent work has demonstrated that a particular set of surface markers of inflammatory and differentiation-related processes, including interleukin (IL)-1α, interleukin 1 receptor (IL-1R)A, IL-8, keratin K1/K10, involucrin, human serum albumin, total protein, histamine, and stratum corneum lipids, reflect pathological changes in the skin of patients with seborrheic dermatitis/dandruff (Kerr *et al.* 2011). Examination of gene expression in the skin of patients with dandruff shows diminished expression of genes involved in lipid metabolism and increased expression of genes involved in inflammation that is corrected with zinc pyrithione treatment (Mills *et al.* 2012).

TREATMENT

The complex etiology of seborrheic dermatitis accounts for the profusion of therapies currently available. Nonspecific keratolytics are the most commonly used agents followed by topical corticosteroids and anti-inflammatory and antifungal medications. As seborrheic dermatitis is likely caused in part by *Malassezia* spp., sebaceous triglycerides, and individual susceptibility, an antifungal agent should be used (DeAngelis *et al.* 2005). Once considered a first-line therapy, topical corticosteroids have been eclipsed by the use of antimycotic agents (Ford *et al.* 1984). However, some antifungal agents may actually exacerbate seborrheic dermatitis (Peter and Richarz-Barthauer 1995). For infantile seborrheic dermatitis, it is essential to reassure parents of the benign disease course, excellent prognosis, and tendency to clear spontaneously and completely.

General skin care is important, especially in infantile seborrheic dermatitis. Irritating substances and alkaline soaps should be avoided. Overaggressive therapies often produce an eczematous reaction with weeping, crusting, and pruritus. Oatmeal baths, once or twice a day, may be soothing. Loose-fitting clothing is recommended to prevent excessive perspiration when there is involvement beyond the scalp and face.

Many of the older treatment modalities for seborrheic dermatitis involve nonspecific keratolytic agents available without prescription (Gupta *et al.* 2004b). These include selenium sulfide and other sulfur preparations that interact with keratinocytes and result in formation of hydrogen sulfide. Whole coal tar and crude coal tar extract are effective remedies for seborrheic dermatitis, perhaps as effective as selenium sulfide (Garcia *et al.* 1978, Olansky 1980, Fredriksson 1985). Salicylic acid shampoo is useful for removing scale and crust but should be avoided in infants because of irritation and systemic toxicity.

Topical corticosteroids remain a popular therapy for seborrheic dermatitis. Adults with seborrheic dermatitis can use topical steroids once or twice daily, often in addition to a medicated shampoo. For infants, low-potency topical steroids may be used carefully. Removal of scales with mineral oil or shampoo improves the efficacy of topical steroids, but, again, care must be taken to avoid excessive washing and skin irritation. Occasional corticosteroid allergy may complicate seborrheic dermatitis. Patch testing to corticosteroid agents should be explored in those with treatment-resistant dermatitis (Ljubojevic et al. 2010). Recently a moisturizer containing licochalcone, an extract from Glycyrrheiza inflata with anti-inflammatory and antimicrobial effects, was compared with hydrocortisone 1% in the treatment of infantile atopic dermatitis (Wananukul et al. 2011). It showed greater efficacy in the first 3–4 days but was equivalent in effect after 1 week.

A major concern with the use of topical corticosteroids, especially high-potency, is the risk of skin atrophy, telangiectasia, striae distensae, and even adrenal suppression when applying to large areas. Topical calcineurin inhibitors, which also have anti-inflammatory properties, have gained favor in recent years, especially for the face and body folds. The two agents currently available, tacrolimus ointment and pimecrolimus cream, do not cause atrophy of the skin (Meshkinpour et al. 2003, Rigopoulos et al. 2004). One week of daily use is necessary before improvement is seen.

A wide variety of antifungal agents has been used to treat seborrheic dermatitis. Zinc pyrithione has both nonspecific keratolytic and antifungal activity. It is available in a 2% shampoo, 1% shampoo, and a cream formulation (Opdyke et al. 1967, Marks et al. 1985). It also has been combined with crude coal tar extract in a shampoo to improve efficacy (Veien et al. 1980). Clinical trials show zinc to be as effective as selenium sulfide in treating seborrheic dermatitis of the scalp (Fredriksson 1985). Zinc pyrithione shampoo has been shown to deliver therapeutic levels of the active agent not only to the skin surface but also to malassezia yeasts in the follicular infundibulum (Schwartz et al. 2011).

The 'azole' antifungals are effective for seborrheic dermatitis. Some azoles, including ketoconazole, itraconazole, and bifonazole, also possess anti-inflammatory activity. Although many formulations are available, ketoconazole 2% shampoo is the most widely used product for scalp disease. Ketoconazole 2% cream is as effective as hydrocortisone 1% cream used once daily for seborrheic dermatitis of the face, scalp, and body (Stratigos et al. 1988). However, ketoconazole shampoo appears more effective than cream for the scalp (Carr et al. 1987). The shampoo formulation also has a prophylactic effect when used once weekly (Peter and Richarz-Barthauer 1995).

Other antifungal agents that have been used to treat seborrheic dermatitis include ciclopirox olamine, a broad-spectrum antifungal agent with effectiveness against Malassezia spp., with an additional anti-inflammatory effect. It is available as a shampoo, cream, or gel. The gel formulation contains ciclopirox as a free acid instead of the olamine salt, and may be the most effective vehicle in treating lesions in the scalp (Aly et al. 2003). Terbinafine, another antifungal agent, has also proven to be an effective treatment for seborrheic dermatitis (Cassano et al. 2002).

Although 'off-label,' oral antifungal therapy has been advocated for patients with widespread seborrheic dermatitis. Ketoconazole 200 mg daily for 4 weeks (Ford et al. 1984), itraconazole 200 mg daily for 7 days (Shemer et al, 2008), and terbinafine 250 mg daily for 4 weeks (Scaparro et al. 2001) have all dramatically improved clinical signs of seborrheic dermatitis. Patients taking these drugs must be monitored for hepatotoxicity.

Seborrheic dermatitis associated with neurological disease often improves when the underlying disorder is treated successfully. Unlike other patients with seborrheic dermatitis, those with Parkinson disease often have increased sebum production that decreases with L-dopa therapy. It is believed that L-dopa restores depleted melanocyte-stimulating hormone (MSH)-inhibiting factor in patients with Parkinson disease, which results in decreased sebum production. Patients with lithium-responsive mood disorders report improved seborrheic dermatitis (Christodoulou and Vareltzides 1978, Sandyk and Kay 1990), although this claim has been disputed (Christodoulou et al. 1983).

CONCLUSION

Seborrheic dermatitis is a complex skin disorder that has eluded clear understanding. The relationships between varying causative factors and between the adult and infantile forms remain imprecise. It appears that infantile seborrheic dermatitis is most closely related to abnormalities in fatty acid metabolism, and has an excellent prognosis. The adult form appears to result from an interplay of fatty acid metabolism, *Malassezia* spp., and individual susceptibility factors, including variations in the immune response. Ongoing research is needed to advance our understanding of seborrheic dermatitis.

CHAPTER 19

THE HISTOPATHOLOGY OF ECZEMA

Cynthia M. Magro, A. Neil Crowson, Molly E. Dyrsen, and Martin C. Mihm Jr

INTRODUCTION

The word 'eczema' derives its meaning from the Greek 'boiling over'. The term was adopted in earlier times from the blistering that occurs in acute hypersensitivity reactions. Use of the word *eczema* has been greatly criticized for its imprecision and a lack of understanding of the full breadth of the concept. Indiscriminate use of the term by clinicians to describe a variety of diseases that are similar to eczema (eg, pityriasis rubra pilaris, inflammatory pityriasis rosea, and small plaque parapsoriasis) has clouded a precise definition of the term.

It is appropriate, therefore, to review the origin of the term, the spectrum of the disorder, and its application to clinical disease in order to understand the histomorphological spectrum of conditions that fall under the designation of eczema. The term 'eczema,' or 'eczematous dermatitis,' is not specific and is applied variably to intrinsic (ie, atopic) dermatitis, to contact reactions (including those centered on the eccrine apparatus such as dyshidrotic eczema, alternatively named *pompholyx* and *miliaria*), to asteatotic eczema (winter itch or eczema craquelé), and to an array of hypersensitivity dermatitides that manifest an eczematous component clinically and histomorphologically.

The focus of this chapter, ostensibly, is histomorphology. However, we also consider the pathophysiology and give an abbreviated synopsis of the salient clinical features of eczema.

The histomorphological spectrum of eczema is best considered in the context of the clinical phases of allergic contact dermatitis. The presentation of acute contact dermatitis is that of a blistering lesion which is usually erythematous and always pruritic, and exhibits prominent vesicles. If the contactant antigen persists, the lesion becomes more erythematous, and patch- to plaque-like with smaller vesicles. As the plaque persists and enters the subacute phase, the lesion crusts and becomes a weeping, chapped, and highly pruritic area. Persistence of the antigen, sometimes by remaining in the epidermal layers of the skin for a protracted time or by being persistently introduced from an external source (eg, chromates in shoe dermatitis), results in the appearance of a more sharply demarcated plaque. The lesion is dusky red, scaly, and pruritic with no vesiculation. This progression describes the appearance of the lichenified plaque stage.

Unfortunately, as the classification schemes for dermatitis are historically and not pathogenically based, the term 'eczema' can be applied to conditions that are due to both intrinsic and extrinsic factors. Thus, each form or cause of dermatitis may have its own specific clinical presentation.

Other appellations such as *nummular* (or *discoid*) *eczema* are a reflection of specific clinical features as opposed to cause. With respect to nummular eczema, the lesions are, as one would expect, coin-shaped and show central clearing of scaling. This form of dermatitis is seen in females and males in the fifth to sixth decades of life as well as in young females in the second and third decades, and reflects a variety of provoking factors. Nummular eczema begins as a vesicular plaque but can progress to a chronic plaque of dermatitis showing variable fibrosis, depending on how often and for how long the patient has rubbed the lesions. Nummular eczema may, however, also be a manifestation of an atopic diathesis (Karvonen 2001).

In some disorders, the presentation, for example, of a bullous disorder, such as bullous pemphigoid, is preceded by what clinically appears as vesicular eczema. The bullous dermatoses are differentiated by the presence of eosinophils at the dermoepidermal junction, as well as by direct and indirect immunofluorescence techniques that aid in diagnosis (Razzaque Ahmed 1984).

Frequent in cold, dry climates, *asteatotic eczema* is considered to be a multifactorial disorder related to reduced sebum production and changes in keratinization and lipid content. It typically affects older people, who manifest dry, scaly areas of acral parts, sometimes in a crisscross pattern. Some patients with a generalized form of asteatotic eczema have an underlying malignancy. Others, particularly males in the fourth to seventh decades, manifest a widespread itchy eruption of erythematous, sometimes oozing, papules and plaques, which may manifest as discoid or lichenified lesions with or without an urticarial phase, in concert with persistent lesions of the penis and scrotum, defining the so-called *Sulzberger–Garbe syndrome* (Goepel 1959).

The id reaction case is a form of sensitization in which distant lesions occur, cognate to a primary infective site in the case of certain forms of viral, fungal, or bacterial infection, or to a primary hypersensitivity site in the case of prior contact sensitization. Various provocative or causal factors, when known, give specific pathophysiological import to the designations, eg, a *tuberculid* is an inflammatory process at a distant, sterile site, which is cognate to a primary infection of the gut or lung by *Mycobacterium* spp. (Choudhri *et al.* 1994). A *fungid* will reflect an inflammatory response distant to a site of a deep, or more commonly a superficial, fungal infection such as a dermatophytosis. Finally, a *bacterid* is characterized by an inflammatory process at a sterile site distant from a bacterial infection, usually arising in oropharyngeal, respiratory, gastrointestinal, or cutaneous sites, which could be designated infectious id panniculitis when involving subcutaneous fat (Magro *et al.* 2008).

GENERAL OVERVIEW OF THE HISTOMORPHOLOGY

Lesions of dermatitis go through defined stages. Acute dermatitis manifests extensive spongiosis with migration of acute and chronic inflammatory cells into the epidermis from the superficial vascular plexus, unaccompanied by significant thickening or acanthosis of the epidermis (**Figs 19.1–19.3**). Subacute dermatitis manifests a more conspicuous acanthosis of the epidermis with a shift from a neutrophil-predominant infiltrate to one rich in lymphocytes and/or eosinophils (**Fig 19.4**).

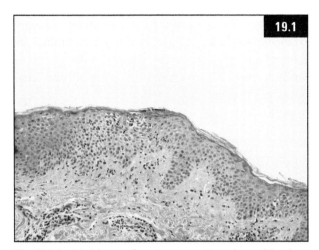

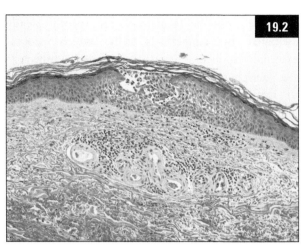

Fig 19.1 In this biopsy of acute eczematous dermatitis, the epidermis is of normal thickness. There is spongiosis with exocytosis of lymphocytes into the epidermis. Incipient Langerhans cell-rich vesicles are present in the superficial layers of the epidermis.

Fig 19.2 In this biopsy of acute eczematous dermatitis, the epidermis is unaltered in thickness. There are Langerhans cell-rich microabscesses present within the epidermis. The superficial dermis shows a glomeruloid congery of vessels reflecting the location of this biopsy from the lower extremity.

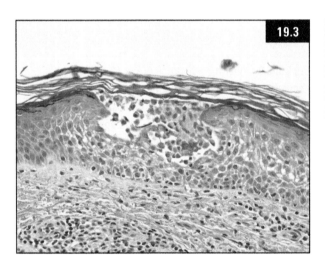

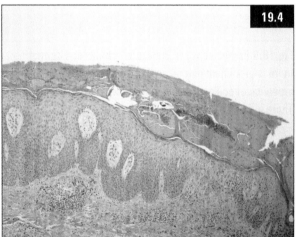

Fig 19.3 In this case of acute eczematous dermatitis, there is a distinct intraepidermal vesicle composed almost exclusively of Langerhans cells. The Langerhans cells have a distinctive appearance (note the reniform kidney-bean-shaped nucleus, its eccentric disposition within the cell, and the rather abundant lightly eosinophilic cytoplasm).

Fig 19.4 This biopsy of subacute eczematous dermatitis shows an irregular psoriasiform hyperplasia. The granular cell layer is mildly increased. The epidermis is surmounted by a scale containing serum, blood, and neutrophils. There is focal exocytosis of lymphocytes into the epidermis. A moderately dense lymphocytic infiltrate is present around vessels of the superficial dermis.

These immune reactions are prototypically mediated by Langerhans cells, which process externally applied antigens or those derived through the peripheral bloodstream, and present them to lymphocytes (**Figs 19.5–19.7**). This form of immune reaction defines the type-IV (delayed-type hypersensitivity or a cell-mediated immune) reaction. Its histomorphological hallmarks are identified by Langerhans cell-rich vesicles present in the epidermis with accompanying spongiosis, lymphocytic, and eosinophilic exocytosis.

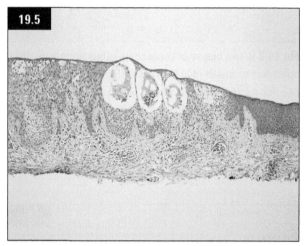

Fig 19.5 In this biopsy of subacute eczematous dermatitis, there is prominent epithelial hyperplasia. Most striking is the presence of coalescing Langerhans cell–rich microvesicles. There is fairly extensive spongiosis noted as well.

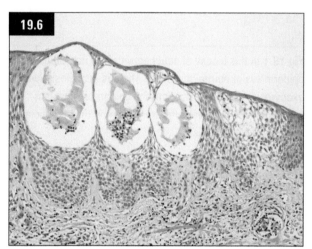

Fig 19.6 A higher magnification of **Fig 19.5** reveals Langerhans vesicles that reflect delayed hypersensitivity. The vesicles are composed of a combination of CD4 T cells, Langerhans cells, and eosinophils. Also apparent in this photomicrograph is prominent spongiosis.

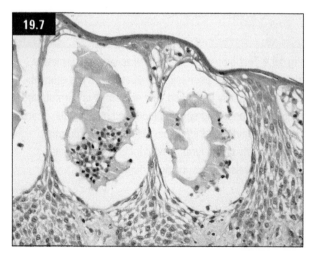

Fig 19.7 A higher magnification of **Fig 19.6** shows the characteristic intraepidermal components in an acute and subacute eczematous dermatitis. The main intraepidermal cellular constituents are eosinophils, Langerhans cells, and lymphocytes. The Langerhans cells are easily distinguished from the lymphocytes by virtue of a less condensed chromatin, the reniform quality to the nucleus, and its eccentric disposition within the cells.

Over time, the degree of acanthosis increases and the degree of spongiosis and inflammation diminishes to produce chronic dermatitis. In this particular setting, lesions are typically psoriasiform with regular elongation and thinning of rete ridges, but with thickening of the suprapapillary plates and diminished inflammation. Lichen simplex chronicus connotes a form of chronic dermatitis in which there is vertical fibrosis (namely *collagen*) laid down alongside elongated rete ridges as a function of persistent rubbing (**Fig 19.8**). The discriminating morphological distinction between subacute eczematous dermatitis and lichen simplex chronicus is the presence of inflammatory cells in the epidermis. If one observes changes of chronicity such as acanthosis and hyperkeratosis, but with supervening vesiculation and exocytosis of inflammatory cells, the designation of subacute eczematous dermatitis is used. If one sees changes of chronicity, but without any migration of inflammatory cells in the epidermis, then the designation is that of lichen simplex chronicus. If the patient persistently irritates and scratches a given site of lichen simplex chronicus, the epidermis can become so markedly acanthotic with contributions from the adnexal structures (the pilosebaceous units and the eccrine straight ducts) that lobules of rather banal squamous epithelium are present in the papillary and/or reticular dermis in a fashion that mimics squamous cell carcinoma. This hyperproliferative form of eczema is termed 'prurigo nodularis.'

During the course of acute dermatitis, formation of spongiotic vesicles causes transmigration of plasma to the epidermal surface to form a scale crust that often contains inflammatory cells. As a component of the hypersensitivity response, fluids such as plasma may leak out of superficial dermal capillaries into

Fig 19.8 In lesions of lichen simplex chronicus, the dermal papillae collagen assumes a vertical orientation to the long axis of the epidermis. Note the lack of exocytosis of lymphocytes into the epidermis.

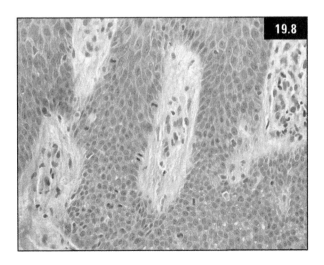

the papillary dermis to produce edema. As epidermal turnover increases, parakeratosis may be seen, and the granular cell layer may diminish in thickness. In lesions of acute and subacute eczematous dermatitis, the extent of intracorneal serum entrapment is more prominent compared with lesions of chronic eczematous dermatitis.

THE HISTOMORPHOLOGY OF DISTINCTIVE FORMS OF ECZEMA

ATOPIC ECZEMA
CLINICAL FEATURES AND PATHOPHYSIOLOGY
Some clinicians use the term 'eczema' to refer to atopic dermatitis, which is a disorder that frequently has its onset in infancy and childhood and is accompanied by an atopic diathesis comprising allergies to various exogenous triggers, rhinitis, and nasal polyps, and an itchy rash that preferentially affects the antecubital and popliteal fossae. Pathogenically, the disorder is due to a complex interaction between the environment and a genetic predisposition that has yet to be fully elucidated, eg, children who are breastfed for a long duration have a lower incidence of childhood atopic dermatitis, but this effect is modified by maternal allergic status (Snijders et al. 2007). Specific mitochondrial haplogroups have been associated with atopic dermatitis (Raby et al. 2007), perhaps suggesting a basis for the common association between maternal atopy and childhood atopic dermatitis. Susceptibility loci have been identified on the long arms of chromosomes 1, 3, 5, 11, 13, and 17 (Chien et al. 2007, Enomoto et al. 2007). There is a common haplotype of the COL29A1 gene located at 3q21, which codes for a novel epidermal collagen, seen in patients with atopic dermatitis; the outer layer of the epidermis lacks this collagen, which could compromise skin integrity and function and contribute to the pathogenesis of atopic dermatitis (Söderhall et al. 2007).

Similarly, specific haplotypes of 5q31-33, which code for T-helper type 2 (Th2) cytokines including interleukin (IL)-3, -4, -5, and -11, are seen in patients with atopic dermatitis (Lipozencić and Wolf 2007). Hyperfunctioning or increased numbers of specific T-helper lymphocytes of the Th2 subset also play a role in the acute phase; these lymphocytes elaborate IL-4 and IL-5 which promote tissue eosinophilia and hyperimmunoglobulinemia E. The chronic phase is dominated by Th1/Th0 lymphocytes and the secretion of interferon (IFN)-γ, IL-12, and granulocyte–macrophage colony-stimulating factor (GM-CSF) (Lipozencić and Wolf 2007). Elevated levels of IL-18 (Park do and Youn 2007) and high age-specific IgE levels (Hon et al. 2007) correlate with the severity of atopic dermatitis, further corroborating the proposed Th1/Th2 imbalance.

With respect to the skin lesions, these manifest as areas of scaling, lichenification, fissuring of palms and soles, vesiculation, and secondary changes such as hyper- or hypopigmentation, excoriation, and bacterial superinfection. This process can appear as early as 2 months of age and in infants involves the head and neck areas, whereas the preferential involvement in the childhood years is the flexural areas. In adults, a wide distribution may be seen. Denny lines are thickened longitudinal grooves in the lower eyelid area due to persistent rubbing and are a telltale clue to an underlying atopic diathesis.

HISTOPATHOLOGY
Atopic eczema is usually apparent clinically based on the chronicity of the lesions and their characteristic distribution. In some instances, however, the patient may present with widespread eczema to the point of erythroderma. Biopsies are frequently performed in this setting because of the clinical concern of cutaneous T-cell lymphoma. Both cutaneous T-cell lymphoma and atopic eczema may have a similar presentation when adults are affected. In both, the dermatitis is typically of years' duration, pruritus can be striking, and the quality of the lesions is similar, specifically scaly erythematous plaques involving truncal and other sun-protected areas. In classic atopic eczema, there may be a relative dearth of inflammatory cells. The overwhelming morphology is one dominated by epidermal changes of chronicity, including epidermal hyperplasia, hyperkeratosis, and vertically oriented superficial fibroplasias (Figs 19.9 and 19.10).

Nevertheless, there are cases in which a fairly exuberant inflammatory cell infiltrate may be present. In such cases, the distinction from cutaneous T-cell lymphoma may be difficult. There are helpful clues,

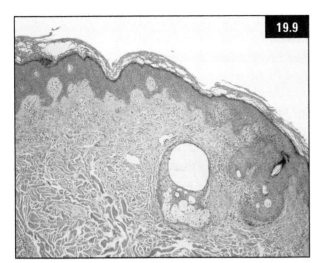

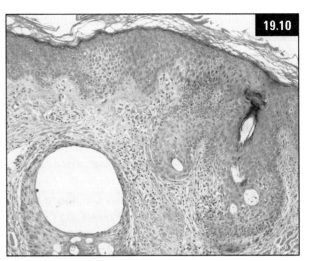

Fig 19.9 In atopic eczema, the changes can be relatively subtle. Often the one aspect of the histomorphology could be simply that of lichen simplex chronicus. However, in this particular biopsy there is some degree of spongiosis with very mild exocytosis of lymphocytes into the epidermis. As well, in atopic eczema, it is quite common to see folliculocentricity of the eczematous response. Note the spongiosis of the outer root sheath epithelium with exocytosis of lymphocytes into the follicle. As a point of reiteration, it is relatively uncommon in classic lesions of atopic eczema to see an exuberant prominent lymphocytic infiltrate within the dermis. Similarly, it is uncommon to see extensive intraepidermal vesiculation with extensive eosinophilic spongiosis. All of the previously mentioned features would point more toward an allergic eczematous dermatitis.

Fig 19.10 This is a higher magnification of **Fig 19.9**, which highlights the relatively subtle qualities that one can encounter in atopic eczema – those of modest spongiosis, slight epidermal hyperplasia, and focal lymphocytic exocytosis typically of low density and often with follicular accentuation.

however, which could define potential morphological discriminators of atopic eczema from cutaneous T-cell lymphoma. If there is prominent inflammation, the pattern of migration in the epidermis is often a directed one in the setting of atopic eczema. There is preferential migration of inflammatory cells to involve the suprapapillary plates, hair follicles, and acrosyringium. The collagen assumes a vertical orientation instead of the classic laminated parallel pattern seen in cutaneous T-cell lymphoma. Although spongiosis can be seen in cutaneous T-cell lymphoma, the presence of supervening Langerhans cell-rich vesicles is characteristic for atopic eczema and is less common in the setting of cutaneous T-cell lymphoma, but there are eczematous variants of cutaneous T-cell lymphoma.

In atopic eczema, the pattern of intraepidermal inflammation should not constitute features of true interface dermatitis. Specifically, seeing foci of lymphocyte tagging along the dermal–epidermal junction would be highly unusual and should prompt concern about evolving cutaneous T-cell lymphoma, or suggest an alternative cause for the dermatosis in question. In cutaneous T-cell lymphoma, lymphocytes typically colonize the basal layer of the epidermis without supervening destructive changes of classic, immunologically mediated, interface dermatitis.

As for cytomorphology, a few cerebriform lymphocytes can be seen in the lesions of atopic eczema. However, if there are significant numbers of intermediate-to-larger cerebriform lymphocytes in the epidermis, and especially if they exceed the atypia of those cells present in the dermis, then the concern is of course that one is dealing with cutaneous T-cell lymphoma.

As a final point, any case of chronic, recalcitrant dermatitis showing a pattern compatible with eczema with prominent inflammation should prompt investigation into a possible recent inciting trigger, whether a drug or a contactant. Patients with an underlying atopic diathesis are genetically predisposed to launching excessive T-cell-driven responses to various exogenous triggers. Although one could surmise that a recent exacerbation of atopic eczema could be part of the variant inflammatory cycle seen in atopy, one should carefully consider an additional exogenous factor as a potential precipitant.

ALLERGIC CONTACT DERMATITIS
CLINICAL FEATURES AND PATHOPHYSIOLOGY

The allergic contact reaction is a form of delayed-type hypersensitivity (cell-mediated immunity/Gell and Combs type IV immune reaction) and is affected by sensitized antigen-specific T lymphocytes. The cytokine release initiating the inflammatory response in both allergic and irritant contact dermatitis is similar, although these processes are mediated by adaptive and innate immunity, respectively (Fyhrquist-Vanni et al. 2007). Hapten and irritant exposure causes epidermal keratinocytes to secrete tumor necrosis factor-α (TNF-α) and IL-1α, dendritic cells to produce IL-1β, and natural killer cells and lymphocytes to secrete IFN-γ. What is unique to allergic contact dermatitis is, however, the hapten presentation by Langerhans cells. Langerhans cells initially process a hapten secondary to topical application and migrate to the lymph nodes, where they present the hapten to naïve T cells. The T cells become activated, clonally expand, and those that express cutaneous lymphocyte-associated antigen can return to the vascular bed in the skin compartment where the hapten was originally processed by Langerhans cells (Fyhrquist-Vanni et al. 2007).

TNF-α induces keratinocytes to secrete the chemokine CCL-27, which also recruits skin-homing T cells (Kanda and Watanabe 2007). When their numbers and activity are sufficient to produce a cytokine milieu capable of effecting local injury to the skin in which they were first recruited, an allergic contact reaction occurs. The sensitization phase typically takes 14–28 days but can occur in as few as 4 days (Kwan 2004); the elicitation phase occurs over the subsequent 1–2 days required to generate the cytokine burden capable of effecting injury.

The exanthematous cutaneous response can be primary, ie, at the site of the original topical application, or distant to it. The latter is referred to as an *id reaction*. It is therefore expected that the histomorphology of the id reaction and allergic contact dermatitis appear identical, although, most characteristically, the id response corresponds to the morphological concept of an acute eczematous response.

HISTOPATHOLOGY

The morphology goes through the characteristic acute, subacute, and chronic patterns as described above. Minor variances occur when the antigen is processed primarily through adnexal structures, resulting in prominent lymphocytic exocytosis within the follicle or acrosyringium. If the process represents photoallergic dermatitis, there is typically a brisk angiocentric lymphocytic infiltrate most prominent superficially with some dissipation as the base of the infiltrate is approached.

In some cases of photoallergic dermatitis, there may be supervening changes of phototoxicity. Hallmarks include suprabasilar dyskeratosis, mitoses above the basal layer of the epidermis, architectural disarray and dysmaturation of the epidermis, irregular melanization of the epidermis, and the presence of apoptotic cells and melanin pigment within the stratum corneum. As keratinocyte and melanocyte injury occur, pigment incontinence results in uptake of melanin by histiocytes in the papillary dermis (ie, postinflammatory hyperpigmentation).

IRRITANT CONTACT DERMATITIS

CLINICAL FEATURES AND PATHOPHYSIOLOGY

Irritant contact dermatitis is a response to various forms of cytotoxic cell injury that is not mediated by adaptive immunological mechanisms. A variety of compounds, when applied to the skin surface, can provoke an irritant contact dermatitis. Notwithstanding the foregoing, a decrease in epidermal Langerhans cells and an increase in the corresponding population of the dermis (Mikulowska and Falck 1994) suggest epidermal migration of antigen-processing cells with subsequent activation of T lymphocytes (Brand *et al.* 1995). Direct toxic injury to keratinocytes can result in their release of immune-response modifiers such as tumor necrosis factor (Lisby *et al.* 1995) and, particularly in psoriatic skin, the release of IL-8 with subsequent recruitment of neutrophils into the inflamed epidermis (Szepietowski *et al.* 2001).

Irritant contact dermatitis occurs at sites where an irritant compound or substance comes in direct contact with the skin. Thus, one can see it, for example, on the hands of workers who handle fiberglass or other chemical products. Unlike an allergic eczematous dermatitis, an id response to the irritant does not usually occur. In almost all cases, the process is localized to the sites of topical application.

HISTOPATHOLOGY

In classic irritant contact dermatitis, features of nonimmunologically mediated epidermal injury are seen. Hence, necrolytic changes that affect the superficial layers of the epidermis are common (**Fig 19.11**). At times, one can see individual cell necrosis without lymphocyte satellitosis around the

Fig 19.11 In this biopsy, irritant epidermal changes due to external trauma (ie, scratching) are seen. Not uncommonly in lesions of eczematous dermatitis there are supervening changes attributable to external trauma induced by pruritus. In this photomicrograph, there is a prominent hypereosinophilic necrolytic alteration of the epidermis due to scratching. Note the entrapped red cells within the epidermis.

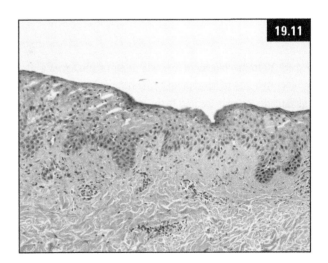

necrotic keratinocyte. There is a secondary influx of neutrophils into the epidermis with eventual localization of neutrophils in the stratum corneum. Seeing Langerhans cell–rich vesicles, prominent lymphocytic exocytosis, and conspicuous tissue eosinophilia suggests a supervening component of a true allergic reaction. With chronicity, there are changes of epidermal hyperplasia and hyperkeratosis. In more acute phases, conspicuous spongiosis can be seen, although unlike true allergic contact dermatitis, the spongiosis is paucicellular apart from neutrophil migration.

As irritant contact dermatitis may be superimposed upon allergic contact reactions, the distinction between the two can be difficult. Photoinduced injury can be superimposed and in fact is a form of contact dermatitis of the irritant type. In this setting, one looks for features of photoirritation and adaptation including large, atypical, suprabasilar 'sunburn' cells,

irregular melanization of the epidermis, melanin pigment in the stratum corneum, and features of melanocyte activation. The latter includes an increase in number and size of the melanocytes with the development of prominent melanin-laden dendrites.

FOLLICULAR ECZEMA
CLINICAL FEATURES

Particularly in Japanese patients, eczematous dermatitides may be localized to follicular structures. This process is termed 'follicular eczema' and is held in some populations as being a manifestation of an underlying atopic diathesis. Perifollicular papules are typically seen on the trunk and extremities in Asian people and people of African descent. Follicular eczema can be recognized both clinically and under the microscope. In follicular eczema, spongiotic change and exocytosis of the inflammatory cells are

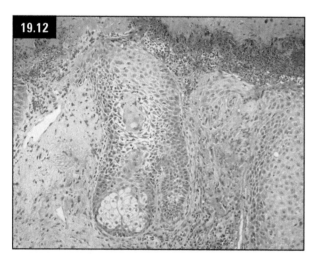

Fig 19.12 In this biopsy of follicular eczema, the surface is ulcerated due to scratching from pruritus. The residual dermatosis leading to the pruritus is, however, morphologically identifiable. In particular, there is prominent spongiosis of the outer root sheath epithelium of the hair follicle, with exocytosis of lymphocytes into the follicle defining the morphological changes – so-called *follicular eczema*. Follicular eczema may be part of the manifestation of the atopic diathesis and/or could be attributable to an allergic contact dermatitis and/or an eczematous drug reaction.

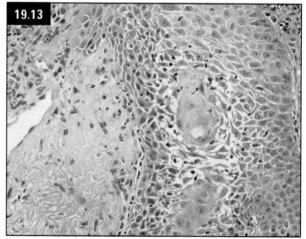

Fig 19.13 In this high-power photomicrograph of follicular eczema, the influx of inflammatory cells into the outer root sheath epithelium is observed with attendant spongiosis. It should be emphasized that a mononuclear cell dominant infiltrate in the follicle may be one of the earliest manifestations of eosinophilic folliculitis, which, in essence, is a form of follicular eczema but with an unusual predominance of eosinophils within the follicle reflective of a Th2 immune deregulatory state.

present within and around follicular structures (**Figs 19.12** and **19.13**).

SEBORRHEIC DERMATITIS

CLINICAL FEATURES

Seborrheic dermatitis is an idiopathic condition that affects the scalp, face, upper chest, and back, sometimes with extension to flexural areas. Lesions are described as having a greasy or scaly red or red–brown morphology that manifests as sharply demarcated patches mimicking psoriasis. The lesions are also often associated with dandruff. Clinically, there is an association of seborrheic dermatitis with human immunodeficiency virus (HIV) infection, while an occasional patient will have coexistent Parkinson syndrome, myocardial infarction, a seizure disorder, obesity, alcoholism, malnutrition, or malabsorption (Schwartz *et al.* 2006).

One thinks of seborrheic dermatitis as a lesion that shows overlapping features between a spongiotic dermatitis as described above and psoriasis. With respect to the latter, a neutrophil-containing, parakeratotic scale crust overlies a deficient granular cell layer in an epidermis in which a spongiform pustulation may be seen (**Fig 19.14**). Capillaries may be ectatic and directly abut the basement membrane zone of the overlying superpapillary plates as in psoriasis. Spongiotic changes with entrapped serum in the scale and tissue eosinophilia may, however, supervene. In the setting of HIV infection, a peculiar interface injury may be seen along with dermal-based plasma cells, often in an angiocentric array. Patients may have coexistent eosinophilic folliculitis comprising eosinophil- or neutrophil-rich pustules within the follicular infundibulum or isthmus (Magro and Crowson 2000). Any form of impetiginized

Fig 19.14 Seborrheic dermatitis can be viewed as an interesting overlap between a subacute eczematous reaction and psoriasis. Therefore, in this photomicrograph, one observes features of a psoriatic diathesis primarily in the context of granular cell layer diminution and an overlying confluent parakeratotic scale. However, at variance with psoriasis is the presence of small Langerhans cell–rich microvesicles in the epidermis, and the fact that the cells within the dermis that focally infiltrate the epidermis are mononuclear cells as opposed to neutrophils. That said, in many lesions of seborrheic dermatitis, one can see neutrophil-imbued parakeratosis with spongiform pustulation, typically localized to the follicular ostia and perifollicular epidermis.

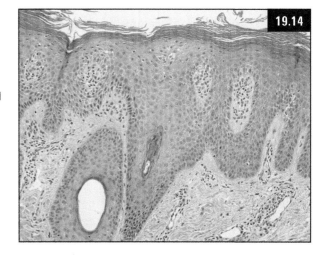

eczema can have a neutrophil-rich scale crust and thereby mimic seborrheic dermatitis. Another important differential diagnosis from both a clinical and a histomorphological perspective is one of lupus erythematosus with features of a supervening psoriatic diathesis.

DIFFERENTIAL DIAGNOSIS

If the clinical history suggests infection, special stains for spirochetes or fungi should exclude important considerations in the differential diagnosis such as secondary syphilis or tinea. Clinical history provides an important clue to a figurate erythema, pityriasis rosea, contact dermatitis, or drug eruption. With respect to the latter considerations, figurate erythemas typically have a superficial and deep sleeve-like perivascular lymphoid infiltrate that may or may not be associated with a spongiotic intraepidermal process, whereas pityriasis rosea comprises mounds of parakeratin overlaying a mildly spongiotic-appearing epidermis; this, in turn, overlies a massively edematous papillary dermis. Drug reactions are typified by an overlap of features between different forms of dermatitis including eczema, psoriasis, and idiopathic lichenoid reactions. But ultimately a drug history is always necessary to confirm the diagnostic consideration. With respect to HIV infection, such patients are said to show a greater density of plasma cells in the infiltrate.

DYSHIDROTIC ECZEMA
CLINICAL FEATURES

Dyshidrotic eczema or pompholyx is held by some observers to be merely a form of contact dermatitis of the hands and soles comprising tense vesicles, often affecting the sides of the digits, the palms, or the soles. The terminology reflects the fact that at one time, this condition was thought to be caused by abnormal sweating because the lesions are, in some cases, centered on eccrine straight ducts and acrosyringes. Dyshidrotic eczema is associated with vesicles and severe pruritus. In most patients the disorder spontaneously regresses but recurs quickly

and is self-limited. In some patients it becomes chronic, giving rise to weeping, hyperkeratotic hand eczema, of which dyshidrotic eczema is one cause. The history of prior pruritic vesicles can be a clue to the cause in some affected patients who present with the chronic form of the disease. Any patient presenting with dyshidrotic eczema should, however, have patch testing to elucidate potential inciting triggers (Jain et al. 2004).

Although an autosomal dominant form of dyshidrotic eczema has been localized to 18q22 in a large Chinese family (Chen et al. 2006), most patients appear to have relevant contact allergies, with cosmetic and hygiene products being the most common cause followed by metal exposure and mycosis (Guillet et al. 2007). Pompholyx has been induced by intravenous immunoglobulin therapy in several cases (Llombart et al. 2007), reported after endoscopic thoracic sympathectomy to treat intractable palmar hyperhidrosis (Niinai et al. 2004), and observed in some HIV+ patients upon initiation of highly active antiretroviral treatment.

HISTOPATHOLOGY

In addition to the common features of spongiotic dermatitis, dyshidrotic eczema shows several clues to diagnosis at a light microscopic level. First is the acral location, with a dense orthohyperkeratotic scale. The second clue is the striking spongiosis with formation of large intraepidermal vesicles that may be near acrosyringes and/or eccrine straight ducts but do not involve them directly (**Figs 19.15** and **19.16**).

ECZEMATOUS DRUG REACTIONS
CLINICAL FEATURES

The eczematous form of drug reaction is one of the more common manifestations of drug reactions. Patients manifest a spongiotic dermatitis that can be symmetrical, localized, or generalized; the more severe inflammatory reaction typically occurs at the site of the first sensitization.

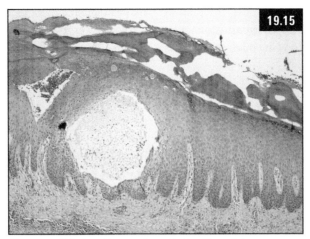

Fig 19.15 This is a biopsy of acral skin. One of the characteristic hallmarks of dyshidrotic eczema is the presence of intraepidermal vesicles composed of Langerhans cells, lymphocytes, and several eosinophils. In addition, the epidermis surrounding the vesicle shows spongiosis with lymphocytic exocytosis. Superficially, the epidermis has a hypereosinophilic quality owing to a necrolytic change caused by scratching.

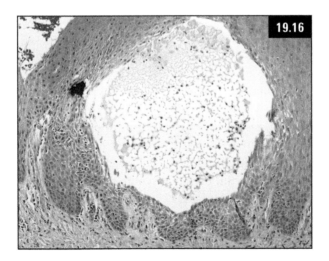

Fig 19.16 Higher magnification of the intraepidermal component shows the composition of the vesicle as being predominated by mononuclear cells including lymphocytes and Langerhans cells as well as adjacent prominent spongiosis. Unlike palmar plantar pustulosis, which potentially would be a clinically diagnostic consideration, the epidermis, instead of being permeated by neutrophils, exhibits lymphocytic exocytosis.

HISTOPATHOLOGY

Skin biopsy shows an eczematous dermatitis of acute, chronic, or subacute morphology in which eosinophils are often numerous.

DIFFERENTIAL DIAGNOSIS

It is impossible to distinguish the eczematous drug reaction from other forms of spongiotic dermatitis. One helpful clue is to see the overlap of otherwise prototypic idiopathic dermatoses such as a lichenoid tissue reaction or urticaria. In our experience, the collision of different prototypic inflammatory morphologies is often a clue to a drug-based etiology.

ERYTHRODERMA AND EXFOLIATIVE DERMATITIS

Erythroderma implies diffuse reddening of the skin with a scaling eruption and can be called *exfoliative dermatitis* when scaling becomes pronounced. Drugs are the most common cause of erythroderma followed by generalized atopic dermatitis, pityriasis rubra pilaris, erythrodermic psoriasis, and cutaneous T-cell lymphoma. There also is a distinctive form of prelymphomatous T-cell dyscrasia that falls under the term 'idiopathic erythroderma.' It can be difficult to distinguish these pathogenic causes of erythroderma under the microscope.

CLINICAL FEATURES

The entire cutaneous surface can be involved by a scaling, erythematous macular eruption. In some cases, there are islands of spared normal skin that can be a clue to pityriasis rubra pilaris or to hematoerythrodermia, the latter associated with acute and chronic leukemias. Control of fluid and electrolyte balance can be impaired in severe erythrodermic states, associated with temperature dysregulation and, in some cases, with cardiac failure. Uncommon causes of erythroderma include contact dermatitis, stasis dermatitis, scabies, lichen planus, pemphigus foliaceus, lamellar ichthyosis, and hypereosinophilic syndrome, which is most commonly related to an eosinophilic myeloproliferative and T-cell dyscrasia. A substantial minority of cases of erythroderma will remain idiopathic. So-called idiopathic erythroderma may eventuate into Sézary syndrome.

HISTOPATHOLOGY

Typically, erythroderma manifests as a dermatitis which may be acute, subacute, or chronic/psoriasiform. Typically, pityriasis rubra pilaris has a specific histomorphology, namely a 'checkerboard' pattern of ortho- and parakeratosis that alternates in vertical and horizontal planes above a thickened epidermis, manifesting a psoriasiform pattern of hyperplasia with preservation or accentuation of the granular cell layer.

The dermal infiltrate in pityriasis rubra pilaris is sparse. When eosinophils are seen in the dermis, possibilities include a drug-based etiology, or atopy; when atypical lymphoid cells colonize the epidermis, the main diagnostic considerations are a lymphomatoid drug eruption, idiopathic erythroderma, and Sézary syndrome. If the process is of recent onset and the patient is on one or more drugs with immune dysregulating properties, then strong consideration should be given to a lymphomatoid drug eruption. Conversely, if the process is a more recalcitrant form of progressive erythroderma that has persisted for years, then one must strongly consider an evolving T-cell dyscrasia, whether in the context of idiopathic erythroderma or Sézary syndrome.

In both idiopathic erythroderma and Sézary syndrome, clonality can be seen along with certain phenotypic abnormalities including losses of CD7 and CD62L. Only biopsies of lesional tissue from Sézary syndrome patients will significantly overexpress CD158k/KIR3DL2 transcripts by reverse transcription polymerase chain reaction. Biopsies from lesional tissue of erythrodermic inflammatory conditions will not, suggesting a unique molecular marker of Sézary syndrome (Ortonne *et al.* 2008). The peripheral blood parameters are still critical, specifically regarding the CD4:CD8 ratio, and any phenotypic abnormalities amidst circulating T cells. A recently introduced diagnostic tool is CD27 expression on peripheral blood lymphocytes. Patients with Sézary syndrome have significantly higher expressions of the CD4+ CD27+ CD45RA− central memory T-cell subset, whereas patients with idiopathic erythroderma have increased CD4+ CD27− CD45RA− effector memory T-cell levels (Fierro *et al.* 2008). There are very specific peripheral blood criteria that allow one to render a diagnosis of Sézary syndrome. Multiple biopsies may be required to make the distinction (Walsh *et al.* 1994, Vasconcellos *et al.* 1995).

STASIS DERMATITIS
CLINICAL FEATURES
The term 'stasis dermatitis' is applied to an eczematous process of the lower extremities, typically in middle-aged females or elderly males, and is attributed to incompetent perforating veins with impaired venous return. A component of forward-based profusion (ie, arterial) impairment is suggested in stasis dermatitis, its exaggerated nodular plaque-like variant (acroangiodermatitis), and the corresponding ischemic dermopathy which may be associated with it (lipodermatosclerosis). The inner aspect of the ankles and the inner aspect of the foreleg are often the first to be involved (Gourdin and Smith 1993). Scaling, erythema, and edema with a brownish discoloration to the skin are typical. Lesions may ulcerate and dilated varicose veins are often evident by clinical examination. Scarring and atrophy will eventually occur.

HISTOPATHOLOGY
Superimposed on acute, subacute, or chronic dermatitis, stasis dermatitis shows prominent congeries of small dermal blood vessels surrounded by fibrous tissue and an inflammatory reaction. Variable hemorrhage including extravasation of erythrocytes and accumulation of perivascular hemosiderophages are additional clues to the process. Involvement of the panniculus is characterized by a form of fat necrosis termed 'lipomembranous fat necrosis' and is held to have an ischemic basis.

DIFFERENTIAL DIAGNOSIS
When lesions are ulcerated, granulation tissue is prominent in the lower extremities; therefore, any cause of ulceration can produce a morphology that mimics stasis dermatitis. Acroangiodermatitis is mimicked by Kaposi sarcoma but can be distinguished because Kaposi sarcoma is characteristically more infiltrative in its pattern of growth and shows endothelial mitoses, cytologic atypia, phagocytosis of

red blood cells within the cytoplasm of endothelia, and interstitial plasma cells.

PITYRIASIS ALBA
CLINICAL FEATURES
Children may manifest a hypopigmented scaly macular dermatitis termed 'pityriasis alba' in which depigmentation of the skin through postinflammatory pigment loss results in pale discoloration. Many of the patients are atopic children between the ages of 3 and 16 years, who manifest one or several hypopigmented macules on the face, trunk, or extremities. The lesions have indistinct borders and a fine scale (ie, pityriasis) and may manifest a follicular-based component as atopy often does. Studies have demonstrated a direct correlation between pityriasis alba and the amount of sun exposure, lack of sunscreen use, and frequency of bathing (Lin and Janniger 2005). Although no effective treatment has yet been established, the lesions do resolve with time.

HISTOPATHOLOGY
Pityriasis alba manifests as mild eczematous alterations cognate to any subacute dermatitis and, if the underlying basis is atopy, eosinophils and a folliculocentric inflammatory component may be prominent. Melanophages are often present in the papillary dermis and, as a sequela of inflammatory injury, the melanocytes may show reduced activity with shrunken dendrites and diminished pigmentation.

DIFFERENTIAL DIAGNOSIS
The clinical considerations include tinea versicolor and vitiligo, the latter characterized histologically by a loss of melanocytes, and the former by colonization of the cornified layer by *Pityrosporum* spp. These yeasts are easily demonstrable in most cases in routinely stained material, where the fungal hyphae and spores stain with hematoxylin.

PITYRIASIS ROSEA
CLINICAL FEATURES
Pityriasis rosea is a common, self-limited dermatosis that affects children and middle-aged adults. It may show geographic clustering (ie, army barracks) and

increased prevalence in the fall and winter, which have been held to suggest a virally based etiology. A prodrome of malaise, headaches, and/or fever can precede the skin lesions, further suggesting a possible viral cause. An association with human herpesvirus HHV-7 has been shown, but is controversial. Various other viral and bacterial causes have been ruled out. The role of autoimmunity is currently under investigation because some patients with pityriasis rosea have T-lymphocytotoxic antibodies and/or significantly elevated levels of antinuclear antibodies (Chuh et al. 2005).

Patients often develop a salmon-colored macular 'herald patch' in the middle of the chest before dissemination of the eruption in a symmetric 'Christmas tree' distribution down the trunk onto the extremities. Individual lesions manifest a salmon-colored morphology with a scale likened to cigarette paper owing to its fine character and peripheral disposition. Oral lesions are seen in roughly one patient in ten (Vidimos and Camisa 1992).

So-called atypical pityriasis rosea manifests as vesicular, purpuric, urticarial, or pustular lesions. The face, axillae, and groin are affected in pityriasis rosea inversus, whereas the shoulders and hips are involved in limb–girdle pityriasis rosea. Associated pruritus, pain, and burning sensation are seen in pityriasis rosea irritata. Pityriasis rosea with large plaques is termed 'pityriasis rosea gigantea of Darier.' Mucous membrane involvement has also been reported. A pityriasiform drug eruption can be seen in a setting of therapy with gold, barbiturates, and angiotensin-converting enzyme inhibitors (Magro et al. 2002).

HISTOPATHOLOGY

The main morphological features of pityriasis rosea are those of an eczematous dermatitis in which mounds of parakeratin-containing plasma occur over areas of epidermal injury and spongiosis, associated in some cases with multinucleation of keratinocytes and hemorrhage. The papillary dermis is edematous and contains a modest perivascular lymphoid infiltrate that shows exocytosis. Individual cell necrosis in the epidermis, with colloid bodies in the papillary dermis, is accompanied by areas of hemorrhage. Eosinophils may be seen, and there may be a component of mild

interface injury. The parakeratotic scale may form an oblique or upward angle likened to a teapot spout and called a *teapot scale*, but this is by no means a specific or constant feature. On occasion, one sees multinucleated keratinocytes lacking viral cytopathic change. The atypical forms may show a heavier infiltrate with more abundant hemorrhage.

DIFFERENTIAL DIAGNOSIS

The differential diagnosis of striking papillary dermal edema includes polymorphous light eruption, erythema multiforme, Sweet syndrome, and pyoderma gangrenosum. The differential diagnosis of an eczematous dermatitis with individual cell necrosis and hemorrhage, ie, a pityriasiform dermatitis, includes pityriasis lichenoides, pityriasiform drug eruptions, and viral exanthemas. Pityriasis lichenoides has two variants: a chronic and an acute one. In pityriasis lichenoides chronica confluent parakeratotic scales overlie an acanthotic epidermis. In pityriasis lichenoides et varioliformis acuta (PLEVA), the scale is patchy in character and there is an intense superficial and deep wedge-shaped infiltrate with abundant hemorrhage and keratinocyte necrosis. Both conditions are a form of clonal lymphoid dyscrasia (Magro et al. 2002, 2003); neither has the striking papillary dermal edema or the patchy character of lymphocyte migration of pityriasis rosea. Pityriasiform drug eruptions tend to occur in older people and thus solar elastosis of dermal collagen may be present; tissue eosinophilia is more abundant and papillary dermal edema is typically less striking. Small plaque parapsoriasis (ie, digitate dermatosis or persistent superficial dermatitis) is another form of lymphoid dyscrasia that can mimic pityriasis rosea but tends to be seen in older people who manifest persistent papules, unlike the self-limited dermatosis of pityriasis rosea. Histologically, small plaque parapsoriasis shows a similar pattern of spongiosis with areas of parakeratosis overlaying the epidermal injury, but also tends to lack the papillary dermal edema of pityriasis rosea.

Guttate psoriasis is a form of eruptive psoriasis that typically manifests clustered papules on the trunk and extremities, seen as a psoriasiform diathesis under the microscope with neutrophil-rich parakeratotic mounds overlying the epidermis, which shows a deficient granular cell layer. The characteristic tortuous ectatic capillaries of psoriasis are present even if, due to the typically sudden onset of the eruption, a psoriasiform pattern of epidermal hyperplasia is not identified. Hemorrhage and keratinocyte necrosis are atypical of guttate psoriasis and, thus, the distinction for pityriasis rosea is typically easy. As is usually the case with spongiotic dermatitis, a superficial fungal infection merits consideration, and special stains for fungi are appropriate.

GIANOTTI–CROSTI SYNDROME (PAPULAR ACRODERMATITIS OF CHILDHOOD)

CLINICAL FEATURES

Similar to pityriasis rosea, Gianotti–Crosti syndrome is a manifestation of a systemic viral illness, although the evidence for this construction is more compelling in the case of Gianotti–Crosti syndrome. In particular, hepatitis B, A, and C, and Epstein–Barr virus (EBV) infection have been associated with this distinctive acral papular eruption. Other implicated viruses include Cocksackie virus, cytomegalovirus, echovirus, poliovirus, respiratory syncytial virus, and parainfluenza. It has been reported in children after immunizations with the live attenuated viruses, including the oral polio (Erkek *et al.* 2001) and measles/mumps/rubella (MMR) (Velangi and Tidman 1998), and after inactivated vaccines for hepatitis A (Monastirli *et al.* 2007) and B (Karakaş *et al.* 2007), Japanese encephalitis (Kang and Oh 2003), diphtheria/tetanus/acellular pertussis, and *Haemophilus influenzae* b (Hib) (Murphy and Buckley 2000). It has also been reported after inactivated influenza immunization in an adult (Cambiaghi *et al.* 1995).

Typically affecting infants and young children, Gianotti–Crosti syndrome manifests as an eruption of nonitchy red papules involving the face, buttocks, and acral parts, sparing the trunk, in an eruption that lasts 3–4 weeks or longer. Other symptomatology specific to the implicated microbial pathogen may be present, such as lymphadenopathy and pharyngitis in the case of EBV, or hepatomegaly and/or jaundice in the setting of hepatitis. The latter is uncommon because most patients do not have severe hepatic injury and most cases do not progress to chronic hepatitis.

HISTOPATHOLOGY

Similar to most viral eczanthemas, lesions of Gianotti–Crosti syndrome manifest as a sparse-to-moderate superficial perivascular and lymphocytic inflammatory process associated with variable spongiosis and, in some cases, acanthosis and parakeratosis. These features are not specific and can be seen in a variety of viral eczanthemas and spongiotic dermatitides of diverse causes.

DIFFERENTIAL DIAGNOSIS

As expected, other viral eczanthemas, drug reactions, and superficial fungal reactions can mimic this picture.

SMALL-PLAQUE PARAPSORIASIS

CLINICAL FEATURES

Parapsoriasis has two forms: small-plaque and large-plaque. Although there is some controversy over this issue, it appears that the large-plaque variety is a precursor to patch-stage lesions of mycosis fungoides (Sehgal *et al.* 2007). The small-plaque variant, alternately termed 'superficial persistent dermatitis' or 'chronic superficial dermatitis,' rarely if ever progresses to mycosis fungoides. Chronic, superficial, persistent dermatitis or small-plaque parapsoriasis is considered with the spongiotic dermatitides. Typically starting in adulthood, patients manifest erythematous round-to-oval scaly patches 1–2 cm in diameter on the trunk or extremities. With an oval contour, they have the approximate size and shape of fingerprints taken from the distal phalanges and, thus, the alternative appellation for this condition is 'digitate dermatosis.' Lesions may be larger on the lower extremities; the face, palms, and soles are typically spared. An older lesion may, when compressed from the sides, show a wrinkling of a fine, cigarette-paper-like scale. Lesions may be more prominent in winter and tend to disappear in the summer.

HISTOPATHOLOGY

This is a form of subacute or chronic dermatitis that shows slight acanthosis of the epidermis surmounted by parakeratosis, with a modest superficial perivascular lymphocytic infiltrate showing slight exocytosis. The horizontal wiry fibrosis of the collagen table typical of large-plaque parapsoriasis is not seen, nor is there haphazard and continuous colonization of the epidermis as in patch-size mycosis fungoides. Lymphoid atypia and Pautrier microabscesses are absent. One of the most striking features of small-plaque parapsoriasis is the large confluent nature of the parakeratotic scale, typically surmounting a relatively normal-appearing stratum corneum with a preserved granular cell layer. In such cases, there is a dearth of inflammation.

DIFFERENTIAL DIAGNOSIS

A variety of chronic and subacute spongiotic dermatitides can produce this picture. Pityriasis lichenoid chronica tends to produce a more band-like infiltrate and less spongiosis whereas drug eruptions typically have a more pronounced tissue eosinophilia.

POLYMORPHOUS ERUPTION OF PREGNANCY

CLINICAL FEATURES

The most common dermatosis of the gravid state, pruritic urticarial papules and plaques of pregnancy (PUPPP), has an incidence of 1 in 20 pregnancies and manifests as pruritic papules and urticarial plaques, sometimes with superimposed vesicles, in and near abdominal striae (Alcalay and Wolf 1988). It usually develops in the last few weeks of pregnancy and may spread to the extremities or become generalized. Periumbilical sparing and spontaneous resolution are characteristic. The association of this eruption with large babies, twin and triplet pregnancies, and increased maternal weight gain raises the possibility that it relates somehow to excessive abdominal distension (Elling et al. 2000, Rudolph et al. 2006).

HISTOPATHOLOGY

Superficial perivascular lymphocytic or lymphocytic and eosinophilic infiltrates with a nondescript appearance, accompanied in a third of cases by exocytosis and spongiosis, are characteristic. Fibroblast proliferation is an infrequent concomitant (Alcalay and Wolf 1988). Leukocyte debris may be present, but there is no vascular fibrin deposition to suggest a leukocytoclastic vasculitis. Although usually nonreactive by direct immunofluorescent testing, lesions of PUPPP may show granular IgM, IgA, or C3 deposition at the dermoepidermal junction and/or in

blood vessels (Zurn et al. 1992, Aronson et al. 1998), suggesting a delayed-type hypersensitivity reaction or possibly an immune complex contribution to the pathogenesis (Alcalay and Wolf 1988, Zurn et al. 1992, Aronson et al. 1998). Analysis of serum hormone levels in one series showed a significant drop in cortisol levels in patients with PUPPP versus normal pregnant control patients (Vaughan Jones et al. 1999). Enhanced progesterone receptor expression in lesional as opposed to nonlesional keratinocytes also suggests the possibility that the hormones have a role to play (Borrego et al. 1999).

DIFFERENTIAL DIAGNOSIS

The differential diagnosis of PUPPP includes atopic dermatitis, dermal hypersensitivity reactions to drugs, contactants, and arthropod bites, and herpes (pemphigoid) gestationis. Most hypersensitivity reactions cannot reliably be distinguished from PUPPP because of their nondescript histomorphology. Pemphigoid gestationis can occur at any time during pregnancy, and is often raised as a clinical consideration. Lesions frequently show subepidermal blisters accompanied by eosinophils in the epidermis, at tips of dermal papillae, and in a perivascular disposition, associated with focal necrosis of basal layer keratinocytes and colloid body formation. Tissue eosinophilia is quantitatively greater in pemphigoid gestationis than in PUPPP (Borrego et al. 1999).

Circulating antibasement membrane IgG is demonstrable by indirect immunofluorescence in 25% of herpes gestationis patients, associated invariably with linear C3 deposition along the dermoepidermal junction and, in 50% of cases, with a similar pattern of IgG deposition (Alcalay and Wolf 1988, Murray 1990). As the linear dermoepidermal junction deposition of C3 and IgG that characterizes herpes gestationis is not seen in PUPPP, direct immunofluorescence testing is a valuable adjunct in making this important distinction.

Herpes gestationis is associated with increased fetal morbidity and may require systemic steroid therapy, whereas PUPPP are self-limited eruptions with no associated fetal morbidity (Alcalay and Wolf 1988, Murray 1990, Sherard and Atkinson 2001). A less problematic concern is that of pruritic folliculitis of pregnancy which manifests a follicular-based eruption characterized histologically by a neutrophilic folliculitis (Borrego 2000).

TRANSIENT ACANTHOLYTIC DERMATOSIS (GROVER DISEASE)

CLINICAL FEATURES

Grover disease was originally defined as a transient, self-limited, acantholytic process that typically affects the front and back of the chest, with occasional lesions on the back or thighs of middle-aged to elderly males. In some cases it may be quite persistent. The cause is not known, but it is included in the consideration of spongiotic dermatitis because multiple forms of acantholysis may be seen in this entity, including spongiotic acantholysis. There appears to be an association with UV light exposure, because eruptions or exacerbations of lesions have occurred after prolonged sun exposure, vacationing in a sunny area, and sunburn from a sunlamp. Grover disease has been considered a reaction to excessive heat and sweating, and associated with ionizing radiation. The medications sulfadoxine–pyrimethamine and recombinant human IL-4 have also been implicated in the development of Grover disease. Oral lesions are rare, as are vesicles and bullae (Parsons 1996). In consequence, the differential diagnosis is that of 'itchy red bump disease,' namely pityrosporum folliculitis, and insect-bite reactions.

HISTOPATHOLOGY

In addition to the spongiotic form of acantholysis, which is admittedly unusual but causes the inclusion of Grover disease and consideration of spongiotic dermatitis, the more common acantholytic patterns are a Darier-like pattern, a Hailey–Hailey-like pattern, and a pemphigus-like pattern. The Darier-like pattern comprises columns of parakeratin-containing corps ronds and grains surmounting an area of suprabasilar acantholysis, often with a small dell, whereas the Hailey–Hailey-like pattern produces acantholysis of virtually the full thickness of the epidermis. The pemphigus-like pattern has a more circumscribed suprabasilar acantholytic morphology. Unlike any of the three prototypic acantholytic disorders that it mimics, Grover disease typically shows smaller foci of acantholysis, which are multiple at any biopsy. A telltale clue is the presence of more than one acantholytic process in a given biopsy. Eosinophils, perivascular lymphoid infiltrate, and dermal hemorrhage may complete the picture.

DIFFERENTIAL DIAGNOSIS

The differential diagnosis includes the prototypic acantholytic process as described above, all separable by the criteria mentioned.

ERYTHEMA TOXICUM NEONATORUM

CLINICAL FEATURES

A common self-limiting disorder in newborn infants, *toxic erythema* may reflect either a form of self-limited graft-versus-host-like reaction from maternal fetal lymphocyte transfer (Bassukas 1992) or a function of viscosity of the newborn extracellular matrix (Stone 1990).

Affecting up to 50% of newborn infants within 12 h of birth and resolving typically in a spontaneous fashion in 2–7 days, infants manifest erythematous macules or papules, associated in 10% of cases with pustule formation. Lesions vary in size and number and tend to involve the trunk preferentially and less often the face, as well as the proximal thighs. Peripheral blood eosinophilia may be seen (Schwartz and Janniger 1996).

HISTOPATHOLOGY

Although the pustular lesions show subcorneal involvement in the territory of the hair follicle, which is striking, often contain eosinophils, and call to mind eosinophilic folliculitis, the macular lesions produce a nonspecific histomorphology comprising dermal edema and a perivascular lymphocytic and eosinophilic infiltrate (**Fig 19.17** overleaf). When papules are biopsied, that morphology is accompanied by neutrophils and/or eosinophils in the outer ridges of the hair follicle structures.

DIFFERENTIAL DIAGNOSIS

An important distinction must be made, namely, with incontinentia pigmenti. Although eosinophils may be seen in the epidermis of erythema neonatorum the process is typically folliculocentric. In addition, in incontinentia pigmenti, there is conspicuous dyskeratosis involving the mid- and upper layers of the epidermis. Miliaria shows a neutrophil-rich pustule that forms typically within the acrosyringium; a more detailed description of miliaria is given below.

MILIARIA

CLINICAL FEATURES AND HISTOPATHOLOGY

The rashes of miliaria are held to reflect abnormalities and/or blockage of acrosyringes and can be subdivided into *eccrine* or *apocrine miliaria*. Further subdivision depends on the theoretical location of the blockade within the eccrine apparatus. Blocking the superficial acrosyrinx produces *miliaria crystalline* and *miliaria rubra*, in which pustular spongiotic microvesicles are noted within the intraepidermal portion of the sweat duct. In addition to pustulation based on the acrosyrinx, a subcorneal vesicle filled with fluid and neutrophils is commonly seen (Straka *et al.* 1991).

In the setting of *miliaria crystalline*, the clinical concomitant is that of 1- to 2-mm vesicles filled with clear fluid and unaccompanied by erythema; these are asymptomatic lesions that occur typically on the trunk (Arpey *et al.* 1992). *Miliaria rubra* or prickly heat rash produces 1- to 2-mm erythematous papules and vesicles on the trunk and groin associated with a prickly sensation. The pathophysiology may involve production of toxins by coagulase-negative staphylococci which damage the ductal epithelium (Mowad *et al.* 1995).

The third type of miliaria, *miliaria profunda*, is also termed 'tropical anhidrotic asthenia;' it is seen in military personnel serving in the tropics and is held to represent a blockade of the lower acrosyrinx that results in a loss of a capacity to sweat and, so, to control temperature and electrolytes (Kirk *et al.* 1996). The corresponding histology shows involvement not only of the acrosyrinx but also of the eccrine coil with a lymphocytic infiltrate and dermal edema.

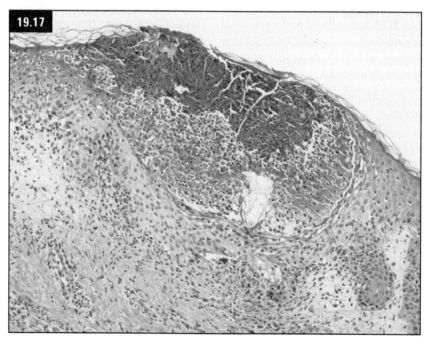

Fig 19.17 Erythema neonatorum can be viewed as neonatal eosinophilic folliculitis. One observes a striking inflammatory response centered on a small follicle. The follicular infiltrate includes numerous eosinophils, neutrophils, Langerhans cells, and lymphocytes.

CHAPTER 20

ERYTHRODERMIC/EXFOLIATIVE DERMATITIS

Daniel H. Parish, Noah Scheinfeld, and Jane M. Grant-Kels

Exfoliative erythroderma is an uncommon, widespread dermatitis of varying etiology, often with scaling and continuous exfoliation involving 90% or more of the total skin surface area (Rothe *et al.* 2000, 2005, Berth-Jones 2002). Affected patients often present with malaise, shivering, and chills as a result of altered thermoregulation from widespread vasodilation, itching, pain, alopecia, and painful fissuring of the palms (**Fig 20.1**) and soles. The clinical course may be complicated by sepsis, high-output heart failure, hypoalbuminemia with edema (**Fig 20.2**), and other metabolic abnormalities, so recognition and appropriate management are vital. Erythroderma usually results from a chronic pre-existing dermatosis, lymphomatous infiltration of the skin, a reaction to a drug, or uncommonly

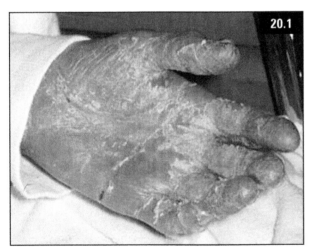

Fig 20.1 Painful fissuring of the hands in a patient with Sézary syndrome. (Reprinted from Rothe *et al.* 2005. © 2005 with permission from Elsevier.)

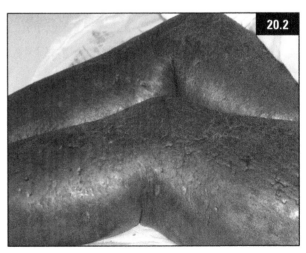

Fig 20.2 Extensive edema and fissuring in a woman with erythroderma from advanced mycosis fungoides.

as a paraneoplastic phenomenon (Grant-Kels *et al.* 2007). The most common causes are psoriasis (23%) (**Figs 20.3** and **20.4**), atopic dermatitis and other spongiotic dermatoses (20%), drug-induced hypersensitivity reactions (15%), and cutaneous T-cell lymphoma (5%), although this varies somewhat in different clinical series. In approximately 20% of cases no underlying cause can be identified (idiopathic erythroderma).

Rarer causes of erythroderma in adults include: (1) other spongiotic dermatoses such as seborrheic dermatitis, allergic contact dermatitis, and stasis dermatitis, (2) pityriasis rubra pilaris (4%), (3) immunobullous diseases especially pemphigus foliaceous, (4) infections such as crusted (Norwegian) scabies (**Fig 20.5**) or HIV disease, (5) graft-versus-host disease (GVHD), (6) lichen planus, (7) sarcoidosis, (8) collagen vascular diseases, eg, dermatomyositis and lupus erythematosus, (9) chronic actinic dermatitis, and (10) underlying neoplasms (paraneoplastic).

As pre-existing skin diseases cause more than half the cases of erythroderma, it is important to inquire about any history of previous conditions such as psoriasis or atopic dermatitis, and to identify exacerbating factors that might have triggered erythroderma, eg, a patient with stable plaque psoriasis might give a history of a burn during phototherapy or having started a new medication such as propranolol. That said, it is also important to investigate alternative causes unrelated to the primary dermatosis because patients with pre-existing psoriasis have been reported with erythroderma from malignancy and drugs.

Exfoliative erythroderma (EE) may result from direct infiltration of the skin by a cutaneous T-cell lymphoma (CTCL) or be caused by an underlying visceral tumor. Erythrodermic mycosis fungoides as opposed to Sézary syndrome lacks hematological involvement. The term 'Sézary syndrome' specifically implies significant involvement of the peripheral blood with malignant atypical lymphocytes in addition to erythrodermic mycosis fungoides (leukemic phase of mycosis fungoides [MF]). Recent work suggests there may be fundamental differences between MF and

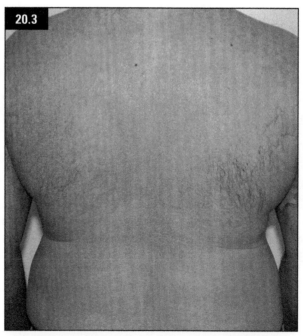

Fig 20.3 Psoriatic erythroderma. (Courtesy of UCONN Department of Dermatology collection c/o Dr Justin Finch.)

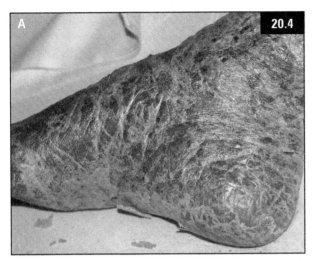

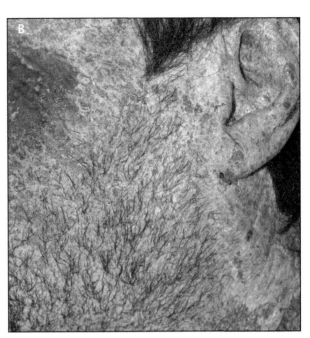

Fig 20.4 Psoriatic erythroderma: in this patient the cause of the erythroderma is suggested by the silvery scaling seen here on (A) the feet and (B) the face.

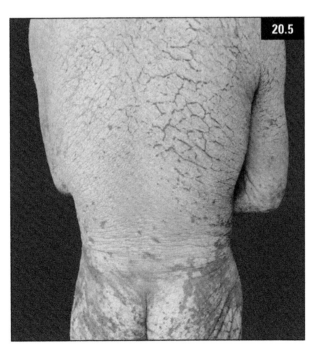

Fig 20.5 Extensive crusted scabies causing erythroderma. (Reprinted from Ekmekci and Koslu 2006 with permission.)

Sézary syndrome with the latter being a malignancy of central memory T cells and MF a malignancy of skin-resident, effector, memory T cells (Campbell *et al.* 2010). Sézary syndrome is typically accompanied by lymphadenopathy and hepatomegaly (Kotz *et al.* 2003).

The diagnosis of Sézary syndrome is established if more than 20% of circulating lymphocytes are identified as Sézary cells on a peripheral smear or by flow cytometry. The presence of fewer than 10% Sézary cells (<10% circulating lymphocytes) is considered nonspecific because it has occasionally been reported in association with atopic dermatitis, psoriasis, lichen planus, discoid lupus erythematosus, and parapsoriasis (Harmon *et al.* 1996). Large Sézary cells easily recognizable on peripheral blood films are found in only 20% of cases of Sézary syndrome. Diagnosis of Sézary syndrome by peripheral smear may be problematic in patients with small (<12 μm)

or intermediate size (12–14 μm) Sézary cells (Russell-Jones and Whittaker 2000) (**Fig 20.6**).

Certain clinical features favor a diagnosis of Sézary syndrome over that of erythrodermic MF. These include extreme pruritus and prominent involvement of the head, neck, palms, and soles. Patients with longstanding Sézary syndrome may have a painful fissured palmoplantar keratoderma and leonine facies (**Fig 20.7**) or alopecia (**Fig 20.8**) from lymphomatous cutaneous infiltration of the face or scalp.

Other malignancies can cause exfoliative erythroderma as well. Adult T-cell leukemia/lymphoma (ATLL) is a neoplastic disease caused by human T-lymphotropic virus type 1 (HTLV-1), an RNA retrovirus (Matutes 2007). Erythroderma may occur with ATLL from massive infiltration of leukemic cells in the skin. Other reticuloendothelial neoplasms, such as acute and chronic leukemia, and less commonly internal visceral malignancies (eg, carcinoma of the colon, lung, prostate thyroid,

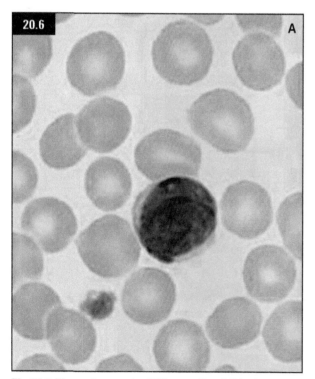 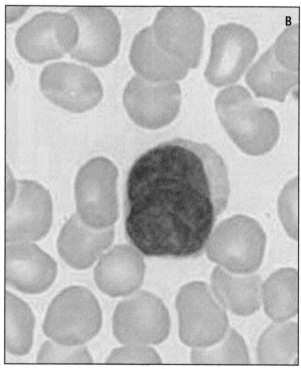

Fig 20.6 Photomicrograph of (A) a small and (B) a large Sézary cell on blood smear from different patients with Sézary syndrome. Note relative cell sizes in relationship to the size of an erythrocyte which is about 7 μm in diameter. (Photograph courtesy of Georges Flandrin, MD, Paris, France.)

fallopian tube, larynx, and esophagus), can also cause erythroderma (Rosen *et al.* 1979). On occasion, erythroderma can be the presenting sign of the underlying malignancy. Kokturk *et al.* (2004) reported the case of a 74-year-old male who developed recalcitrant seborrheic dermatitis that evolved into erythroderma as a paraneoplastic manifestation of lung carcinoma (Kokturk *et al.* 2004).

Medications are a common cause of erythroderma. Over 100 different drugs, including physician-prescribed medications, over-the-counter preparations, herbal supplements, and homeopathic agents, have been implicated. Usually, medication-induced erythroderma develops abruptly and progresses over a short period of time; thankfully, once the culprit drug has been identified and eliminated, the eyrthroderma usually resolves fairly rapidly. On the other hand, certain drugs such as antibiotics, anticonvulsants, dapsone, and others can cause erythroderma in the context of the *drug*

hypersensitivity syndrome. These reactions are accompanied by fever, edema, lymphadenopathy, organomegaly, abnormal renal and liver function, leukocytosis, and eosinophilia, and often do not develop until 2–6 weeks after the introduction of the medication. DRESS syndrome (drug reaction with eosinophilia and systemic symptoms) refers to the aforementioned type of drug hypersensitivity when accompanied by eosinophilia. Erythroderma from these agents may persist for months after discontinuation of the culprit drug, and result in liver failure and hypothyroidism. It cannot be overemphasized how important it is to obtain an accurate and detailed history of medication and supplement use in evaluating and treating the erythrodermic patient. Management can be quite complicated when the patient is receiving multiple medications for diabetes, hypertension, or tuberculosis, where stopping a medication may cause complications.

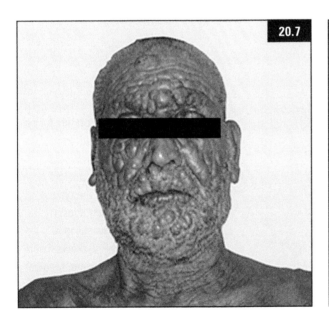

Fig 20.7 Sézary syndrome presenting with *leonine facies.* (Reprinted from Nassem *et al.* 2009. © 2009 Nassem *et al.* and the Australasian College of Dermatologists with permission from John Wiley & Sons.)

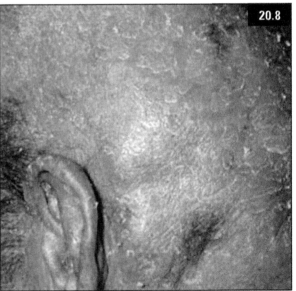

Fig 20.8 Diffuse alopecia in a patient with chronic idiopathic erythroderma. (Reprinted from Rothe *et al.* 2005. © 2005, with permission from Elsevier.)

PEDIATRIC AND NEONATAL ERYTHRODERMA

Erythroderma in children and in the neonatal period can be caused by: psoriasis, atopic dermatitis, seborrheic dermatitis, drug reactions, infections (especially staphylococcal scalded skin syndrome), congenital ichthyoses such as bullous and nonbullous congenital ichthyosiform erythroderma, Netherton syndrome (**Fig 20.9**), and various immunodeficiency syndromes.

Some reports in the literature suggest that erythroderma in young people is most commonly caused by seborrheic dermatitis and genodermatoses. In a case series of 42 children in Iraq, etiologies for erythroderma included seborrheic dermatitis (21.4%), atopic dermatitis (14.3%), different types of ichthyoses (31.5%), psoriasis (4.7%), pityriasis rubra pilaris (2.4%), staphylococcal scalded skin syndrome (7.14%), Netherton syndrome (4.7%), and immune deficiency syndromes (4.8%) (Al-Dhalimi 2007). In 9.5% of the patients the cause of the erythroderma remained undetermined. Biopsies obtained in 29 patients showed nonspecific histopathology in 58.7% of the specimens reviewed. The underlying etiology could be established histopathologically in only 41.3% of the patients.

Sarkar *et al.* (1999) reported on 17 children with erythroderma in India with a median age of 3.3 years. The erythroderma was caused by drugs (29%), genodermatoses (18%), psoriasis (18%), staphylococcal scalded skin syndrome (18%), atopic dermatitis 12%, and in one patient, infantile seborrheic dermatitis coexisting with dermatophytosis.

Infectious causes of neonatal erythroderma include staphylococcal scalded skin syndrome, toxic shock syndrome, and congenital cutaneous candidiasis. Congenital cutaneous candidiasis is caused by an ascending infection involving the amnion. A resulting widely distributed macular, papular, and pustular eruption can evolve into erythroderma (Glassman and Muglia 1993).

Children with erythroderma and fever are at risk for hypotension and shock (Byer and Bachur 2006). In a study of 56 patients aged 19 years or less, who presented to an emergency department with fever of 38°C or more and erythroderma (defined as a

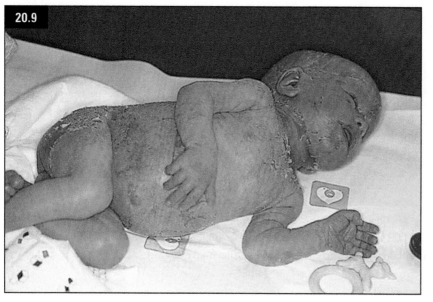

Fig 20.9 Exfoliative erythroderma in a neonate with Netherton syndrome. In the first weeks of life, the erythroderma is not specific. Often, the typical circumflex linear ichthyosis appears several weeks later. (Reprinted from Pruszkowski *et al.* 2000. © 2000 American Medical Association. All rights reserved.)

persistent, nonpatchy, diffuse erythema or 'sunburn erythema'), 18% presented with hypotension. Of the remaining patients who were normotensive on arrival in the emergency department, a third developed shock and many required vasopressors. The most important predictors of incipient toxic shock syndrome were age 3 years or more, ill appearance, elevated creatinine, and hypotension on presentation. In addition, the presence of vomiting and identification of a focal bacterial source were also important predictors of shock. Thus, the acute appearance of erythroderma in children with fever should be considered an emergency necessitating hospital admission.

EPIDEMIOLOGY

Erythroderma remains rare worldwide and incidence rates tend to vary in different geographic areas, eg, there was an incidence of 35 cases of erythroderma per 100 000 outpatients at a dermatology clinic in the Indian subcontinent, whereas the Netherlands reported an incidence of 0.9 per 100 000 cases (Sehgal *et al.* 2004). The variability in presentation and nonuniform reporting procedures may contribute to this difference in incidence rates. In general, erythroderma in adults is more common in males whereas, in children, females are more likely to be affected.

The proportion of cases attributable to a given cause varies with the patient population studied. In young adults, the leading cause is medications. The cause also varies by country. In a study from South Africa, atopic dermatitis (23.9%), psoriasis (23.9%), and drug reactions (22.5%) were the most common causes of erythroderma (Morar *et al.* 1999). However, in the HIV-positive group, drug reactions (40.6%) caused most cases and the most common causative drug identified was ethambutol (30.8%).

EVALUATION

A detailed and comprehensive past medical history, including previous illnesses, use of oral and topical medications and supplements, as well as sunlight/ultraviolet light exposure, is essential in identifying the underlying causative condition or trigger of erythroderma. Patients should be asked about a personal or family history of psoriasis, atopic dermatitis or other manifestations of atopy, possible risk factors for HIV or HTLV-1 infection, swollen glands, and weight loss.

Multiple skin-punch biopsies are the most helpful laboratory test performed. As approximately a third of the biopsies submitted will fail to reveal the diagnostic features of the underlying etiology of the erythroderma, multiple biopsies are required. Any single biopsy has only a 50% chance of revealing diagnostic pathology.

Other laboratory findings are not especially helpful in defining the underlying etiology for EE. Patients with erythroderma of any cause may have leukocytosis, lymphocytosis, eosinophilia, anemia, elevated erythrocyte sedimentation rates, C-reactive proteins, increased serum IgE, elevated creatinine levels, elevated uric acid, decreased serum protein levels, and hypoalbuminemia. However, patients with abnormal serum protein electrophoresis with a polyclonal elevation in the γ-globulin region may have an underlying myeloproliferative disorder that manifests as erythroderma.

Patients with atopic dermatitis can have elevated IgE levels. Leukemia as the cause for erythroderma can be diagnosed by complete blood counts, peripheral smear examination, and bone marrow studies. Assessing blood for circulating Sézary cells can make the diagnosis of this syndrome only if the Sézary cells are identified in large and certain quantities. Immunophenotyping of skin lymphocytes and gene rearrangement studies can also be helpful in differentiating a possible malignant lymphoproliferative disorder. A skin scraping with oil can be helpful for diagnosis of scabies and should be performed.

CLINICAL MANIFESTATIONS AND SYMPTOMS

Exfoliative erythroderma starts with erythematous patches that become confluent, covering the greater part of the cutaneous surface. Desquamation or shedding occurs usually 2–6 days after the onset of erythema. The quality of the desquamation can be variable and can appear as fine flakes or large sheets of skin (**Figs 20.10** and **20.11**). Erythrodermic scale often possesses a white to yellow hue and is generally fine. Thick scale can develop in the scalp, although this might be a manifestation of psoriasis or seborrheic dermatitis. Larger scales may be seen in more acute cases and also on the palms and soles. Pruritus related to erythroderma is near constant and can be intolerable.

Erythrodermic skin can develop a shiny look as a result of epidermal thinning. Progressive edema secondary to the cutaneous inflammation and gradual lichenification of the skin can result in tightening of the skin, which may limit range of motion and cause pain on movement. Eyelid swelling may result in ectropion. Impaired epidermal integrity can lead to yellow or straw-colored serosanguineous exudation that causes dressings and clothing to adhere to the skin. Once erythroderma takes on a more chronic course, the hair and nails also become affected and may both begin to shed. Nails become ridged and brittle, and splinter hemorrhages are commonly seen. Patients with Sézary syndrome may have total loss of body hair (Bi *et al.* 2011).

At times, clinical clues to the etiology of the underlying erythroderma may be recognized among the generalized erythema and desquamation, eg, typical psoriatic plaques with silvery scales may still be evident on physical examination (see **Fig 20.4**). Classic lichenified lesions in the antecubital and popliteal fossae may suggest underlying atopic dermatitis. As erythroderma usually does not involve mucosal surfaces, lesions of the buccal mucosa along with violaceous papules may point to an underlying lichen planus. Salmon-colored erythroderma with islands of sparing, follicular papules, and palmoplantar keratoderma are suggestive of pityriasis rubra pilaris. Lymphadenopathy, organomegaly, and fever, along with a history of recently starting a new drug, should direct the clinician to explore a possible drug-related etiology.

Alternatively, lymphadenopathy along with leonine facies (see **Fig 20.7**) and alopecia should warrant suspicion for CTCL. Collarettes of scales and flaccid blisters suggest underlying superficial pemphigus. Muscle weakness, heliotrope sign, Gottron papules, poikiloderma, and periungual telengiectasis hint at underlying dermatomyositis.

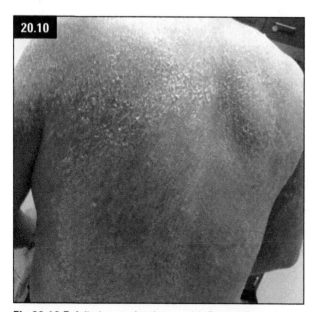

Fig 20.10 Exfoliative erythroderma with fine scaling.

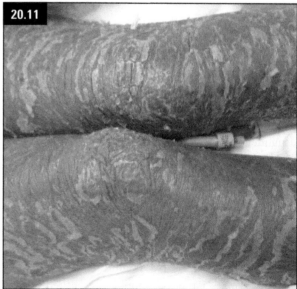

Fig 20.11 Psoriatic erythroderma with large scales.

SYSTEMIC COMPLICATIONS

The body goes into a catabolic state in patients with exfoliative erythroderma, often leading to weight loss. It is thought that displacement of albumin into the skin and loss of albumin from the shedding skin accounts for hypoalbuminemia and subsequent peripheral edema (Parving *et al.* 1976). Dilation of dermal blood vessels and shunting of blood into the skin causes heat loss and dysregulation of core body temperature, chills, and shivering. The increased blood flow to the skin can also lead to high-output cardiac failure and tachycardia (Shuster 1963). As a result of the ineffective epidermal protective layer, there is increased loss of fluids, leading to fluid and electrolyte imbalances, similar to those that occur in burn patients. Stress on the heart and lungs can lead to systemic collapse, especially in older patients. Finally, increased susceptibility to cutaneous bacterial colonization may result in sepsis.

HISTOPATHOLOGY

Histopathological evaluation of multiple skin biopsies of patients with EE may provide critical information to help pinpoint the precise etiology. A study investigating the accuracy of histopathological diagnosis in erythroderma performed by four dermatopathologists found a mean accuracy of 53% (range 48–66%) (Walsh *et al.* 1994). Histopathological examination was effective in identifying underlying psoriasis, spongiotic dermatitis, and CTCL as the cause to a much greater extent than in identifying drug eruptions and pityriasis rubra pilaris. The study also concluded that epidermotropism might be mistaken for inflammatory interface changes of drug eruptions rather than a clue to CTCL, and vice versa.

Many nonspecific histological features can be identified in a biopsy of erythroderma, including hyperkeratosis, parakeratosis, epidermal hyperplasia, and chronic inflammation. These features are nondiagnostic and can mask the diagnostic features of the underlying disease entity causing the erythroderma. Although certain changes may suggest a specific diagnosis, serial biopsies may be necessary to arrive at a definitive diagnosis. Vacuolar changes and diffusely dispersed necrotic keratinocytes, along with perivascular inflammation and the presence of eosinophils, are all characteristics of drug-induced erythroderma.

An interface dermatitis without eosinophils and with increased mucin in the dermis is consistent with an underlying collagen vascular disease. Interface dermatitis with satellite cell necrosis in the appropriate clinical setting suggests that a diagnosis of possible GVHD be explored. Psoriasis characteristically displays regular epidermal hyperplasia with elongation of rete ridges, hyperkeratosis with confluent parakeratosis, loss of the granular layer, spongiform pustules, neutrophils in the stratum corneum, and dilated and tortuous papillary blood vessels. Epidermal hyperplasia with horizontal and vertical alternating orthokeratosis and parakeratosis, with some dilated plugged follicular infundibula, suggests pityriasis rubra pilaris rather than psoriasis. Atopic dermatitis may show spongiosis and eosinophils within a superficial lymphocytic perivascular infiltrate. The same histopathology may occur in allergic contact dermatitis so correlation of histological findings and clinical history is important.

Other histopathological patterns may be encountered as well. Spongiotic dermatitis in association with parakeratosis and neutrophils at the lips of follicular ostia suggests seborrheic dermatitis. Atypical mononuclear cells, singly along the basal cell layer and in groups within the epidermis unassociated with significant spongiosis but often with a lichenoid infiltrate, suggest the possibility of CTCL. Intraepidermal bullae with acantholysis indicate pemphigus, whereas subepidermal bullae and eosinophilic spongiosis suggest pemphigoid. Direct immunofluorescence is recommended in these cases.

MALIGNANCIES AND NONDERMATOLOGICAL DISEASES AS CAUSES OF ERYTHRODERMA

In various series and case reports erythroderma has been reported in association with malignancies other than CTCL. Nicolis and Helwig (1973) reported cases associated with Hodgkin disease, non-Hodgkin lymphoma, leukemia, and carcinoma of the prostate, lung, thyroid, and liver.

Additional cases with visceral neoplasms have included melanoma, ovarian, breast, rectal, and mammary carcinoma (Thestrup-Pedersen *et al.* 1988), laryngeal carcinoma (Faure *et al.* 1985), esophageal cancer (Deffer *et al.* 1985), prostate carcinoma (Momm *et al.* 2002), renal carcinoma (Tebbe *et al.* 1991), fallopian tube carcinoma (Axelrod *et al.* 1988), and malignant histiocytosis (Patrizi *et al.* 1990). In general, association with visceral neoplasm is much less common than association with lymphoreticular malignancy.

Further cancer screening evaluation should be performed according to the most recent age-appropriate guidelines.

Erythrodermic reactions are also observed in a variety of immunological disorders such as hypogammaglobulinemia, GVHD, and Di George syndrome. Therefore a clinical history and evaluation of the patient's immune status should be considered.

Erythroderma has also been reported in patients with HIV infection in various populations. HIV/AIDS was the cause of erythroderma in 4.6% of cases in a series from Nairobi, Kenya (Munyao *et al.* 2007). As HIV-infected patients have a high frequency of drug eruptions and other dermatoses, these diagnoses should be ruled out before blaming the HIV infection itself. HIV infection was common among erythroderma patients in a series from South Africa; among these, 40.6% were associated with a drug, 25% with psoriasis, 6.3% with Reiter disease, 12.5% with seborrheic dermatitis, and 3.13% with pityriasis rubra pilaris (Morar *et al.* 1999). Occasionally, AIDS patients experience erythroderma during conversion from HIV to AIDS. Thus HIV polymerase chain reaction (PCR) testing is essential if there is a reason to suspect a seroconversion reaction (Sehgal and Srivastava 2006). The link between AIDS and erythroderma highlights a possible immunological imbalance and/or disturbance, serving as a trigger, causing the downstream dermatological manifestations of inflammation, erythema, and scaling.

Presumed idiopathic exfoliative erythroderma cases require repeat skin biopsies sequentially over time in addition to other studies, because a later diagnosis of a specific condition has been identified in up to half of such patients. Multiple biopsies are a critical component in establishing the primary etiology in these erythroderma patients.

PATHOPHYSIOLOGY

A variety of cutaneous and systemic diseases can manifest as exfoliative erythroderma. Although the exact mechanism of erythrodermic reactions is unknown, it is currently thought that a complicated interaction of adhesion molecules, cytokines, interleukins, and tumor necrosis factor (TNF) results in increased rates of epidermal turnover, contributing to the red and rapidly peeling skin. However, Sigurdsson *et al.* (2000) failed to find specific expression patterns of adhesion molecules in various underlying skin conditions that eventually led to the erythroderma. Thus the final common mechanism that leads to an erythrodermic reaction has not been fully elucidated.

IgE levels may be elevated in erythroderma, particularly when the underlying cause is atopic dermatitis. However, the IgE marker alone is not a diagnostic tool, because IgE production might also be evident in psoriasis (via a secondary mechanism) and also in hyper-IgE syndrome (via decreased interferon-γ production).

In erythroderma, epidermal cells migrate through the epidermis faster and mature faster than in normal skin, resulting in premature loss of proteins and vitamins. This contributes to some of the systemic manifestations of the disease and nutritional deficits, which must be addressed in these patients.

Although linked to an immunological disturbance, the exact immunological mechanism leading to erythroderma is currently unknown. As mechanisms of underlying etiologies that can lead to erythroderma become elucidated, however, they provide a glimpse into potential routes via which erythrodermic reactions may develop and thus be therapeutically halted, eg, atopic dermatitis, which is one cause of erythroderma, has recently been shown to be highly linked to the peroxisome proliferator-activated receptor γ (PPAR-γ). Dahten et al. (2007) have demonstrated an increased PPAR-γ expression in patients with atopic dermatitis. These PPAR receptors act as transcription factors and convert external environmental cues into internal signals, affecting cellular response. As a result treatments based on development of ligands for PPAR-γ may be promising therapeutically for EE due to atopic dermatitis in the future.

TREATMENT

In general patients with symptomatic EE are hospitalized. Whether a patient needs to be hospitalized depends on age, underlying medical condition, presence of fever, chills, pain, metabolic abnormalities, and the presumed underlying etiology. Those patients with compromised cardiovascular status, respiratory problems, and possible infection definitely require inpatient therapy.

Treatment of erythroderma is twofold: (1) amelioration of its potentially acute life-threatening complications and (2) therapy of the underlying cause. Thus, when a patient advances to EE, stabilization with fluids and electrolytes along with patient comfort is the key goal. In the hospitalized patient, analgesia, wet dressings, bland emollients (eg, petroleum jelly), and systemic corticosteroids (if underlying psoriasis is not suspected) are recognized therapies to help reduce inflammation and stabilize the patient (Anderson and Loeffel 1970). With increased protein loss, nutritional supplementation is essential.

The role of oral steroids for treatment of erythroderma is not clear. In particular, the use of oral steroids is considered by most clinicians to be contraindicated in psoriasis even if the psoriasis has evolved to the erythrodermic stage. Topical corticosteroids along with emollients have been the mainstay of topical treatment in the treatment of erythroderma from various causes, including atopic dermatitis. Although topical tacrolimus has been considered, the risk of absorption in erythrodermic

patients with impaired barrier function and widespread involvement precludes its use. Successful treatment of recalcitrant, erythroderma-associated pruritus with etanercept has been reported (Querfeld et al. 2004).

It is recommended that drugs that might have precipitated the erythroderma be identified and discontinued immediately. A diet high in protein that exceeds normal caloric requirements should also be instituted along with folate supplementation.

It is extremely important to make an accurate etiological diagnosis. Use of inappropriate treatments can have disastrous consequences such as flare of CTCL with immunosuppressive agents and anti-TNF biologics (Adams et al. 2004, Lafaille et al. 2009, Quéreux et al. 2010). Psoriatic erythroderma is responsive to methotrexate, acitretin, cyclosporine (ciclosporin), mycophenolate mofetil, and some biologics such as infliximab alone or in combination with methotrexate (Rongioletti et al. 2003, Heikkilä et al. 2005, Lewis et al. 2006). Unfortunately, most recommendations are based on individual case reports and small case series. Infliximab and cyclosporine have been recommended in appropriate patients where a rapid response is deemed necessary (Rosenbach et al. 2010). Recently ustekinumab proved efficacious in two patients with psoriatic erythroderma resistant to anti-TNF therapy (Santos-Juanes et al. 2010).

Exfoliative erythroderma due to CTCL may be treated with topical steroids, PUVA (psoralen + ultraviolet A), electron beam, systemic chemotherapy, extracorporeal photo(chemo)therapy, interferon-α, bexarotene, or denileukin diftitox. Atopic dermatitis is generally responsive to a course of systemic steroids or other systemic medications including methotrexate, cyclosporine, and mycophenolate mofetil. Azathioprine has also on occasion proved helpful but has a very slow onset of action. Pityriasis rubra pilaris is generally responsive to systemic retinoids, methotrexate, and infliximab (Müller et al. 2008).

Based on the notion that wound healing is favored by a wet as opposed to a dry environment, the use of wet-wrap treatments has been advocated (Oranje et al. 2006). Dry skin has lost its normal functional and physiological integrity, contributing to increased water evaporation from lesions, decreased sebaceous gland secretions, and reduced protection from the environment. Affected areas are predisposed to barrier invasion by microorganisms, decreased threshold for inflammation, and chronic wound-like conditions. Wet dressings aid in maintaining moisture and serve to cool the skin, which can lead to anti-inflammatory and antipruritic effects (Oranje *et al.* 2006). There are several variations in technique for wet-wrap treatments, including single- or double-layer wraps, and the addition of creams and ointments as adjuncts to the wraps. Each of these variations of wet-wrap treatment has similar success; however, the addition of ointment has sometimes been associated with an increased risk of folliculitis. It is common to incorporate topical corticosteroids along with wet-wrap dressings. Dilution of the topical corticosteroids together with patient education about appropriate utilization of wet-wrap treatments help to greatly decrease risk of adverse events.

The patient optimally should be kept in a warm and humid environment. Skin care should be gentle and topical irritants must be avoided. Symptomatic treatments include antihistamines for the pruritus, leg elevation, and diuretics for persistent leg edema. Systemic antibiotics are sometimes used to reduce colonization but are generally reserved for secondary infections.

PROGNOSIS

The outcome of erythroderma depends on the original cause and the underlying health of the patient. Drug-induced erythroderma usually appears suddenly and clears rapidly with discontinuation of the causative drug. The exception to this is erythroderma due to a severe drug hypersensitivity reaction (DRESS syndrome), as has been reported secondary to some antibiotics, anticonvulsants, and allopurinol. This hypersensitivity reaction develops within 2–6 weeks after the medication was initiated and may persist for weeks after discontinuation of the medication. Erythroderma due to psoriasis or a spongiotic dermatitis usually clears within several weeks to months but can be chronic. Approximately 15% of cases of erythrodermic psoriasis recur. Erythrodermic CTCL and erythroderma associated with an underlying malignancy are often persistent and refractory to treatment. Idiopathic erythroderma, especially in older male patients, is likely to evolve into CTCL.

Early case series of erythroderma reported a significant death rate but more recent studies have reported better overall survival (Rothe *et al.* 2000). Most deaths have been related to pneumonia, cardiac failure, sepsis, and especially lymphoproliferative malignancy. Deaths in erythroderma patients have also been reported in patients with underlying pemphigus, severe drug eruptions, or idiopathic erythroderma.

SEQUELAE OF ERYTHRODERMA

A number of alterations in the skin can result from erythroderma. Postinflammatory hyper- and hypopigmentation occur, particularly in patients of color. A distinctive nail abnormality, *shoreline nails*, in which a transverse line of discontinuity is preceded by a transverse band of leukonychia, has been described in patients with drug-induced erythroderma (Shelley and Shelley 1985). An abnormality of keratinization causing leukonychia is followed by matrix arrest which causes the transverse line.

In psoriatic individuals, nail dystrophy after erythroderma is common. In addition, the inflammation and edema in the periorbital region may result in ectropion and epiphora (Thomson and Berth-Jones 2009). Erythroderma not uncommonly involves the scalp, with 25% of patients developing alopecia. Rare cases of eruptive seborrheic keratoses have been described in patients with erythroderma (Flugman *et al.* 2001, Sahin *et al.* 2004). These may resolve with improvement of the erythroderma.

CONCLUSION

Exfoliative erythroderma is a potentially life-threatening reaction caused by a number of inflammatory, neoplastic, and infectious skin and systemic diseases. Prompt diagnosis of the underlying cause is essential for successful treatment. Morbidity and mortality are dependent on the promptness of treatment, the underlying etiology, and the underlying health of the patient.

In healthy adults, mortality is low. In children the potential mortality rate is higher, especially in those whose disease is due to a genetic defect. As with many other diseases in dermatology, the exact molecular pathogenesis remains to be defined. As the manifestations of erythroderma are well known to dermatologists but poorly appreciated by other specialists, dermatological input in the care of these patients is mandatory.

Clinical suggestions

1. Assess and treat erythrodermic patients for signs of temperature dysregulation (usually manifested by chills), peripheral edema, cardiovascular decompensation, lymphadenopathy, hepatosplenomegaly, and sepsis (with blood cultures). With increased protein loss, nutritional supplementation with a diet high in protein which exceeds normal caloric requirement is indicated.
2. Look for subtle signs or pre-existing dermatoses (eg, nail changes of psoriasis or pityriasis rubra pilaris) and obtain multiple skin biopsies.
3. The patient should optimally be kept in a warm and humid environment. Symptomatic treatments include antihistamines for the pruritus, leg elevation, and diuretics for persistent leg edema.
4. Adequate analgesia, gentle local skin-care measures such as wet dressings or oatmeal baths followed by bland emollients (eg, petroleum jelly), and low- to moderate-potency topical corticosteroids should be instituted.
5. Discontinue any drugs that are possibly implicated in causing the erythroderma.
6. Specific interventions with systemic corticosteroids, acitretin, infliximab, methotrexate, or other agents will be determined by the underlying condition.

CHAPTER 21

PRIMARY IMMUNODEFICIENCY DISEASES

Adam Friedman, Manju Chacko Dawkins, and Donald Rudikoff

INTRODUCTION

Primary immunodeficiency diseases (PIDs) comprise more than 130 usually monogenic genetic disorders which influence the development and/or function of the immune system (Notarangelo 2010). Although some primary immune defects are detected in adulthood, others characteristically present in infancy and early childhood with recurrent, atypical, and recalcitrant infections, often accompanied by mucocutaneous manifestations, diarrhea, and failure to thrive (Berron-Ruiz *et al.* 2000, Sillevis Smitt *et al.* 2005, Notarangelo 2010). Not only is early recognition vital for treatment, affecting patient survival and quality of life, but it also alerts clinicians to the need for genetic counseling, identification of asymptomatic carriers, and prenatal testing in family members.

Cutaneous findings include abscesses, petechiae/purpura, telangiectasias, granulomas, chronic candidal infections, angioedema, lupus-like findings, pigmentary changes, seborrhea-like dermatitis, and eczematous eruptions (Paller 2005). Eczematous eruptions in some cases meet standard criteria for atopic dermatitis and in other cases are atypical with seborrheic and other non-specific features.

Four diseases that regularly present with an atopic-like eczema are Wiskott–Aldrich syndrome (WAS), hyper-IgE syndrome (HIES), Omenn syndrome, and immune dysregulation, polyendocrinopathy, enteropathy, X-linked syndrome (IPEX) (*Table 21.1*). So-called *atopiform dermatitis* has also been reported less frequently with selective IgA deficiency, selective IgM deficiency, X-linked agammaglobulinemia, X-linked immunodeficiency with hyper-IgM, ataxia telangiectatica, Shwachman syndrome, and chronic granulomatous disease (Saurat *et al.* 1985, Bos 2002).

Dermatologists play a special role in recognizing cutaneous signs and symptoms that indicate severe underlying systemic illnesses. This is especially relevant for PIDs, which can present in the fragile infant population. This chapter reviews the most important PIDs associated with atopic-like dermatitis or eczema, including clinical presentation, pathophysiology, diagnostic work-up, and management, with the hope of facilitating early diagnosis and appropriate management. Patients with severe PIDs should be cared for by immunologists experienced in their management at tertiary care centers with active hemopoietic cell transplantation programs.

Table 21.1   Primary immunodeficiency disease syndromes with eczematous dermatitis

CONDITION	GENETIC BASIS	AGE AT PRESENTATION	CUTANEOUS FINDINGS
Wiskott–Aldrich syndrome	X-linked recessive; mutations in the *WASP* gene	First days of life	Patient presents with petechiae and bruising Eczematous eruption develops after 1–2 months of life
Hyper-IgE syndrome	Autosomal dominant and sporadic types → mutation in STAT3 gene Autosomal recessive form → *TyK2* and *DOCK8* mutations	Between end of week 1 up to 3 months	Presents as a pustular eruption Characteristic facies: asymmetry, prominent brow and supraorbital ridge, broad nasal bridge, wide, fleshy nasal tip, and rough skin with prominent pores Eczema Cold abscesses
Omenn syndrome	Autosomal recessive; hypomorphic mutations in recombinase genes *RAG-1* and *RAG-2*	At birth	Presentation: unique generalized erythroderma with features of a subacute eczema and associated desquamation Alopecia universalis may be present Diffuse lymphadenopathy is a key feature Exaggerated skinfolds
Immune dysregulation, polyendocrinopathy, enteropathy, X-linked syndrome (IPEX)	X-linked recessive; mutation in *FOXP3* gene	Infancy (first 4 months of life)	Generalized eczematous eruption → exfoliative erythroderma Cheilitis Urticaria Alopecia universalis

COMMON INFECTIONS

Encapsulated bacteria:
Streptococcus pneumoniae,
Hemophilus influenzae, and
Neisseria meningitidis
Various clinical forms:
furunculosis, conjunctivitis,
otitis media and externa,
sinusitis, pneumonia,
meningitis, and septicemia

Recurrent staphylococcal skin
and soft-tissue infection
Candidiasis
Pseudomonas aeruginosa and
Aspergillus spp. pneumonia
TYK2 → BCG lymphadenitis
(one case)
DOCK8 → viral infections

Staphylococcal sepsis or
Gram-negative enteric bacterial
sepsis associated with
episodes of infectious diarrhea

Recurrent infections more
associated with the need
for indwelling catheters and
immunosuppressive therapy

ASSOCIATED CLINICAL FEATURES

Ophthalmological: hemorrhagic
complications
ENT: gingival bleeding and palatal
petechiae
Hematological: hemolytic anemia,
vasculitis, non-Hodgkin lymphoma
Renal: nephritis
Gastrointestinal (GI): hematochezia,
inflammatory bowel disease

Musculoskeletal: scoliosis, osteoporosis,
craniosynostosis, hemivertebrae, short
limbs, spina bifida, bifid rib
Dental: retained primary teeth owing to
failure of root resorption, noneruption of
permanent teeth, or double rows of teeth
and high arched palate
Vascular: coronary artery tortuosity or
dilation in 70%, coronary aneurysms in
37%, lacunar infarctions
Neurological: Chiari type 1
malformations
Pulmonary: recurrent pneumonia,
pneumatoceles

Failure to thrive
GI: hepatomegaly

Endocrine: diabetes, hypothyroidism,
hyperthyroidism
GI: watery diarrhea, autoimmune
hepatitis
Heme: hemolytic anemia, neutropenia,
thrombocytopenia
Renal: rapidly progressive
glomulonephritis

LABORATORY FEATURES

Elevated immunoglobulin E (IgE)
Thrombocytopenia
Small platelets on peripheral smear

Elevated circulating levels of IgE
>2000 IU/ml
Eosinophilia

Elevated white cell count (WBC)
Elevated IgE
Eosinophilia
Hypogammaglobulinemia

Increased IgE
Increased IgA
Neutropenia, thrombocytopenia
Absence of FOXP3 cells in the
lamina propria and lymphoid
aggregates in intestinal biopsy

Before discussing specific clinical syndromes, it is important to mention the factors that should alert the clinician to the possible presence of immunodeficiency (Box 21.1). Most of these relate to the presence of infections that are atypical, recurrent, chronic, or unresponsive to antibiotic therapy. Failure to thrive, chronic diarrhea, and a positive family history should raise the clinician's index of suspicion.

WISKOTT–ALDRICH SYNDROME

Wiskott–Aldrich syndrome (WAS) is a well-recognized triad of eczema, bleeding diathesis, and recurrent infections, although the complete triad occurs in only 27% of patients (Sullivan *et al.* 1994). With X-linked recessive inheritance, WAS typically occurs in males whereas females act as asymptomatic carriers. The full-blown syndrome can occur rarely in females, however, when the X-chromosome carrying the normal WASP gene is inactivated, leaving the

---

Box 21.1   Warning signs for a primary immunodeficiency disease (PID)

- Infections with atypical presentation, opportunistic organisms, or serious chronic course
- Six or more episodes of otitis media within 1 year
- Antibiotic treatment of bacterial infections for ≥2 months without effect
- Two or more episodes of pneumonia in 1 year
- Failure to thrive, chronic diarrhea
- Persistent oral thrush after 6–12 months of age
- Recurrent deep organ or skin abscesses
- Recurrent serious infections (eg, meningitis, cellulitis, osteomyelitis, sepsis)
- Family history of PID

Reprinted with permission from Sillevis Smitt *et al.* (2005).

WASP-mutated allele active (Andreu *et al.* 2003). WAS is uncommon, with an incidence estimated at 1 in 100 000 births (Puck and Candotti 2006). The spectrum of WAS-related disorders has been expanded to include chronic or intermittent X-linked thrombocytopenia (XLT), a milder variant of WAS, and X-linked neutropenia (Thrasher 2009).

CLINICAL PRESENTATION

Typically a patient affected with WAS presents in the first days of life with petechiae, bruising, and bloody diarrhea resulting from a decreased platelet count and dysfunctional undersized platelets (microthrombocytopenia). Prolonged bleeding after circumcision sometimes unmasks the bleeding tendency (Peacocke and Siminovitch 1992).

Eczema, basically indistinguishable from atopic dermatitis, appears in the first 2 months of life. It may be mild and localized but sometimes severe and resistant to topical therapy. Ophthalmological manifestations may occur including eyelid eczema, dandruff-like flakes on the eyelid margin (scurf), eyelash debris (collars), and dry eye (Rescigno and Dinowitz 2001). Ocular hemorrhagic complications such as subconjunctival hemorrhage, hyphema (blood in the anterior chamber), and vitreous hemorrhage can occur and require prompt ophthalmological consultation. Oral manifestations include gingival bleeding and palatal petechiae (Boraz 1989). Purpura and petechiae typically improve as the child ages. By 5–6 months of age, when residual maternal antibodies have disappeared, the child becomes increasingly susceptible to encapsulated bacteria, such as *Streptococcus pneumoniae*, *Hemophilus influenzae*, and *Neisseria meningitidis*. Infection presents in various forms including furunculosis, conjunctivitis, otitis media and externa, sinusitis, pneumonia, meningitis, and septicemia. Over time, T-cell function deteriorates, enhancing susceptibility to viruses such as molluscum contagiosum and herpes simplex virus, including acyclovir (aciclovir)-resistant forms (St Geme *et al.* 1962, Saijo *et al.* 1998).

Approximately 80% of patients with WAS suffer from atopic-like dermatitis, although it may not be present at the time of initial diagnosis (Sullivan *et al.* 1994). Distribution typically includes the face, upper arms, and back, with relative sparing of the abdomen

(Krivit and Good 1959). The scalp and flexural surfaces may be involved, and sometimes eczema may be diffuse or generalized with widespread lichenification (**Figs 21.1** and **21.2**) (Paller 2003).

A high proportion of WAS patients have elevated IgE levels (Buckley and Fiscus 1975) and urticaria, food allergies, and asthma can be seen, in addition to atopic dermatitis (Imai *et al.* 2004). Patients who have absent or defective WAS protein are more likely to have severe eczema (Imai *et al.* 2004). Furthermore, approximately 40% of WAS patients develop autoimmune disease, including hemolytic anemia, vasculitis, nephritis, immune thrombocytopenia (ITP), and inflammatory bowel disease (Sullivan *et al.* 1994).

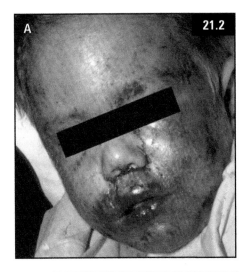

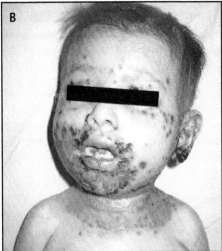

Fig 21.2 Wiskott–Aldrich syndrome: (A) a young child with erosive, eczematous lesions of the cheeks, chin and forehead. (Courtesy of UCONN Dermatology Residency Collection c/o Dr Justin Finch.) (B) Erythematous, desquamative, plaque-like lesions on the entire body, including the scalp; hemorrhagic lesions on the mucosal sites; and candidiasis on the tongue. (Courtesy of M. Davutoglu. Reprinted from Davutoglu *et al.* 2009.)

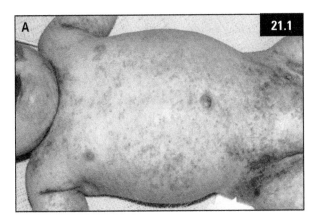

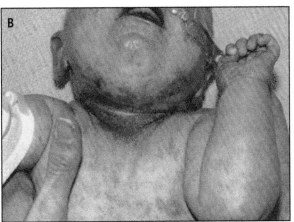

Fig 21.1 Wiskott–Aldrich syndrome: scaly erythematous plaques, predominantly over the head and neck, maceration in flexural regions, and scattered petechiae diffusely over the body. (Reprinted from Moore *et al.* 2007 with permission from John Wiley & Sons.)

Tumors, mostly of lymphoreticular origin, affect roughly a fifth of patients, probably as a result of cytotoxic lymphocyte (CTL) dysfunction (De Meester *et al.* 2010). Non-Hodgkin lymphomas are most common and unfortunately often affect the brain and extranodal sites, leading to a poor prognosis (Cotelingam *et al.* 1985, Shcherbina *et al.* 2003).

PATHOPHYSIOLOGY

WAS is caused by mutations in the *WASP* gene, which encodes WAS protein (WASp), a key regulator of actin polymerization in hemopoietic cells. It is a multifunctional cytoskeletal regulator involved in cell mobility, cell–cell interaction, immune regulation, cell signaling, and cytotoxicity required for induction of normal antibody function, T-cell responses and platelet production, and homeostasis (Orange *et al.* 2004, Albert *et al.* 2011). The gene for WASp is localized to Xp11.22-23 and consists of 12 exons which encode a 502-amino acid (53-kDa) protein. About 300 mutations have been identified to date throughout the gene and include basepair substitutions, insertions, and deletions. Revertent somatic mosaicism is apparently not uncommon in patients with WAS and usually involves T lymphocytes (Wada and Candotti 2008).

WAS is characterized by immunodeficiency and autoimmunity associated with impaired T-helper type 1 (Th1) immunity alongside intact Th2 immunity, all resulting from WASp deficiency (Taylor *et al.* 2010). WASp is necessary for the transcriptional regulation of the Th1 regulator gene at the chromatin level and also plays a selective, post-transcriptional role in Th2 effector function (Morales-Tirado *et al.* 2010, Taylor *et al.* 2010). It is also important for the formation of immunological synapses between T lymphocytes and antigen-presenting cells (APCs), and is needed for downstream signaling, ultimately resulting in interleukin (IL)-2 secretion after T-cell receptor (TCR) engagement with CD28 (Albert *et al.* 2011).

DIAGNOSIS

As early diagnosis is necessary for appropriate treatment and prophylaxis, WAS should be suspected when a male infant presents with a bleeding diathesis and eczema. The presence of thrombocytopenia ($<70\ 000$ platelets/mm^2) and small platelet size (<2 standard deviations [SD] below the mean for the laboratory) on peripheral smear should suggest a WAS-related syndrome (Filipovich *et al.* 2001). The diagnosis can be firmly established by the presence of the aforementioned platelet abnormalities in combination with the finding of a mutation in WASP DNA, or absent WASP mRNA on gene mutation analysis and absent WASp (Conley *et al.* 1999). Prospective parents with a known family history should receive genetic counseling and be advised that the syndrome can be detected prenatally by chorionic villous sampling or amniocentesis.

MANAGEMENT

Although stem-cell transplantation is the only curative therapy for classic WAS, with 5-year survival rates over 80% using donor cells from HLA-identical siblings and HLA-matched unrelated donors transplanted into recipients aged less than 5 years, this may not be feasible due to the lack of a suitable donor (Conley *et al.* 2003, Yarmohammadi and Cunningham-Rundles 2008). In such cases, management approaches vary widely from center to center (Conley *et al.* 2003). Treatment is often focused on treating infections with antibiotics and antiviral drugs, and preventing infection using antibiotic or antiviral prophylaxis. Prophylaxis against *Pneumocystis jiroveci* (formerly *carinii*) with trimethoprim–sulfamethoxazole is instituted at some centers on all patients and at others is rarely used (Conley *et al.* 2003). Likewise, intravenous immunoglobulin (IVIG) therapy is frequently but not universally used at all centers.

Eczema is often severe and recalcitrant to most therapeutic regimens, especially in those with absent or defective WASp. Topical therapy with corticosteroids may be helpful but systemic steroids are sometimes required (Bienemann *et al.* 2007). Systemic agents used for the treatment of atopic dermatitis such as cyclosporine (ciclosporin), mycophenolate, and azathioprine should not be used for eczema associated with WAS because of the risk of lymphoreticular malignancy. Likewise, topical tacrolimus, although effective, should be used with caution and only for short periods of time given the recent concerns over its potential to induce lymphoma. Milk and other potential food allergens can be eliminated from the diet on a trial basis to observe for improvement. Eczema often waxes and wanes without an apparent trigger and some patients seem to improve during antibiotic therapy. Lymphadenopathy is common and often the consequence of superinfection. The clinician should always be on the lookout for malignancy given its high incidence in WAS.

Platelet transfusions are restricted to treatment of serious bleeds such as those in the brain or gastrointestinal (GI) tract. Blood products are best irradiated and should be cytomegalovirus (CMV)-negative. Aspirin, which interferes with platelet function, should not be used (Ochs and Thrasher 2006).

Hemopoietic cell transplantation is the only curative therapy for WAS and is the standard of care (Ochs *et al.* 2009). It is recommended that transplantation be performed in WAS patients who have an HLA-matched sibling donor. The procedure may be done at any age, but results have been best when performed before age 5. Outcomes for patients with unmatched donors have not been as positive, so the decision to transplant depends on disease severity, age, and other factors (Filipovich *et al.* 2001). Both myeloid and lymphoid engraftment are required to correct the major manifestations of WAS, thus necessitating the use of myeloablative conditioning regimens (Ochs *et al.* 2009). The small percentage of patients rejecting their initial transplant (approximately 10%) usually can be retransplanted successfully (Ochs *et al.* 2009). Interestingly, reports indicate that the eczema improves dramatically after transplantation (Saurat 1985). A recent paper suggests that hemopoietic stem cell transplantation with genetically modified hemopoietic stem cells may be effective (Boztug *et al.* 2010).

Use of splenectomy varies widely among treatment centers (Conley *et al.* 2003). Splenectomy can increase platelet number and size, and generally ameliorates the requirement for platelet transfusions, although immune thrombocytopenia may occur later (Litzman *et al.* 1996). As a result of the risk of septicemia and the requirement for lifelong antibiotic prophylaxis after splenectomy, it is best avoided in children who in the future may undergo or who have already received hemopoietic cell transplantation (Ochs *et al.* 2009).

However it is the treatment of choice for significantly thrombocytopenic patients who cannot receive bone marrow transplantation.

HYPER-IGE SYNDROME (JOB SYNDROME)

Hyper-IgE syndrome (HIES) is an immunoregulatory disorder, which in its classic form is characterized by elevated circulating levels of immunoglobulin E (IgE) >2000 IU/ml, frequent bacterial infections such as staphylococcal abscesses, recurrent cyst-forming pneumonia, and chronic eczematous dermatitis, which begin early in life (Grimbacher *et al.* 2005). Autosomal dominant, sporadic, and autosomal recessive forms of HIES are recognized.

The disease entity was first reported by Davis *et al.* (1966) as Job syndrome in two red-haired girls with recurrent staphylococcal infections and severe eczematous dermatitis associated with eosinophilia. Both had eczema soon after birth, persistent weeping lesions on the ears and face, and *cold* abscesses, so called because they lacked surrounding warmth, erythema, and tenderness. The definition was subsequently expanded to include: severe eczema; recurrent cutaneous, pulmonary and joint abscesses; growth retardation; exaggerated immediate hypersensitivity reactions associated with markedly elevated serum IgE levels and eosinophilia; dental abnormalities; scoliosis; joint hyperextensibility; frequent bone fractures; and distinctive facial features (Buckley *et al.* 1972, Grimbacher *et al.* 1999).

Autosomal dominant/sporadic HIES is caused by dominant-negative mutations in the human signal transducer and activator of transcription 3 (*STAT3*) gene on chromosome 17q21; besides eczema, sinopulmonary infections, and elevated serum IgE levels, it manifests a number of connective-tissue, skeletal, and vascular abnormalities (Minegishi *et al.* 2007, Freeman and Holland 2010). Autosomal recessive HIES is caused by mutations in the tyrosine kinase 2 (*Tyk2*) gene (Minegishi and Karasuyama 2008) and the dedicator of cytokinesis 8 (*DOCK8*) gene (Engelhardt *et al.* 2009). A single case of HIES caused by *Tyk2* deficiency has been described in the literature and some have questioned whether *Tyk2* deficiency should be considered a form of HIES or a distinct disease entity (Minegishi *et al.* 2006, Woellner *et al.* 2007). The patient was a 22-year-old Japanese male with atopic dermatitis starting at 1 month of age who developed multiple recurrent infections including otitis media, sinusitis, pneumonias, skin abscesses, BCG lymphadenitis, molluscum contagiosum, herpes simplex, and oral candidiasis.

Patients with *DOCK8* deficiency develop elevated IgE, eczema, skin and sinopulmonary infections associated with severe cutaneous viral infections such as warts, molluscum contagiosum, serious herpes simplex virus or herpes zoster infections, and a predisposition to squamous cell carcinoma and other malignancies at a young age (Zhang *et al.* 2009).

CLINICAL PRESENTATION

Infections usually begin during the first 3 months of life, but papulopustules may be present by the end of week 1 (**Fig 21.3**). Not infrequently, affected infants present with a vesicular eruption of the face or scalp and may show evidence of candidal infections (Eberting *et al.* 2004). Almost two-thirds of patients meet the diagnostic criteria of atopic dermatitis (Eberting *et al.* 2004). Multiple warm and tender staphylococcal furuncles occur, most commonly around the face (Erlewyn-Lajeunesse 2000). Young children may develop *cold* abscesses and infected flexural eczema resulting in *autoeczematization* and further spread (**Fig 21.4**). Cold abscesses are large, nontender, fluctuant masses that are pathognomonic of but not essential to the diagnosis of HIES (Erlewyn-Lajeunesse 2000).

Identifiable facial features in older children include asymmetry, prominent brow, and supraorbital ridge (frontal bossing), giving the impression of deep-set eyes, broad nasal bridge, wide, fleshy nasal tip, mild prognathism, and rough skin with prominent pores (**Figs 21.5** and **21.6a**) (Borges *et al.* 1998, Grimbacher *et al.* 1999). Postauricular eczema is characteristic and cold abscesses continue to occur (**Fig 21.6b**).

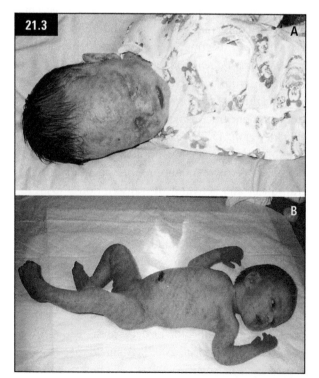

Fig 21.3 The newborn rash of hyper-IgE syndrome began on the face of this 5-day-old infant (A) and progressed to involve most of the body by age 2 weeks (B). Newborn face and scalp involvement often begins as pink papules which develop into pustules within a few days. Oozing is often present. (Reprinted from Eberting *et al.* 2004. © 2004 American Medical Association. All rights reserved.)

Fig 21.4 (A) Characteristic staphylococcal 'cold' abscess in 18-month-old patient with hyper-IgE syndrome. (Reprinted from DeWitt *et al.* 2006 with permission from Elsevier.) (B) Dermatitis of the antecubital fossa; pictured here is a typical distribution for atopic dermatitis before treatment with antistaphylococcal therapy. (Reprinted from Eberting *et al.* 2004. © 2004 American Medical Association. All rights reserved.)

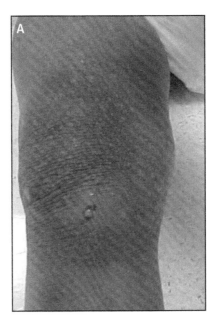

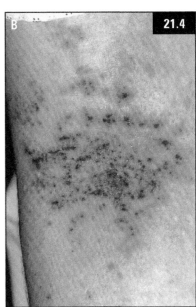

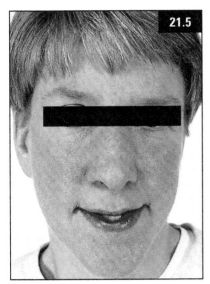

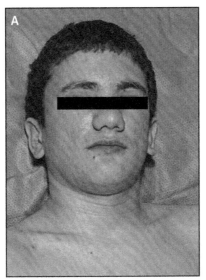

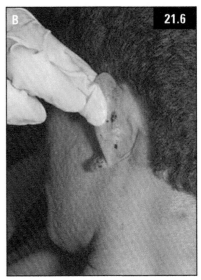

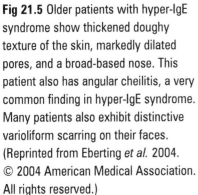

Fig 21.5 Older patients with hyper-IgE syndrome show thickened doughy texture of the skin, markedly dilated pores, and a broad-based nose. This patient also has angular cheilitis, a very common finding in hyper-IgE syndrome. Many patients also exhibit distinctive varioliform scarring on their faces. (Reprinted from Eberting *et al.* 2004. © 2004 American Medical Association. All rights reserved.)

Fig 21.6 A 15-year-old hyper-IgE syndrome patient: (A) stereotypic facies include prominent forehead, broadened nasal bridge, increased alar and outer canthal distance, and coarsening of skin. (B) Cold abscess (seen at the nape in this patient), retroauricular fissuring, and pitted scarring of the face are common cutaneous findings. (Reprinted from DeWitt *et al.* 2006 with permission from Elsevier.)

In addition to coarse facies, patients may have skeletal abnormalities and osteopenia resulting in fractures (O'Connell *et al.* 2000, Chamlin *et al.* 2002). Skeletal abnormalities include scoliosis, osteoporosis, craniosynostosis, hemivertebrae, short limbs, spina bifida, bifid rib, and Blount disease, a nonrachitic bowing of the legs (Heimall *et al.* 2010).

Dental abnormalities include retained primary teeth owing to failure of root resorption, noneruption of permanent teeth or double rows of teeth, and high arched palate (**Fig 21.7**) (Grimbacher *et al.*

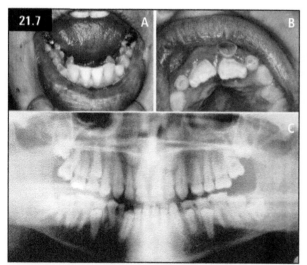

Fig 21.7 Failure of dental exfoliation in patients with the hyper-IgE syndrome. (A) Lower canines of 11-year-old patient; (B) upper central incisor and high palate of 8-year-old patient. Persistent deciduous teeth required extraction in both individuals. (C) Panoramic radiograph of 23-year-old patient revealing retention of five primary teeth with unresorbed roots. The eruption of four upper and lower premolars has been blocked by retained primary teeth, and a retained deciduous right lower canine can be seen behind and lateral to its erupted permanent counterpart. In contrast, timely removal of unshed primary teeth in the upper left quadrant of the patient's mouth (upper right) allowed normal eruption of the premolars. (Reprinted from Grimbacher *et al.* 1999. © 1999 Massachusetts Medical Society.)

1999). Vascular and brain abnormalities are also common in HIES caused by *STAT3* deficiency. They include coronary artery tortuosity or dilation in 70% of patients, coronary aneurysms in 37%, lacunar infarctions, Chiari type 1 malformations, and infectious complications (Freeman *et al.* 2007, 2011).

PATHOGENESIS

Before the discovery that heterozygous mutations in *STAT3* caused autosomal dominant HIES, many investigations focused on the immunological abnormalities of the syndrome. The most consistent laboratory abnormality is a very high serum IgE level, typically above 2000 IU/µl (Freeman and Holland 2010). IgE levels may be normal in early infancy, subsequently increase to very high levels in late infancy/early childhood, and, in at least one study, decrease and approach normal levels in the fourth or fifth decade of life in about a quarter of patients (Grimbacher *et al.* 1999, Chamlin *et al.* 2002). The eosinophil count is typically elevated as well, but there is no obvious correlation of eosinophil counts, IgE levels, and disease severity (Freeman and Holland 2010). IgE expression in patients with HIES is maximally activated, with high constitutive levels that do not increase further with IL-4 stimulation (Garraud *et al.* 1999).

Various studies have had conflicting results regarding cytokine dysregulation in HIES. Th1/Th2 imbalances, such as reduced sensitivity to IL-12/IL-18 stimulation associated with decreased interferon (IFN)-γ production by T cells, predominance of Th0 lymphocytes, and increased IL-13 production by T cells have been reported but none appears to be the critical abnormality (Rodriguez *et al.* 1998, Presotto *et al.* 1999, Borges *et al.* 2000, Chehimi *et al.* 2001, Gudmundsson *et al.* 2002, Netea *et al.* 2005). Another reported abnormality comprises intermittent defects of neutrophil chemotaxis, possibly as a result of reduced expression of receptors for chemoattractants (Hill *et al.* 1974, Mintz *et al.* 2010). The most critical immune abnormality that has been identified to date is impaired differentiation and deficiency of Th17 cells in HIES (Ma *et al.* 2008, Milner *et al.* 2008).

As autosomal dominant HIES is a multisystem disorder not confined to the immune system and has diverse manifestations involving the skin, connective tissue, skeletal system, and vascular tissue, it had previously been suspected that the genetic defect might involve a cytokine signaling molecule involving multiple pathways. STAT proteins are intimately involved with cytokine receptor signaling and defects in the production of STAT3 can be expected to affect multiple cytokines, including IL-6, IL-10, IL-17, IL-21, and IL-22, with which it is associated (Heimall et al. 2010). STAT3- null mice die during embryogenesis (Takeda et al. 1997).

Human STAT3 mutations result in dysfunctional protein of normal length with dominant negative activity but the alternate unaffected allele produces normal STAT3. Homodimerization of STAT3 molecules occurs such that autosomal dominant HIES patients have reduced levels (about 25%) of normally functioning STAT3 activity (Tangye et al. 2009). This results in deficiency of Th17 cells, impaired IL-10 production, increased bone resorption, and probably deficient antigen-specific plasma cells (Tangye et al. 2009). Deficiency of Th17 cells is likely responsible for cutaneous staphylococcal infections and mucocutaneous candidal infections (Conti et al. 2009, Cho et al. 2010). Interestingly staphylococcal infections are largely confined to the skin and lungs. A possible explanation for this is that human keratinocytes and bronchial epithelial cells are dependent on the synergistic action of Th17 cytokines and classic proinflammatory cytokines for their production of antistaphylococcal factors, including neutrophil-recruiting chemokines and antimicrobial peptides (Minegishi et al. 2009).

DIAGNOSIS

The rash of HIES must be differentiated from atopic dermatitis, other immunodeficiencies presenting with eczematoid eruptions such as WAS, neonatal eosinophilic pustular folliculitis, erythema toxicum neonatorum, neonatal herpes and other pustular disorders of the newborn, and Netherton syndrome. Patients with Netherton syndrome often have erythroderma at birth and develop hair abnormalities, most commonly trichorrhexis invaginata. The more common neonatal pustular disorders are usually transient and unlikely to be confused with HIES.

Although the eruption of HIES often meets the criteria for atopic dermatitis, it most commonly presents with a pustular eruption (Chamlin et al. 2002, Eberting et al. 2004). Areas of initial involvement include the face, axillae, upper trunk, extremities, and diaper area. Diaper area involvement usually does not occur in atopic dermatitis. In HIES, skin rashes usually begin in the first year of life and may be evident by 1 or 2 weeks (Erlewyn-Lajeunesse 2000, Chamlin et al. 2002). Atopic dermatitis usually presents at age 2 months or more when the infant is able to scratch. HIES skin infections are more severe than those of atopic dermatitis, often with abscess formation. Although patients with atopic dermatitis are usually colonized with Staphylococcus aureus, infections are usually mild, typically impetiginized eczema or folliculitis, and rarely disseminate (Van Eendenburg et al. 1991). Frank abscesses are unusual in atopic dermatitis patients.

Whereas patients with exogenous atopic dermatitis often have a personal or family history of atopy including respiratory allergy, this is uncommon in patients with HIES. It must of course be remembered that atopic dermatitis is extremely common whereas HIES is rare.

An underlying immunodeficiency syndrome should be suspected when a patient presents with severe, persistent, pruritic dermatitis with atypical distribution of lesions, with little response to first-line treatment. The main clinical guidelines for the diagnosis of HIES (apart from laboratory evaluation) are pustular eruption in infancy, severe eczema with an atypical distribution, chronicity, and lack of responsiveness to treatment (Grimbacher et al. 2005). An IgE level more than 2 SD higher than normal limits is highly suggestive and merits genetic testing. Histopathology usually demonstrates an eosinophilic folliculitis and/or eosinophilic spongiotic dermatitis.

Additional work-up includes computed tomography (CT) of the lungs because of the high incidence (approximately 80%) of patients with HIES who develop pneumatoceles (lung cysts) secondary to recurrent pulmonary infections. These lesions can become superinfected with organisms such as Pseudomonas aeruginosa and Aspergillus spp. Bronchopulmonary fistulas must also be delineated.

Furthermore, CT of the paranasal sinuses is indicated to evaluate for sinus disease (Erlewyn-Lajeunesse 2000).

A recent study identified seven key findings, highly specific for atopic dermatitis HIES: (1) abscesses of internal organs, (2) severe infections, (3) pneumatoceles, (4) nail and mucocutaneous candidiasis, (5) bone fractures, (6) scoliosis, and (7) a positive family history of HIES (Schimke et al. 2010).

TREATMENT

Treatment of HIES includes oral antibiotics, local care, and surgical incision and drainage of abscesses – the goal being to reduce morbidity and prevent complications. Antimicrobial treatment decreases the likelihood of pneumonia and its sequelae, improves the dermatitis, and reduces the formation of abscesses (Freeman and Holland 2010). Dilute bleach baths have been shown to be useful in the treatment of atopic dermatitis to reduce staphylococcal colonization, and may benefit HIES patients with recurrent abscesses. Chronic candidiasis of the nails and mucous membranes can be effectively controlled by oral antifungal agents. IVIG and subcutaneous immunoglobulin have been used anecdotally but there are no controlled clinical trials supporting its use. Omalizumab, a recombinant humanized anti-IgE antibody, was also reported in a case report to improve the eczematous eruption of HIES (Bard et al. 2008).

Despite earlier unsuccessful attempts at improving HIES symptoms with bone marrow transplantation, a recent paper suggests that hemopoietic stem cell transplantation may reverse complications of autosomal dominant STAT3-deficient HIES (Goussetis et al. 2010). Likewise, in DOCK8 deficiency, which often has a poor prognosis with central nervous system bleeding and infarction and tendency to malignancy, improved prognosis has been reported after hemopoietic stem cell transplantation (Bittner et al. 2010, Gatz et al. 2011).

OMENN SYNDROME

Gilbert S. Omenn (1965) was the first to describe a distinct hereditary entity that demonstrated reticuloendotheliosis with eosinophilia in several individuals from an inbred American family of Irish extraction. Clinical findings included pruritic skin lesions, fever, lymphadenopathy, anemia, eosinophilia, and chronic diarrhea. This description from 1965 served as the foundation for multiple clinical case reports, all demonstrating the aforementioned clinical hallmarks of an autosomal recessive form of severe combined immunodeficiency (SCID) titled Omenn syndrome (Barth et al. 1972, Gelfand et al. 1984, Jouan et al. 1987, Schwarz et al. 1999). A survey of the literature suggested that the syndrome is best described as a clinical entity presenting during the first 8 weeks of life with a combination of erythroderma, hepatosplenomegaly, and lymphadenopathy (Aleman et al. 2001).

CLINICAL PRESENTATION

Patients with Omenn syndrome generally present at birth or in the first weeks of life with a unique generalized erythroderma, with features of a subacute eczematous reaction pattern (Fig 21.8) (Puzenat et al. 2007). Unlike most cases of eczematous dermatitis, there is progression to desquamation and edema caused by shifts in oncotic pressures, which result from insensible protein loss via the skin and gut (de Saint-Basile et al. 1991). There may be diffuse alopecia including absence of eyebrows and eyelashes (Fig 21.9) (Tatli et al. 2007). The severe dermatitis may be complicated by staphylococcal sepsis or Gram-negative enteric bacterial sepsis associated with episodes of infectious diarrhea. As with other forms of SCID, life-threatening infections with common viral, bacterial, and fungal pathogens generally follow, and chronic diarrhea and infection lead to failure to thrive. Of note, diffuse lymphadenopathy is a distinguishing feature separating Omenn syndrome from most other SCID variants in which lymphadenopathy and hepatomegaly are uncommon (Aleman et al. 2001).

PATHOPHYSIOLOGY

Until recently, Omenn syndrome was considered a distinct subtype of SCID that, unlike conventional

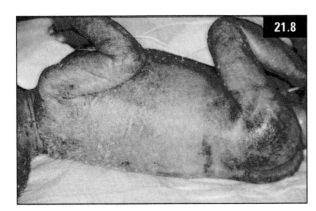

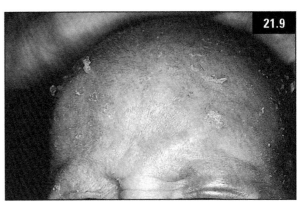

Fig 21.8 Erythroderma in a baby with Omenn syndrome. (Reprinted with permission from Sillevis Smitt *et al.* 2005.)

Fig 21.9 Generalized scaling erythroderma with infiltrated thick folds and alopecia of the eyelashes in a neonate with Omenn syndrome. (Reprinted with permission from Pruszkowski *et al.* 2000.)

SCID, was characterized by enlarged lymphoid tissue, severe erythroderma, increased IgE levels, and eosinophilia (Villa *et al.* 2008). Most cases of Omenn syndrome are caused by hypomorphic mutations in recombinase genes *RAG-1* and *RAG-2*, which decrease the efficiency of variable diversity joining (VDJ) recombination; this, in turn, impairs the development of mature T and B cells (Villa *et al.* 1998, 2008, Corneo *et al.* 2001). The few residual T-cell clones that develop escape negative selection and expand in the periphery, eventually causing autoimmune reactions (Cavadini *et al.* 2005). The expansion of this 'survivor' oligoclonal Th2 cell population also results in the production of elevated levels of Th2 cytokines such as IL-4 and IL-5 which mediate high IgE levels and eosinophilia. Notably these changes occur only in patients with hypomorphic *RAG-1* and *RAG-2* mutations but not with *deleterious* (inactivating) mutations that cause more severe SCID (Villa *et al.* 2008).

It has also been noted that Omenn syndrome can occur with a number of other distinct genetic defects defining *leaky* SCIDs, such as mutations in RNA component of mitochondrial RNA processing endoribonuclease, adenosine deaminase, IL-2 receptor-γ, IL-7 receptor-α, ARTEMIS, and DNA ligase 4 (Villa *et al.* 2008).

DIAGNOSIS

Omenn syndrome should be suspected in infants presenting with exfoliative erythroderma at birth or in the early neonatal period, accompanied by diffuse alopecia, lymphadenopathy, hepatosplenomegaly, recurrent infections, failure to thrive, elevated white count with eosinophilia, hypogammaglobulinemia, and raised IgE levels (Hoeger and Harper 1998). It should be differentiated from Netherton syndrome, neonatal GVHD (Graft–versus–host disease) in infants with T-cell deficiency or after intrauterine maternofetal transfusion, and other causes of neonatal erythroderma or SCID (Scheimberg *et al.* 2001). Exaggerated skinfolds, alopecia of the scalp, eyelashes, and eyebrows, and widespread lymphadenopathy, although not absolutely specific, support the diagnosis. Histological features suggesting Omenn syndrome or neonatal GVHD include keratinocyte necrosis with satellite lymphocytes and significant epidermal and dermal lymphocytic infiltration (**Fig 21.10**) (Pruszkowski *et al.* 2000).

Patients with Omenn syndrome have decreased or absent CD19+ B cells in most variants, and depressed humoral immunity, except for elevated IgE levels, but may have variable (often increased) numbers of activated CD45Ro+, HLA-DR+ circulating T cells (Kato *et al.* 2006, Villa *et al.* 2008). Patients reported with variant Omenn syndrome resulting from mutations in the RNase mitochondrial RNA-processing (*RMRP*) gene causing cartilage hair hypoplasia (CHH), adenosine deaminase deficiency, or mutations of DNA ligase 4 all presented with lymphopenia or low T-cell count (Roifman *et al.* 2006, 2008, Grunebaum *et al.* 2008). Rare cases of Omenn syndrome associated with Artemis mutations have had elevated or decreased total lymphocyte counts (Ege *et al.* 2005, Mancebo *et al.* 2011). SCID with maternal T-cell engraftment (GVHD), a condition that can clinically overlap Omenn syndrome, has similar histological findings and similar elevation of activated T lymphocytes. As a result of the wide variety of immune defects that can cause Omenn syndrome, patients should be referred to an immunologist experienced in the management of immunodeficiencies. It is vital that primary practitioners are not misled by possibly normal lymphocyte counts and appreciate the profound immunodeficiency.

MANAGEMENT

Patients with Omenn syndrome should undergo hemopoietic cell transplantation. Gomez *et al.* (1995) evaluated the outcome of allogeneic bone marrow transplantation (BMT) in nine consecutive patients with Omenn syndrome treated between 1980 and 1989, and concluded that both HLA-identical and haploidentical BMT can cure Omenn syndrome, provided that parenteral nutrition and immunosuppressive therapy are given before transplantation. Mazzolari *et al.* (2005) reported on 11 patients who underwent a total of 15 hemopoietic stem cell transplantations (HSCTs) beginning at a mean age of 8.4 months. The overall mortality rate was 18.2%. Nine of 11 patients were alive and immunoreconstituted 30–146 months after transplantation, nine with normal T-cell function, and eight with normal antibody production. Currently, stem cell transplantation from matched unrelated donors after myeloablative regimens with busulfan

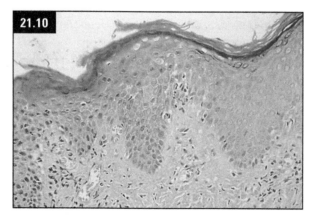

Fig 21.10 Biopsy specimen from a patient with Omenn syndrome showing lymphocytic infiltration of the dermis and necrotic keratinocytes with satellite lymphocytes. (Reprinted with permission from Pruszkowski *et al.* 2000.)

and cyclophosphamide has dramatically improved the otherwise dismal prognosis of these patients, with reported survival rates >80% (Villa *et al.* 2008).

In the case of patients for whom a suitable donor is not available, immunosuppression with cyclosporine (ciclosporin) and the downregulation of IL-4 and IL-5 with interferon-γ is effective for managing the associated dermatitis and lymphadenitis. Topical tacrolimus has also been reported anecdotally to be helpful for the dermatitis of Omenn syndrome (Faaij *et al.* 2010). Broad-spectrum antibiotics are frequently required to treat the invasive infections stemming from both *S. aureus* and Gram-negative enteric bacteria. Prophylactic antimicrobial therapy is often warranted. The use of IVIG for immune replacement therapy has been variably successful in further decreasing the risk of infections in these patients (Thampakkul and Ballow 2001). Nutritional supplementation is mandatory to replace insensible losses caused by the exfoliative dermatitis.

IMMUNE DYSREGULATION, POLYENDOCRINOPATHY, ENTEROPATHY, X-LINKED SYNDROME

Immune dysregulation, polyendocrinopathy, enteropathy, X-linked syndrome (IPEX) is a primary immune deficiency syndrome with autoimmune manifestations resulting in GI disturbances, endocrine disorders (mostly diabetes and thyroid abnormalities), and dermatitis that is usually eczematous (Torgerson and Ochs 2007). First described by Powell *et al.* (1982) as an X-linked syndrome of diarrhea, polyendocrinopathy, and fatal infections in male infants, presumably of immune origin, it is now known to be caused by mutations in the Forkhead box protein 3 (*FOXP3*) gene resulting in markedly decreased or absent FOXP+ T-regulatory cells. In addition to GI disease, autoimmune endocrinopathies involving the pancreas and thyroid, and dermatitis, IPEX patients also develop autoimmune hematological disorders, food allergies, renal disease, hepatitis, and severe infections, such as sepsis, meningitis, pneumonia, and osteomyelitis (Torgerson and Ochs 2007). Death is common before age 2 in the absence of immunosuppressive therapy or BMT. There are, however, milder phenotypes, such as those with the *V408M* mutation of the *FOXP3* gene which have prolonged survival (still alive at age 12–15 years) (Rubio-Cabezas *et al.* 2009).

CLINICAL PRESENTATION

The syndrome usually presents in infancy with watery, mucoid, or bloody diarrhea that is exacerbated when the child is weaned from breast milk to formula (Torgerson and Ochs 2007). The various manifestations usually occur sequentially rather than simultaneously (Wildin and Freitas 2005). Failure to thrive may require parenteral nutrition. Type 1 diabetes occurs in the first year of life. It is treatment-resistant, may be present at birth, and rarely may present with diabetic ketoacidosis (Torgerson and Ochs 2007). Autoimmune thyroid disease results in hypothyroidism more commonly than hyperthyroidism. Other autoimmune manifestations include Coombs-positive hemolytic anemia, autoimmune thrombocytopenia and neutropenia, renal disease varying from mild

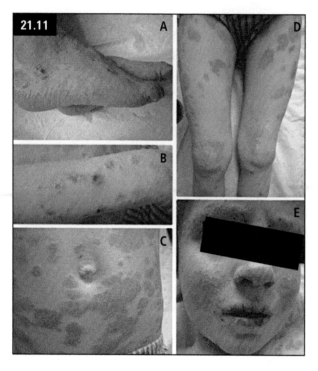

Fig 21.11 Clinical aspects of cutaneous involvement in children with immune dysregulation, polyendocrinopathy, enteropathy, X-linked syndrome (IPEX) syndrome. (A) Eczematiform involvement of extremities with lichenified pruriginous plaques, (B) eczema–prurigo, (C,D) extensive cutaneous involvement in a boy with diffuse psoriasiform plaques, and (E) atopic dermatitis with involvement of convexities of the face and severe bleeding cheilitis. (Reprinted with permission from Halabi-Tawil *et al.* 2009. © 2009 John Wiley & Sons.)

changes to rapidly progressive glomerulonephritis, and autoimmune hepatitis (Torgerson and Ochs 2007). However, lymphadenopathy and hepatosplenomegaly are uncommon.

Severe systemic infections are more likely the result of impaired skin and gut barriers, catheters, central lines, immunosuppressive drug regimens and malnutrition than any particular intrinsic immune dysfunction (Wildin and Freitas 2005). Patients with one variant of IPEX may present with severe allergies to milk and other foods but without endocrinopathy or cytopenia (Torgerson *et al.* 2007).

Eczematous eruptions occur in most patients (70% in one series), usually in the first 4 months of life (median 1.5 months) (Halabi-Tawil *et al.* 2009). Dermatitis is often widespread and severe with erythematous, exudative plaques or lichenified areas which in some patients evolve into exfoliative erythroderma (Halabi-Tawil *et al.* 2009) (**Fig 21.11**). Psoriasiform dermatitis, severe cheilitis with

fissuring, urticaria, bullae, alopecia universalis, and nail changes may also occur (Nieves *et al.* 2004).

Most patients with IPEX have marked increases in serum IgE concentration and more than half of them have elevated IgA levels (Torgerson and Ochs 2007). Although T-cell subsets are otherwise normal, FOXP3+ T-regulatory cells are strikingly decreased or absent, accounting for the characteristic autoimmune manifestations.

PATHOPHYSIOLOGY

IPEX is the human analog of the lethal X-linked recessive disorder mouse *scurfy*, in which affected males have scaly skin, diarrhea, GI bleeding, lymphadenopathy, and hematological abnormalities; scurfy mice die within 4 weeks of birth (Bennett *et al.* 2001, Wildin *et al.* 2001). Scurfy is caused by mutations in the *Foxp3* gene, which encodes a highly conserved protein, scurfin; human IPEX is caused by mutations in *FOXP3* (the human analog of *Foxp3*), which is a transcription factor and critical regulator of CD4+ CD25+ regulatory T-cell development and function (Fontenot *et al.* 2003). *FOXP3* expression is mostly restricted to these CD4+ CD25+ FOXP3+ T-regulatory cells (Torgerson and Ochs 2007), which modulate effector T-cell function, B-cell development, susceptibility of plasma cells to apoptosis, and the persistence of humoral autoimmunity (Leonardo *et al.* 2010, Jang *et al.* 2011). However, the idea that IPEX is simply a result of loss of peripheral tolerance and unbridled autoimmunity, as a result of absent FOXP3+ regulatory cells, is probably an oversimplification. Different point mutations in *FOXP3* may manifest as IPEX with varying degrees of severity, but there is no clear-cut phenotypic correlation with the various mutations so far identified. Patients with IPEX syndrome may also have detectable levels of CD4+ CD25+ FOXP3+ T-regulatory cells, and it may be that *FOXP3* mutations cause a variety of biological abnormalities with dysfunction of these cells and effector cells (Bacchetta *et al.* 2006). Moreover, different environmental, genetic, and epigenetic factors probably play a role in disease variability (d'Hennezel *et al.* 2009). Importantly, another major subtype of T-regulatory cells, IL-10-producing type 1 regulatory T (Tr1) cells, is unaffected by *FOXP3* mutations and might play a supplemental role in suppressing autoimmunity (Passerini *et al.* 2011).

DIAGNOSIS

Intractable diarrhea in a male infant, especially in the presence of an eczematous skin rash, villous atrophy on intestinal biopsy, and failure to thrive, should strongly suggest the diagnosis of IPEX (Torgerson and Ochs 2007). The presence of other features of IPEX such as type 1 diabetes, hypothyroidism, Coombs-positive hemolytic anemia, leukopenia, thrombocytopenia, and elevated IgE levels make the diagnosis even more likely. Absence of immunostaining for FOXP3 cells in the lamina propria and lymphoid aggregates in intestinal biopsy specimens are highly suggestive of severe IPEX (Heltzer *et al.* 2007). Diagnosis should be confirmed by genetic testing for *FOXP3* mutant alleles and, if negative, may suggest an IPEX-like syndrome such as CD25 deficiency (Caudy *et al.* 2007).

TREATMENT

Young males with IPEX require aggressive supportive therapy, including insulin and thyroid replacement, red cell and platelet transfusions, and parenteral nutrition (Torgerson and Ochs 2007). A number of immunosuppressive agents have been used including cyclosporine, tacrolimus, methotrexate, corticosteroids, infliximab, and rituximab; however, the best agent so far has been sirolimus, which lacks the nephrotoxicity of the calcineurin inhibitors (Bindl *et al.* 2005, Yong *et al.* 2008).

HSCT is currently considered the most promising treatment for IPEX. Patients in early case reports using high-intensity conditioning regimens usually died of transplant-related causes (Burroughs *et al.* 2010). More recently, stable, long-term engraftment of hemopoietic cells has been accomplished using a lower-intensity conditioning regimen, thus offering hope that this procedure may help patients with this deadly condition.

CONCLUSION

Congenital or primary immune deficiencies may present with the dermatological manifestation of eczema, sometimes indistinguishable from atopic dermatitis and at other times atypical. It is important for practitioners to have a high index of suspicion when confronted with eczematous children who also have evidence of recurrent infections, hematological abnormalities, persistent diarrhea, failure to thrive, and other atypical features. Many such children have previously been misdiagnosed as only having severe atopic dermatitis, resulting in a delay in necessary treatment. Early diagnosis of PID and consultation with an immunologist allow appropriate management, genetic counseling, and in some patients the opportunity for timely hemopoietic cell transplant that may be lifesaving.

CHAPTER 22

HIV INFECTION AND ATOPIC DERMATITIS

Adam Friedman, Donald Rudikoff, and Francis Iacobellis

INTRODUCTION

Patients with HIV infection often have dry skin, prurigo nodularis, eosinophilic folliculitis, *pruritic papular eruption of AIDS*, exaggerated insect-bite reactions, and other skin disorders, usually as a result of immune dysregulation. Some dermatologists have noted new adult-onset atopic dermatitis in patients with HIV infection, typical flexural lichenification, or sometimes other patterns of lichenification, and other reports have suggested an association of childhood atopic dermatitis onset or worsening with HIV infection (Ball and Harper 1987).

For HIV-infected patients who do develop such atopiform dermatitis, the question arises whether it is truly atopic dermatitis and, if it is, is its onset related to the HIV infection or is it simply occurring coincidentally. Might HIV-induced immune dysregulation increase the likelihood of true atopy either by immune perturbations or by affecting the cutaneous skin barrier and facilitating antigen penetration? The prevalence of atopic dermatitis is high in childhood, averaging around 17% in various studies, so that a small increase in the number of cases of atopic dermatitis in HIV-infected patients compared with normal individuals might be difficult to detect. On the other hand, the low prevalence of adult-onset atopic dermatitis might allow easier detection of cases that might be related to HIV infection.

Onset of atopic dermatitis in adulthood has traditionally been considered uncommon but this concept has recently been questioned. The proportion of cases of atopic dermatitis beginning after age 18–21 has been reported as 13.6% (age ≥21) in Singapore (Tay *et al.* 1999) and 9% in Australia (age ≥20) (Bannister and Freeman 2000). Moreover, adult-onset atopic dermatitis patients have been reported to have atypical presentations, some with nonflexural involvement, nummular lesions, prurigo-like lesions, and follicular patterns (Ozkaya 2005). Unfortunately, studies of adult-onset atopic dermatitis have not reported HIV status. If atopic or atopiform dermatitis can occur as a result of HIV infection, one might expect that this would be reflected in case series of HIV-related dermatoses in adults and children (Ball and Harper 1987).

Most case series of cutaneous manifestations of HIV infection in adults and children fail to reflect an expected increase in frequency of atopic dermatitis. One study demonstrated a prevalence of 'unclassified eczema' in approximately 10% of this patient population (Supanaranond *et al.* 2001). Knowing that the prevalence of atopic dermatitis in a non-HIV-infected population is also approximately 10–17%, one might assume from these data that there is no significant difference in the prevalence between the general population and HIV patients.

HIV-ASSOCIATED ATOPY

Atopic dermatitis and other manifestations of atopy such as sinusitis, asthma, elevated IgE levels, hyper-IgE syndrome, eosinophilia, and T-helper type 1/type 2 (Th1/Th2) imbalances have in fact all been described in adults and children with HIV infection, suggesting a possible predilection for atopic disorders in these patients (Ball and Harper 1987, Israël-Biet *et al.* 1992, Ellaurie *et al.* 1995, Koutsonikolis *et al.* 1996, Bacot *et al.* 1997, Corominas *et al.* 2000). Investigators have also examined the association between elevated IgE levels in HIV-infected children and adults and disease severity and progression (Vigano *et al.* 1955, Koutsonikolis *et al.* 1996). Some studies in adults and children revealed an increased prevalence of atopic disease in HIV-infected patients compared with the general population, but other studies do not support this supposition.

Bronchial asthma may be more prevalent in the male HIV population. Ellaurie *et al.* (1995) found that wheezing occurred in 27% of patients and sinusitis in 8%. One study offered that approximately 29% of HIV-infected individuals have atopic manifestations, ranging from chronic pruritic rashes to eczematous eruptions (Lin and Lazarus 1995). Many of the patients who reported histories of atopic dermatitis also reported either a personal or a family history of allergic rhinitis and asthma. Sample *et al.* (1990) found that patients with AIDS have elevated IgE levels and positive radioallergosorbent tests (RASTs) for a panel of environmental allergens.

On the other hand, Bowser *et al.* (2007) found a prevalence of atopy (52%) and pattern of aeroallergen sensitivity in perinatally HIV-infected children comparable to that of the general US population of children.

IGE ELEVATION AND EOSINOPHILIA IN HIV-INFECTED PATIENTS

Although IgE elevation in atopic dermatitis patients has been associated with atopic responses to food allergens and aeroallergens, this may not be the case in patients with HIV infection. Current thinking is that elevated IgE levels in HIV infection are mostly due to direct effects of the virus. Two HIV-1 proteins, gp120 and Tat, trigger the release of cytokines interleukin (IL)-4 and IL-13, critical for Th2 polarization from human Fcε-receptor-I-positive (FcεRI+) cells (mast cells, basophils, dendritic cells), and this causes elevation of IgE levels (Marone *et al.* 2000). Moreover, HIV-1-shed gp120 virions closely resemble allergens that bind to IgE molecules bound to FcεRI+ cells, resulting in synthesis and release of IL-4 (Becker 2004). Thus HIV infection might be considered an *allergic disease* with gp120 as the *allergen*.

Some investigators have directed their focus toward eosinophilia and a variety of shared atopic manifestations (Paganelli *et al.* 1991, Skiest and Keiser 1997). Although there are those who argue that elevated IgE levels did not correlate with allergic disease in the setting of HIV infection (Bacot *et al.* 1997, Tubiolo *et al.* 1997, Bowser *et al.* 2007), there is substantial evidence that HIV-associated eosinophilia does correlate with the development of skin disease and perhaps more prominent HIV infection (Sanchez-Borges *et al.* 1993, Skiest and Keiser 1997).

Also relevant is the known prevalence of dry skin in HIV-infected patients. The question arises as to whether a damaged skin barrier could be present and predispose patients to antigen penetration and atopic manifestations, as has been proposed in patients with atopic dermatitis. It is thought that abnormal barrier function in atopic dermatitis patients as a result of filaggrin mutations and ceramide abnormalities allows antigen penetration and favors the development of a Th2-dominant immune response. A further Th2 inflammatory response then causes further barrier dysfunction and results in a vicious cycle of inflammation and barrier abnormalities (Elias and Steinhoff 2008, Elias *et al.* 2008). It is thought that HIV infection can cause a Th2-dominant immune milieu which can suppress barrier function recovery, ceramide synthesis, and filaggrin synthesis (Klein *et al.* 1997, Hatano *et al.* 2005, Howell *et al.* 2007, Kurahashi *et al.* 2008).

Hypothesizing that a Th2 milieu in HIV-infected patients might provoke barrier dysfunction, Gunathilake *et al.* (2010) looked at transepidermal water loss (TEWL) in HIV-infected patients with no previous history of atopy, who were negative for two common filaggrin mutations that might influence barrier function. They found a threefold increase of TEWL in nonxerotic skin of HIV patients. In patients with HIV-associated xerotic eczema there was an even greater increase in TEWL as well as an increased pH compared with nonxerotic skin.

DIAGNOSIS

The diagnosis of atopic dermatitis in an immunocompetent host is made on the basis of a primary feature: pruritus, a chronic relapsing dermatitis manifested by lichenification in *flexural* areas in adults and older children. The diagnosis is strengthened by a personal or family history of atopic diseases and an elevated IgE level, which is found in approximately 80% of immunocompetent atopic dermatitis patients. In the immunosuppressed patient, there are many overlapping signs and symptoms that can befuddle the diagnostician. In particular, eczematous eruptions of various presentations occur in HIV patients, most often in individuals with a CD4 count <200, but also as a result of immune reconstitution.

There are many reasons for this. HIV patients often have other cutaneous diseases, which have as the immunological core a Th2 dominance, such as eosinophilic folliculitis (Rodwell and Berger 2000). Scratching and rubbing eosinophilic folliculitis could result in lichenification which could be confused with atopic dermatitis.

As mentioned above HIV-infected patients also have an impaired skin barrier. Scratching dry, itchy skin and staphylococcal colonization and infection are also likely to impair barrier function. Many HIV patients are known to scrub vigorously with strong, alkaline-based, antibacterial soaps in an attempt to diminish staphylococcal colonization. This further compromises and damages the skin barrier. Moreover, a number of HIV-positive patients are psychologically traumatized by the infection and can develop obsessive–compulsive hand and body washing in an attempt to psychologically rid themselves of the disease (Iacobellis F, 2011, personal observation). This adds insult to the injury of barrier disruption. Finally, many protease inhibitors, primarily *indinavir*, can cause secondary xerosis of the skin, another compromising factor of skin barrier disruption.

Among HIV-infected patients presenting with atopic-like dermatitis, some have a personal or family history of atopy such as asthma or seasonal allergic rhinitis, but many never had childhood eczema (Rudikoff D, 2002, personal observation). There is often diffuse xerosis and areas of flexural and extensor lichenification on the arms, legs, and neck (**Figs 22.1–22.3**). Linear crusted erosions indicative of excoriations may be prominent and secondary cutaneous infections (**Fig 22.4**) and prurigo nodularis are common. As xerosis and prurigo are so common and often associated with the areas of lichenification, determining a definitive diagnosis in the HIV-positive patient is often difficult.

Pruritic papular eruptions and papular urticaria may themselves give manifestations suggestive of atopy. Thus, it would be inaccurate to classify a clinical entity, resulting from underlying papular urticaria or pruritic papular eruption that has become lichenified from rubbing, as true atopic dermatitis despite the clinical resemblance. Specific diagnostic criteria would be helpful in these cases and should be determined in the future.

DIFFERENTIAL DIAGNOSIS OF HIV-ASSOCIATED ATOPIC DERMATITIS

Pruritic eruptions in HIV-infected patient, comprise two main groups: eruptions with scaling, and conditions in which general pruritus with minimal or no primary lesion is present (Chen and Cockerell 2003) (*Table 22.1*). Scaly eruptions include lichen simplex chronicus, acquired ichthyosis, seborrheic dermatitis, psoriasis, Reiter disease, chronic actinic dermatitis, crusted scabies, some drug eruptions, and cutaneous T-cell lymphoma (CTCL). Pruritus without rash can occur from underlying systemic disorders such as renal insufficiency, cholestatic liver disease, thyroid disorders, Hodgkin disease, or non-Hodgkin lymphoma. Xerosis and scabies commonly cause pruritus and may have a paucity of primary skin lesions. Drug eruptions are another common cause of pruritus, and finally papular eruptions such as eosinophilic folliculitis and papular eruption of HIV are a source of severe itching. Any eruption with eczematous changes or lichenification might conceivably be mistaken for atopic dermatitis.

Xerosis is one of the most common skin manifestations of HIV disease that can cause itching. It can be generalized or confined to the extremities and, when severe, may be resistant to treatment. Severe xerosis over the anterior legs may be indistinguishable from acquired ichthyosis. Acquired ichthyosis seen

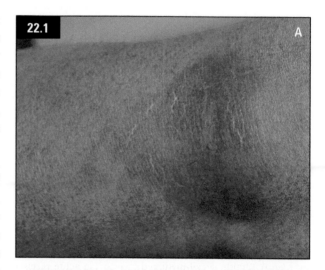

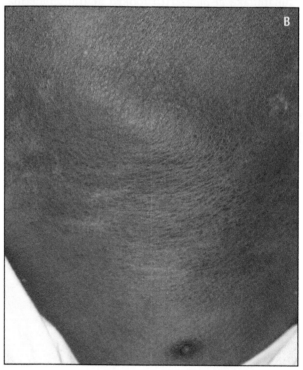

Fig 22.1 (A) Scaly plaques in the popliteal fossa of an HIV-infected male with a CD4 count of 91, total eosinophil count of 1700, and a positive family history of asthma (brother). (B) Eczematous and lichenoid changes on the trunk of an HIV-infected male.

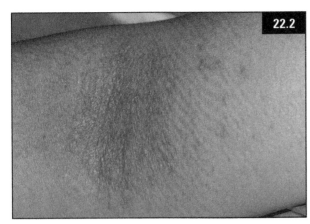

Fig 22.2 Erythematous, eczematous involvement of the antecubital fossa of an HIV-infected patient.

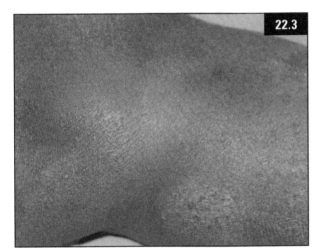

Fig 22.3 Dry, scaly, eczematous patches and plaques on the thigh and calf of a patient with AIDS.

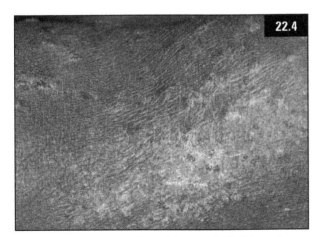

Fig 22.4 HIV-infected patient with secondarily infected flexural eczema and lichenification and crusted papules.

at extremely low CD4 counts sometimes portends an underlying lymphoma. Xerosis or xerotic eczema may occasionally be mistaken for atopic dermatitis if there is secondary lichenification from rubbing or scratching.

Seborrheic dermatitis occurs in most HIV-infected patients, often in an exaggerated fashion (**Fig 22.5**). In addition to the usual areas of involvement, such as the scalp and hair-bearing surfaces of the face, patients with HIV often have involvement on the chest, as well as intertriginous and anogenital areas, which can be difficult to treat. Plaque-like facial lesions have been seen in more extreme cases of HIV disease. Characterized by a greasy appearing scale and flaking it is rarely mistaken for atopic dermatitis.

The prevalence of psoriasis in the HIV-infected population is not increased but its presentation may differ from that seen in HIV-seronegative patients. There are two variations of psoriasis in this population. If the onset of psoriasis predates seroconversion, the lesions are usually those of *garden variety* plaque

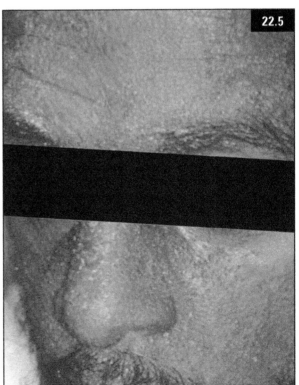

Fig 22.5 Severe seborrheic dermatitis of the face.

Table 22.1 Differential diagnosis of eczematous and pruritic eruptions in patients with HIV infection

CONDITION	CLINICAL FEATURES
Atopiform dermatitis	Flexural or extensor lichenification and eczematous changes
Xerotic eczema	Generalized dry-appearing skin, especially on the extensor aspects of the extremities
Seborrheic dermatitis	Greasy, erythematous scaling of the nasolabial area, eyebrows, beard area, scalp, chest, and back. May involve the entire face, axillae, and groin
Psoriasis	Garden variety psoriasis; acral psoriasis with reactive arthritis and severe nail changes, inverse psoriasis, sebopsoriasis, rupioid psoriasis, and overlap of psoriasis presentations may occur
Prurigo nodularis	Hyperkeratotic nodules with central hypopigmentation and peripheral hyperpigmentation typically involve the extremities, and sometimes the trunk
Pruritic papular eruption of AIDS	Pruritic excoriated papules usually present on the arms and legs. May represent several entities or be part of a spectrum of disease that includes eosinophilic folliculitis (Junqueira Magalhães Afonso et al. 2012)
Eosinophilic folliculitis	Extremely pruritic papules surmounted by pustules typically appear on the scalp, forehead, cheeks, behind the ears, neck, upper chest and back, and proximal arms. Lesions are usually excoriated
Acquired ichthyosis	Resembles ichthyosis vulgaris with polygonal 'fish-like,' scales especially on the extensor aspect of the legs, sparing the flexures. May be associated with lymphoma and other malignancy
Crusted scabies	'Dirty' grayish-brown hyperkeratotic scaling may be widespread causing erythroderma or may be confined to elbows, knees, and genital area. Unlike typical scabies it may involve the face and scalp
Cutaneous T-cell lymphoma (CTCL) and pseudo-CTCL	Mycosis fungoides rarely occurs in patients with HIV disease. Scaly patches with 'smudgy' borders involve non-sun-exposed areas such as the buttocks and thighs; may be more widespread. Pseudo-CTCL, a lymphoproliferative disorder, may present with erythematous patches, plaques, or tumors, or mimic Sézary syndrome
Drug eruption	Severe maculopapular drug eruptions are common in patients with HIV infection and usually involve the face, trunk, and proximal extremities
Photosensitivity reaction	Hyper- or hypopigmentation and lichenoid or eczematous lesions involving sun-exposed areas of the face, including the lower lip and ears, neck, and dorsa of the hands
Dermatophyte infection	Dermatophyte infections, although not more common in HIV-infected individuals, may occasionally be widespread and atypical looking

psoriasis. If the psoriasis is flexural and mild, it might be mistaken for atopic dermatitis.

If the onset of psoriasis occurs after HIV seroconversion, an inverse pattern of psoriasis can be seen with extensive recalcitrant plaques in the anogenital area, inguinal folds, fingers, and often on the palms and soles. Thick rupioid lesions may occur (**Fig 22.6**). The acral pattern of psoriasis may be accompanied by psoriatic arthritis and nail dystrophy. Reiter syndrome, classically a triad of arthritis, conjunctivitis, and urethritis, occurs in patients with HIV disease and can rarely be confused with atopic dermatitis. Of interest is recent work suggesting that genetic variants that are protective against HIV may predispose to psoriasis (Chen *et al.* 2012).

Several photosensitivity disorders have been reported in patients with HIV infection. Some HIV-infected patients develop a lichenoid photosensitivity eruption, which when chronic can present with lesions extending beyond sun-exposed areas. The more usual presentation is confined to the face, back of the neck, and dorsal aspect of the hands (**Fig 22.7**). Skin biopsy often reveals a lichenoid dermatitis with increased eosinophils, sometimes accompanied by a peripheral eosinophilia and elevated IgE.

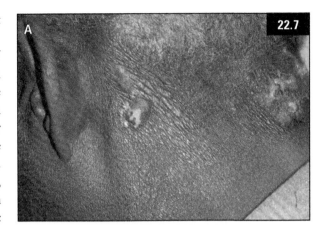

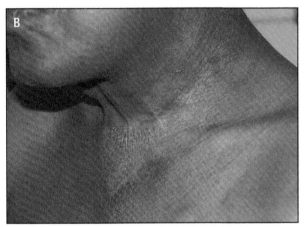

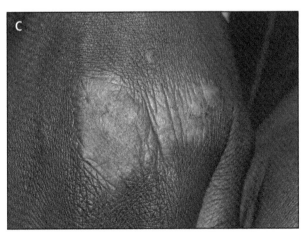

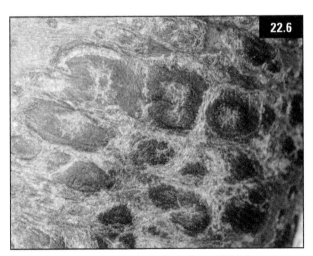

Fig 22.6 Rupioid lesions of psoriasis in an HIV-infected patient.

Fig 22.7 (A) Lichenoid photoeruption of HIV. There is photo-distributed hyperpigmentation, lichenification and pruriginous lesions with hypopigmentation. Note hyperpigmentation of the sun-exposed superior helix. (B) Lichenoid photoeruption with involvement of the 'V' of the neck. (C) Lichenoid photoeruption on sun-exposed dorsa of hands with lichenification.

Chronic actinic dermatitis, comprising actinic reticulosis and photosensitive eczema, can also occur in association with HIV disease. It is characterized by scaly eczematous lesions that evolve into thickened plaques on the dorsal aspect of the hands and neck, which may extend to nonphotoexposed areas (Hawk and Magnus 1979). Histological changes resemble chronic eczema or may suggest cutaneous lymphoma. Patients with HIV infection may also be taking photosensitizing drugs such as sulfamethoxazole–trimethoprim or using photosensitizers such as those found in colognes and perfumes. Most of these photosensitivity reactions can be differentiated from atopic dermatitis by their photodistribution but on occasion the distinction may not be that obvious.

Dermatophyte infections may be exaggerated in HIV-seropositive patients and can sometimes be confused with atopic dermatitis. These may manifest as dry scaly patches extending from the buttocks (**Fig 22.8**), tinea pedis extending to the dorsa of the feet, or lichenified or prurigo nodularis lesions on the shins resulting from picking, scratching, and rubbing of fungal folliculitis (Majocchi granuloma). KOH examination, cultures, and biopsy will identify fungal hyphae.

Scabies is common in the HIV population and its presentation is usually no different from that seen in HIV-seronegative individuals. In severely immunosuppressed individuals (CD4 count <200), scabies can present as a generalized scaling with

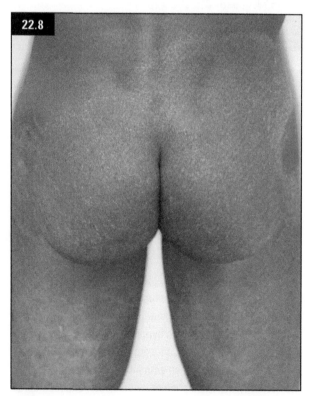

Fig 22.8 Tinea corporis in an HIV-infected male. Sharply demarcated, extensive scaly patches involving the buttocks, thighs, and lower back.

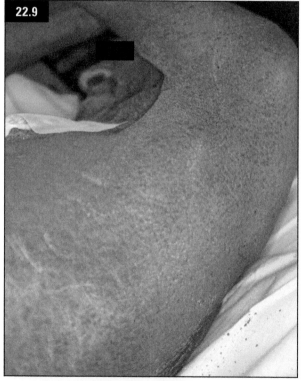

Fig 22.9 Crusted scabies in a patient with AIDS. Note dry, brownish-gray papules and scaly plaques.

minimal pruritus (**Fig 22.9**), and sometimes with numerous papules on the trunk mimicking prurigo nodularis. This presentation, crusted scabies, might be confused with atopic dermatitis. Identification of mites in skin scrapings is diagnostic.

Drug eruptions can be included in the differential diagnosis of many dermatoses. They are particularly common in HIV-infected patients, especially those being treated for *Pneumocystis jiroveci* infections with sulfa-based drugs. Most drug eruptions in HIV patients are morbilliform and originate in the groin and genital area. Tissue eosinophilia is common. In cases of chronic pruritic drug eruptions, lichen simplex chronicus and prurigo nodularis may occur and be confused with atopic dermatitis. A careful drug history and previous reactions to therapy are warranted.

Adult kwashiorkor can present as mild discoloration, dryness, and pallor of the skin and can be confused with atopic dermatitis. When associated with HIV, kwashiorkor is part of a wasting syndrome that can be seen terminally and has a poor prognosis. Obvious signs of malnutrition, wasting, and irregular bands of pigmentation of hair – the so-called flag sign – are aids to diagnosis.

Non-Hodgkin lymphomas including CTCLs occur with HIV disease. Mycosis fungoides is uncommon in this setting. The patch stage of the mycosis fungoides presents as scaly, poorly defined patches distributed on the thighs, trunk, and extremities. Lichenification may sometimes occur but the presence of typical patches with *smudgy* borders usually makes differentiation from atopic dermatitis straightforward. Pseudo-CTCL resembling mycosis fungoides has also been reported in association with HIV infection (Wilkins *et al.* 2006).

Eosinophilic folliculitis is one of the most common, perhaps the most common, pruritic eruptions of HIV disease. Although the lesions can be numerous, erythematous, and urticarial, they can also be nondescript and sparse but still associated with severe pruritus. In addition to the numerous eosinophils in the skin biopsy, a distinguishing feature of eosinophilic folliculitis is the location of skin lesions in the vast majority of patients on the upper body, head, and neck (**Fig 22.10**). Scratching and picking of these extremely pruritic lesions may

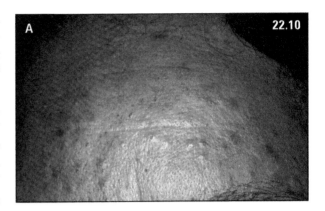

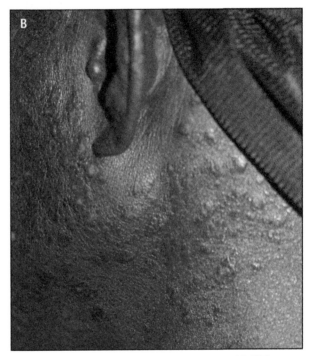

Fig 22.10 Eosinophilic folliculitis in a patient with HIV infection. Note excoriated hyperpigmented papules on the (A) forehead, and (B) neck and cheek. Eosinophilic folliculitis typically occurs in patients with low CD4 counts but may occur on institution of antiretroviral therapy as a result of the immune reconstitution inflammatory syndrome (IRIS). Constant scratching and rubbing can cause lichenification.

result in a clinical picture that can be confused with atopiform dermatitis of HIV disease (**Fig 22.11**).

There is also a spectrum of nondescript pruritic papular disorders that occur in the HIV patient usually with CD4 counts <200. Some consider these nondescript lesions a variant of prurigo nodularis; others use the term 'red itchy bump disease.' Underlying systemic disorders such as uremia, hepatic dysfunction, and lymphoma can also cause pruritus, as can neuronal involvement with the virus causing paraesthesias and itching. All of these disorders, when rubbed and scratched, may result in lichenification suggesting atopic dermatitis.

THERAPY

Treatment of eczematous eruptions in patients with HIV infection is similar to treatment in non-HIV-infected patients with the exception that systemic immunosuppressive agents such as cyclosporine (ciclosporin), mycophenolate mofetil, azathioprine, and methotrexate are generally avoided. Moreover, treatment with topical tacrolimus or pimecrolimus should be undertaken cautiously in patients with immunosuppression. Both agents, according to their package inserts, 'should not be used in immunocompromised adults and children.' On the other hand, a recent study investigating the use of topical pimecrolimus in the treatment of seborrheic dermatitis in HIV-infected patients demonstrated efficacy with no negative effect on CD4 and CD8 lymphocyte counts and HIV viral load (de Moraes *et al.* 2007). Topical tacrolimus 0.1% has demonstrated efficacy in the treatment of HIV-associated eosinophilic folliculitis (Toutous-Trellu *et al.* 2005).

Treatment approaches usually rely on topical corticosteroid preparations and topical emollients. A potent topical corticosteroid may be used followed by a lower-potency preparation as the condition improves or a short course of a topical corticosteroid followed by a maintenance regimen of emollients (Hoare *et al.* 2000).

Sodium hypochlorite (bleach) baths have recently shown efficacy in the treatment of children with atopic dermatitis (Huang *et al.* 2009). As patients with HIV infection may be colonized with *Staphylococcus aureus*, using bleach baths in patients with folliculitis or weeping lesions would make sense. A short course of antistaphylococcal antibiotics may be helpful at the start of treatment.

CONCLUSION

Patients with HIV infection are known to have dry skin and a variety of skin conditions related to their immunosuppression. There is some evidence that HIV-infected patients may develop a dermatitis that could be said to be atopiform in its clinical presentation. Whether the development of such cases of atopiform dermatitis is coincidental or related to the immune perturbations and barrier abnormalities of HIV infection remains to be elucidated.

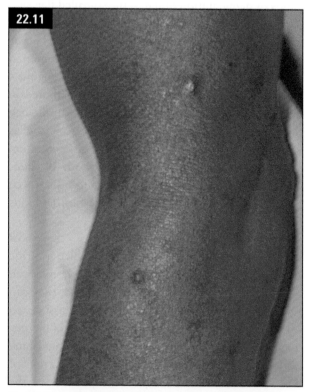

Fig 22.11 Prurigo lesions and eczematous patches in the same patient as in **Fig 22.8**.

CHAPTER 23

ICHTHYOSIS VULGARIS

Jessica Simon and Robert Buka

The term 'ichthyosis,' derived from the ancient Greek root ι χ θ υ ς (ichthys) meaning 'fish', is used to describe a heterogeneous group of keratinization disorders characterized by generalized scaling of the skin. Ichthyosis vulgaris (IV) is the most common form of ichthyosis. It has been considered to be inherited as an autosomal dominant trait but recent work on the role of filaggrin gene (*FLG*) mutations in this condition suggests that it is inherited in a 'semi-dominant' manner in which one *FLG* mutation causes a mild phenotype, but two mutations (either homozygous or compound heterozygous) lead to a more pronounced expression of the disorder (Oji and Traupe 2009). Recently another genetic locus for ichthyosis vulgaris in two Chinese families was found on chromosome 10q22.3-q24.2 (Liu *et al.* 2008). There was no association of their ichthyosis with the filaggrin gene.

On rare occasions, ichthyosis can be acquired in adulthood with associated internal disease, malignancy, and the use of certain medications. Both acquired and hereditary forms can be clinically and histologically indistinguishable (Okulicz and Schwartz 2003). This chapter discusses the hereditary form of IV and its association with atopic presentations.

PATHOPHYSIOLOGY AND GENETICS

The scaling in ichthyosis is not attributed to epidermal hyperproliferation as in lamellar ichthyosis and epidermolytic hyperkeratosis, but is instead caused by abnormal desquamation. The abnormal retention of stratum corneum cells can be explained by a defect in the 'bricks-and-mortar model' proposed by Peter Elias more than two decades ago (Shwayder and Ott 1991). The bricks representing protein-enriched corneocytes are composed of keratins, keratohyalin, and a stratum corneum envelope which collectively function to promote water retention. These components are surrounded by a lipid-rich mortar or matrix which also functions as a barrier to water loss. A disturbance in the interactions between these 'bricks' and 'mortar' leads to defective desquamation. This has been connected with an increased persistence of desmosomes in IV stratum corneum (Elsayed-Ali *et al.* 1992).

Profilaggrin (PF), a high-molecular-weight precursor of filaggrin, is synthesized in the granular layer of the epidermis and is a major component of keratohyalin granules (Okulicz and Schwartz 2003). Profilaggrin normally undergoes a succession of post-translational modifications and is converted to filaggrin, a protein that helps aggregate keratin intermediate filaments in the lower stratum corneum (Nirunsuksiri *et al.* 1998). Filaggrin is subsequently proteolized into free amino acids which play a major role in water-binding properties of the upper stratum corneum (Fleckman *et al.* 1993, Nirunsuksiri *et al.* 1998). Expression of profilaggrin is reduced or absent in the epidermis of IV patients and correlates with a reduction of keratohyalin granules on electron microscopy and clinical severity of the disorder (Sybert *et al.* 1985).

Two mechanisms have been postulated as causing IV: function mutations that may occur throughout the *FLG* genes or a defect in post-transcriptional regulation that leads to decreased stability of profilaggrin mRNA. Both mechanisms show how a defect in the gene for profilaggrin, a precursor of filaggrin, can lead to reduced filaggrin synthesis, subsequently impairing the ability to retain water in the stratum corneum.

Genetic linkage has been established between IV and markers in the epidermal differentiation complex (EDC) on chromosome 1q21 (Compton *et al.* 2002). The EDC is a cluster of genes that encode for several epidermal structural proteins including filaggrin. Several mutations (*2282del4*, *R501X*, *3702delG*) in the *FLG* gene have been identified as a cause of IV in European populations. Heterozygotes exhibit a mild phenotype with incomplete penetrance, whereas homozygotes with such mutations have severe ichthyosis, suggesting a semi-dominant inheritance pattern (Sandilands *et al.* 2006, Smith *et al.* 2006).

Two of the more prevalent null mutations described above (*R501X* and *2282del4*) in IV are also significant risk factors for atopic dermatitis (AD) and have also been associated with AD-associated asthma in European studies (Sandilands *et al.* 2007). Different sets of filaggrin mutations associated with AD and IV have been described in Asian populations (Akiyama 2010).

EPIDEMIOLOGY AND CLINICAL MANIFESTATIONS

Ichthyosis vulgaris occurs worldwide in all races and affects males and females equally (Rabinowitz and Esterly 1994). Incidence is approximately 1:250 in the general population, although this figure is probably an underestimate due to decreased reporting of milder cases and varying degrees of penetrance within families (Shwayder and Ott 1991, Okulicz and Schwartz 2003).

The condition manifests clinically as symmetric scaling of the skin primarily involving the extensor extremities, with involvement favoring the arms and lower legs (**Figs 23.1** and **23.2**). The flexures are usually spared. Although less frequent, the trunk may also be involved with bran-like scales, especially on the back (**Fig 23.3**). Scales are small, fine, and irregular, often giving the skin a rough texture with colors ranging from white to brown (Rabinowitz and Esterly 1994, Okulicz and Schwartz 2003).

Clinical scaling usually appears after age 3 months with most cases apparent by age 5. Symptoms generally improve with age and vary tremendously with temperature and humidity (Rabinowitz and Esterly 1994, Okulicz and Schwartz 2003).

Warmer climates and increased humidity account for symptom improvement in the summer months. This is also evident in areas of the body with increased

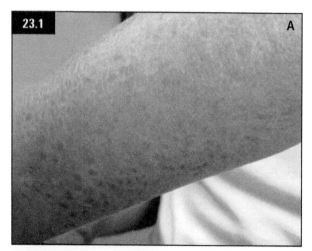 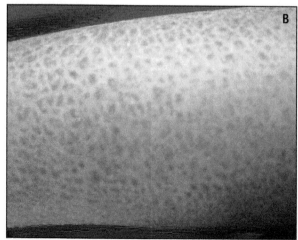

Fig 23.1 (A) Ichthyosis vulgaris involving the arms of a child with hyperpigmented polygonal scales. (B) Close-up showing hyperpigmented scales separated by a zone of lighter skin.

humidity, explaining the sparing of flexor surfaces and the skin under diapers. Although the face is usually spared in adults, presumably as a result of increased sebaceous secretions, the cheeks and forehead of young children may be involved (**Fig 23.4**) (Shwayder and Ott 1991, Okulicz and Schwartz 2003).

Ichthyosis vulgaris is also often associated with hyperlinear palms and soles (**Fig 23.5**), dry skin resulting in pruritus, and other common dermatological conditions such as keratosis pilaris and atopic manifestations, including eczema, asthma, and hayfever (Rabinowitz and Esterly 1994). About 50% of patients have concomitant AD that can mask the typical scales of IV (Rabinowitz and Esterly 1994).

Should biopsy be considered necessary, it should be taken from areas of hyperkeratosis such as the lateral shin which contains thick scale (Feinstein *et al.* 1970, Ziprkowski and Feinstein 1972). Histological examination often reveals a basket-weave hyperkeratotic stratum corneum and a diminished or absent granular layer (Feinstein *et al.* 1970). Ultrastructural studies show diminished or absent keratohyalin granules within the granular layer (Anton-Lamprecht and Hofbauer 1972).

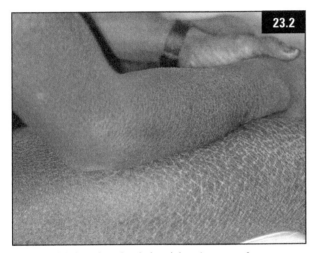

Fig 23.2 Ichthyosis vulgaris involving the arms, forearms, and thighs of an adult. The flexures are spared.

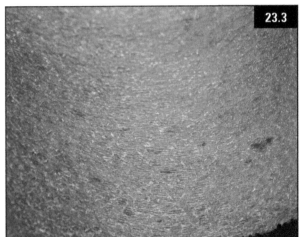

Fig 23.3 Bran-like scale on the trunk of a teenager with ichthyosis vulgaris.

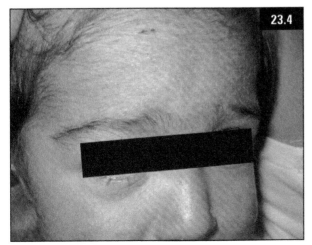

Fig 23.4 Mild forehead scaling in a child with ichthyosis vulgaris.

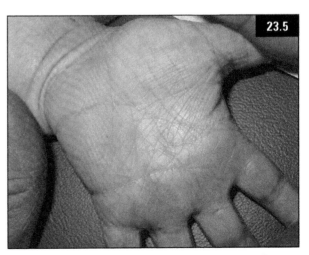

Fig 23.5 Filaggrin deficiency results in hyperlinear palms.

DIFFERENTIAL DIAGNOSIS

Ichthyosis vulgaris must be differentiated from other ichthyotic conditions such as the less common X-linked ichthyosis, lamellar ichthyosis, and acquired ichthyosis. Unlike ichthyosis vulgaris, X-linked ichthyosis frequently has dark scaling of the neck and face causing a 'dirty' appearance (**Fig 23.6**) and the flexures are often involved (**Fig 23.7**). Whereas children with IV are normal at birth, those with lamellar ichthyosis are often born with a collodion membrane (**Fig 23.8**) and develop thick plate-like scales (**Fig 23.9**). Acquired ichthyosis may be indistinguishable from IV but generally occurs in adults associated with underlying disease such as Hodgkin disease, other lymphomas, sarcoidosis, leprosy, and hypothyroidism (Okulicz and Schwartz 2003, Patel *et al.* 2006) (*Table 23.1*).

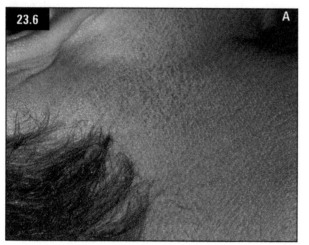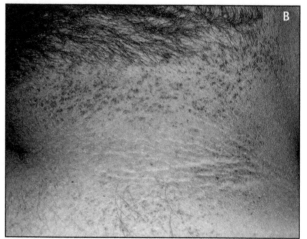

Fig 23.6 Dark scales causing a *dirty neck* appearance in (A) a teenage patient and (B) an older adult with X-linked ichthyosis.

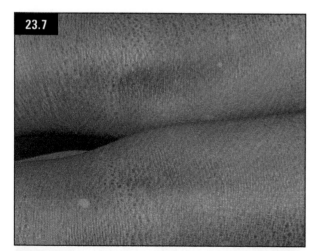

Fig 23.7 Involvement of the popliteal fossae in a teenager with X-linked ichthyosis. Ichthyosis vulgaris typically spares the flexures.

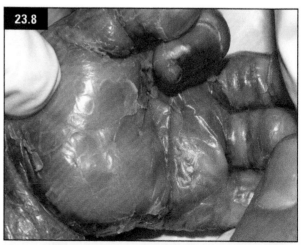

Fig 23.8 Collodion membrane on the hands of a baby with lamellar ichthyosis. Infants with ichthyosis vulgaris have normal skin at birth.

Fig 23.9 Thick plate-like scales in lamellar ichthyosis.

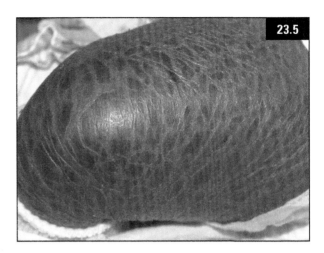

Table 23.1   Clinical features of acquired ichthyosis compared with ichthyosis vulgaris

	ICHTHYOSIS VULGARIS	ACQUIRED ICHTHYOSIS
Onset	Early childhood – mild childhood cases may worsen and later be confused with acquired ichthyosis	Adult onset
Genetics	Positive family history (atopic dermatitis) Associated with filaggrin mutations, and possibly other genes Heterozygous → mild disease Homozygous or compound heterozygous → more severe disease	Not hereditary
Clinical appearance	Symmetrical, large, plate-like scales on extensor surfaces of legs and arms. Whitish branny scales on trunk	May appear identical to ichthyosis vulgaris
Histopathology	Compact orthohyperkeratosis with diminished or absent granular layer, usually with absence of inflammatory cell infiltrate	Indistinguishable from ichthyosis vulgaris; however, ichthyosiform sarcoidosis often shows noncaseating granulomas and ichthyosiform mycosis fungoides shows malignant infiltrate
Associated conditions	Atopic dermatitis, asthma, allergic rhinitis	Malignancies (Hodgkin lymphoma, mycosis fungoides, Kaposi sarcoma, others) Sarcoidosis Hypothyroidism Leprosy HIV and HTLV-1 disease Metabolic disease Drugs

MANAGEMENT

The epidermis of patients with IV exhibits decreased pliability and water-retentive properties resulting in a defective barrier. Adequate hydration increases pliability and facilitates desquamation of the stratum corneum, by increasing hydrolytic enzyme activity and assisting mechanical desquamative forces (Shwayder and Ott 1991, Okulicz and Schwartz 2003, Rubeiz and Kibbi 2003). The goal of therapy in IV is to alleviate symptoms of the disease through hydration, lubrication, and keratolysis (Rubeiz and Kibbi 2003). α-Hydroxy acids such as lactic, glycolic, or pyruvic acids hydrate the skin and promote desquamation by causing disaggregation of cells in the lower stratum corneum. When used twice a day, in a 12% ammonium lactate lotion or compounded at a concentration of 5–10% in a suitable vehicle, lactic acid has been shown to be more effective than petrolatum-based creams (Shwayder and Ott 1991, Okulicz and Schwartz 2003, Rubeiz and Kibbi 2003).

Keratolytics such as salicylic acid in 1–6% concentrations promote scale removal by inducing keratinocyte disaggregation in the upper stratum corneum (Rubeiz and Kibbi 2003). Urea-containing creams in lower concentrations (10–20%) have humectant properties that improve pliability of the stratum corneum. Propylene glycol sheds thick skin on hydration, by establishing a water gradient and facilitating water movement through the stratum corneum (Shwayder and Ott 1991), but its widespread use is precluded by common allergic and irritant reactions. Topical retinoids such as tretinoin and tazarotene increase epidermal cell turnover and mitosis, reduce cohesiveness of keratinized cells, and suppress keratin synthesis, and have been used in certain severe forms of congenital ichthyosis (Okulicz and Schwartz 2003, Rubeiz and Kibbi 2003). Although tretinoin or tazarotene might be of some theoretical benefit, side effects such as irritation and flares of concomitant AD make them a poor choice for the treatment of IV patients (Rubeiz and Kibbi 2003).

A recent case study reported the successful use of combined therapy with ammonium lactate and a *physiological* lipid-based barrier-repair eruption (Epiceram) in the treatment of IV (Bellew and Del Rosso 2010).

CONCLUSION

The prognosis of IV is excellent, improving significantly with age. IV remains, however, a significant source of psychological distress and discomfort in affected patients, especially when associated with other common dermatological conditions such as xerosis or AD. Although significant advances in the discovery of associated mutations and molecular defects increased understanding of the pathophysiology of IV, only modest progress has been made in treatment paradigms within the last few decades. Effective symptomatic management without significant adverse effects remains a priority in ongoing research.

CHAPTER 24

LEGAL ASPECTS OF ATOPIC DERMATITIS

Daniel H. Parish and Noah Scheinfeld

INTRODUCTION

When the senior author of this chapter (NS) was in his first week at Harvard Law School, *l'enfant terrible* of the leftist critical legal studies movement looked out at the horseshoe of 140 students in the room and snickered, 'You're all wondering: where is the Marxism in all this? Really now, you do not need to be a Marxist to realize that economics informs all aspects of the law and human life.'

Really now, you do not need to be a lawyer to understand that, just as the field of medicine abuts deeply and profoundly on human health, law, which defines the economic and social interface of man and his fellows, abuts strongly on the practice of medicine.

Questions of life and death are the most critical at the intersection of law and medical practice. However, even diseases marked only by morbidity and not mortality fit into a legal framework. Atopic dermatitis presents fewer legal questions and complications than does organ transplantation, but both generate litigation (Mathias 1989, Ruzicka *et al.* 1991, Williams 2000, Marks *et al.* 2002, Goldberg 2007).

Dermatology can intersect with a variety of legal areas including administrative law, tort law, product liability law, disability law, and law governed by the Federal Trade Commission. Most articles discussing the legal aspects of dermatology and dermatological practice understandably focus on dermatological surgery or issues relating to cancer diagnosis, especially melanoma (Goldberg 2007). Indeed, it is possible to publish a textbook on the topic without reference to legal matters, and to our knowledge there has never been a chapter written regarding legal issues associated with atopic dermatitis.

Diagnosis and treatment of atopic dermatitis can have many legal implications for patients and their physicians. Atopic dermatitis treatment and diagnosis do not frequently lead to medical malpractice claims; a missed diagnosis of atopic dermatitis will typically have fewer consequences than will a missed diagnosis of melanoma, yet litigation does occur. Legal aspects of atopic dermatitis are more likely to involve such areas of the law as employment, disability, workers' compensation, tort law, family law, and rarely criminal law. This chapter surveys these legal aspects.

EMPLOYMENT AND BENEFITS LAW

The most significant interface of atopic dermatitis and the law relates to employment and benefits law, such as workers' compensation, Social Security, veterans' benefits, and employment discrimination. In these cases, the dermatologist or other physician is likely to be called on as an expert or a treating physician to support or contest a claim for benefits.

WORKERS' COMPENSATION

Throughout most of the industrialized world, systems of workers' compensation have evolved by which employees can be compensated for injury or illness that has occurred as a consequence of employment, without regard to whether the employee or employer is at fault. In the USA, each state has its own workers' compensation laws and, although these regulations have similarities, they vary from state to state.

Most skin-related workers' compensation cases involve contact dermatitis, and useful criteria have been developed to evaluate such cases (Mathias 1989, Marks *et al.* 2002). The same criteria used to evaluate the extent of an impairment caused by a skin disease can apply to cases of atopic dermatitis (Marks *et al.* 2002).

The more complicated questions become those of cause. It is more difficult to assess whether a workplace exposure or event can be proven to have precipitated an atopic dermatitis flare, eg, a patient with an underlying history of severe atopic dermatitis flares, who worked as an investigator for the state department of labor, claimed that she had new flares as a consequence of her exposure to temperature fluctuations, wind, and dust while traveling for her job (*Hughes v Department of Labor and Industry* 1992). The court found that the atopic dermatitis clearly predated her current position, and was not caused by her current employment, and that the conditions that the patient claimed to have caused the exacerbations were not unique to her employment.

Employment law litigation allows or rejects the establishment of a workplace connection to an exacerbation based on factors specific to the claimant's employment and not from generic environmental factors (*Wheeler v Boise* 1985, *Bodish v Fischer* 1965, *Dednam v American Machine and Foundry* 1963). In addition, where a flare is clearly connected to workplace exposure, disability cannot be shown if the atopic dermatitis is successfully treated and the patient can find new work (*Harris vs Board of Supervisors LSU* 1984). Conversely, employers also may use a patient's atopic dermatitis history to show that an alleged case of occupational contact dermatitis was in fact an exacerbation of pre-existing atopic dermatitis that had nothing to do with the employment, although the burden to bring forth this evidence may rest with the employer (*Kilgore v Daugherty* 1983).

As with patients with contact dermatitis, it would be advisable to urge patients prone to severe atopic dermatitis flares to avoid 'wet' work or other environments known to cause flares.

SOCIAL SECURITY AND PRIVATE INSURANCE BENEFITS

Patients may claim disability and be entitled to Social Security benefits or private employment insurance because of extensive atopic dermatitis. A patient may obtain Social Security benefits if his disease meets or exceeds the severity of the relevant impairment listing. If the individual is not engaged in 'substantial gainful activity' as a consequence of this disease and cannot perform other work existing in the national economy, he should be awarded disability benefits (*Masterson v Barnhart* 2002).

The law allows patients with psoriasis, atopic dermatitis, and dyshidrosis to qualify for disability, if they have 'extensive lesions, including involvement of the hands and feet, which impose a marked limitation of function and which are not responding to prescribed treatment' (20 CFR 404). The mere fact that a patient has had a disease for years does not mean that it has failed to respond to treatment, where evidence shows disease was merely episodic with treatment response (*Masterson v Barnhart* 2002). Interestingly, atopic dermatitis and asthma are often listed as comorbidities in claims for Social Security benefits without being the primary reason asserted for disability (*Eback v Chater* 1996, *Penn v Sullivan* 1990).

In Social Security benefit cases, the so-called *treating physician rule* applies and dictates that administrative law judges are to accord special deference to the physician who is actually taking care of the benefits claimant. The treating physician rule at issue here was originally developed by federal appellate courts as a means to control disability determinations by administrative law judges under the Social Security Act, and is now a regulatory rule (Maccaro 1993).

Patients may also seek disability benefits for severe atopic dermatitis that interferes with their life activities and prevents them from working under private insurance plans. Such plans are generally governed by federal law under the Employee Retirement Income and Security Act (ERISA) (29 USC). There are two important differences to note between ERISA claims and social security benefit claims. First, determinations of the employment plan administrator are reviewed fairly deferentially if challenged in court and can only be reversed if deemed 'arbitrary and capricious.' Second, the treating physician rule does not apply, and no special weight is given to the treating physician's opinion (*Black and Decker Disability Plan v Nord* 2003). Thus, in a case where a patient had received benefits and long-term disability for atopic dermatitis affecting the feet and hands, the plan administrator was within his discretion to terminate those benefits after the company presented new evidence from a reviewing dermatologist who specialized in occupational dermatology and opined that the impairment was only about 10% and that the patient should simply avoid wet work and prolonged walking (*Sparkman v Prudential* 2006). The reviewing court indicated that it was permissible to rely on this opinion over that of the treating (nondermatologist) physician, especially where there was evidence that the patient also had not seen the treating physician for some time.

VETERANS' BENEFITS

The Veterans' Administration must pay disability compensation for a 'disability resulting from a personal injury suffered or disease contracted in the line of duty, or for aggravation of a pre-existing injury suffered or disease contracted in the line of duty, in the active military, naval or air service' (38 USC 2005a, 2005b). Proof of a claim thus requires three elements: (1) medical evidence of a current disability, (2) lay or medical evidence of a disease or injury in service, and (3) medical evidence of a link between the current disability and the in-service injury or disease (*Caluza v Brown* 1995). The standards for veterans trying to establish this so-called 'service connection' for an illness or disability are comparatively lenient in that all reasonable doubts about the information to be resolved are in the veteran's favor (38 CFR 2006, 18 USC).

Under federal regulations, the determination of the percentage of disability depends on the extent of the atopic dermatitis. The particular regulations that govern the extent of a disability can be found at 38 CFR § 4.118 diagnostic codes 7800–7806. Although the diagnostic code 7806 deals specifically with 'dermatitis or eczema,' it can be appropriate to consider disability under either that code or under those from 7800 through 7805, which deal with scars and scarring, depending on the nature of skin problem at issue (*Dries v Principi* 2001). Code 7806 bases disability on the extent of the body affected by disease or the need for constant systemic therapy. 'Itching constant' was eliminated as a criterion for disability in 2002. Determination of this disability, which is a finding based on medical evidence, is to be done by the Board of Veterans' Appeals – it is an administrative proceeding – and not in a subsequent court case appealing such decision (*Elkins v Gober* 2000).

Although the standards for establishing a disability are low, they are not always surmounted, eg, temporary exacerbation shortly after induction was not an *increase in disability* or *aggravation in service* within the meaning of section 1153 which qualifies for disability (*Anderson v Brown* 1995). In addition, a patient is required to do more than simply submit his own opinion that his medical condition is related to his military service. Thus, a patient who served in Vietnam and had been diagnosed with atopic dermatitis in 1988 could not link his disease to Agent Orange exposure without a statutory presumption or medical evidence of a service connection for this condition. As the court noted, the veteran 'as a layperson, is not competent to testify that his skin problems resulted from Agent Orange exposure or other service-related disease or injury … . The absence of a medical opinion that there is a nexus between the appellant's service and his skin condition renders both of the appellant's claims not well grounded' (*Thomas v Brown* 1996). In the particular case of claims for illnesses associated with Agent Orange, the diagnosis of atopic dermatitis (as opposed to chloracne or other acneiform lesions) typically serves to defeat a veteran's claims of a service connection (Title Redacted 1999).

WORKPLACE ACCOMMODATION

The Americans with Disabilities Act protects individuals with disabilities from discrimination in employment and requires that certain employers (those with a minimum number of employees) make reasonable accommodations to permit an employee with a disability to continue working. A disability is defined as a 'physical or mental impairment that substantially limits one or more of the major life activities' (42 USC). Despite the prevalence of atopic dermatitis, there have been relatively few reported cases involving claims under the Americans with Disabilities Act.

In the context of the workplace, the fact that impairment limits an employee's ability to perform only one job does not constitute a disability under the Americans with Disabilities Act. Thus, a corrections officer with atopic dermatitis who was capable of performing other related work for her employer, even if limited in some aspects of her position, was not considered disabled for the purposes of the statute (*Sharp v Abate* 1995). Alternatively, a plaintiff who claimed that his eczema limited his ability to sleep well and interfered with other aspects of his life was unable to show that it was a disability within the meaning of the act that would require his employer to give him longer breaks between shifts and to limit his overtime, which the employer considered to be an essential part of the employment (*Verhoff v Time Warner Cable* 2006). An employer is also permitted to discriminate under certain circumstances against an employee who has atopic dermatitis that is exacerbated by latex gloves (even if he or she does not have latex allergy). If wearing such gloves is deemed necessary for employment and there is no evidence that the disease rendered her disabled, there is no violation of the Americans with Disabilities Act (*Franklin v Ingalls Memorial Hospital* 2002).

TORT LAW: MEDICAL MALPRACTICE, PRODUCT LIABILITY, AND OTHER INJURY CLAIMS

MEDICAL MALPRACTICE

Atopic dermatitis appears to provide an infrequent source of malpractice claims. Although the disease can be disfiguring and difficult to live with, improper treatment and missed diagnosis do not typically create severe or lasting damage. In the literature, the number of malpractice claims against dermatologists and for skin diseases remains well below those against other physicians. Within that realm, malpractice suits most commonly relate to malignant neoplasms and failure to diagnose (Glusac 2003, Lydiatt 2004, Read and Hill 2005).

A Physicians' Insurance Association of America report titled, 'A Risk Management Review of Malpractice Claims: Dermatology, 2001 Edition,' included malpractice claim data self-reported by the more than 20 member companies to the Association. The Association's data encompassed a 17-year period (1985–2001), and included information from a total compilation of 189 712 claims and suits for all insured providers. This report focused on the specialty of dermatology, and compared its experience with 27 other specialties and cumulative figures for all specialties. Contact dermatitis and other eczemas were involved in 99 cases or 9% of the dermatology cases in which insurers were involved (Read and Hill 2005).

Nevertheless, some malpractice cases do present. As an historical matter, physicians, who in the days before corticosteroids treated atopic dermatitis patients with radiation therapy, were targets of lawsuits alleging complications and negligence that left many patients burned, and, in at least one instance, led to limb amputation (*Kenney v La Grone* 1936, *McCoy v Buck* 1926, *Vaughan v Oliver* 1926, *Street v Hodgson* 1921, *Hayes v Lufkin* 1920, *Hamilton v Harris* 1920, *Hunter vs Burroughs* 1918, *Waddle vs Sutherland* 1930). The advent of corticosteroids, however, gave dermatologists and other physicians a generally safe and reliable treatment that made extreme adverse effects much rarer and lawsuits infrequent.

Treatment missteps nevertheless remain a potential legal landmine. As corticosteroids are the standard treatment, and treatment can be chronic, failure to monitor their use over the long term can lead to a lawsuit when untoward adverse effects occur. Thus, in one instance, a patient who had used oral steroids for 9 years and developed glaucoma sued his internist for failing to monitor him. Although the jury found the physician, an internist, negligent in filling prescriptions without seeing the patient and writing for amounts in excess of what the patient needed, it also found that the patient's use of doses far beyond what had been prescribed and his failure to come to office visits were intervening causes that made the physician not liable (*Stilloe v Contini* 1995). Similarly, patients who come in for treatment for one part of their body may be inclined to self-medicate by applying steroids to another part of the body when similar lesions arise. The use of inappropriately potent steroids can, of course, cause problems, and physicians must warn patients that an ointment that 'magically' clears a lesion on the arm would not be appropriate for the face.

Given its prevalence, however, atopic dermatitis can also provide the excuse for a patient to ask the dermatologist about another skin issue, which must be pursued if evaluated and can lead to legal liability on its own. In one case, a patient sought treatment for a flare of atopic dermatitis but also asked his dermatologist about a growing mole that the dermatologist then biopsied. The mole was reported as a nonmalignant nevus. During a subsequent visit 30 months later, again for an eczema flare, the patient pointed out a lump under his left arm for which the dermatologist referred the patient to his internist. Subsequent biopsy of the lump revealed it to be a metastatic melanoma, and the patient died soon after. A malpractice case followed, which the court ultimately dismissed for failure to have been filed within the statute of limitations. The patient's family was not allowed to claim that there had been continuous treatment for the condition from the time of the first biopsy to the second (*Trimper v Jones* 2007). The case nevertheless serves as a reminder

that a physician must carefully identify the scope of a patient's treatment in a given situation and adhere to it.

Another area of potential litigation with atopic dermatitis is adrenal suppression from inappropriate (usually long-term) use of high-potency topical steroids for atopic or other dermatitides (Kubetin 2003, Ault 2005, Skin-Cap 2008) (*Perkins and Perkins v Walker* 1987). Many case reports exist that relate class I steroid use (clobetasol propionate) to adrenal suppression, bone pathology, and other serious adverse effects. A lawsuit was successfully waged against a dermatologist who prescribed months of topical high-potency corticosteroids for chronic hand dermatitis which led to adrenal suppression, osteoporosis, and sequelae from the osteoporosis, including damage to the spine. The issue of adrenal suppression from long-term topical steroid use in a psoriatic patient was a legal issue in a surgical case involving proper preoperative preparation. A product named Skin-Cap, which was supposed to contain natural remedies and zinc and instead contained high-potency steroids, prompted the US Food and Drug Administration (FDA) to ban its sale and resulted in a class action lawsuit against its maker.

In sum, ultra-high-potency corticosteroid creams (class I corticosteroids) should be used with care. Practitioners should note that almost all side effects to topical corticosteroids (and most litigation involving corticosteroids) have been linked to long-term use of class I corticosteroids. Short-term use of topical corticosteroids should not prompt special warning but, for long-term use of class I steroids, a written patient handout is useful as well as discussion with patients documented in the medical chart. In addition, although no lawsuits to the author's knowledge have been linked to topical corticosteroids, it is prudent to mention the existence of the 'black box' warning to patients, to avoid callbacks at the very least and the possibility of litigation at worst. It is also prudent to provide patient handouts for systemic corticosteroids and systemic agents that are used off-label to treat atopic dermatitis.

PRODUCT LIABILITY

Legal issues in product liability and atopic dermatitis can be divided into two groups: those in which a treatment for atopic dermatitis is alleged to be unsafe, and those in which another product is alleged to have exacerbated atopic dermatitis.

As the lower-potency steroids that are the mainstay of treatment for atopic dermatitis have very favorable adverse effect profiles, and those adverse effects that do occur tend not to occur suddenly, they present little problem. Thus, the number of cases of pediatric hypothalamic–pituitary axis disruption – perhaps the most serious adverse consequence of corticosteroid use – from 1970 to 2003 amounted to just 22.

On the other hand, the immunomodulators, tacrolimus and pimecrolimus, which serve as second-line therapies for atopic dermatitis, have generated recent litigation over their possible association with certain cancers, especially in the wake of the FDA issuing 'black box' warnings for the drugs in 2005. Claims in the USA are largely against drug companies, and legal issues have focused on the adequacies of warnings and issues of pre-emption – whether and to what degree a federal statute, regulation, or agency ruling (here from the FDA) trumps any state law or suit filed under that state law. Two courts have ruled that the fact that the FDA had approved the drugs but had not reached any conclusions about any links between calcineurin inhibitors and cancer risks in children did not prevent claims under state law for 'failure to warn' from proceeding (*Perry v Novartis* 2006, *Weiss v Fujisawa* 2006a). Specifically, the FDA approval of the drugs as 'safe and effective' under 21 USC § 355(a) did not pre-empt claims for behavior during the time before the black box warning, when the FDA had not made conclusive findings about a cancer link to calcineurin inhibitors. The underlying claims in each case hinge on the proposition that atopic dermatitis is a relatively mild disease and that, as one court ruled, 'the cancer risk allegedly posed by [the calcineurin inhibitors] appears to vastly outweigh the benefit of treating eczema' (*Weiss vs Fujisawa* 2006b). There has been much criticism of this warning, and the legal climate that it has generated, as well as the reality of the increased cancer risk, but the warning and the legal problems remain (Aaronson 2006, Fleischer 2006).

There is also litigation surrounding non-pharmaceutical products that plaintiffs allege dangerously exacerbate or cause atopic dermatitis. Although there is no reason to doubt the reality and severity of the underlying disease noted in these situations, many of the cases of medical claims of causation seem to border on the frivolous, eg, in one case parents alleged that synthetic sheets caused a severe exacerbation of their child's atopic dermatitis, leading to permanent physical injury and disfigurement. It is worth noting that the plaintiff's experts who attempted to establish the connection with atopic dermatitis were not dermatologists or even general medical practitioners but, rather, a physiatrist who had no professional experience treating anyone with atopic dermatitis or asthma and a child psychologist (*Israel v Spring Industries* 2006). Likewise, the plaintiff's failure to secure an expert with medical or dermatological training led to the exclusion of evidence that a rash after exposure to polychlorinated biphenyls and dioxin might be chloracne and not the plaintiff's underlying atopic dermatitis, as asserted by appropriate experts for the defense (*Mancuso v Consolidated Edison* 1999).

Similarly, a plaintiff who had atopic dermatitis claimed a severe exacerbation after using a particular shampoo. She was not entitled to prevail on a duty-to-warn claim or strict liability for manufacture of a dangerous product because there had been just three verifiable allergic reactions from the sale of 225 million tubes. This did not show that the product was dangerous or that a warning was needed (*Mountain v Procter and Gamble* 1970).

In at least one case, however, the plaintiffs prevailed at the trial, and the appellate court upheld a claim of exacerbation of atopic dermatitis secondary to mold exposure. A pediatric allergist in the case had opined that mold would not exacerbate atopic dermatitis, whereas a dermatologist thought it would. Damages against the home builder were affirmed (*Chenniliaro v Kaufman et al.* 1994).

Misdiagnosis of allergic contact dermatitis as atopic dermatitis may complicate questions of product liability and the issue of statute of limitations. Under general rules, a statute of limitations will be suspended or 'tolled' if some legal disability prevents a patient from reasonably uncovering the facts necessary to initiate a lawsuit within the allotted time, eg, a dental office worker likely misdiagnosed as having a flare of atopic dermatitis in 1988 (after a history of the disease) was later diagnosed as having a latex allergy in 1996 (after she saw a program on latex allergy and raised the issue with her physician). She was permitted to maintain her suit against the manufacturer because she could not reasonably have discovered her latex allergy until that later date, given the 1988 diagnosis (*Salemme v Aero-Med* 2004); a similar issue and conclusion were obtained in an almost identical case involving a nursing student (*Zamboni v Aladan* 2004). On the other hand, where the evidence belied the claim that a patient was told she had dermatitis and only later determined it to be latex allergy, the statute of limitations was not tolled, and the claim was dismissed (*Hughes v Allegiance Healthcare* 2001).

GENERAL TORT LAW – OTHER ALLEGED INJURIES

Above and beyond the realm of malpractice, claims that tortuous conduct caused or exacerbated atopic dermatitis have arisen outside the realm of malpractice law. A patient's history of atopic dermatitis will usually function as a defense against a claim that some recent exposure caused the patient's dermatitis (*Gibbs v Riverwalk Cruise Lines* 1992). Similarly, when arguments are made that intentional infliction of emotional distress exacerbated an underlying condition, that exacerbation must be tied directly to the tortuous conduct with no other related cause (*Langeslag v KYMN* 2003), a fairly strict standard. At least one published case, however, records an action allowed to proceed for a recurrence of atopic dermatitis after an especially traumatic event (an airline hijacking) (*Herman v TWA* 1972).

FAMILY AND CRIMINAL LAW: PEDIATRICS AND CHILD CUSTODY, NEGLECT, AND ABUSE

The prevalence of atopic dermatitis among children and the bitterness of family custody disputes bring about misunderstandings about the disease. The unfortunate reality of child sexual abuse is, of course, the subject of legal issues. In these situations, the role of physician will often be as a treating physician or expert to clarify what is and is not atopic dermatitis, and what is and is not appropriate handling and care of the disease by a parent or guardian.

The care of atopic dermatitis frequently becomes an issue in child abuse and neglect cases, as well as in custody battles. In one case that serves as an example of many of these issues, one parent alleged that the other had sexually abused a child based on signs of vaginal irritation that may or may not have been atopic dermatitis (*Whitworth v Whitworth* 2007). A previous diagnosis of eczema had led child protective service agents to determine that the allegation of abuse was not founded. On the other hand, the father's mother, who had intervened to seek custody of her grandchild, alleged that the investigation into the matter initiated by the birth mother had caused stress significant enough to exacerbate the daughter's atopic dermatitis, a claim that was also rejected.

In some custody cases, parents and guardians have raised the mere development of atopic dermatitis as evidence of parental neglect (*Miller v Rieser* 1994). More often, however, one side will claim failure on the part of the other to treat atopic dermatitis or follow a physician's recommendations (In re *Kaisson* 2006, *New Jersey Division of Youth and Family Services v SNJ* 2006), especially if the atopic dermatitis has become superinfected (*MP v JJT Sr* 2005). They may claim this as evidence of neglect that should lead to termination or limitation of parental or guardian rights. Courts have in fact terminated rights where a child is known to have severe atopic dermatitis and asthma, and the guardian or parent has demonstrated neglect in handling the condition appropriately as a caregiver (In the Interest of NVD 2003).

Claims of stress-induced atopic dermatitis flares have also been used to challenge visitation schedules and parental rights (*Mann v Mann* 2001). One parent used his child's atopic dermatitis to his advantage in a custody proceeding, by noting that he and his new wife were so attentive to his children's asthma and atopic dermatitis that they had stopped smoking so as not to aggravate the conditions (*Ray v Ray* 2002).

On the other hand, misperceptions about atopic dermatitis on the part of parents can lead to inappropriate behavior by a caregiver (such as refusing to let a child attend school) that has also resulted in reduction or termination of custody (In the Interest of RHL 2003). The mere failure of atopic dermatitis to improve under a parent's care should not, however, lead to termination of parental rights, in the absence of evidence of gross neglect. As one court noted, 'the subject of proper medical treatment for eczema is not within the realm of common knowledge and everyday experience' (In re *MD* 2000).

In child sexual abuse cases, defendants will often claim that the only reason they touched, examined, or applied lotion to a minor in a sensitive area was to treat or monitor his or her atopic dermatitis (*Family Independence Agency v Jelinek* 2005, *State vs Rose* 1982). Likewise, defendants have offered the defense that genital irritation represented atopic dermatitis and was not evidence of child sexual abuse (*State v Martin* 2004). Defendants have asserted more generally that marks on a victim were the result of atopic dermatitis and not beatings (*State v Noil* 2001). In all of these cases, it is the factual determination of the nature of a rash or disease, as clarified by a medical expert, rather than any particular legal rules, that will usually determine the outcome of a case.

PRISONERS' RIGHTS

Atopic dermatitis is sometimes a subject of complaint in prisoner *pro se* petitions seeking a civil rights action under 42 USC section 1983 for deliberate indifference to medical conditions. Under this statute prisoners will accuse prison authorities, and occasionally but less commonly physicians, of violating their Eighth Amendment right to be free from cruel and unusual punishment by not properly addressing their atopic dermatitis (*Sledge v Kooi* 2007, *Jackson v Clowers* 2003). Most such cases fail, both because they are typically factually deficient and because the level of care required to meet the 'deliberate indifference' standard is not especially high. An issue that engenders grievances in prisons is the lack of access to specialist care and restricted drug formularies. In some states, court-appointed monitors have their prison healthcare being administered under a court-appointed monitor. It is overseen prison healthcare.

CONCLUSIONS

There are many potential legal scenarios that involve patients with atopic dermatitis or their caregivers. This chapter has covered many, but not all, legal aspects particular to atopic dermatitis. It is based on US case law and is intended only to raise the physician's awareness of possible legal issues. The chapter does not pretend, nor is it intended, to be a comprehensive source of legal advice. Moreover, regulations vary from state to state, as well as from country to country.

There are likely to be cases that involve denial of payment, private insurance companies, or government insurance agencies for phototherapy or expensive medications used by dermatologists but deemed experimental.

Although atopic dermatitis does not present the more pervasive threat of medical malpractice that other aspects of dermatological practice might, it does arise in a wide variety of legal contexts, especially but not exclusively those related to employment law and benefits that may require dermatological expertise to settle disputes.

TABLE OF CASES

18 USC 5107

20 CFR 404, Subpt. P, App.1 Listing of Impairments

29 USC § 1132

38 CFR 3.102 (2006)

38 USC 1110 (2005a)

38 USC 1131 (2005b)

42 USC § 12102(2)(A)

Anderson v Brown, 8 Vet.App. 145, 1995 WL 495416 (Vet.App. 1995)

Black and Decker Disability Plan v Nord, 538 U.S. 822 (2003)

Bodish v Fischer, Inc., 133 N.W.2d 867 (Iowa 1965)

Caluza v Brown, 7 Vet. App. 498 (1995)

Chenniliaro v Kaufman and Broad Home Systems of Louisiana, Inc., 636 So.2d 246 (La.App. 1994)

Dednam v American Machine and Foundry Co., 363 S.W.2d 419 (Ark. 1963)

Dries v Principi, 18 Vet.App. 5 (2001)

Eback v Chater, 94 F.3d 410 (8th Cir. 1996)

Elkins v Gober, 229 F.3d 1369 (Fed.Cir. 2000)

Family Independence Agency v Jelinek, 2005 WL 1160221 (Mich.App. 2005)

Franklin v Ingalls Memorial Hospital, 2002 WL 643367 (N.D.Ill. 2002)

Gibbs v Riverwalk Cruise Lines, Inc., 2 Fla. J.V.R.A. (8)8, 1992 WL 1473687 (Fla.Dist.Ct. 1992)

Hamilton v Harris, 223 S.W. 533 (Tex.Civ. App. 1920)

Harris v Board of Supervisors of LSU, Agricultural and Mechanical College, 451 So.2d 1293 (La. App. 1984)

Hayes v Lufkin, 179 N.W. 1007 (Minn. 1920)

Herman v Trans World Airlines, Inc., 337 N.Y.S.2d 827, A.D.2d 850 (N.Y.App. 1972)

Hughes v Dept. of Labor and Industry, 833 P2d 1099 (Mont. 1992)

Hughes v Allegiance Healthcare Corp., 152 F.Supp.2d 667 (E.D.Pa. 2001)

Hunter v Burroughs, 96 S.E. 360 (Va. 1918)

In re Kaisson C, 2006 WL 2349046, (Conn. Super. 2006)

In re MD, 758 A.2d 27 (D.C. 2000)

In the Interest of NVD, 102 S.W.3d 268 (Tex. Ct.App. 2003)

In the Interest of RHL, 272 Ga.App. 10, 611 S.E.2d 700 (Ga.App. 2003)

Israel v Spring Industries, 2006 WL 3196956 (E.D.N.Y. 2006)

Jackson v Clowers, 83 Fed.Appx. 990 (10th Cir. 2003)

Kenney v La Grone, 93 Tex.Civ.App. 397 398 (Tex. Civ.App. 1936)

Kilgore v Daugherty, Admin. Bur. Workers' Comp. Loarin App. No., C.A.No.3451 (Ohio Bd.Work. App. June 1, 1983)

Langeslag v KYMN Inc., 664 N.W.2d 860 (Minn. 2003)

Mancuso v Consolidated Edison Co. of New York, 56 F.Supp.2d 391 (S.D.N.Y. 1999), affirmed in relevant part, vacated in part, 216 F.3d 1072 (2d Cir. 2000)

Mann v Mann, 798 So.2d 24 (Fla.App. 2001)

Masterson v Barnhart, 309 F.3d 237 (5th Cir. 2002)

McCoy v Buck, 160 46 (Ind.App. 1926)

Miller v Rieser, 446 S.E.2d 233 (Ga.App. 1994)

Mountain v Procter and Gamble Co., 312 F.Supp. 534 (E.D.Wisc. 1970)

MP v JJT Sr, 2005 WL 3592722 (Del.Fam.Ct 2005)

New Jersey Division of Youth and Family Services v S.N.J., 2006 WL 1419399 (N.J.Super. 2006)

Penn v Sullivan, 896 F.2d 313 (8th Cir. 1990)

Perkins S and Perkins G, Appellants, v John R. Walker, Appellee (1987)

Perry v Novartis Pharmaceutical Corp., 456 F.Supp.2d 786 (E.D.Pa. 2006)

Ray v Ray, 83 S.W.3d 726 (2002)

Salemme v Aero-Med, Ltd., 2004 WL 2550423 (Mass.Super 2004)

Sharp v Abate, 887 F.Supp. 695 (S.D.N.Y. 1995)

Sledge v Kooi, 2007 WL 951447 (N.D.N.Y. 2007)

Sparkman v Prudential Ins. Corp. of Amer., 427 F.Supp.2d 1117 (D.Utah 2006)

State v Martin, 2004 WL 2340121 (Ohio.App. 2004)

State v Noil, 807 So.2d 295 (La.App. 2001)

State v Rose, 324 N.W.2d 894 (S.Dak. 1982)

Stilloe v Contini, 623 N.Y.S.2d 213 (N.Y.App. 1995)

Street v Hodgson, 115 A. 27 (Md.App. 1921)

Thomas v Brown, (Vet.App. 1996)

Title Redacted, Bd.Vet.App. 9933070, 1999 WL 33879333 (Bd.Vet.App. 1999)

Trimper v Jones, 829 N.Y.S.2d 786 (N.Y.App. 2007)

Vaughan v Oliver, 3 Tenn.App. 559 (Tenn.App. 1926)

Verhoff v Time Warner Cable, Inc., 2006 WL 3304179 (N.D.Ohio 2006)

Waddle v Sutherland, 120 So. 201 (Miss. 1930)

Weiss v Fujisawa, 464 F.Supp.2d 666 (E.D.Ky. 2006a)

Weiss v Fujisawa Pharmaceutical Co., 2006 WL 3533072 (E.D.Ky. 2006b)

Wheeler v Boise Cascade Corp., 298 Or. 452, 693 P.2d 632 (Or. 1985)

Whitworth v Whitworth, – S.W.3d –, 2007 WL 852544 (Tex.App. 2007)

Zamboni v Aladan Corp., 304 F.Supp.2d 218 (D.Mass. 2004)

REFERENCES

CHAPTER 1

Ackerknecht EH (1982). Diathesis: the word and the concept in medical history. *Bulletin of the History of Medicine*, **56**: 317–325.

Ackerman AB, Ragaz A (1982). A plea to expunge the word 'eczema' from the lexicon of dermatology and dermatopathology. *Archives of Dermatological Research*, **272**: 407–420

Agnes M (2006). *Webster's New World College Dictionary*. Webster's New World, Cleveland.

Anonymous (1881). Report of Societies – Annual meeting of the American Medical Association. *The Boston Medical and Surgical Journal*, **104**: 469–470.

Anonymous (1898). Abortion dangerous in England. *New England Medical Monthly*, **17**(1): 191.

Baer RL, ed. (1955). The development of the concept of atopic dermatitis. In: *Atopic Dermatitis*, New York University Press, New York, pp. 1–9.

Baer RL (1982). No–the word 'eczema' should not be expunged but be retained for the time being. *The American Journal of Dermatopathology*, **4**: 327–328.

Bateman T (1817). *Delineations of Cutaneous Diseases*, Longman, Hurst, Rees, Orme & Brown, London, plate XXXVII.

Bateman T (1836). In: Thomson AT (ed.), *A Practical Synopsis of Cutaneous Diseases According to the Arrangement of Dr. Willan*, 8th edn, Longman, Rees, Orme, Brown, Green & Longman, London, pp. 108, 305, 311.

Beeson B, Pierre FR (1930). Pierre Francois Rayer 1793–1867. *Archives of Dermatology and Syphilology*, **22**: 893–897.

Besnier ME (1892). Première note et observations préliminaires pour servir d'introduction à l'étude des prurigos diathésiques (dermatites multiformes prurigineuses chroniques exacerbantes et paroxystiques, du type du prurigo de Hebra). *Bulletin de la Société française de dermatologie et de syphiligraphie*, **3**: 267–280.

Black MM (2003). The Neil Smith memorial lecture: John Laws Milton. The founder of St John's Hospital for diseases of the skin. *Clinical and Experimental Dermatology*, **28**: 89–91.

Blackfan KD (1916). Cutaneous reaction from proteins in eczema. *American Journal of Diseases of Children*, **11**: 441–454.

Bos JD (2002). Atopiform dermatitis. *British Journal of Dermatology*, **147**: 426–429.

Bos JD, Brenninkmeijer EE, Schram ME, Middelkamp-Hup MA, Spuls PI, Smitt JH (2010). Atopic eczema or atopiform dermatitis. *Experimental Dermatology*, **19**: 325–331.

Brocq L (1896). Papular affections. In: Stedman TL (ed.), *An International Encyclopedia of Modern Medical Science by Leading Authorities of Europe and America*, Vol 5, *Diseases of the Skin*, William Wood, New York, pp. 326–343.

Brocq L, Jacquet L 1891 Notes pour servir a l'histoire des neurodermites. Du lichen circumscriptus des anciens auteurs, ou lichen simplex chronique de M. Le Dr. E. Vidal. *Annales de Dermatologie et de Syphilographie* **2**: 634.

Browne EA (1870). Detached notes on eczema. *The Liverpool Medical and Surgical Reports*, **4**: 71–84.

Bulkley LD (1881). *Eczema and Its Management; A Practical Treatise Based on the Study of Three Thousand Cases of the Disease*, G.P. Putnam's Sons, New York, p. 1.

Bulkley LD (1882). *Eczema and Its Management: A Practical Treatise Based on the Study of Two Thousand Five Hundred Cases of the Disease*, Putnam Sons, New York, pp. 19–20.

Caillault C, Blake RH (1861). *A Practical Treatise on Diseases of the Skin in Children: from the French of Caillault*, Churchill, London, p. 2.

Chaucer G (2006). *Canterbury Tales*, Prestwick House.

Clayton DE, Coca AF (1929). The skin as a shock tissue. *Bulletin of the New York Academy of Medicine*, **5**: 223–231.

Crissey JT, Parish LC (1981). The legacy of Aetius. In: Crissey JT, Parish LC (eds), *The Dermatology and Syphilology of the Nineteenth Century*, Praeger, New York, pp. 332–351.

Crissey JT, Parish LC (1998). Two hundred years of dermatology. *Journal of the American Academy of Dermatology*, **39**: 1006.

De Benedetto A, Agnihothri R, McGirt LY, *et al.* (2009). Atopic dermatitis: A disease caused by innate immune defects? *Journal of Investigative Dermatology*, **129**: 14–30.

Dickinson MD (1891). Eczema in the Jew – original translations from the French. *Weekly Medical Review*, **24**: 329–330.

Dotz W, Jean Paul M (1979). His life, cutaneous disease, death, and depiction by Jacques Louis David. *American Journal of Dermatopathology*, **1**: 247–250.

Elias PM, Steinhoff M (2008). 'Outside-to-inside' (and now back to 'outside') pathogenic mechanisms in atopic dermatitis. *Journal of Investigative Dermatology*, **128**: 1067–1070.

Farhi D, Taïeb A, Tilles G, Wallach D (2010). The historical basis of a misconception leading to undertreating atopic dermatitis (eczema): facts and controversies. *Clinical Dermatology*, **28**: 45–51.

Goddard JA (1670). Discourse, setting forth the unhappy Condition of the Practice of Physick in London, and offering some means to put it into a better; for the Interests of Patients, no less, or rather much more, than of Physicians. John Martyn & James Alestry, London, reprinted in: 1746 Harleian Miscellany: or, a collection of scarce, curious and entertaining pamphlets and tracts, as well in manuscript as in print found in the late Earl of Oxford's libary, Vol VIII, Osborne, London.

Hand WD (1980). *Magical Medicine: The Folkloric Component of Medicine in the Folk Belief, Custom and Ritual of the Peoples of Europe and America*, University of California Press, Berkeley, p. 189.

Hanifin JM (2002). Atopiform dermatitis: do we need another confusing name for atopic dermatitis? *British Journal of Dermatology*, **147**: 430–432.

Hardy A, Piffard HG (1868). *The Dartrous Diathesis*, Moorhead, Simpson & Bond, New York, p. 2.

Hazen HH (1915). *Diseases of the Skin*, CV Mosby, St Louis, p. 249.

Hebra F (1868). *On Diseases of the Skin, including the Exanthemata*, Vol 2 (translated by Fagge CH, Pye-Smith PH), The New Sydenham Society, London, pp. 119, 267–268.

Heimann WJ (1916). A critical review of eczema and dermatitis with an analysis of a group of cases. *Journal of Cutaneous Diseases*, **34**: 259–284.

Highman WJ (1921). *Dermatology: The Essentials of Cutaneous Medicine*, Macmillan, New York, p. 5.

Hyde JN (1904). The passing of eczema (editorial). *Journal of Cutaneous Diseases including Syphilis*, **22**: 30S.

Jackson SH (1792). *Dermato-pathologia: or practical observations from some new thoughts on the pathology and proximate cause of diseases of the true skin and its emanations, the rete mucosum and cuticle, etc. (with an appendix and remarks on scurvy)*, Robson Johnson, London.

Kaposi M (1895). *Pathology and Treatment of Diseases of the Skin* (translated by Johnston JC),

William Wood, New York, pp. 346–347.

Kerley CG (1919). *Practice of Pediatrics*, WB Saunders, Philadelphia, p. 593.

Kershaw I (2008). *Hitler: A Biography*, Norton, New York, p. 380.

Leider M (1982). Comments by the Consultant Editor on the controversy about eczema. *American Journal of Dermatopathology*, **4**: 339–341.

Liang JH (1988). *A Handbook of Traditional Chinese Dermatology*, Blue Poppy Press, Boulder, p. 22.

Mier PD (1975). Earliest description of the atopic syndrome? *British Journal of Dermatology*, **92**: 359.

Montefiore SS (2005). *Stalin: The Court of the Red Tsar*, First Vintage Books, New York, p. 190.

Morris M (1909). *Diseases of the Skin*, William Wood, New York, p. 255.

Morris M (1912). Prurigo, pruriginous eczema and lichenification. *British Medical Journal*, **1**: 1469–1474.

Mysticus (1920). Jean Paul Marat: Free Mason and friend of the people. *The New Age Magazine*, **28**: 507–511.

Neligan JM (1866). *A Practical Treatise on Diseases of the Skin*, Lea, Philadelphia, p. 114.

Nexmand PH (1948). *Clinical Studies of Besnier's Prurigo*, Rosenkilde & Bagger, Copenhagen.

Nolosco MA (2004). *Physician Heal Thyself: Medical Practitioners of Eighteenth-Century New York*, Peter Lang, New York, p. 4.

Patalay R, Leslie KS, Levell NJ (2008). Robert Willan and the age of enlightenment. *International Journal of Dermatology*, **47**: 297–300.

Pye-Smith PH (1893). *An Introduction to the Study of Diseases of the Skin*, Lea Brothers, Philadelphia, PA, p. 342.

Ravogli A (1918). Dermatological notes 1 – eczema. *The American Journal of Clinical Medicine*, **25**: 421–424.

Rayer P (1833). *Treatise on Diseases of the Skin* (translated by Dickinson WB), John Churchill, London, p. 86.

Rayer P (1835). *Traité des maladies de la peau* [atlas]. Baillière, Paris.

Rydström J (2003). *Sinners and Citizens – Bestiality and Homosexuality in Sweden, 1880–1950*, University of Chicago Press, Chicago, pp. 189–190.

Schamberg JF (1908), Eczema. *Diseases of the skin and the eruptive fevers*, W.B. Saunders, p. 71.

Schuttelaar ML, Vermeulen KM, Drukker N, Coenraads PJ (2010). A randomized controlled trial in children with eczema: nurse practitioner vs. dermatologist. *British Journal of Dermatology*, **162**: 162–170.

Sulzberger MB (1939). The treatment of infantile eczema from the point of view of the dermatologist. *Journal of the American Medical Association*, **112**: 38–45.

Sulzberger MB (1982). Eczema viewed from the perspective of 60 years' experience. *American Journal of Dermatopathology*, **4**: 337–338.

Sulzberger MB, Goodman J (1936). The relative importance of specific skin hypersensitivity in adult atopic dermatitis. *Journal of the American Medical Association*, **106**: 1000–1003.

Sulzberger MB, Witten VH (1952). The effect of topically applied compound F in selected dermatoses. *Journal of Investigative Dermatology*, **19**: 101–102.

Sutton RL (1916). *Diseases of the Skin*, Mosby, St Louis, p. 195.

Taïeb A, Wallach D, Tilles G (2006). The history of atopic eczema/dermatitis. In: Ring J, Przybilla B, Ruzicka T (eds), *Handbook of Atopic Eczema*, 2nd edn, Springer-Verlag, Berlin, pp. 10–20.

Talbot FB (1918). Eczema in childhood. *Medical Clinics of North America*, **1**: 985.

Tilbury Fox W (1879). *Skin Diseases: Their Description, Pathology, Diagnosis, and Treatment*, William Wood, New York, p. 163.

Tilles G, Wallach D (1999). Robert Willan and the French Willanists. *British Journal of Dermatology*, **140**: 1122–1126.

Turner D (1731). *De Morbis Cutaneis. A Treatise of Diseases Incident to the Skin*, Walthoe, Wilkin, Bonwicke, Birt, Ward & Wicksteed, London.

Unna PG (1903). The history of eczema in the last century in England. The oration delivered at the annual meeting and congress of the Dermatological Society of Great Britain and Ireland. In: Shillitoe A, Warde WB (eds), *Transactions of the Dermatological Society of Great Britain and Ireland (1902–1903)*, Vol 9, Lewis, London, pp. 6–29.

Van Harlingen A (1889). Eczema. In: Keating JM (ed.), *Cyclopedia of the Disease of Children*, Vol 2, JB Lipincott, Philadelphia, p. 71.

Vickers HR (1952). The problem of the pathogenesis of endogenous eczema. *British Journal of Dermatology*, **64**: 225–230.

Wallach D, Coste J, Tilles G, Taïeb A (2005). The first images of atopic dermatitis: an attempt at retrospective diagnosis in dermatology. *Journal of the American Academy of Dermatology*, **53**: 684–689.

Walzer A (1929). Allergy in skin disease: Discussion. *Bulletin of the New York Academy of Medicine*, **5**: 243–252.

White JC (1870). On the pathology of eczema (letter). *American Journal of Syphilography and Dermatology*, **1**: 282–283, 385.

White JC (1881). Some of the causes of infantile eczema and the importance of mechanical restraint in its treatment. *Boston Medical and Surgical Journal*, **105**: 365–368.

Wigley JE (1953). The everlasting eczema; a retrospect. *Australasian Journal of Dermatology*, **2**: 5–10.

Willan R (1808). *On Cutaneous Diseases*, Johnson, London.

Wilson E (1857). Eczema infantile. In: Wilson E (ed.), *On Diseases of the Skin*, 4th American edn, Blanchard & Lea, Philadelphia, pp. 171–181.

Wilson E (1878). *Cleopatra's Needle: With Brief Notes on Egypt and Egyptian Obelisks*, Brain, London.

Wilson E (1881). *The Egypt of the Past*, Kegan Paul & Trench, London.

Witten VH, Amler AB, Sulzberger MB, Desanctis AG (1954). Hydrocortisone ointment in the treatment of infantile eczema. *American Medical Association – American Journal of Diseases of Children*, **87**: 298–304.

CHAPTER 2

Akiyama M (2010). FLG mutations in ichthyosis vulgaris and atopic eczema: spectrum of mutations and population genetics. *British Journal of Dermatology*, **162**: 472–477.

Baurecht H, Irvine AD, Novak N, *et al.* (2007). Toward a major risk factor for atopic eczema: meta-analysis of filaggrin polymorphism data. *Journal of Allergy and Clinical Immunology*, **120**: 1406–1412.

Beck H-I, Hagdrup HK (1987). Atopic dermatitis, house dust mite allergy and month of birth. *Acta Dermato-Venereologica (Stockholm)*, **67**: 448–451.

Behrendt H, Krämer U, Dolgner R, *et al.* (1993). Elevated levels of total serum IgE in East German children: atopy, parasites, or pollutants? *Allergology Journal*, **2**: 31–40.

Ben-Gashir MA, Seed PT, Hay RJ (2002). Are quality of family life and disease severity related in childhood atopic dermatitis? *Journal of the European Academy of Dermatology and Venereology*, **16**: 455–462.

Ben-Gashir MA, Seed PT, Hay RJ (2004). Predictors of atopic dermatitis severity over time. *Journal of the American Academy of Dermatology*, **50**: 349–356.

Björkstén B (1999). The intrauterine and postnatal environment. *Journal of Allergy and Clinical Immunology*, **104**: 1119–1127.

Björkstén B (2000). Perinatal events in relation to sensitization in the human. *American Journal of Respiratory and Critical Care Medicine*, **162**: S105–S107.

Bobák M, Koupilová I, Williams HC, *et al.* (1995). Prevalence of asthma, atopic eczema and hay fever in five Czech towns with different levels of air pollution. *Epidemiology*, **6**: S35.

Böhme M, Svensson A, Kull I, Nordvall SL, Wahlgren CF (2001). Clinical features of atopic dermatitis at 2 years of age: a prospective, population-based case-control study. *Acta Dermato-Venereologica*, **81**: 193–197.

Boyle RJ, Bath-Hextall FJ, Leonardi-Bee J, Murrell DF, Tang ML (2009). Probiotics for the treatment of eczema: a systematic review. *Clinical and Experimental Allergy*, **39**: 1117–1127.

Brehler RB, Luger TA (2001). Atopic dermatitis: the role of *Pityrosporum ovale*. *Journal of the European Academy of Dermatology and Venereology*, **15**: 5–6.

Brenninkmeijer EE, Schram ME, Leeflang MM, Bos JD, Spuls PI (2008). Diagnostic criteria for atopic dermatitis: a systematic review. *British Journal of Dermatology*, **158**: 754–765.

Burney PGJ, Chinn S, Rona RJ (1990). Has the prevalence of asthma increased in children? Evidence from the national study of health and growth 1973–86. *British Medical Journal*, **300**: 1306–1310.

Burrel-Morris C, Williams HC (2000). Atopic dermatitis in migrant populations. In: Williams HC (ed.), *Atopic Dermatitis. The Epidemiology, Causes and Prevention of Atopic Eczema*, Cambridge University Press, Cambridge, pp. 169–182.

Chalmers DA, Todd G, Saxe N, *et al.* (2007). Validation of the UK working party diagnostic criteria for atopic eczema in a Xhosa-speaking African population. *British Journal of Dermatology*, **156**: 612.

Chen H, Common JE, Haines RL, *et al.* (2011). Wide spectrum of filaggrin-null mutations in atopic dermatitis highlights differences between Singaporean Chinese and European populations. *British Journal of Dermatology*, **165**: 106–114.

Colloff MJ (1992). Exposure to house dust mites in homes of people with atopic dermatitis. *British Journal of Dermatology*, **127**: 322–327.

Currie JM, Wright RC, Miller OG (1971). The frequency of warts in atopic patients. *Cutis*, **8**: 243–245.

Daud LR, Garralda ME, David TJ (1993). Psychosocial adjustment in preschool children with atopic eczema. *Archives of Disease in Childhood*, **69**: 670–676.

Devereux G, Seaton A, Barker RN (2001). *In utero* priming of allergen-specific helper T cells. *Clinical and Experimental Allergy*, **31**: 1686–1695.

Dimich-Ward H, Chow Y, Chung J, Trask C (2006). Contact with livestock – a protective effect against allergies and asthma? *Clinical and Experimental Allergy*, **36**: 1122–1129.

Dotterud LK, Odland ØJ, Falk ES (2001). Atopic diseases among schoolchildren in Nikel, Russia, an Arctic area with heavy air pollution. *Acta Dermato-Venereologica*, **81**: 198–201.

Droste JHJ, Wieringa MH, Weyler JJ, *et al.* (2000). Does the use of antibiotics in early childhood increase the risk of asthma and allergic disease? *Clinical and Experimental Allergy*, **30**: 1547–1553.

Eigenmann PA, Sicherer SH, Borkowski TA, Cohen BA, Sampson HA (1998). Prevalence of IgE-mediated food allergy among children with atopic dermatitis. *Pediatrics*, **101**: 1–6.

Emerson RM, Williams HC, Allen BR (1998). Severity distribution of atopic dermatitis in the community and its relationship to secondary referral. *British Journal of Dermatology*, **S139**: 73–76.

Emerson RM, Charman CR, Williams HC (2000). The Nottingham Eczema Severity Score: preliminary refinement of the Rajka and Langeland grading. *British Journal of Dermatology*, **142**: 288–297.

Farooqi IS, Hopkin JM (1998). Early childhood infection and atopic disorder. *Thorax*, **53**: 927–932.

Feeney MA, Murphy F, Clegg AJ, Trebble TM, Sharer NM, Snook JA (2002). A case-control study of childhood environmental risk factors for the development of inflammatory bowel disease. *European Journal of Gastroenterology and Hepatology*, **14**: 529–534.

Fergusson DM, Horwood LJ (1994). Early solid food diet and eczema in childhood: a 10-year longitudinal study. *Pediatric Allergy and Immunology*, **5**: 44–47.

Finlay AY, Khan GK (1994). Dermatology Life Quality Index (DLQI): a simple practical measure for routine clinical use. *Clinical and Experimental Dermatology*, **19**: 210–216.

Flohr C (2003). Dirt, worms, and atopic dermatitis. *British Journal of Dermatology*, **148**: 871–877.

Flohr C, Johansson SGO, Wahlgren CF, et al. (2004). How atopic is atopic dermatitis? *Journal of Allergy and Clinical Immunology*, **114**: 150–158.

Forsyth J, Ogston S, Clark A, Florey C, Howie P (1993). Relation between early introduction of solid food to infants and their weight and illnesses during the first 2 years of life. *British Medical Journal*, **306**: 1572–1576.

Friedmann PS (1999). Dust mite avoidance in atopic dermatitis. *Clinical and Experimental Dermatology*, **24**: 433–437.

Fung WK, Lo KK (2000). Prevalence of skin disease among school children and adolescents in a student health service centre in Hong Kong. *Pediatric Dermatology*, **17**: 440–446.

Giwercman C, Halkjaer LB, Jensen SM, Bønnelykke K, Lauritzen L, Bisgaard H (2010). Increased risk of eczema but reduced risk of early wheezy disorder from exclusive breastfeeding in high-risk infants. *Journal of Allergy and Clinical Immunology*, **125**: 866–871.

Godfrey KM, Barker DJP, Osmond C (1994). Disproportionate fetal growth and raised IgE concentration in adult life. *Clinical and Experimental Allergy*, **24**: 641–648.

Golding J, Peters TJ (1987). The epidemiology of childhood eczema 1987. A population-based study of associations. *Paediatric and Perinatal Epidemiology*, **1**: 67–79.

Gu H, Chen XS, Chen K, et al. (2001). Evaluation of diagnostic criteria for atopic dermatitis: validity of the criteria of Williams et al. in a hospital setting. *British Journal of Dermatology*, **145**: 428–433.

Haileamlak A, Lewis SA, Britton J, et al. (2005). Validation of the International Study of Asthma and Allergies in Children (ISAAC) and U.K. criteria for atopic eczema in Ethiopian children. *British Journal of Dermatology*, **152**: 735–741.

Halkjaer LB, Loland L, Buchvald FF, et al. (2006). Development of atopic dermatitis during the first 3 years of life: the Copenhagen prospective study on asthma in childhood cohort study in high-risk children. *Archives of Dermatology*, **142**: 561–566.

Hanifin JM (1992). *Atopic Eczema*. In: Marks RM (ed.), *Eczema*, Martin Dunitz, London, p. 77.

Hanifin JM, Rajka G (1980). Diagnostic features of atopic eczema. *Acta Dermato-Venereologica (Stockholm)*, **92**: 44–47.

Hanifin JM, Reed ML (2007). Eczema Prevalence and Impact Working Group. A population-based survey of eczema prevalence in the United States. *Dermatitis*, **18**: 82–91.

Harris JM, Cullinan P, Williams HC, et al. (2001). Environmental associations with eczema in early life. *British Journal of Dermatology*, **144**: 795–802.

Harris JM, Williams HC, White C (2007). Early allergen exposure and atopic eczema. *British Journal of Dermatology*, **156**: 698–704.

Harrop J, Chinn S, Verlato G, et al. (2007). Eczema, atopy and allergen exposure in adults: a population-based study. *Clinical and Experimental Allergy*, **37**: 526–535.

Hennekens CH, Buring JE (1987). *Epidemiology in Medicine*, Little, Brown, Boston.

Hoare C, Li Wan PA, Williams HC (2000). A systematic review of treatments for atopic eczema. *Health Technology Assessment*, **4**: 1–203.

Holden CA, Parish WE (1998). Atopic dermatitis. In: Champion RH, Burton JL, Burns DA, Breathnach SM (eds), *Textbook of Dermatology*, 6th edn, Blackwell Science, Oxford, p. 681.

Igawa K, Nishioka K, Yokozeki H (2007). Odontogenic focal infection could be partly involved in the pathogenesis of atopic dermatitis as exacerbating factor. *International Journal of Dermatology*, **46**: 376–379.

Ip S, Chung M, Raman G, et al. (2007). Breastfeeding and maternal and infant health outcomes in developed countries. *Evidence Report – Technology Assessment (Full Report)*, **153**: 1–186.

Johnke H, Vach W, Norberg LA, et al. (2005). A comparison between criteria for diagnosing atopic eczema in infants. *British Journal of Dermatology*, **153**: 352–358.

Kalyoncu AF, Selçuk ZT, Enünlü T, et al. (1999). Prevalence of asthma and allergic diseases in primary school children in Ankara, Turkey: Two cross-sectional studies, five years apart. *Pediatric Allergy and Immunology*, **10**: 261–265.

Karmaus W, Botezan C (2002). Does a higher number of siblings protect against the development of allergy and asthma? A review. *Journal of Epidemiology and Community Health*, **56**: 209–217.

Karmaus W, Kuehr J, Kruse H (2001). Infections and atopic disorders in childhood and organochlorine exposure. *Archives of Environmental Health*, **56**: 485–492.

Kjaer HF, Eller E, Høst A, Andersen KE, Bindslev-Jensen C (2008). The prevalence of allergic diseases in an unselected group of 6-year-old children. The DARC birth cohort study. *Pediatric Allergy and Immunology*, **19**: 737–745.

Kjellman B, Petterson R, Hyensjö B (1982). Allergy among school children in a Swedish county. *Allergy*, **37**: S5.

Kjellman M (1981). Effect on parental smoking on IgE-levels in children. *The Lancet*, **i**: 933.

Kölmel KF, Compagnone D (1988). Melanoma and atopy. *Deutsche Medizinische Wochenschrift*, **113**; 69–71.

Kramer M, Chalmers B, Hodnett E, et al. (2001). Promotion of Breastfeeding Intervention Trial (PROBIT): a randomized trial in the Republic of Belarus. *Journal of the American Medical Association*, **285**: 413–420.

Kull I, Wickman M, Lilja G, Nordvall SL, Pershagen G (2002). Breastfeeding and allergic disease in infants - a prospective birth cohort study. *Archives of Disease in Childhood*, 87: 478–481.

Langan SM, Williams HC (2006). What causes worsening of eczema? A systematic review. *British Journal of Dermatology*, 155: 504–514.

Laughter D, Istvan JA, Tofte SJ, Hanifin JM (2000). The prevalence of atopic dermatitis in Oregon schoolchildren. *Journal of the American Academy of Dermatology*, 43: 649–655.

Lawson V, Lewis-Jones MS, Finlay AY, Reid P, Owens RG (1998). The family impact of atopic dermatitis: the Dermatitis Family Impact Questionnaire. *British Journal of Dermatology*, 138: 107–113.

Lee J, Seto D, Bielory L (2008). Meta-analysis of clinical trials of probiotics for prevention and treatment of pediatric atopic dermatitis. *Journal of Allergy and Clinical Immunology*, 121: 116–121.

Lee YL, Li CW, Sung FC, Yu HS, Sheu HM, Guo YL (2007). Environmental factors, parental atopy and atopic eczema in primary-school children: a cross-sectional study in Taiwan. *British Journal of Dermatology*, 157: 1217–1224.

Lee YL, Su HJ, Sheu HM, Yu HS, Guo YL (2008). Traffic-related air pollution, climate, and prevalence of eczema in Taiwanese school children. *Journal of Investigative Dermatology*, 128: 2412–2420.

Lehtonen EP, Holmberg-Marttila D, Kaila M (2003). Cumulative prevalence of atopic eczema and related skin symptoms in a well-baby clinic: a retrospective cohort study. *Pediatric Allergy and Immunology*, 14: 405–408.

Lewis SA (2000). Animals and allergy. *Clinical and Experimental Allergy*, 30: 153–157.

Linos E, Raine T, Alonso A, Michaud D (2007). Atopy and risk of brain tumors: a meta-analysis. *Journal of the National Cancer Institute*, 99: 1544–1550.

Lowe AJ, Hosking CS, Bennett CM, *et al.* (2007) Skin prick test can identify eczematous infants at risk of asthma and allergic rhinitis. *Clinical and Experimental Allergy*, 37: 1624–1631.

Macaubas C, Prescott SL, Venaille TJ, Holt BJ (2000). Primary sensitization to inhalant allergens. *Pediatric Allergy and Immunology*, 13(suppl): 9–11.

McKeever TM, Lewis SA, Smith C, Hubbard R (2002). The importance of prenatal exposures on the development of allergic disease: A British cohort study using the West Midlands General Practice Database. *American Journal of Respiratory and Critical Care Medicine*, 166: 827–832.

McNally N, Phillips D (2000). Geographical epidemiology of atopic dermatitis. In: Williams HC (ed.), *Atopic Dermatitis: The Epidemiology, Causes and Prevention of Atopic Dermatitis*, Cambridge University Press, Cambridge, pp. 113–124.

McNally NJ, Williams HC, Phillips DR (2001). Atopic eczema and the home environment. *British Journal of Dermatology*, 145: 730–736.

Majamaa H, Isolauri E (1996). Evaluation of the gut mucosal barrier: evidence for increased antigen transfer in children with atopic eczema. *Journal of Allergy and Clinical Immunology*, 97: 985–990.

Mancini AJ, Kaulback K, Chamlin SL (2008). The socioeconomic impact of atopic dermatitis in the United States: a systematic review. *Pediatric Dermatology*, 25: 1–6.

Mar A, Tam M, Jolley D, Marks R (1999). The cumulative incidence of atopic dermatitis in the first 12 months among Chinese, Vietnamese, and Caucasian infants born in Melbourne, Australia. *Journal of the American Academy of Dermatology*, 40: 597–602.

Marks M, Kilkenny M, Plunkett A, Merlin K (1999). The prevalence of common skin conditions in Australian school students: 2. Atopic dermatitis. *British Journal of Dermatology*, 140: 468–473.

Mihrshahi S, Ampon R, Webb K, *et al.* (2007). The association between infant feeding practices and subsequent atopy among children with a family history of asthma. *Clinical and Experimental Allergy*, 37: 671.

Montgomery SM, Ehlin AG, Sparen P, Björkstén B, Ekbom A (2002). Childhood indicators of susceptibility to subsequent cervical cancer. *British Journal of Cancer*, 87: 989–993.

Morar N, Willis-Owen SA, Moffatt MF, Cookson WO (2006). The genetics of atopic dermatitis. *Journal of Allergy and Clinical Immunology*, 118: 24–34.

Mortimer MJ, Kay J, Gawkrodger DJ, *et al.* (1993). The prevalence of migraine in atopic children: an epidemiological study in general practice. *Headache*, 33: 427–431.

Mortz CG, Lauritsen JM, Bindslev-Jensen C, Andersen KE (2001). Prevalence of atopic dermatitis, asthma, allergic rhinitis, and hand and contact dermatitis in adolescents. The Odense Adolescence Cohort Study on atopic diseases and dermatitis. *British Journal of Dermatology*, 144: 523–532.

Neame RL, Berth-Jones J, Kurinczuk JJ, Graham-Brown RAC (1995). Prevalence of atopic dermatitis in Leicester: a study of methodology and examination of possible ethnic variation. *British Journal of Dermatology*, 132: 772–77.

Norris PG, Schofield O, Camp RDR (1988). A study of the role of house dust mite in atopic eczema. *British Journal of Dermatology*, 118: 435–440.

Odhiambo J, Williams H, Clayton T, Robertson C, Asher MI, and the ISAAC Phase Three Study group (2009) Global variations in prevalence of eczema symptoms in children from ISAAC Phase Three. *Journal of Allergy and Clinical Immunology*, 124: 1251–1258.

Ong PY, Ohtake T, Brandt C, *et al.* (2002). Endogenous antimicrobial peptides and skin infections in atopic dermatitis. *New England Journal of Medicine*, 347: 1151–1160.

Palmer CN, Irvine AD, Terron-Kwiatkowski A, *et al.* (2006). Common loss-of-function variants of the epidermal barrier protein filaggrin are a major predisposing factor for atopic dermatitis. *Nature Genetics*, 38: 441–446.

Perzanowski MS, Miller RL, Thorne PS, *et al.* (2006). Endotoxin in inner-city homes: associations with wheeze and eczema in early childhood. *Journal of Allergy and Clinical Immunology*, 117: 1082–1089.

Peters TJ, Golding J (1987). The epidemiology of childhood eczema. II. Statistical analyses to identify independent early predictors. *Paediatric and Perinatal Epidemiology*, 1: 80–94.

Popescu CM, Popescu R, Williams H, Forsea D (1998). Community validation of the United Kingdom diagnostic criteria for atopic dermatitis in Romanian schoolchildren. *British Journal of Dermatology*, **138**: 436–442.

Prescott SL, Macaubas C, Holt BJ, *et al.* (1998). Transplacental priming of the human immune system to environmental allergens: universal skewing of initial T cell responses toward the Th2 cytokine profile. *Journal of Immunology*, **160**: 4730–4737.

Purvis DJ, Thompson JM, Clark PM, *et al.* (2005). Risk factors for atopic dermatitis in New Zealand children at 3.5 years of age. *British Journal of Dermatology*, **152**: 742–749.

Reichtová E, Ciznár P, Prachar V, Palkoviková L, Veningerová M (1999). Cord serum immunoglobulin E related to environmental contamination of human placentas with organochlorine compounds. *Environmental Health Perspectives*, **107**: 895–899.

Ricci G, Patrizi A, Baldi E, Menna G, Tabanelli M, Masi M (2006). Long-term follow-up of atopic dermatitis: retrospective analysis of related risk factors and association with concomitant allergic diseases. *Journal of the American Academy of Dermatology*, **55**: 765–771.

Riedel F (1991). Environmental pollution and atopy. In: Ruzicka T, Ring J, Pryzbilla B (eds), *Handbook of Atopic Eczema*, Springer-Verlag, London, pp. 319–322.

Rodríguez E, Baurecht H, Herberich E, *et al.* (2009). Meta-analysis of filaggrin polymorphisms in eczema and asthma: robust risk factors in atopic disease. *Journal of Allergy and Clinical Immunology*, **123**: 1361–1370.

Roguedas AM, Machet L, Fontes V, *et al.* (2004). Atopic dermatitis: which are the diagnostic criteria used in medical literature? *Annales de Dermatologie et de Syphiligraphie*, **131**: 161–164.

Ruiz RG, Kemeny DM, Price JF (1992). Higher risk of infantile atopic dermatitis from maternal atopy than from paternal atopy. *Clinical and Experimental Allergy*, **22**: 762–766.

Rystedt I (1980). Long-term follow-up in atopic dermatitis. *Acta Dermato-Venereologica (Stockholm)*, suppl 114: 117–120.

Sanchez-Borges M, de Orozco A, Arellano S, *et al.* (1986). Preventive role of atopy in lung cancer. *Clinical Immunology and Immunopathology*, **41**: 314–319.

Sangsupawanich P, Chongsuvivatwong V, Mo-Suwan L, Choprapawon C (2007). Relationship between atopic dermatitis and wheeze in the first year of life: analysis of a prospective cohort of Thai children. *Journal of Investigational Allergology and Clinical Immunology*, **17**: 292–296.

Schäfer T, Dirschedl P, Kunz B, Ring J, Überla K (1997). Maternal smoking during pregnancy and lactation increases the risk for atopic eczema in the offspring. *Journal of the American Academy of Dermatology*, **36**: 550–556.

Schäfer T, Heinrich J, Wjst M, *et al.* (1999). Indoor risk factors for atopic eczema in school children from East Germany. *Environmental Research*, **81**: 151–158.

Schmitt J, Langan S, Williams HC (2007). What are the best outcome measurements for atopic eczema? A systematic review. *Journal of Allergy and Clinical Immunology*, **120**: 1389–1398.

Schoetzau A, Filipiak-Pittroff B, Koletzko S, *et al.* (2002). Effect of exclusive breastfeeding and early solid food avoidance on the incidence of atopic dermatitis in high-risk infants at 1 year of age. *Pediatric Allergy and Immunology*, **13**: 234–242.

Schultz Larsen F (1993). The epidemiology of atopic dermatitis. In: Burr ML (ed.), *Epidemiology of Clinical Allergy*, Karger, Basel pp. 9–28.

Schultz Larsen F, Diepgen T, Svensson A (1996).Clinical criteria in diagnosing atopic dermatitis: the Lillehammer criteria 1994. *Acta Dermato-Venereologica (Stockholm)*, **96**: 115–119.

Seaton A, Godden William Wood, New York DJ, Brown KM (1994). Increase in asthma: a more toxic environment or a more susceptible population? *Thorax*, **49**: 171–174.

Sherriff A, Golding J, and the Alspac Team (2002). Hygiene levels in a contemporary population cohort are associated with wheezing and atopic eczema in preschool infants. *Archives of Disease in Childhood*, **87**: 26–29.

Smidesang I, Saunes M, Storrø O, *et al.* (2008). Atopic dermatitis among 2-year olds; high prevalence, but predominantly mild disease – the PACT study, Norway. *Pediatric Dermatology*, **25**: 13–8.

Strachan DP (1989). Hay fever, hygiene, and household size. *British Medical Journal*, **299**: 1259–1260.

Strachan DP (2000). Family size, infection and atopy: the first decade of the 'hygiene hypothesis'. *Thorax*, **55**: S2-S10.

Stranegård Ö, Stranegård I-L (1978). T lymphocyte numbers and function in human IgE-mediated allergy. *Immunological Reviews*, **41**: 149–170.

Svejgaard E (1986). Epidemiology and clinical features of dermatomycoses and dermatophytoses. *Acta Dermato-Venereologica (Stockholm)*, **121**: 19–26.

Tanaka K, Miyake Y, Arakawa M, Sasaki S, Ohya Y (2007). Prevalence of asthma and wheeze in relation to passive smoking in Japanese children. *Annals of Epidemiology*, **17**: 1004–1010.

Tanaka Y, Tanaka M, Anan S, Yoshida H (1989). Immunohistochemical studies on dust mite antigen in positive reaction site of patch test. *Acta Dermato-Venereologica (Stockholm)*, **144**: 93–96.

Tay YK, Kong KH, Khoo L, Goh CL, Giam YC (2002). The prevalence and descriptive epidemiology of atopic dermatitis in Singapore school children. *British Journal of Dermatology*, **146**: 101–106.

Tupker RA, De Monchy JG, Coenraads PJ, Homan A, van der Meer JB (1996). Induction of atopic dermatitis by inhalation of house dust mite. *Journal of Allergy and Clinical Immunology*, **97**: 1064–1070.

van Reijsen FC, Felius A, Wauters EA, Bruijnzeel-Koomen CA, Koppelman SJ (1998). T-cell reactivity for a peanut-derived epitope in the skin of a young infant with atopic dermatitis. *Journal of Allergy and Clinical Immunology*, **101**: 207–209.

Vickers CFH (1980). The natural history of atopic eczema. *Acta Dermato-Venereologica (Stockholm)*, suppl 92: 113–115.

von Mutius E (2002). Environmental factors influencing the development and progression of pediatric asthma. *The Journal of Allergy and Clinical Immunology*, **109**: S525–532.

von Mutius E, Fritzsch C, Weiland SW, *et al.* (1992). Prevalence of asthma and allergic disorders among children in united Germany: a descriptive comparison. *British Medical Journal*, **305**: 1395–1399.

von Mutius E, Martinez FD, Fritzsch C, et al. (1994). Skin reactivity and number of siblings. *British Medical Journal*, 308: 692–695.

Waite DA, Eyles EF, Tonkin SL, et al. (1980). Asthma prevalence in Tokelauan children in two environments. *Clinical and Experimental Allergy*, 10: 71–75.

Warner JA, Miles EA, Jones AC, et al. (1994). Is deficiency of interferon gamma production by allergen targeted cord blood cells a predictor of atopic dermatitis? *Clinical and Experimental Allergy*, 24: 423–430.

Werner S, Buser K, Kapp A, Werfel T (2002). The incidence of atopic dermatitis in school entrants is associated with individual life-style factors but not with local environmental factors in Hannover, Germany. *British Journal of Dermatology*, 147: 95–104.

Williams H, Robertson C, Stewart A, et al. (1999). Worldwide variations in the prevalence of symptoms of atopic eczema in the international study of asthma and allergies in childhood. *The Journal of Allergy and Clinical Immunology*, 103: 125–138.

Williams H, Stewart A, von Mutius E, Cookson B, Anderson HR and the International Study of Asthma and Allergies in Childhood (ISAAC) Phase One and Three Study groups (2008). Is eczema really on the increase worldwide? *Journal of Allergy and Clinical Immunology*, 121: 947–954.

Williams HC (1992). Is the prevalence of atopic dermatitis increasing? *Clinical and Experimental Dermatology*, 17: 385–391.

Williams HC (1999). Diagnostic criteria for atopic dermatitis: where do we go from here? *Archives of Dermatology*, 135: 583–586.

Williams HC (2000a). Epidemiology of atopic dermatitis. *Clinical and Experimental Dermatology*, 25: 522–529.

Williams HC (2000b). What is atopic dermatitis and how should it be defined in epidemiological studies? In: Williams HC (ed.), *Atopic Dermatitis: The Epidemiology, Causes and Prevention of Atopic Dermatitis*, Cambridge University Press, Cambridge, pp. 3–24.

Williams HC, Flohr C (2006). How epidemiology has challenged 3 prevailing concepts about atopic dermatitis. *Journal of Allergy and Clinical Immunology*, 118: 209–213.

Williams HC, Strachan DP (1998). The natural history of childhood eczema: observations from the 1958 birth cohort study. *British Journal of Dermatology*, 139: 834–839.

Williams HC, Wüthrich B (2000). The natural history of atopic dermatitis. In: Williams HC (ed.), *Atopic Dermatitis: The Epidemiology, Causes and Prevention of Atopic Dermatitis*, Cambridge University Press, Cambridge pp. 41–59.

Williams HC, Strachan D, Hay RJ (1992). Eczema and family size. *Journal of Investigative Dermatology*, 98: 601.

Williams HC, Pottier A, Strachan D (1993). Are viral warts seen more commonly in children with eczema? *Archives of Dermatology*, 129: 717–721.

Williams HC, Strachan DP, Hay RJ (1994). Childhood eczema: disease of the advantaged? *British Medical Journal*, 308: 1132–1135.

Williams HC, Pembroke AC, Forsdyke H, et al. (1995a). London-born black Caribbean children are at increased risk of atopic dermatitis. *Journal of the American Academy of Dermatology*, 32: 212–217.

Williams HC, Forsdyke H, Boodoo G, Hay RJ, Burney PGF (1995b). A protocol for recording the sign of visible flexural dermatitis. *British Journal of Dermatology*, 133: 941–949.

Wolkewitz M, Rothenbacher D, Löw M, et al. (2007). Lifetime prevalence of self-reported atopic diseases in a population-based sample of elderly subjects: results of the ESTHER study. *British Journal of Dermatology*, 156: 693–697.

Worm M, Forschner K, Lee HH, et al. (2006). Frequency of atopic dermatitis and relevance of food allergy in adults in Germany. *Acta Dermato-Venereologica*, 86: 119–122.

Worth RM (1962). Atopic dermatitis among Chinese infants in Honolulu and San Francisco. *Hawaii Medical Journal*, 22: 31–34.

Wüthrich B (1989). Epidemiology of the allergic diseases: are they really on the increase? *International Archives of Allergy and Immunology*, 90: 3–10.

Xu B, Järvelin MR, Pekkanen J (1999). Prenatal factors and occurrence of rhinitis and eczema among offspring. *Allergy*, 54: 829–836.

Yamada E, Vanna AT, Naspitz CK, Solé D, International Study of Asthma and Allergies in Childhood (ISAAC) (2002). Validation of the written questionnaire (eczema component) and prevalence of atopic eczema among Brazilian children. *Journal of Investigational Allergology and Clinical Immunology*, 12: 34–41.

Yang YW, Tsai CL, Lu CY (2009). Exclusive breastfeeding and incident atopic dermatitis in childhood: a systematic review and meta-analysis of prospective cohort studies. *British Journal of Dermatology*, 161: 373–383.

Yazdanbakhsh M, Kremsner PG, van Ree R (2002). Allergy, parasites, and the hygiene hypothesis. *Science*, 296: 490–494.

Yura A, Shimizu T (2001). Trends in the prevalence of atopic dermatitis in school children: longitudinal study in Osaka Prefecture, Japan, from 1985 to 1997. *British Journal of Dermatology*, 145: 966–993.

CHAPTER 3

Ackerman AB (1979). Subtle clues to histopathologic findings from gross pathology (clinical lesions). Collarettes of scales as signs of spongiosis. *American Journal of Dermatopathology*, 1: 267–272.

Allison DS, El-Azhary RA, Calobrisi SD, Dicken CH (2002). Pityriasis rubra pilaris in children. *Journal of the American Academy of Dermatology*, 47: 386–389.

Amato L, Berti S, Chiarini C, Fabbri P (2005). Atopic dermatitis exclusively localized on nipples and areolas. *Pediatric Dermatology*, 22: 64–66.

Andrews MD, Burns M (2008). Common tinea infections in children. *American Family Physician*, 77: 1415–1420.

Aoyama H, Tanaka M, Hara M, Tabata N, Tagami H (1999). Nummular eczema: an addition of senile xerosis and unique cutaneous reactivities to environmental aeroallergens. *Dermatology*, 199: 135–139.

Bannister MJ, Freeman S (2000). Adult-onset atopic dermatitis. *Australasian Journal of Dermatology*, 41: 225–228.

Beltrani VS, Beltrani VP (1997). Contact dermatitis. *Annals of Allergy, Asthma and Immunology*, 78: 160–173.

Blessmann Weber M, Sponchiado de Avila LG, Albaneze R, Magalhães de Oliveira OL, Sudhaus BD, Cestari TF (2002). Pityriasis alba: a study of pathogenic factors. *Journal of the European Academy of Dermatology and Venereology*, 16: 463–468.

Böhme M, Svensson A, Kull I, Wahlgren CF (2000). Hanifin's and Rajka's minor criteria for atopic dermatitis: which do 2-year-olds exhibit? *Journal of the American Academy of Dermatology*, 43(5 Pt 1): 785–792.

Bos JD (2002). Atopiform dermatitis. *British Journal of Dermatology*, 147: 426–429.

Bos JD, Van Leent EJ, Sillevis Smitt JH (1998). The millennium criteria for the diagnosis of atopic dermatitis. *Experimental Dermatology*, 7: 132–138.

Braun-Falco O (2000). *Dermatology*, Springer, Berlin, pp. 493–503.

Bruckner AL, Weston WL, Morelli JG (2000). Does sensitization to contact allergens begin in infancy? *Pediatrics*, 105: e3.

Bulkley LD (1881). *Eczema and Its Management; A Practical Treatise Based on the Study of Three Thousand Cases of the Disease*, Putnam, New York, pp. 38–40.

Burk C, Hu S, Lee C, Connelly EA (2008). Netherton syndrome and trichorrhexis invaginata – a novel diagnostic approach. *Pediatric Dermatology*, 25: 287–288.

Chen CH, Lin YT, Wen CY (2009). Quantitative assessment of allergic shiners in children with allergic rhinitis. *Journal of Allergy and Clinical Immunology*, 123: 665–671, 671 e1–6.

Cohen DE, Heidary N (2004). Treatment of irritant and allergic contact dermatitis. *Dermatologic Therapy*, 17: 334–340.

de Berker DA, Paige DG, Ferguson DJ, Dawber RP (1995). Golf tee hairs in Netherton disease. *Pediatric Dermatology*, 12: 7–11.

DiGiovanna JJ, Robinson-Bostom L (2003). Ichthyosis: etiology, diagnosis, and management. *American Journal of Clinical Dermatology*, 4: 81–95.

Du Toit G (2005). Clinical allergy images: the atopic syndrome. *Current allergy and Clinical Immunology*, 18: 22–23.

Fisch RO, Tsai MY, Gentry WC Jr (1981). Studies of phenylketonurics with dermatitis. *Journal of the American Academy of Dermatology*, 4: 284–290.

Foti C, Bonifazi E, Casulli C, Bonamonte D, Conserva A, Angelini G (2005). Contact allergy to topical corticosteroids in children with atopic dermatitis. *Contact Dermatitis*, 52: 162–163.

Gibbs NF (2004). Juvenile plantar dermatosis. Can sweat cause foot rash and peeling? *Postgraduate Medicine*, 115: 73–75.

Griffiths WA (1980). Pityriasis rubra pilaris. *Clinical and Experimental Dermatology*, 5: 105–112.

Griffiths WA (1992). Pityriasis rubra pilaris: the problem of its classification. *Journal of the American Academy of Dermatology*, 26: 140–142.

Hainer BL (2003). Dermatophyte infections. *American Family Physician*, 67: 101–108.

Halabi-Tawil M, Ruemmele FM, Fraitag S, et al. (2009). Cutaneous manifestations of immune dysregulation, polyendocrinopathy, enteropathy, X-linked (IPEX) syndrome. *British Journal of Dermatology*, 160: 645–651.

Hanifin JM, Rajka G (1980). Diagnostic features of atopic dermatitis. *Acta Dermato-Venereologica Supplement (Stockholm)*, 92: 44–47.

Hebert A, Mays S (1996). Atopic dermatitis in infancy. *Dermatological Therapy*, 1: 61–74.

Hellgren L, Mobacken H (1969). Nummular eczema – clinical and statistical data. *Acta Dermato-Venereologica*, 49: 189–196.

Hicks MI, Elston DM (2009). Scabies. *Dermatologic Therapy*, 22: 279–292.

Hunter HL, McKenna KE, Edgar JD (2008). Eczema and X-linked agammaglobulinaemia. *Clinical and Experimental Dermatology*, 33: 148–150.

Illi S, von Mutius E, Lau S, et al. (2004). The natural course of atopic dermatitis from birth to age 7 years and the association with asthma. *Journal of Allergy and Clinical Immunology*, 113: 925–931.

Jacob SE, Steele T (2007). Avoiding formaldehyde allergic reactions in children. *Pediatric Annals*, 36: 55–56.

Katz KA, Mahlberg MJ, Honig PJ, Yan AC (2005). Rice nightmare: Kwashiorkor in 2 Philadelphia-area infants fed Rice Dream beverage. *Journal of the American Academy of Dermatology*, 52(5 suppl 1): S69–72.

Krol AB, Krafchik B (2006). The differential diagnosis of atopic dermatitis in childhood. *Dermatologic Therapy*, 19: 73–82.

La Grenade L, Manns A, Fletcher V, et al. (1998). Clinical, pathologic, and immunologic features of human T-lymphotrophic virus type I-associated infective dermatitis in children. *Archives of Dermatology*, 134: 439–444.

Lee HJ, Ha SJ, Ahn WK, et al. (2001). Clinical evaluation of atopic hand-foot dermatitis. *Pediatric Dermatology*, 18: 102–106.

Lynch PJ (2004). Lichen simplex chronicus (atopic/neurodermatitis) of the anogenital region. *Dermatologic Therapy*, 17: 8–19.

Mahé A, Meertens L, Ly F, et al. (2004). Human T-cell leukaemia/lymphoma virus type 1-associated infective dermatitis in Africa: a report of five cases from Senegal. *British Journal of Dermatology*, 150: 958–965.

Mark BJ, Slavin RG (2006). Allergic contact dermatitis. *Medical Clinics of North America*, 90: 169–185.

Maverakis E, Fung MA, Lynch PJ, et al. (2007). Acrodermatitis enteropathica and an overview of zinc metabolism. *Journal of the American Academy of Dermatology*, 56: 116–124.

Menni S, Piccinno R, Baietta S, Ciuffreda A, Scotti L (1989). Infantile seborrheic dermatitis: seven-year follow-up and some prognostic criteria. *Pediatric Dermatology*, 6: 13–15.

Mevorah B, Frenk E, Wietlisbach V, Carrel CF (1988). Minor clinical features of atopic dermatitis. Evaluation of their diagnostic significance. *Dermatologica*, 177: 360–364.

Militello G, Jacob SE, Crawford GH (2006). Allergic contact dermatitis in children. *Current Opinion in Pediatrics*, 18: 385–390.

Morris A, Rogers M, Fischer G, Williams K (2001). Childhood psoriasis: a clinical review of 1262 cases. *Pediatric Dermatology*, 18: 188–198.

Naldi L, Rebora A (2009). Clinical practice. Seborrheic dermatitis. *New England Journal of Medicine*, 360: 387–396.

Nashan D, Faulhaber D, Ständer S, Luger TA, Stadler R (2007). Mycosis fungoides: a dermatological masquerader. *British Journal of Dermatology*, **156**: 1–10.

Neville EA, Finn OA (1975). Psoriasiform napkin dermatitis – a follow-up study. *British Journal of Dermatology*, **92**: 279–285.

Nichols KM, Cook-Bolden FE (2009). Allergic skin disease: major highlights and recent advances. *Medical Clinics of North America*, **93**: 1211–1224.

Nnoruka EN (2004). Current epidemiology of atopic dermatitis in south-eastern Nigeria. *International Journal of Dermatology*, **43**: 739–744.

Powell J (2000). Increasing the likelihood of early diagnosis of Netherton syndrome by simple examination of eyebrow hairs. *Archives of Dermatology*, **136**: 423–442.

Primo JR, Brites C, Oliveira M de F, Moreno-Carvalho O, Machado M, Bittencourt AL (2005). Infective dermatitis and human T cell lymphotropic virus type 1-associated myelopathy/tropical spastic paraparesis in childhood and adolescence. *Clinical Infectious Diseases*, **41**: 535–554.

Rudikoff D, Lebwohl M (1998). Atopic dermatitis. *Lancet*, **351**: 1715–1721.

Rudikoff D, Akhavan A, Cohen SR (2003). Color atlas: eczema. *Clinics in Dermatology*, **21**:101–108.

Rudzki E, Samochocki Z, Rebandel P (1994). Frequency and significance of the major and minor features of Hanifin and Rajka among patients with atopic dermatitis. *Dermatology*, **189**: 41–6.

Samimi SS, Siegfried E, Belsito DV (2004). A diagnostic pearl: the school chair sign. *Cutis*, **74**: 27–28.

Simpson EL, Thompson MM, Hanifin JM (2006). Prevalence and morphology of hand eczema in patients with atopic dermatitis. *Dermatitis*, **17**: 123–127.

Singh G (1973). Atopy in lichen simplex (neurodermatitis circumscripta). *British Journal of Dermatology*, **89**: 625–627.

Sulzberger MB (1955). Atopic dermatitis: its clinical and histologic picture. In: Baer RL (ed.), *Atopic Dermatitis*, New York University Press, New York, pp. 11–42.

Tay YK, Khoo BP, Goh CL (1999). The profile of atopic dermatitis in a tertiary dermatology outpatient clinic in Singapore. *International Journal of Dermatology*, **38**: 689–692.

Tilly JJ, Drolet BA, Esterly NB (2004). Lichenoid eruptions in children. *Journal of the American Academy of Dermatology*, **51**: 606–624.

Treadwell PA (2008). Eczema and infection. *Pediatric Infectious Disease Journal*, **27**: 551–552.

Uehara M (1981). Infraorbital fold in atopic dermatitis. *Archives of Dermatology*, **117**: 627–629.

Weismann K, Hoyer H (1985). Serum alkaline phosphatase and serum zinc levels in the diagnosis and exclusion of zinc deficiency in man. *American Journal of Clinical Nutrition*, **41**: 1214–1219.

Werchniak AE, Storm CA, Dinulos JG (2004). Hyperpigmented patches on the tongue of a young girl. *Archives of Dermatology*, **140**: 1275–1280.

Williams HC, Burney PG, Hay RJ, *et al.* (1994). The U.K. working party's diagnostic criteria for atopic dermatitis. I. Derivation of a minimum set of discriminators for atopic dermatitis. *British Journal of Dermatology*, **131**: 383–396.

Wise F, Sulzberger MB (1933). Other eczematous eruptions. In: Wise F, Sulzberger MB (eds.), *Yearbook of Dermatology and Syphilology*, Yearbook Publishers, Chicago, pp. 38–39.

Zoli V, Silvani S, Vincenzi C, Tosti A (2006). Allergic contact cheilitis. *Contact Dermatitis*, **54**: 296–297.

CHAPTER 4

Abramovits W, Cockerell C, Stevenson LC, Goldstein AM, Ehrig T, Menter A (2005). PsEma – a hitherto unnamed dermatologic entity with clinical features of both psoriasis and eczema. *Skinmed*, **4**: 275–281.

Alibert JL (1818). *Précis théorique et pratique des maladies de la peau*, Crapart, Caille et Ravier, Paris.

Bach JF (2002). The effect of infections on susceptibility to autoimmune and allergic diseases. *New England Journal of Medicine*, **347**: 911–920.

Baker AM, Johnson DG, Levisky JA, *et al.* (2003). Fatal diphenhydramine intoxication in infants. *Journal of Forensic Science*, **48**: 425–428.

Berth-Jones J, Damstra RJ, Golsch S, *et al.* (2003). Twice weekly fluticasone propionate added to emollient maintenance treatment to reduce risk of relapse in atopic dermatitis: randomised, double blind, parallel group study. *British Medical Journal*, **326**: 1367.

Braae Olesen A, Thestrup-Pedersen K (2000). The 'old mother' hypothesis. In: Williams HC (ed.), *Atopic Dermatitis: The Epidemiology, Causes and Prevention of Atopic Eczema*, Cambridge University Press, New York, pp. 148–154.

Bråbäck L, Hjern A, Rasmussen F (2004). Trends in asthma, allergic rhinitis and eczema among Swedish conscripts from farming and non-farming environments. A nationwide study over three decades. *Clinical and Experimental Allergy*, **34**: 38–43.

Breuer K, Haussler S, Kapp A, Werfel T (2002). *Staphylococcus aureus*: colonizing features and influence of an antibacterial treatment in adults with atopic dermatitis. *British Journal of Dermatology*, **147**: 55–61.

Bulkley LD (1913). *Diet and Hygiene in Diseases of the Skin*, PB Hoeber, New York, p. 125.

Bustos GJ, Bustos D, Bustos GJ, Romero O (1995). Prevention of asthma with ketotifen in preasthmatic children: a three-year follow-up study. *Clinical and Experimental Allergy*, **25**: 568–573.

Centers for Disease Control and Prevention (2008). *Smallpox vaccination and adverse events training module*, Centers for Disease Control and Prevention, Atlanta. Available at: www.bt.cdc.gov/training/smallpoxvaccine/reactions/ec_vac.html (accessed October 12, 2011).

Chiang C, Eichenfield LF (2006). Quantitative measurement of bathing and moisturizer induced changes in skin hydration in atopic dermatitis subjects. *Society for Investigative Dermatology*, abstract 212.

Chiang C, Eichenfield L (2009). Quantitative assessment of combination bathing and moisturizing regimens on skin hydration in atopic dermatitis. *Pediatric Dermatology*, **26**: 273–278.

Cork MJ, Robinson DA, Vasilopoulos Y, *et al.* (2006). New perspectives on epidermal barrier dysfunction in atopic dermatitis: gene–environment interactions. *Journal of Allergy and Clinical Immunology*, **118**: 3–21.

David TJ, Ewing CI (1988). Atopic eczema and preterm birth. *Archives of Diseases in Childhood*, **63**: 435–436.

Davis LR, Marten RH, Sarkany I (1961). Atopic eczema in European and Negro West Indian infants in London. *British Journal of Dermatology*, 73: 410–414.

Diepgen TL (2000). Is the prevalence of atopic dermatitis increasing? In: Williams HC (ed.), *Atopic Dermatitis: The Epidemiology, Causes and Prevention of Atopic Eczema*, Cambridge University Press, Cambridge, pp. 96–109.

Diepgen TL (2002). Early treatment of the atopic child study group. Long-term treatment with cetirizine of infants with atopic dermatitis: a multi-country, double-blind, randomized, placebo-controlled trial (the ETAC trial) over 18 months. *Pediatric Allergy and Immunology*, 13: 278–286.

Eichenfield LF, Hanifin JM, Luger TA, Stevens SR, Pride HB (2003). Consensus conference on pediatric atopic dermatitis. *Journal of the American Academy of Dermatology*, 49: 1088–1095.

Ellis CN, Drake LA, Prendergast MM, *et al.* (2002). Cost of atopic dermatitis and eczema in the United States. *Journal of the American Academy of Dermatology*, 46: 361–370.

Ewing CI, Ashcroft C, Gibbs AC, Jones GA, Connor PJ, David TJ (1998). Flucloxacillin in the treatment of atopic dermatitis. *British Journal of Dermatology*, 138: 1022–1029.

Flohr C, Williams HC (2006). Epidemiology of atopic dermatitis. In: Harper J, Oranje AP, Prose NS (eds), *Textbook of Pediatric Dermatology*, Blackwell Publishing, Oxford, pp. xxii, 2251, lxx.

Fortunov RM, Hulten KG, Hammerman WA, Mason EO Jr, Kaplan SL (2007). Evaluation and treatment of community-acquired *Staphylococcus aureus* infections in term and late-preterm previously healthy neonates. *Pediatrics*, 120: 937–945.

Franck LS, Quinn D, Zahr L (2000). Effect of less frequent bathing of preterm infants on skin flora and pathogen colonization. *Journal of Obstetric and Gynecologic Neonatal Nursing*, 29: 584–589.

Gdalevich M, Mimouni D, David M, Mimouni M (2001). Breastfeeding and the onset of atopic dermatitis in childhood: a systematic review and meta-analysis of prospective studies. *Journal of the American Academy of Dermatology*, 45: 520–527.

Golding J, Peters TJ (1987). The epidemiology of childhood eczema: I. A population based study of associations. *Paediatric Perinatology and Epidemiology*, 1: 67–79.

Gong JQ, Lin L, Lin T, *et al.* (2006). Skin colonization by *Staphylococcus aureus* in patients with eczema and atopic dermatitis and relevant combined topical therapy: a double-blind multicentre randomized controlled trial. *British Journal of Dermatology*, 155: 680–687.

Hachem JP, Man MQ, Crumrine D, *et al.* (2005). Sustained serine proteases activity by prolonged increase in pH leads to degradation of lipid processing enzymes and profound alterations of barrier function and stratum corneum integrity. *Journal of Investigative Dermatology*, 125: 510–520.

Hanifin J, Gupta AK, Rajagopalan R (2002). Intermittent dosing of fluticasone propionate cream for reducing the risk of relapse in atopic dermatitis patients. *British Journal of Dermatology*, 147: 528–537.

Hanifin JM, Rajka G (1980). Diagnostic features of atopic dermatitis. *Acta Dermato-Venereologica*, 92(suppl): 44–47.

Hauk PJ, Hamid QA, Chrousos GP, Leung DY (2000). Induction of corticosteroid insensitivity in human PBMCs by microbial superantigens. *Journal of Allergy and Clinical Immunology*, 105: 782–787.

Henderson CA (1995). The prevalence of atopic eczema in two different villages in rural Tanzania. *British Journal of Dermatology*, 133 (supp 45.): 50–53.

Hepburn DJ, Aeling JL, Weston WL (1996). A reappraisal of topical steroid potency. *Pediatric Dermatology*, 13: 239–245.

Higuchi K, Hara J, Okamoto R, Kawashima M, Imokawa G (2000). The skin of atopic dermatitis patients contains a novel enzyme, glucosylceramide sphingomyelin deacylase, which cleaves the N-acyl linkage of sphingomyelin and glucosylceramide. *Biochemical Journal*, 3: 747–756.

Honig PJ, Frieden IJ, Kim HJ, Yan AC (2003). Streptococcal intertrigo: an underrecognized condition in children. *Pediatrics*, 112: 1427–1429.

Horii KA, Simon SD, Liu DY, Sharma V (2007). Atopic dermatitis in children in the United States, 1997–2004: visit trends, patient and provider characteristics, and prescribing patterns. *Pediatrics*, 120: e527–e534.

Huang X, Tanojo H, Lenn J, Deng CH, Krochmal L (2005). A novel foam vehicle for delivery of topical corticosteroids. *Journal of the American Academy of Dermatology*, 53(1 suppl 1): S26–S38.

Iikura Y, Naspitz CK, Mikawa H, *et al.* (1992). Prevention of asthma by ketotifen in infants with atopic dermatitis. *Annals of Allergy*, 68: 233–236.

Isogai R, Matsukura A, Aragane Y, *et al.* (2002). Quantitative analysis of bikunin-laden mast cells in follicular eruptions and chronic skin lesions of atopic dermatitis. *Archives of Dermatological Research*. 294: 387–392.

Kay J, Gawkrodger DJ, Mortimer MJ, Jaron AG (1994). The prevalence of childhood atopic eczema in a general population. *Journal of the American Academy of Dermatology*, 30: 35–39.

Kerkhof M, Koopman LP, van Strien RT, *et al.* (2003). Risk factors for atopic dermatitis in infants at high risk of allergy: the PIAMA study. *Clinical and Experimental Allergy*, 33: 1336–1341.

Kezic S, Kemperman PM, Koster ES, *et al.* (2008). Loss-of-function mutations in the filaggrin gene lead to reduced level of natural moisturizing factor in the stratum corneum. *Journal of Investigative Dermatology*, 128: 1604.]

Kimata H (2008). Kaposi's varicelliform eruption associated with the use of tacrolimus ointment in two neonates. *Indian Journal of Dermatology, Venerology and Leprology*, 74: 262–263.

Laubereau B, Brockow I, Zirngibl A, *et al.* (2004). Effect of breast-feeding on the development of atopic dermatitis during the first 3 years of life – results from the GINI-birth cohort study. *Journal of Pediatrics*, 144: 602–607.

Laughter D, Istvan JA, Tofte SJ, Hanifin JM (2000). The prevalence of atopic dermatitis in Oregon schoolchildren. *Journal of the American Academy of Dermatology*, 43: 649–655.

Leyden JJ, Marples RR, Kligman AM (1974). *Staphylococcus aureus* in the lesions of atopic dermatitis. *British*

Journal of Dermatology, 90: 525–530.

Li LB, Goleva E, Hall CF, Ou LS, Leung DY (2004). Superantigen-induced corticosteroid resistance of human T cells occurs through activation of the mitogen-activated protein kinase kinase/extracellular signal-regulated kinase (MEK-ERK) pathway. Journal of Allergy and Clinical Immunology, 114: 1059–1069.

McKenzie AW, Stoughton RB (1962). Method for comparing percutaneous absorption of steroids. Archives of Dermatology, 86: 611–614.

McNally N, Phillips D (2000). Social factors and atopic dermatitis. In: Williams HC (ed.), Atopic Dermatitis: The Epidemiology, Causes and Prevention of Atopic Eczema, Cambridge University Press, Cambridge, pp. 139–147.

Mancini AJ (2004). Skin. Pediatrics, 113(4 suppl): 1114–1119.

Mills CM, Srivastava ED, Harvey IM, et al. (1994). Cigarette smoking is not a risk factor in atopic dermatitis. International Journal of Dermatology, 33: 33–34.

Mortz CG, Lauritsen JM, Bindslev-Jensen C, Andersen KE (2001). Prevalence of atopic dermatitis, asthma, allergic rhinitis, and hand and contact dermatitis in adolescents. The Odense adolescence cohort study on atopic diseases and dermatitis. British Journal of Dermatology, 144: 523–532.

Neame RL, Berth-Jones J, Kurinczuk JJ, Graham-Brown RA (1995). Prevalence of atopic dermatitis in Leicester: a study of methodology and examination of possible ethnic variation. British Journal of Dermatology, 132: 772–777.

Netchiporouk E, Cohen BA (2012). Recognizing and managing eczematous id reactions to molluscum contagiosum virus in children. Pediatrics, 129: e1072–1075.

Nonprescription Drugs Advisory Committee and the Dermatologic and Ophthalmic Drugs Advisory Committee (2005a). Topical Corticosteroids: HPA Axis Suppression and Cutaneous Effects. Available at: www.fda.gov/ohrms/dockets/ac/05/slides/2005–4099S1_03_FDA-Cook_files/frame.htm (accessed October 12, 2011).

Nonprescription Drugs Advisory Committee and the Dermatologic and Ophthalmic Drugs Advisory Committee (2005b). Dermatologic Corticosteroids. Available at: www.fda.gov/ohrms/dockets/ac/05/slides/2005–4099S1_02_FDA-Koenig_files/frame.htm (accessed October 12, 2011).

Olesen AB, Ellingsen AR, Olesen H, Juul S, Thestrup-Pedersen K (1997). Atopic dermatitis and birth factors: historical follow up by record linkage. British Medical Journal, 314: 1003–1008.

Ong PY, Ohtake T, Brandt C, et al. (2002). Endogenous antimicrobial peptides and skin infections in atopic dermatitis. New England Journal of Medicine, 347: 1151–1160.

Palmer CN, Irvine AD, Terron-Kwiatkowski A, et al. (2006). Common loss-of-function variants of the epidermal barrier protein filaggrin are a major predisposing factor for atopic dermatitis. Nature Genetics, 38: 441–446.

Peat JK, van den Berg RH, Green WF, Mellis CM, Leeder SR, Woolcock AJ (1994). Changing prevalence of asthma in Australian children. British Medical Journal, 308: 1591–1596.

Peserico A, Städtler G, Sebastian M, Fernandez RS, Vick K, Bieber T (2008). Reduction of relapses of atopic dermatitis with methylprednisolone aceponate cream twice weekly in addition to maintenance treatment with emollient: a multicentre, randomized, double-blind, controlled study. British Journal of Dermatology, 158: 801–807.

Peters TJ, Golding J (1987). The epidemiology of childhood eczema: II. Statistical analyses to identify independent early predictors. Paediatric Perinatology and Epidemiology, 1: 80–94.

Quinn D, Newton N, Piecuch R (2005). Effect of less frequent bathing on premature infant skin. Journal of Obstetric, Gynecologic, and Neonatal Nursing, 34: 741–746.

Schäfer T, Dirschedl P, Kunz B, Ring J, Uberla K (1997). Maternal smoking during pregnancy and lactation increases the risk for atopic eczema in the offspring. Journal of the American Academy of Dermatology, 36: 550–556.

Schultz Larsen F (1993). The epidemiology of atopic dermatitis. In: Burr ML (ed.), Epidemiology of Clinical Allergy, Basel, New York, pp. 9–28.

Siklar Z, Bostanci I, Atli O, Dallar Y (2004). An infantile Cushing syndrome due to misuse of topical steroid. Pediatric Dermatology, 21: 561–563.

Snijders BE, Thijs C, Dagnelie PC, et al. (2007). Breastfeeding duration and infant atopic manifestations, by maternal allergic status, in the first 2 years of life (KOALA study). Journal of Pediatrics, 151: 347–351, 351.e1–2.

Spergel JM, Paller AS (2003). Atopic dermatitis and the atopic march. Journal of Allergy and Clinical Immunology, 112(6 suppl): S118-S127.

Steffensen FH, Sørensen HT, Gillman MW, et al. (2000). Low birth weight and preterm delivery as risk factors for asthma and atopic dermatitis in young adult males. Epidemiology, 11: 185–188.

Strachan DP (1989). Hay fever, hygiene, and household size. British Medical Journal, 299: 1259–1260.

Suh LM, Honig PJ, Yan AC (2006). Methicillin-resistant Staphylococcus aureus skin abscesses in a pediatric patient with atopic dermatitis: a case report. Cutis, 78: 113–116.

Suh LM, Coffin S, Leckerman KH, et al. (2008) Methicillin-resistant Staphylococcus aureus colonization in children with atopic dermatitis. Pediatric Dermatology, 25: 528–534.

Tilles G, Wallach D, Taïeb A (2007). Topical therapy of atopic dermatitis: controversies from Hippocrates to topical immunomodulators. Journal of the American Academy of Dermatology, 56: 295–301.

Turner KJ, Rosman DL, O'Mahony J (1974). Prevalence and familial association of atopic disease and its relationship to serum IgE levels in 1,061 school children and their families. International Archives of Allergy and Immunology, 47: 650–664.

Werner S, Buser K, Kapp A, Werfel T (2002). The incidence of atopic dermatitis in school entrants is associated with individual life-style factors but not with local environmental factors in Hannover, Germany. British Journal of Dermatology, 147: 95–104.

Williams HC, Strachan DP, Hay RJ (1994). Childhood eczema: disease of the advantaged? British Medical Journal, 308: 1132–1135.

Williams HC, Pembroke AC, Forsdyke H, Boodoo G, Hay RJ, Burney PG (1995). London-born black

Caribbean children are at increased risk of atopic dermatitis. *Journal of the American Academy of Dermatology*, 32: 212–217.

Wüthrich B (1999). Clinical aspects, epidemiology, and prognosis of atopic dermatitis. *Annals of Allergy, Asthma and Immunology*, 83: 464–470.

CHAPTER 5

Andoh T, Nishikawa Y, Yamaguchi-Miyamoto T, Nojima H, Narumiya S, Kuraishi Y (2007). Thromboxane A2 induces itch-associated responses through TP receptors in the skin in mice. *Journal of Investigative Dermatology*, 127: 2042–2047.

Bell JK, McQueen DS, Rees JL (2004). Involvement of histamine H4 and H1 receptors in scratching induced by histamine receptor agonists in Balb C mice. *British Journal of Pharmacology*, 142: 374–380.

Bernstein JE, Swift R (1979). Relief of intractable pruritus with naloxone. *Archives of Dermatology*, 115: 1366–1367.

Bigliardi PL, Stammer H, Jost G, Rufli T, Büchner S, Bigliardi-Qi M (2007). Treatment of pruritus with topically applied opiate receptor antagonist. *Journal of the American Academy of Dermatology*, 56: 979–988.

Bíró T, Tóth BI, Marincsák R, Dobrosi N, Géczy T, Paus R (2007). TRP channels as novel players in the pathogenesis and therapy of itch. *Biochimica et Biophysica Acta*, 1772: 1004–1021.

Boguniewicz M (2005). Atopic dermatitis: beyond the itch that rashes. *Immunology and Allergy Clinics of North America*, 25: 333–451.

Bohm-Starke N, Hilliges M, Brodda-Jansen G, Rylander E, Torebjörk E (2001). Psychophysical evidence of nociceptor sensitization in vulvar vestibulitis syndrome. *Pain*, 94: 177–183.

Bromm B, Scharein E, Darsow U, Ring J (1995). Effects of menthol and cold on histamine-induced itch and skin reactions in man. *Neuroscience Letters*, 187: 157–160.

Chamlin SL, Kao J, Frieden IJ, *et al.* (2002). Ceramide-dominant barrier repair lipids alleviate childhood atopic dermatitis: changes in barrier function provide a sensitive indicator of disease activity. *Journal of the American Academy of Dermatology*, 47: 198–208.

Charlesworth EN, Beltrani VS (2002). Pruritic dermatoses: overview of etiology and therapy. *American Journal of Medicine*, 113(suppl 9A): 25S–33S.

Cork MJ, Robinson DA, Vasilopoulos Y, *et al.* (2006). New perspectives on epidermal barrier dysfunction in atopic dermatitis: gene–environment interactions. *Journal of Allergy and Clinical Immunology*, 118: 3–21.

Darsow U, Drzezga A, Frisch M, *et al.* (2000). Processing of histamine-induced itch in the human cerebral cortex: a correlation analysis with dermal reactions. *Journal of Investigative Dermatology*, 115: 1029–1033.

Davidson S, Zhang X, Yoon CH, Khasabov SG, Simone DA, Giesler GJ Jr (2007). The itch-producing agents histamine and cowhage activate separate populations of primate spinothalamic tract neurons. *Journal of Neuroscience*, 27: 10007–10014.

Dawn A, Yosipovitch G (2006a). Treating itch in psoriasis. *Dermatologic Nursing*, 18: 227–233.

Dawn A, Yosipovitch G (2006b). Butorphanol for treatment of intractable pruritus. *Journal of the American Academy of Dermatology*, 54: 527–531.

Dawn A, Papoiu AD, Chan YH, Rapp SR, Rassette N, Yosipovitch G (2009). Itch characteristics in atopic dermatitis: results of a web-based questionnaire. *British Journal of Dermatology*, 160: 642–644.

Denda M (2002). New strategies to improve skin barrier homeostasis. *Advanced Drug Delivery Reviews*, 54(suppl 1): S123–S130.

Devillers AC, Oranje AP (2006). Efficacy and safety of 'wet-wrap' dressings as an intervention treatment in children with severe and/or refractory atopic dermatitis: a critical review of the literature. *British Journal of Dermatology*, 154: 579–585.

Dijkstra D, Stark H, Chazot PL, *et al.* (2008). Human inflammatory dendritic epidermal cells express a functional histamine H4 receptor. *Journal of Investigative Dermatology*, 128: 1696–1703.

Dillon SR, Sprecher C, Hammond A, *et al.* (2004). Interleukin 31, a cytokine produced by activated T cells, induces dermatitis in mice. *Nature Immunology*, 6: 114.

Dou YC, Hagströmer L, Emtestam L, Johansson O (2006). Increased nerve growth factor and its receptors in atopic dermatitis: an immunohistochemical study. *Archives of Dermatological Research*, 298: 31–37.

Drake LA, Fallon JD, Sober A (1994). Relief of pruritus in patients with atopic dermatitis after treatment with topical doxepin cream. The Doxepin Study Group. *Journal of the American Academy of Dermatology*, 31: 613–616.

Drzezga A, Darsow U, Treede R D, *et al.* (2001). Central activation by histamine-induced itch: analogies to pain processing: a correlational analysis of O-15 H_2O positron emission tomography studies. *Pain*, 92: 295–305.

Dunford PJ, Williams KN, Desai PJ, Karlsson L, McQueen D, Thurmond RL (2007). Histamine H_4 receptor antagonists are superior to traditional antihistamines in the attenuation of experimental pruritus. *Journal of Allergy and Clinical Immunology*, 119: 176–183.

Dunteman E, Karanikolas M, Filos KS (1996). Transnasal butorphanol for the treatment of opioid-induced pruritus unresponsive to antihistamines. *Journal of Pain and Symptom Management*, 12: 255–260.

El-Khalawany MA, Hassan H, Shaaban D, Ghonaim N, Eassa B (2013). Methotrexate versus cyclosporine in the treatment of severe atopic dermatitis in children: a multicenter experience from Egypt. *European Journal of Pediatrics*, 172(3) 351-356.

Fjellner B, Hägermark O (1982). Potentiation of histamine-induced itch and flare responses in human skin by the enkephalin analogue FK-33-824, beta-endorphin and morphine. *Archives of Dermatological Research*, 274: 29–37.

Fjellner B, Hägermark O (1984). The influence of the opiate antagonist naloxone on experimental pruritus. *Acta Dermato-Venereologica*, 64: 73–75.

Freitag G, Höppner T (1997). Results of a postmarketing drug monitoring survey with a polidocanol-urea preparation for dry, itching skin. *Current Medical Research and Opinion*, 13: 529–537.

Grando SA, Kist DA, Qi M, Dahl MV (1993). Human keratinocytes synthesize, secrete, and degrade acetylcholine. *Journal of Investigative Dermatology*, **101**: 32–36.

Grewe M, Vogelsang K, Ruzicka T, Stege H, Krutmann J (2000). Neurotrophin-4 production by human epidermal keratinocytes: increased expression in atopic dermatitis. *Journal of Investigative Dermatology*, **114**: 1108–1112.

Grobe K, Pöppelmann M, Becker WM, Petersen A (2002). Properties of group I allergens from grass pollen and their relation to cathepsin B, a member of the C1 family of cysteine proteinases. *European Journal of Biochemistry*, **269**: 2083–2092.

Groneberg DA, Serowka F, Peckenschneider N, et al. (2005). Gene expression and regulation of nerve growth factor in atopic dermatitis mast cells and the human mast cell line-1. *Journal of Neuroimmunology*, **161**: 87–92.

Gutzmer R, Mommert S, Gschwandtner M, Zwingmann K, Stark H, Werfel T (2009). The histamine H4 receptor is functionally expressed on T(H)2 cells. *Journal of Allergy and Clinical Immunology*, **123**: 619–625.

Hachem JP, Man MQ, Crumrine D, et al. (2005). Sustained serine proteases activity by prolonged increase in pH leads to degradation of lipid processing enzymes and profound alterations of barrier function and stratum corneum integrity. *Journal of Investigative Dermatology*, **125**: 510–520.

Hägermark O (1992). Peripheral and central mediators of itch. *Skin Pharmacology*, **5**: 1–8.

Hägermark O, Strandberg K, Hamberg M (1977). Potentiation of itch and flare responses in human skin by prostaglandins E$_2$ and H$_2$ and a prostaglandin endoperoxide analog. *Journal of Investigative Dermatology*, **69**: 527–530.

Hanifin JM, Rajka G (1980). Diagnostic features of atopic dermatitis. *Acta Dermato-Venereologica Supplementum (Stockholm)*, **92**: 44–47.

Hartmann PM (1999). Mirtazapine: a newer antidepressant. *American Family Physician*, **59**: 159–161.

Heller M, Shin HT, Orlow SJ, Schaffer JV (2007). Mycophenolate mofetil for severe childhood atopic dermatitis: experience in 14 patients. *British Journal of Dermatology*, **157**: 127–132.

Herman SM, Vender RB (2003). Antihistamines in the treatment of dermatitis. *Journal of Cutaneous Medicine and Surgery*, **7**: 467–473.

Heyer G, Ulmer FJ, Schmitz J, et al. (1995). Histamine-induced itch and alloknesis (itchy skin) in atopic eczema patients and controls. *Acta Dermato-Venereologica*, **75**: 348–352.

Heyer G, Vogelgsang M, Hornstein OP (1997). Acetylcholine is an inducer of itching in patients with atopic eczema. *Journal of Dermatology*, **24**: 621–625.

Hon KL, Lam MC, Leung TF, Chow CM, Wong E, Leung AK (2007). Assessing itch in children with atopic dermatitis treated with tacrolimus: objective versus subjective assessment. *Advances in Therapy*, **24**: 23–28.

Hosogi M, Schmelz M, Miyachi Y, Ikoma A (2006). Bradykinin is a potent pruritogen in atopic dermatitis: a switch from pain to itch. *Pain*, **126**: 16–23.

Hsieh JC, Hägermark O, Ståhle-Bäckdahl M, et al. (1994). Urge to scratch represented in the human cerebral cortex during itch. *Journal of Neurophysiology*, **72**: 3004–3008.

Hundley JL, Yosipovitch G (2004). Mirtazapine for reducing nocturnal itch in patients with chronic pruritus: a pilot study. *Journal of the American Academy of Dermatology*, **50**: 889–891.

Ikoma A, Rukwied R, Ständer S, Steinhoff M, Miyachi Y, Schmelz M (2003). Neurophysiology of pruritus: interaction of itch and pain. *Archives of Dermatology*, **139**: 1475–1478.

Ikoma A, Fartasch M, Heyer G, Miyachi Y, Handwerker H, Schmelz M (2004). Painful stimuli evoke itch in patients with chronic pruritus: central sensitization for itch. *Neurology*, **62**: 212–217.

Ikoma A, Handwerker H, Miyachi Y, Schmelz M (2005). Electrically evoked itch in humans. *Pain*, **113**: 148–154.

Ikoma A, Steinhoff M, Ständer S, Yosipovitch G, Schmelz M (2006). The neurobiology of itch. *Nature Reviews Neuroscience*, **7**: 535–547.

Inoue K, Koizumi S, Fuziwara S, Denda S, Inoue K, Denda M (2002). Functional vanilloid receptors in cultured normal human epidermal keratinocytes. *Biochemical and Biophysical Research Communications*, **291**: 124–129.

Ishiuji Y, Coghill RC, Patel T, et al. (2007). Itch-related brain activity in patients with atopic eczema. *Journal of Investigative Dermatology*, **127**: S8. (Abstr.).

Ishiuji Y, Coghill RC, Patel TS, Oshiro Y, Kraft RA, Yosipovitch G (2009). Distinct patterns of brain activity evoked by histamine-induced itch reveal an association with itch intensity and disease severity in atopic dermatitis. *British Journal of Dermatology*, **161**: 1072–1080.

Johanek LM, Meyer RA, Hartke T, et al. (2007). Psychophysical and physiological evidence for parallel afferent pathways mediating the sensation of itch. *Journal of Neuroscience*, **27**: 7490–7497.

Kaufmann R, Bieber T, Helgesen AL, et al. (2006). Onset of pruritus relief with pimecrolimus cream 1% in adult patients with atopic dermatitis: a randomized trial. *Allergy*, **61**: 375–381.

Kirchner A, Stefan H, Schmelz M, Haslbeck KM, Birklein F (2002). Influence of vagus nerve stimulation on histamine-induced itching. *Neurology*, **59**: 108–112.

Klein PA, Clark RA (1999). An evidence-based review of the efficacy of antihistamines in relieving pruritus in atopic dermatitis. *Archives of Dermatology*, **135**: 1522–1525.

Lee CH, Chuang HY, Shih CC, Jong SB, Chang CH, Yu HS (2006). Transepidermal water loss, serum IgE and beta-endorphin as important and independent biological markers for development of itch intensity in atopic dermatitis. *British Journal of Dermatology*, **154**: 1100–1107.

Lee SS, Tan AW, Giam YC (2004). Cyclosporin in the treatment of severe atopic dermatitis: a retrospective study. *Annals Academy of Medicine Singapore*, **33**: 311–313.

Leknes SG, Bantick S, Willis CM, Wilkinson JD, Wise RG, Tracey I (2007). Itch and motivation to scratch: an investigation of the central and peripheral correlates of allergen- and histamine-induced itch in humans. *Journal of Neurophysiology*, **97**: 415–422.

Liu Q, Tang Z, Surdenikova L, et al. (2009). Sensory neuron-specific GPCR Mrgprs are itch receptors mediating chloroquine-induced pruritus. *Cell*, **139**: 1353–1365.

Malekzad F, Arbabi M, Mohtasham N et al. (2009). Efficacy of oral naltrexone on pruritus in atopic eczema: a double-blind, placebo-controlled study. *Journal of the European Academy of Dermatology and Venereology*, **23**: 948–950.

Meggitt SJ, Reynolds NJ (2001). Azathioprine for atopic dermatitis. *Clinical and Experimental Dermatology*, **26**: 369–375.

Meggitt SJ, Gray JC, Reynolds NJ (2006). Azathioprine dosed by thiopurine methyltransferase activity for moderate-to-severe atopic eczema: a double-blind, randomised controlled trial. *Lancet*, **367**: 839–846.

Mendell LM, Albers KM, Davis BM (1999). Neurotrophins, nociceptors, and pain. *Microscopy Research and Technique*, **45**: 252–261.

Metze D, Reimann S, Beissert S, Luger T (1999). Efficacy and safety of naltrexone, an oral opiate receptor antagonist, in the treatment of pruritus in internal and dermatological diseases. *Journal of the American Academy of Dermatology*, **41**: 533–539.

Miyamoto T, Nojima H, Shinkado T, Nakahashi T, Kuraishi Y (2002). Itch-associated response induced by experimental dry skin in mice. *Japanese Journal of Pharmacology*, **88**: 285–292.

Mochizuki H, Tashiro M, Kano M, Sakurada Y, Itoh M, Yanai K (2003). Imaging of central itch modulation in the human brain using positron emission tomography. *Pain*, **105**: 339–346.

Munro CS, Levell NJ, Shuster S, Friedmann PS (1994). Maintenance treatment with cyclosporin in atopic eczema. *British Journal of Dermatology*, **130**: 376–380.

Namer B, Carr R, Johanek LM, Schmelz M, Handwerker HO, Ringkamp M (2008). Separate peripheral pathways for pruritus in man. *Neurophysiology*, **100**: 2062–2069.

Neisius U, Olsson R, Rukwied R, Lischetzki G, Schmelz M (2002). Prostaglandin E2 induces vasodilation and pruritus, but no protein extravasation in atopic dermatitis and controls. *Journal of the American Academy of Dermatology*, **47**: 28–32.

Nilsson HJ, Schouenborg J (1999). Differential inhibitory effect on human nociceptive skin senses induced by local stimulation of thin cutaneous fibers. *Pain*, **80**: 103–112.

Oranje AP, Devillers AC, Kunz B, *et al.* (2006). Treatment of patients with

atopic dermatitis using wet-wrap dressings with diluted steroids and/or emollients. An expert panel's opinion and review of the literature. *Journal of the European Academy of Dermatology and Venereology*, **20**: 1277–1286.

Otsuka A, Honda T, Doi H, Miyachi Y, Kabashima K (2011). An H1-histamine receptor antagonist decreases serum IL-31 levels in patients with atopic dermatitis. *Britsh Journal of Dermatology*, **164**: 455–6.

Patel T, Ishiuji Y, Yosipovitch G (2007a). Nocturnal itch: why do we itch at night? *Acta Dermato-Venereologica*, **87**: 295–298.

Patel T, Ishiuji Y, Yosipovitch G (2007b). Menthol: a refreshing look at this ancient compound. *Journal of the American Academy of Dermatology*, **57**: 873–878.

Paus R, Schmelz M, Bíró T, Steinhoff M (2006). Frontiers in pruritus research: scratching the brain for more effective itch therapy. *Journal of Clinical Investigation*, **116**: 1174–1186.

Pereira U, Boulais N, Lebonvallet N, Pennec JP, Dorange G, Misery L (2010). Mechanisms of sensory effects of tacrolimus on the skin. *British Journal of Dermatology*, **163**: 70–77.

Pfab F, Huss-Marp J, Gatti A, *et al.* (2009). Influence of acupuncture on type I hypersensitivity itch and the wheal and flare response in adults with atopic eczema – a blinded, randomized, placebo-controlled, crossover trial. *Allergy*, **65**: 903–910.

Phan NQ, Bernhard JD, Luger TA, Ständer S (2010). Antipruritic treatment with systemic μ-opioid receptor antagonists: a review. *Journal of the American Academy of Dermatology*, **63**: 680–688.

Raap U, Goltz C, Deneka N, *et al.* (2005). Brain-derived neurotrophic factor is increased in atopic dermatitis and modulates eosinophil functions compared with that seen in nonatopic subjects. *Journal of Allergy and Clinical Immunology*, **115**: 1268–1275.

Raap U, Wichmann K, Bruder M, *et al.* (2008). Correlation of IL-31 serum levels with severity of atopic dermatitis. *Journal of Allergy and Clinical Immunology*, **122**: 421–423.

Rajka G (1969). Latency and duration of pruritus elicited by trypsin in aged patients with itching eczema

and psoriasis. *Acta Dermato-Venereologica*, **49**: 401–403.

Reddy VB, Iuga AO, Shimada SG, LaMotte RH, Lerner EA (2008). Cowhage-evoked itch is mediated by a novel cysteine protease: a ligand of protease-activated receptors. *Journal of Neuroscience*, **28**: 4331–4335.

Reddy VB, Shimada SG, Sikand P, Lamotte RH, Lerner EA (2010). Cathepsin S elicits itch and signals via protease-activated receptors. *Journal of Investigative Dermatology*, **130**: 1468–1470.

Rivard J, Lim HW (2005). Ultraviolet phototherapy for pruritus. *Dermatologic Therapy*, **18**: 344–354.

Rukwied R, Heyer G (1999). Administration of acetylcholine and vasoactive intestinal polypeptide to atopic eczema patients. *Experimental Dermatology*, **8**: 39–45.

Schmelz M (2001). A neural pathway for itch. *Nature Neuroscience*, **4**: 9–10.

Schmelz M, Schmidt R, Bickel A, Handwerker HO, Torebjörk HE (1997). Specific C-receptors for itch in human skin. *Journal of Neuroscience*, **17**: 8003–8800.

Schmelz M, Michael K, Weidner C, Schmidt R, Torebjörk HE, Handwerker HO (2000). Which nerve fibers mediate the axon reflex flare in human skin? *NeuroReport*, 28;**11**: 645–648.

Schmelz M, Schmidt R, Weidner C, Hilliges M, Torebjork HE, Handwerker HO (2003). Chemical response pattern of different classes of C-nociceptors to pruritogens and algogens. *Journal of Neurophysiology*, **89**: 2441–2448.

Schmitt J, Schmitt N, Meurer M (2007). Cyclosporin in the treatment of patients with atopic eczema – a systematic review and meta-analysis. *Journal of the European Academy of Dermatology and Venereology*, **21**: 606–619.

Schram ME, Roekevisch E, Leeflang MM, Bos JD, Schmitt J, Spuls PL(2001). A randomized trial of methotrexate versus azathioprine for severe atopic eczema. *Journal of Allergy and Clinical Immunology*, **128**(2) 353-359.

Schulte-Herbrüggen O, Fölster-Holst R, von Elstermann M, Augustin M, Hellweg R (2007). Clinical relevance of nerve growth factor serum levels in patients with atopic dermatitis and psoriasis. *International Archives of Allergy and Immunology*, **144**: 211–216.

Senba E, Katanosaka K, Yajima H, Mizumura K (2004). The immunosuppressant FK506 activates capsaicin- and bradykinin-sensitive DRG neurons and cutaneous C-fibers. *Neuroscience Research*, **50**: 257–262.

Shelley WB, Arthur RP (1955a). Studies on cowhage (*Mucuna pruriens*) and its pruritogenic proteinase, mucunain. *AMA Archives of Dermatology*, **72**: 399–406.

Shelley WB, Arthur RP (1955b). Mucunain, the active pruritogenic proteinase of cowhage. *Science*, **122**: 469–470.

Shelley WB, Arthur RP (1957). The neurohistology and neurophysiology of the itch sensation in man. *AMA Archives of Dermatology*, **76**: 296–323.

Shenefelt PD (2003). Biofeedback, cognitive–behavioral methods, and hypnosis in dermatology: is it all in your mind? *Dermatologic Therapy*, **16**: 114–122.

Shu X, Mendell LM (1999). Neurotrophins and hyperalgesia. *Proceedings of the National Academy of Sciences of the United States of America – Physical Sciences*, **96**: 7693–7696.

Shu X, Mendell LM (2001). Acute sensitization by NGF of the response of small-diameter sensory neurons to capsaicin. *Journal of Neurophysiology*, **86**: 2931–2938.

Simone DA, Alreja M, LaMotte RH (1991). Psychophysical studies of the itch sensation and itchy skin ('alloknesis') produced by intracutaneous injection of histamine. *Somatosensory and Motor Research*, **8**: 271–279.

Sonkoly E, Muller A, Lauerma AI, et al. (2006). IL-31: a new link between T cells and pruritus in atopic skin inflammation. *Journal of Allergy and Clinical Immunology*, **117**: 411–417.

Ständer S, Luger TA (2003). Antipruritic effects of pimecrolimus and tacrolimus [in German]. *Hautarzt*, **54**: 413–417.

Stefansson K, Brattsand M, Roosterman D, et al. (2008). Activation of proteinase-activated receptor-2 by human kallikrein-related peptidases. *Journal of Investigative Dermatology*, **128**: 18–25.

Steinhoff M, Neisius U, Ikoma A, et al. (2003). Proteinase-activated receptor-2 mediates itch: a novel pathway for pruritus in human skin. *Journal of Neuroscience*, **23**: 6176–6180.

Steinhoff M, Bienenstock J, Schmelz M, Maurer M, Wei E, Bíró T (2006). Neurophysiological, neuroimmunological, and neuroendocrine basis of pruritus. *Journal of Investigative Dermatology*, **126**: 1705–1718.

Stevens SR, Hanifin JM, Hamilton T, Tofte SJ, Cooper KD (1998). Long-term effectiveness and safety of recombinant human interferon gamma therapy for atopic dermatitis despite unchanged serum IgE levels. *Archives of Dermatology*, **134**: 799–804.

Sugimoto M, Arai I, Futaki N, et al. (2007). Putative mechanism of the itch-scratch circle: repeated scratching decreases the cutaneous level of prostaglandin D_2, a mediator that inhibits itching. *Prostaglandins Leukotrienes and Essential Fatty Acids*, **76**: 93–101.

Sugimoto Y, Iba Y, Nakamura Y, Kayasuga R, Kamei C (2004). Pruritus-associated response mediated by cutaneous histamine H3 receptors. *Clinical and Experimental Allergy*, **34**: 456–459.

Sun YG, Chen ZF (2007). A gastrin-releasing peptide receptor mediates the itch sensation in the spinal cord. *Nature*, **448**: 700–703.

Szepietowski JC, Morita A, Tsuji T (2002). Ultraviolet B induces mast cell apoptosis: a hypothetical mechanism of ultraviolet B treatment for uraemic pruritus. *Medical Hypotheses*, **58**: 167–170.

Tanaka A, Arita K, Lai-Cheong JE, Palisson F, Hide M, McGrath JA (2009). New insight into mechanisms of pruritus from molecular studies on familial primary localized cutaneous amyloidosis. *The British Journal of Dermatology*, **161**: 1217–1224.

Tominaga M, Ogawa H, Takamori K (2007). Possible roles of epidermal opioid systems in pruritus of atopic dermatitis. *Journal of Investigative Dermatology*, **127**: 2228–2235.

Toyoda M, Nakamura M, Makino T, Hino T, Kagoura M, Morohashi M (2002). Nerve growth factor and substance P are useful plasma markers of disease activity in atopic dermatitis. *British Journal of Dermatology*, **147**: 71–79.

Tran BW, Papoiu AD, Russoniello CV, et al. (2010). Effect of itch, scratching and mental stress on autonomic nervous system function in atopic dermatitis. *Acta Dermato-Venereologica*, **90**: 354–361.

Urashima R, Mihara M (1998). Cutaneous nerves in atopic dermatitis. A histological, immunohistochemical and electron microscopic study. *Virchows Archive*, **432**: 363–370.

Vergnolle N, Ferazzini M, D'Andrea MR, Buddenkotte J, Steinhoff M (2003). Proteinase-activated receptors: novel signals for peripheral nerves. *Trends in the Neurosciences*, **26**: 496–500.

Vogelsang M, Heyer G, Hornstein O (1995). Acetylcholine induces different cutaneous sensations in atopic and non-atopic subjects. *Acta Dermato-Venereologica*, **75**: 434–436.

Wahlgren CF (1991). Itch and atopic dermatitis: clinical and experimental studies. *Acta Dermato-Venereologica Supplementum (Stockholm)*, **165**: 1–53.

Wahlgren CF, Scheynius A, Hägermark O (1990). Antipruritic effect of oral cyclosporin A in atopic dermatitis. *Acta Dermato-Venereologica*, **70**: 323–329.

Ward L, Wright E, McMahon SB (1996). A comparison of the effects of noxious and innocuous counterstimuli on experimentally induced itch and pain. *Pain*, **64**: 129–138.

Wang H, Papoiu AD, Ishiuji Y, Yosipovitch G, Schmelz M (2010). A study of NGF levels in atopic dermatitis. NGF does not seem to be a reliable marker for severity of atopic dermatitis. *Journal of Investigative Dermatology*, (abstract) Supplement 1. S101.

Yosipovitch G (2004). Dry skin and impairment of barrier function associated with itch – new insights. *International Journal of Cosmetic Science*, **26**: 1–7.

Yosipovitch G, Maibach HI (1997). Effect of topical pramoxine on experimentally induced pruritus in humans. *Journal of the American Academy of Dermatology*, **37**: 278–280.

Yosipovitch G, Xiong GL, Haus E, Sackett-Lundeen L, Ashkenazi I, Maibach HI (1998). Time-dependent variations of the skin barrier function in humans: transepidermal water loss, stratum corneum hydration, skin surface pH, and skin temperature. *Journal of Investigative Dermatology*, 110: 20–23.

Yosipovitch G, Sugeng MW, Chan YH, Goon A, Ngim S, Goh CL (2001). The effect of topically applied aspirin on localized circumscribed neurodermatitis. *Journal of the American Academy of Dermatology*, 45: 910–913.

Yosipovitch G, Goon AT, Wee J, Chan YH, Zucker I, Goh CL (2002). Itch characteristics in Chinese patients with atopic dermatitis using a new questionnaire for the assessment of pruritus. *International Journal of Dermatology*, 41: 212–216.

Yosipovitch G, Duque MI, Fast K, *et al.* (2007). Scratching and noxious heat stimuli inhibit itch in humans: a psychophysical study. *British Journal of Dermatology*, 156: 629–634.

Yu B, Shao Y, Zhang J, *et al.* (2010). Polymorphisms in human histamine receptor H4 gene are associated with atopic dermatitis. *British Journal of Dermatology*, 162: 1038–1043.

CHAPTER 6

Ackerman AB (1978). *Histologic Diagnosis of Inflammatory Skin Diseases*, Lea & Febiger, Philadelphia, pp. 256–258.

Aichberger KJ, Mittermann I, Reininger R, *et al.* (2005). Hom s 4, an IgE-reactive autoantigen belonging to a new subfamily of calcium-binding proteins, can induce Th cell type 1-mediated autoreactivity. *Journal of Immunology*, 175: 1286–1294.

Akdis CA, Akdis M, Simon D, *et al.* (1999a). Role of T cells and cytokines in the intrinsic form of atopic dermatitis. In: Wüthrich B (ed.), *The Atopy Syndrome in the Third Millennium*, Vol 28, *Current Problems in Dermatology*, Karger, Basel, pp. 37–44.

Akdis CA, Akdis M, Simon D, *et al.* (1999b). T cells and T cell-derived cytokines as pathogenic factors in the nonallergic form of atopic dermatitis. *Journal of Investigative Dermatology*, 113: 628–634.

Akdis M, Akdis CA, Weigl L, Disch R, Blaser K (1997). Skin-homing, CLA+ memory T cells are activated in atopic dermatitis and regulate IgE by an IL-13-dominated cytokinepattern: IgG4 counter-regulation by CLA memory T cells. *Journal of Immunology*, 159: 4611–4619.

Akdis M, Trautmann A, Klunker S, *et al.* (2003). T helper (Th) 2 predominance in atopic diseases is due to preferential apoptosis of circulating memory/effector Th1 cells. *FASEB Journal*, 17: 1026–1035.

Allakhverdi Z, Comeau MR, Jessup HK, *et al.* (2007). Thymic stromal lymphopoietin is released by human epithelial cells in response to microbes, trauma, or inflammation and potently activates mast cells. *Journal of Experimental Medicine*, 204: 253–258.

Allen HB, Mueller JL (2011). A novel finding in atopic dermatitis: film-producing *Staphylococcus epidermidis* as an etiology. *International Journal of Dermatology*, 50: 992–993.

Aloe L, Bracci-Laudiero L, Bonini S, *et al.* (1997). The expanding role of nerve growth factor: from neurotrophic activity to immunologic diseases. *Allergy*, 52: 883–894.

Aly R, Maibach HI, Shinefield HR (1977). Microbial flora of atopic dermatitis. *Archives of Dermatology*, 113: 780–782.

Andoh T, Saito A, Kuraishi Y (2009). Leukotriene B(4) mediates sphingosylphosphorylcholine-induced itch-associated responses in mouse skin. *Journal of Investigative Dermatology*, 129: 2854–2860.

Arikawa J, Ishibashi M, Kawashima M, Takagi Y, Ichikawa Y, Imokawa G (2002). Decreased levels of sphingosine, a natural antimicrobial agent, may be associated with vulnerability of the stratum corneum from patients with atopic dermatitis to colonization by *Staphylococcus aureus*. *Journal of Investigative Dermatology*, 119: 433–439.

Armbruster N, Trautmann A, Bröcker EB, Leverkus M, Kerstan A (2009). Suprabasal spongiosis in acute eczematous dermatitis: cFLIP maintains resistance of basal keratinocytes to T-cell-mediated apoptosis. *Journal of Investigative Dermatology*, 129: 1696–1702.

Asano S, Ichikawa Y, Kumagai T, Kawashima M, Imokawa G (2008). Microanalysis of an antimicrobial peptide, beta-defensin-2, in the stratum corneum from patients with atopic dermatitis. *British Journal of Dermatology*, 159: 97–104.

Ashida Y, Denda M (2003). Dry environment increases mast cell number and histamine content in dermis in hairless mice. *British Journal of Dermatology*, 149: 240–247.

Ashida Y, Ogo M, Denda M (2001). Epidermal interleukin-1 alpha generation is amplified at low humidity: implications for the pathogenesis of inflammatory dermatoses. *British Journal of Dermatology*, 144: 238–243.

Badertscher K, Brönnimann M, Karlen S, Braathen LR, Yawalkar N (2005). Mast cell chymase is increased in chronic atopic dermatitis but not in psoriasis. *Archives of Dermatological Research*, 296: 503–506.

Baker BS (2006). The role of microorganisms in atopic dermatitis. *Clinical and Experimental Immunology*, 144: 1–9.

Ballardini N, Johansson C, Lilja G, *et al.* (2009). Enhanced expression of the antimicrobial peptide LL-37 in lesional skin of adults with atopic eczema. *British Journal of Dermatology*, 161: 40–47.

Barberio G, Pajno GB, Vita D, Caminiti L, Canonica GW, Passalacqua G (2008). Does a 'reverse' atopic march exist? *Allergy*, 63: 1630–1632.

Barker JN, Alegre VA, MacDonald DM (1988). Surface-bound immunoglobulin E on antigen-presenting cells in cutaneous tissue of atopic dermatitis. *Journal of Investigative Dermatology*, 90: 117–21.

Behne M, Uchida Y, Seki T, de Montellano PO, Elias PM, Holleran WM (2000). Omega-hydroxyceramides are required for corneocyte lipid envelope (CLE) formation and normal epidermal permeability barrier function. *Journal of Investigative Dermatology*, 114: 185–192.

Berard F, Marty JP, Nicolas JF (2003). Allergen penetration through the skin. *European Journal of Dermatology*, 13: 324–330.

Bieber T, de la Salle H, Wollenberg A, *et al.* (1992). Human epidermal Langerhans cells express the high affinity receptor for immunoglobulin E (Fc epsilon RI). *Journal of Experimental Medicine*, 175: 1285–1290.

Bigliardi-Qi M, Lipp B, Sumanovski LT, Buechner SA, Bigliardi PL (2005). Changes of epidermal mu-opiate receptor expression and nerve endings in chronic atopic dermatitis. *Dermatology*, **210**: 91–99.

Bilsborough J, Leung DY, Maurer M, *et al*. (2006). IL-31 is associated with cutaneous lymphocyte antigen-positive skin homing T cells in patients with atopic dermatitis. *Journal of Allergy and Clinical Immunology*, **117**: 418–425.

Bønnelykke K, Pipper CB, Tavendale R, Palmer CN, Bisgaard H (2010). Filaggrin gene variants and atopic diseases in early childhood assessed longitudinally from birth. *Pediatric Allergy and Immunology*, **21**: 954–961.

Boralevi F, Hubiche T, Léauté-Labrèze C, *et al*. (2008). Epicutaneous aeroallergen sensitization in atopic dermatitis infants – determining the role of epidermal barrier impairment. *Allergy*, **63**: 205–210.

Bos JD (2002). Atopiform dermatitis. *British Journal of Dermatology*, **147**: 426–429.

Bos JD, Meinardi MM (2000). The 500 Dalton rule for the skin penetration of chemical compounds and drugs. *Experimental Dermatology*, **9**: 165–169.

Bos JD, Wierenga EA, Sillevis Smitt JH, *et al*. (1992). Immune dysregulation in atopic eczema. *Archives of Dermatology*, **128**: 1509–1512.

Bos JD, Brenninkmeijer EE, Schram ME, Middelkamp-Hup MA, Spuls PI, Smitt JH (2010). Atopic eczema or atopiform dermatitis. *Experimental Dermatology*, **19**: 325–331.

Boussault P, Léauté-Labrèze C, Saubusse E, *et al*. (2007). Oat sensitization in children with atopic dermatitis: prevalence, risks, and associated factors. *Allergy*, **62**: 1251–1256.

Braathen LR, Førre O, Natvig JB, Eeg-Larsen T (1979). Predominance of T lymphocytes in the dermal infiltrate of atopic dermatitis. *British Journal of Dermatology*, **100**: 511–519.

Brady KB, Levin TL (2007). Necrotizing fasciitis in a young girl with atopic eczema. *Clinical Pediatrics (Philadelphia)*, **46**: 181–183.

Brenninkmeijer EE, Spuls PI, Legierse CM, Lindeboom R, Smitt JH, Bos JD (2008). Clinical differences between atopic and atopiform dermatitis. *Journal of the American Academy of Dermatology*, **58**: 407–414.

Bruynzeel-Koomen C, van Wichen DF, Toonstra J, Berrens L, Bruynzeel PL (1986). The presence of IgE molecules on epidermal Langerhans cells in patients with atopic dermatitis.' *Archives of Dermatological Research*, **278**: 199–205.

Burgess JA, Lowe AJ, Matheson MC, Varigos G, Abramson MJ, Dharmage SC (2009). Does eczema lead to asthma? *Journal of Asthma*, **46**: 429–436.

Candi E, Schmidt R, Melino G (2005). The cornified envelope: a model of cell death in the skin. *Nature Reviews Molecular Cell Biology*, **6**: 328–340.

Caproni M, Torchia D, Antiga E, Volpi W, del Bianco E, Fabbri P (2006). The effects of tacrolimus ointment on regulatory T lymphocytes in atopic dermatitis. *Journal of Clinical Immunology*, **26**: 370–375.

Carmi-Levy I, Homey B, Soumelis V (2011). A modular view of cytokine networks in atopic dermatitis. *Critical Reviews in Allergy and Immunology*, **41**: 245–253.

Casagrande BF, Flückiger S, Linder MT, *et al*. (2006). Sensitization to the yeast *Malassezia sympodialis* is specific for extrinsic and intrinsic atopic eczema. *Journal of Investigative Dermatology*, **126**: 2414–2421.

Cavani A, Ottaviani C, Nasorri F, Sebastiani S, Girolomoni G (2003). Immunoregulation of hapten and drug induced immune reactions. *Current Opinion in Allergy and Clinical Immunology*, **3**: 243–247.

Cheng JF, Ott NL, Peterson EA, *et al*. (1997). Dermal eosinophils in atopic dermatitis undergo cytolytic degeneration. *Journal of Allergy and Clinical Immunology*, **99**: 683–692.

Choi H, Kim S, Kim HJ, *et al*. (2010). Sphingosylphosphorylcholine down-regulates filaggrin gene transcription through NOX5-based NADPH oxidase and cyclooxygenase-2 in human keratinocytes. *Biochemical Pharmacology*, **80**: 95–103.

Church MK, Lowman MA, Robinson C, Holgate ST, Benyon RC (1989). Interaction of neuropeptides with human mast cells. *International Archives of Allergy and Applied Immunology*, **88**: 70–78.

Cooper KD (1994). Atopic dermatitis: recent trends in pathogenesis and therapy. *Journal of Investigative Dermatology*, **102**: 128–137.

Cremona S, Dusi D, Emanuele E, Lossano C (2007). Atopic dermatitis and anxiety: possible role of brain-derived neurotrophic factor (BDNF). *Medical Hypotheses*, **68**: 1419.

Curtiss FR (2007). Atopic march to a dead end or does the theory really have legs? *Journal of Managed Care Pharmacy*, **13**: 810–811.

De Benedetto A, Rafaels NM, McGirt LY, *et al*. (2010). Tight junction defects in patients with atopic dermatitis. *Journal of Allergy and Clinical Immunology*, **127**: 773–786.

Debes GF, Diehl MC (2011). CCL8 and skin T cells – an allergic attraction. *Nature Immunology*, **12**: 111–112.

de Jongh CM, Khrenova L, Verberk MM (2008). Loss-of-function polymorphisms in the filaggrin gene are associated with an increased susceptibility to chronic irritant contact dermatitis: a case-control study. *British Journal of Dermatology*, **159**: 621–627.

de Vries IJ, Langeveld-Wildschut EG, van Reijsen FC, Bihari IC, Bruijnzeel-Koomen CA, Thepen T (1997). Nonspecific T-cell homing during inflammation in atopic dermatitis: expression of cutaneous lymphocyte-associated antigen and integrin alphaE beta7 on skin-infiltrating T cells. *Journal of Allergy and Clinical Immunology*, **100**: 694–701.

de Vries JE, Punnonen J, Cocks BG, de Waal Malefyt R, Aversa G (1993). Regulation of the human IgE response by IL4 and IL13. *Research in Immunology*, **144**: 597–601.

Demehri S, Morimoto M, Holtzman MJ, Kopan R (2009). Skin-derived TSLP triggers progression from epidermal-barrier defects to asthma. *PLoS Biology*, **7**: e1000067.

Denda M, Sato J, Tsuchiya T, Elias PM, Feingold KR (1998). Low humidity stimulates epidermal DNA synthesis and amplifies the hyperproliferative response to barrier disruption: implication for seasonal exacerbations of inflammatory dermatoses. *Journal of Investigative Dermatology*, **111**: 873–878.

Dibbert B, Daigle I, Braun D (1998). Role for Bcl-xL in delayed eosinophil apoptosis mediated by granulocyte-macrophage colony-stimulating factor and interleukin-5. *Blood*, **92**: 778–783.

Dijkstra D, Stark H, Chazot PL, *et al*. (2008). Human inflammatory dendritic epidermal cells express a functional histamine H4 receptor. *Journal of Investigative Dermatology*, **128**: 1696–1703.

Dunstan JA, Hale J, Breckler L, *et al.* (2005). Atopic dermatitis in young children is associated with impaired interleukin-10 and interferon-gamma responses to allergens, vaccines and colonizing skin and gut bacteria. *Clinical and Experimental Allergy*, **35**: 1309–1317.

Eberlein-König B, Schäfer T, Huss-Marp J, *et al.* (2000). Skin surface pH, stratum corneum hydration, trans-epidermal water loss and skin roughness related to atopic eczema and skin dryness in a population of primary school children. *Acta Dermato-Venereologica*, **80**: 188–191.

Ebner S, Nguyen VA, Forstner M, *et al.* (2007). Thymic stromal lymphopoietin converts human epidermal Langerhans cells into antigen-presenting cells that induce proallergic T cells. *Journal of Allergy and Clinical Immunology*, **119**: 982–990.

Eckhart L, Tschachler E (2011). Cuts by caspase-14 control the proteolysis of filaggrin. *Journal of Investigative Dermatology*, **131**: 2173–2175.

Elias PM (1983). Epidermal lipids, barrier function, and desquamation. *Journal of Investigative Dermatology*, **80**(1 suppl): 44s-49s.

Elias PM, Schmuth M (2009). Abnormal skin barrier in the etiopathogenesis of atopic dermatitis. *Current Allergy and Asthma Reports*, **9**: 265–272.

Erickson L, Kahn G (1970). The granular layer thickness in atopy and ichthyosis vulgaris. *Journal of Investigative Dermatology*, **54**: 11–12.

Favre A (1989). Identification of filaggrin in Hassall's corpuscle by histochemical and immunohistochemical methods. *Acta Anatomica (Basel)*, **135**: 71–76.

Feldmeyer L, Werner S, French LE, Beer HD (2010). Interleukin-1, inflammasomes and the skin. *European Journal of Cell Biology*, **89**: 638–644.

Finlay AY, Nicholls S, King CS, Marks R (1980). The 'dry' non-eczematous skin associated with atopic eczema. *British Journal of Dermatology*, **103**: 249–256.

Fitzharris P, Riley G (1999). House dust mites in atopic dermatitis.

International Journal of Dermatology, **38**: 173–175.

Freeny I, Allen H, Puja S (2011). A novel finding in atopic dermatitis. Film-producing *Staphylococcus epidermidis* as an etiology. Abstract. *Journal of the American Academy of Dermatology*, **64**: AB61.

Fujita H, Nograles KE, Kikuchi T, Gonzalez J, Carucci JA, Krueger JG (2009). Human Langerhans cells induce distinct IL-22-producing CD4+ T cells lacking IL-17 production. *Proceeding of the National Academy of Sciences of the United States of America*, **106**: 21795–21800.

Galli SJ, Maurer M, Lantz CS (1999). Mast cells as sentinels of innate immunity. *Current Opinion in Immunology*, **11**: 53–59.

Gallo RL, Leung DYM (2003). Antimicrobial peptides in the skin. *New England Journal of Medicine*, **348**: 361–363.

Geiger E, Magerstaedt R, Wessendorf JH, Kraft S, Hanau D, Bieber T (2000). IL-4 induces the intracellular expression of the alpha chain of the high-affinity receptor for IgE in *in vitro*-generated dendritic cells. *Journal of Allergy and Clinical Immunology*, **105**(1 Pt 1): 150–156.

Gittler JK, Shemer A, Suárez-Fariñas M, *et al.* (2012). Progressive activation of T(H)2/T(H)22 cytokines and selective epidermal proteins characterizes acute and chronic atopic dermatitis. *Journal of Allergy and Clinical Immunology* **130**(6):1344–1354.

Gondo A, Saeki N, Tokuda Y (1986). Challenge reactions in atopic dermatitis after percutaneous entry of mite antigen. *British Journal of Dermatology*, **115**: 485–493.

Goo J, Ji JH, Jeon H, *et al.* (2010). Expression of antimicrobial peptides such as LL-37 and hBD-2 in nonlesional skin of atopic individuals. *Pediatric Dermatology*, **27**: 341–8.

Goujon-Henry C, Hennino A, Nicolas JF (2008). Do we have to recommend not using oat-containing emollients in children with atopic dermatitis? *Allergy*, **63**: 781–782.

Gregory GD, Brown MA (2006). Mast cells in allergy and autoimmunity: implications for adaptive immunity. *Methods in Molecular Biology*, **315**: 35–50.

Grewe M, Gyufko K, Schöpf E, Krutmann J (1994). Lesional

expression of interferon-gamma in atopic eczema. *Lancet*, **343**: 25–26.

Grewe M, Bruijnzeel-Koomen CA, Schöpf E, *et al.* (1998a). A role for Th1 and Th2 cells in the immunopathogenesis of atopic dermatitis. *Immunology Today* **19**: 359–361.

Grewe M, Czech W, Morita A (1998b). Human eosinophils produce biologically active IL-12: implications for control of T cell responses. *Journal of Immunology*, **161**: 415–420.

Grimstad O, Sawanobori Y, Vestergaard C, *et al.* (2009). Anti-interleukin-31-antibodies ameliorate scratching behaviour in NC/Nga mice: a model of atopic dermatitis. *Experimental Dermatology*, **18**: 35–43.

Groneberg DA, Bester C, Grützkau A, *et al.* (2005). Mast cells and vasculature in atopic dermatitis – potential stimulus of neoangiogenesis. *Allergy*, **60**: 90–97.

Grutz G (2005). New insights into the molecular mechanism of interleukin-10-mediated immunosuppression. *Journal of Leukocyte Biology*, **77**: 3–15.

Guttman-Yassky E, Suárez-Fariñas M, Chiricozzi A, *et al.* (2009). Broad defects in epidermal cornification in atopic dermatitis identified through genomic analysis. *Journal of Allergy and Clinical Immunology*, **124**: 1235–1244.e58.

Gutzmer R, Mommert S, Gschwandtner M, Zwingmann K, Stark H, Werfel T (2009). The histamine H4 receptor is functionally expressed on T(H)2 cells. *Journal of Allergy and Clinical Immunology*, **123**: 619–625.

Hachem JP, Man MQ, Crumrine D, *et al.* (2005). Sustained serine proteases activity by prolonged increase in pH leads to degradation of lipid processing enzymes and profound alterations of barrier function and stratum corneum integrity. *Journal of Investigative Dermatology*, **125**: 510–520.

Hachem JP, Roelandt T, Schürer N, *et al.* (2010). Acute acidification of stratum corneum membrane domains using polyhydroxyl acids improves lipid processing and inhibits degradation of corneodesmosomes. *Journal of Investigative Dermatology*, **130**: 500–510.

Hamid Q, Boguniewicz M, Leung DY (1994). Differential *in situ* cytokine gene expression in acute versus chronic atopic dermatitis. *Journal of Clinical Investigation*, 94: 870–876.

Hamid Q, Naseer T, Minshall EM, Song YL, Boguniewicz M, Leung DY (1996). *In vivo* expression of IL-12 and IL-13 in atopic dermatitis. *Journal of Allergy and Clinical Immunology*, 98: 225–231.

Hanifin JM (1990). Phosphodiesterase and immune dysfunction in atopic dermatitis. *Journal of Dermatological Science*, 1: 1–6.

Hanifin JM, Chan SC (1995). Monocyte phosphodiesterase abnormalities and dysregulation of lymphocyte function in atopic dermatitis. *Journal of Investigative Dermatology*, 105(1 suppl): 84S-88S.

Hara J, Higuchi K, Okamoto R, Kawashima M, Imokawa G (2000). High-expression of sphingomyelin deacylase is an important determinant of ceramide deficiency leading to barrier disruption in atopic dermatitis. *Journal of Investigative Dermatology*, 115: 406–413.

Harder J, Dressel S, Wittersheim M, et al. (2010). Enhanced expression and secretion of antimicrobial peptides in atopic dermatitis and after superficial skin injury. *Journal of Investigative Dermatology*, 130: 1355–1364.

Harding CR (2004). The stratum corneum: structure and function in health and disease. *Dermatologic Therapy*, 17(suppl 1): 6–15.

Heckmann M, Heyer G, Brunner B, Plewig G (2002). Botulinum toxin type A injection in the treatment of lichen simplex: an open pilot study. *Journal of the American Academy of Dermatology*, 46: 617–619.

Hennino A, Vocanson M, Toussaint Y, et al. (2007). Skin-infiltrating CD8+ T cells initiate atopic dermatitis lesions. *Journal of Immunology*, 178: 5571–5577.

Henry J, Hsu CY, Haftek M, et al. (2011). Hornerin is a component of the epidermal cornified cell envelopes. *FASEB Journal*, 25: 1567–1576.

Hide M, Tanaka T, Yamamura Y, Koro O, Yamamoto S (2002). IgE-mediated hypersensitivity against human sweat antigen in patients with atopic dermatitis. *Acta Dermato-Venereologica*, 82: 335–340.

Higuchi K, Kawashima M, Takagi Y, et al. (2001). Sphingosylphosphorylcholine is an activator of transglutaminase activity

in human keratinocytes. *Journal of Lipid Research*, 42: 1562–1570.

Hijnen D, Knol EF, Gent YY, et al. (2013) CD8(+) T Cells in the Lesional Skin of Atopic Dermatitis and Psoriasis Patients Are an Important Source of IFN-g, IL-13, IL-17, and IL-22. *Journal of Investigative Dermatology* 133(4): 973–979.

Hill W (1956). *The Treatment of Eczema in Infants and Children*, Mosby, St Louis, pp. 34–35.

Hodeib A, El-Samad ZA, Hanafy H, El-Latief AA, El-Bendary A, Abu-Raya A (2010). Nerve growth factor, neuropeptides and cutaneous nerves in atopic dermatitis. *Indian Journal of Dermatology*, 55: 135–139.

Hoeger PH, Ganschow R, Finger G (2000). Staphylococcal septicemia in children with atopic dermatitis. *Pediatric Dermatology*, 17: 111–114.

Hofer MF, Harbeck RJ, Schlievert PM, Leung DY (1999). Staphylococcal toxins augment specific IgE responses by atopic patients exposed to allergen. *Journal of Investigative Dermatology*, 112: 171–176.

Holleran WM, Takagi Y, Uchida Y (2006). Epidermal sphingolipids: metabolism, function, and roles in skin disorders. *FEBS Letters*, 580: 5456–5466.

Hon KL, Lam MC, Wong KY, Leung TF, Ng PC (2007). Pathophysiology of nocturnal scratching in childhood atopic dermatitis: the role of brain-derived neurotrophic factor and substance P. *British Journal of Dermatology*, 157: 922–925.

Horejs-Hoeck J, Schwarz H, Lamprecht S, et al. (2012). Dendritic cells activated by IFN-γ/STAT1 express IL-31 receptor and release proinflammatory mediators upon IL-31 treatment. *Journal of Immunology*, 188: 5319–5326.

Horsmanheimo L, Harvima IT, Järvikallio A, Harvima RJ, Naukkarinen A, Horsmanheimo M (1994). Mast cells are one major source of interleukin-4 in atopic dermatitis. *British Journal of Dermatology* 131: 348–353.

Hosoi J, Murphy GF, Egan CL, et al. (1993). Regulation of Langerhans cell function by nerves containing calcitonin gene-related peptide. *Nature*, 363: 159–163.

Hoste E, Kemperman P, Devos M, et al. (2011). Caspase-14 is required for filaggrin degradation to natural moisturizing factors in

the skin. *Journal of Investigative Dermatology*, 131: 2233–2241.

Howell MD (2007). The role of human beta defensins and cathelicidins in atopic dermatitis. *Current Opinion in Allergy and Clinical Immunology*, 7: 413–417.

Howell MD, Novak N, Bieber T, et al. (2005). Interleukin-10 downregulates anti-microbial peptide expression in atopic dermatitis. *Journal of Investigative Dermatology*, 125: 738–745.

Howell MD, Kim BE, Gao P, et al. (2007). Cytokine modulation of atopic dermatitis filaggrin skin expression. *Journal of Allergy and Clinical Immunology*, 120: 150–155.

Huang IT, Lin WM, Shun CT, Hsieh ST (1999). Influence of cutaneous nerves on keratinocyte proliferation and epidermal thickness in mice. *Neuroscience*, 94: 965–973.

Hvid M, Johansen C, Deleuran B, Kemp K, Deleuran M, Vestergaard C (2011). Regulation of caspase 14 expression in keratinocytes by inflammatory cytokines – a possible link between reduced skin barrier function and inflammation? *Experimental Dermatology*, 20: 633–636.

Igawa S, Kishibe M, Murakami M, et al. (2011). Tight junctions in the stratum corneum explain spatial differences in corneodesmosome degradation. *Experimental Dermatology*, 20: 53–55.

Ikezawa Z, Komori J, Ikezawa Y, et al. (2010). A role of *Staphylococcus aureus*, interleukin-18, nerve growth factor and semaphorin 3A, an axon guidance molecule, in pathogenesis and treatment of atopic dermatitis. *Allergy, Asthma and Immunology Research*, 2: 235–246.

Illi S, von Mutius E, Lau S (2004). The natural course of atopic dermatitis from birth to age 7 years and the association with asthma. *Journal of Allergy and Clinical Immunology*, 113: 925–31.

Imokawa G (2001). Lipid abnormalities in atopic dermatitis. *Journal of the American Academy of Dermatology*, 45(1 suppl): S29–32.

Imokawa G, Takagi Y, Higuchi K, Kondo H, Yada Y (1999). Sphingosylphosphorylcholine is a potent inducer of intercellular adhesion molecule-1 expression in human keratinocytes. *Journal of Investigative Dermatology*, 112: 91–96.

Ingordo V, D'Andria G, D'Andria C, Tortora A (2002). Results of atopy patch tests with house dust mites in adults with 'intrinsic' and'extrinsic' atopic dermatitis. *Journal of the European Academy of Dermatology and Venereology*, 16: 450–454.

Inoue Y, Aihara M, Kirino M, *et al.* (2010). Interleukin-18 is elevated in the horny layer in atopic dermatitis patients and associated with *Staphylococcus aureus* colonisation. *British Journal of Dermatology*, 164: 560–567.

Islam SA, Chang DS, Colvin RA, *et al.* (2011). Mouse CCL8, a CCR8 agonist, promotes atopic dermatitis by recruiting IL-5+ T(H)2 cells. *Nature Immunology*, 12: 167–177.

Jensen JM, Fölster-Holst R, Baranowsky A, *et al.* (2004). Impaired sphingomyelinase activity and epidermal differentiation in atopic dermatitis. *Journal of Investigative Dermatology*, 122: 1423–1431.

Jeong CW, Ahn KS, Rho NK, *et al.* (2003). Differential in vivo cytokine mRNA expression in lesional skin of intrinsic vs. extrinsic atopic dermatitis patients using semiquantitative RT-PCR. *Clinical and Experimental Allergy*, 33: 1717–1724.

Jeong SK, Kim HJ, Youm JK, *et al.* (2008). Mite and cockroach allergens activate protease-activated receptor 2 and delay epidermal permeability barrier recovery. *Journal of Investigative Dermatology*, 128: 1930–1939.

Johnson HH Jr, Deoreo GA, Lascheid WP, Mitchell F (1960). Skin histamine levels in chronic atopic dermatitis. *Journal of Investigative Dermatology*, 34: 237–238.

Jung K, Schlenvoigt G, Ladwig K, *et al.* (1996). The sweat of patients with atopic dermatitis contains specific IgE antibodies to inhalant allergens. *Clinical and Experimental Dermatology*, 21: 347–350.

Jungersted JM, Scheer H, Mempel M, *et al.* (2010). Stratum corneum lipids, skin barrier function and filaggrin mutations in patients with atopic eczema. *Allergy*, 65: 911–918.

Junghans V, Gutgesell C, Jung T, Neumann C (1998). Epidermal cytokines IL-1beta, TNF-alpha, and IL-12 in patients with atopic dermatitis: response to application of house dust mite antigens. *Journal*

of *Investigative Dermatology*, 111: 1184–1188.

Kägi MK, Wüthrich B, Montano E, Barandun J, Blaser K, Walker C (1994). Differential cytokine profiles in peripheral blood lymphocyte supernatants and skin biopsies from patients with different forms of atopic dermatitis, psoriasis and normal individuals. *International Archives of Allergy and Immunology*, 103: 332–340.

Kasraie S, Niebuhr M, Werfel T (2010). Interleukin (IL)-31 induces pro-inflammatory cytokines in human monocytes and macrophages following stimulation with staphylococcal exotoxins. *Allergy*, 65: 712–721.

Katagiri K, Itami S, Hatano Y, Takayasu S (1997). Increased levels of IL-13 mRNA, but not IL-4 mRNA, are found *in vivo* in peripheral blood mononuclear cells (PBMC) of patients with atopic dermatitis (AD). *Clinical and Experimental Immunology*, 108: 289–294.

Kato T, Takai T, Fujimura T, *et al.* (2009). Mite serine protease activates protease-activated receptor-2 and induces cytokine release in human keratinocytes. *Allergy*, 64: 1366–1374.

Katoh N, Hirano S, Suehiro M, Ikenaga K, Yasuno H (2002). Increased levels of serum tissue inhibitor of metalloproteinase-1 but not metalloproteinase-3 in atopic dermatitis. *Clinical and Experimental Immunology*, 127: 283–288.

Kawagoe J, Takizawa T, Matsumoto J, *et al.* (2002). Effect of protease-activated receptor-2 deficiency on allergic dermatitis in the mouse ear. *Japanese Journal of Pharmacology*, 88: 77–84.

Kerschenlohr K, Decard S, Przybilla B, Wollenberg A (2003). Atopy patch test reactions show a rapid influx of inflammatory dendritic epidermal cells in patients with extrinsic atopic dermatitis and patients with intrinsic atopic dermatitis. *Journal of Allergy and Clinical Immunology*, 111: 869–874.

Kezic S, Kemperman PM, Koster ES, *et al.* (2008). Loss-of-function mutations in the filaggrin gene lead to reduced level of natural moisturizing factor in the stratum corneum. *Journal of Investigative Dermatology*, 128: 2117–2119.

Kim HJ, Kim KM, Koh JY (2010). Sphingosylphosphorylcholine

induces degranulation of mast cells in the skin and plasma exudation in the ears of mice. *Journal of Dermatological Science*, 57: 57–59.

Koga C, Kabashima K, Shiraishi N, Kobayashi M, Tokura Y (2008). Possible pathogenic role of Th17 cells for atopic dermatitis. *Journal of Investigative Dermatology*, 128: 2625–2630.

Koharazawa H, Kanamori H, Takabayashi M, *et al.* (2005). Resolution of atopic dermatitis following allogeneic bone marrow transplantation for chronic myelogenous leukemia. *Bone Marrow Transplantation*, 35: 1223–1224.

Komatsu N, Saijoh K, Kuk C, *et al.* (2007). Human tissue kallikrein expression in the stratum corneum and serum of atopic dermatitis patients. *Experimental Dermatology*, 16: 513–519.

Krien PM, Kermici M (2000). Evidence for the existence of a self-regulated enzymatic process within the human stratum corneum – an unexpected role for urocanic acid. *Journal of Investigative Dermatology*, 115: 414–420.

Kubo A, Nagao K, Yokouchi M, Sasaki H, Amagai M (2009). External antigen uptake by Langerhans cells with reorganization of epidermal tight junction barriers. *Journal of Experimental Medicine*, 206: 2937–2946.

Kusel MM, Holt PG, de Klerk N, Sly PD (2005). Support for two variants of eczema. *Journal of Allergy and Clinical Immunology*, 116: 1067–1072.

Kwiek B, Peng WM, Allam JP, Langner A, Bieber T, Novak N (2008). Tacrolimus and TGF-beta act synergistically on the generation of Langerhans cells. *Journal of Allergy and Clinical Immunology*, 122: 126–132.

Lampinen M, Carlson M, Håkansson LD, Venge P (2004). Cytokine-regulated accumulation of eosinophils in inflammatory disease. *Allergy*, 59: 793–805.

Langeveld-Wildschut EG, Bruijnzeel PL, Mudde GC, *et al.* (2000). Clinical and immunologic variables in skin of patients with atopic eczema and either positive or negative atopy patch test reactions. *Journal of Allergy and Clinical Immunology*, 105: 1008–1016.

Langrish CL, Chen Y, Blumenschein WM, *et al.* (2005). IL-23 drives a pathogenic T cell population that induces autoimmune inflammation. *Journal of Experimental Medicine*, 201: 233–240.

Lee FE, Georas SN, Beck LA (2010). IL-17: important for host defense, autoimmunity, and allergy? *Journal of Investigative Dermatology*, 130: 2540–2542.

Lee HJ, Lee HP, Ha SJ, Byun DG, Kim JW (2000). Spontaneous expression of mRNA for IL-10, GM-CSF, TGF-beta, TGF-alpha, and IL-6 in peripheral blood mononuclear cells from atopic dermatitis. *Annals of Allergy Asthma and Immunology*, 84: 553–558.

Lee SE, Jeong SK, Lee SH (2010). Protease and protease-activated receptor-2 signaling in the pathogenesis of atopic dermatitis. *Yonsei Medical Journal*, 51: 808–822.

Leiferman KM, Ackerman SJ, Sampson HA, Haugen HS, Venencie PY, Gleich GJ (1985). Dermal deposition of eosinophil-granule major basic protein in atopic dermatitis. Comparison with onchocerciasis. *New England Journal of Medicine*, 313: 282–285.

LeMaster AM, Krimm RF, Davis BM, *et al.* (1999). Overexpression of brain-derived neurotrophic factor enhances sensory innervation and selectively increases neuron number. *Journal of Neuroscience*, 19: 5919–5931.

Leon A, Buriani A, Dal Toso R, *et al.* (1994). Mast cells synthesize, store, and release nerve growth factor. *Proceedings of the National Academy of Science USA*, 91: 3739–3743.

Leung DY, Boguniewicz M, Howell MD, Nomura I, Hamid QA (2004). New insights into atopic dermatitis. *Journal of Clinical Investigation*, 113: 651–657.

Li MO, Wan YY, Sanjabi S, Robertson AK, Flavell RA (2006). Transforming growth factor-β regulation of immune responses. *Annual Review of Immunology*, 24: 99–146.

Lin YT, Wang CT, Chiang BL (2007). Role of bacterial pathogens in atopic dermatitis. *Clinical Reviews in Allergy and Immunology*, 33: 167–177.

Liu YJ (2007). Thymic stromal lymphopoietin and OX40 ligand pathway in the initiation of dendritic cell-mediated allergic inflammation.'

Journal of Allergy and Clinical Immunology, 120: 238–244.

Lowe AJ, Carlin JB, Bennett CM, *et al.* (2008). Do boys do the atopic march while girls dawdle? *Journal of Allergy and Clinical Immunology*, 121: 1190–1195.

Luger TA, Beissert S, Schwarz T (1997). The epidermal cytokine network. In: Bos JD (ed.) *Skin Immune System (SRS)*, 2nd edn, CRC Press, Boca Raton, pp. 274–275.

Macfarlane SR, Seatter MJ, Kanke T, Hunter GD, Plevin R (2001). Proteinase-activated receptors. *Pharmacological Reviews*, 53: 245–282.

McGirt LY, Beck LA (2006). Innate immune defects in atopic dermatitis. *Journal of Allergy and Clinical Immunology*, 118: 202–208.

McGrath JA (2008). Filaggrin and the great epidermal barrier grief. *Australasian Journal of Dermatology*, 49(2): 67–73.

McGrath JA, Uitto J (2008). The filaggrin story: novel insights into skin-barrier function and disease. *Trends in Molecular Medicine*, 14: 20–27.S

Maeda K, Yamamoto K, Tanaka Y, Anan S, Yoshida H (1992). House dust mite (HDM) antigen in naturally occurring lesions of atopic dermatitis (AD): the relationship between HDM antigen in the skin and HDM antigen-specific IgE antibody. *Journal of Dermatological Science*, 3: 73–77.

Mallbris L, Carlén L, Wei T, *et al.* (2010). Injury downregulates the expression of the human cathelicidin protein hCAP18/LL-37 in atopic dermatitis. *Experimental Dermatology*, 19: 442–449.

Maretzky T, Scholz F, Köten B, Proksch E, Saftig P, Reiss K (2008). ADAM10-mediated E-cadherin release is regulated by proinflammatory cytokines and modulates keratinocyte cohesion in eczematous dermatitis. *Journal of Investigative Dermatology*, 128: 1737–1746.

Matsumoto M, Sugiura H, Uehara M (2000). Skin barrier function in patients with completely healed atopic dermatitis. *Journal of Dermatological Science*, 23: 178–182.

Matsushima H, Hayashi S, Shimada S (2003). Skin scratching switches immune responses from Th2 to Th1 type in epicutaneously immunized

mice. *Journal of Dermatological Science*, 32: 223–230.

Miajlovic H, Fallon PG, Irvine AD, Foster TJ (2010). Effect of filaggrin breakdown products on growth of and protein expression by *Staphylococcus aureus*. *Journal of Allergy and Clinical Immunology*, 126: 1184–1190.

Miedzobrodzki J, Kaszycki P, Bialecka A, Kasprowicz A (2002). Proteolytic activity of *Staphylococcus aureus* strains isolated from the colonized skin of patients with acute-phase atopic dermatitis. *European Journal of Clinical Microbiology and Infectious Diseases*, 21: 269–276.

Mihm MC Jr, Soter NA, Dvorak HF, Austen KF (1976). The structure of normal skin and the morphology of atopic eczema. *Journal of Investigative Dermatology*, 67: 305–312.

Milovanovic M, Drozdenko G, Weise C, Babina M, Worm M (2010). Interleukin-17A promotes IgE production in human B cells. *Journal of Investigative Dermatology*, 130: 2621–2628.

Miossec P, Korn T, Kuchroo VK (2009). Interleukin-17 and type 17 helper T cells. *New England Journal of Medicine*, 361: 888–898.

Miraglia del Giudice M, Decimo F, Leonardi S, *et al.* (2006). Immune dysregulation in atopic dermatitis. *Allergy and Asthma Proceedings*, 27: 451–455.

Mittermann I, Aichberger KJ, Bünder R, Mothes N, Renz H, Valenta R (2004). Autoimmunity and atopic dermatitis. *Current Opinion in Allergy and Clinical Immunology*, 4: 367–371.

Morizane S, Yamasaki K, Kajita A, *et al.* (2012). T(H)2 cytokines increase kallikrein 7 expression and function in patients with atopic dermatitis. *Journal of Allergy and Clinical Immunology*, (Epublication ahead of print).

Mowad CM, McGinley KJ, Foglia A, Leyden JJ (1995). The role of extracellular polysaccharide substance produced by *Staphylococcus epidermidis* in miliaria. *Journal of the American Academy of Dermatology*, 33(5 Pt 1): 729–733.

Mudde GC, Van Reijsen FC, Boland GJ, de Gast GC, Bruijnzeel PL, Bruijnzeel-Koomen CA (1990). Allergen presentation by epidermal Langerhans cells from patients with atopic dermatitis is mediated by IgE. *Immunology*, 69: 335–341.

Nakahigashi K, Kabashima K, Ikoma A, Verkman AS, Miyachi Y, Hara-Chikuma M (2010). Upregulation of aquaporin-3 is involved in keratinocyte proliferation and epidermal hyperplasia. *Journal of Investigative Dermatology*, 131: 865–73.

Nakanishi K, Yoshimoto T, Tsutsui H, Okamura H (2001). Interleukin-18 regulates both Th1 and Th2 responses. *Annual Review of Immunology*, 19: 423–74.

Namura K, Hasegawa G, Egawa M, et al. (2007). Relationship of serum brain-derived neurotrophic factor level with other markers of disease severity in patients with atopic dermatitis. *Clinical Immunology*, 122: 181–186.

Neis MM, Peters B, Dreuw A, et al. (2006). Enhanced expression levels of IL-31 correlate with IL-4 and IL-13 in atopic and allergic contact dermatitis. *Journal of Allergy and Clinical Immunology*, 118: 930–937.

Nemoto-Hasebe I, Akiyama M, Nomura T, et al. (2009). Clinical severity correlates with impaired barrier in filaggrin-related eczema. *Journal of Investigative Dermatology*, 129: 682–689.

Niessen CM (2007). Tight junctions/adherens junctions: basic structure and function. *Journal of Investigative Dermatology*, 127: 2525–32.

Niggemann B, Reibel S, Wahn U (2000). The atopy patch test (APT) – a useful tool for the diagnosis of food allergy in children with atopic dermatitis. *Allergy*, 55: 281–285.

Nobbe S, Dziunycz P, Mühleisen B, et al. (2011). IL-31 expression by inflammatory cells is preferentially elevated in atopic dermatitis. *Acta Dermato-Venereologica*, [Epub ahead of print].

Noga O, Englmann C, Hanf G, Grützkau A, Seybold J, Kunkel G (2003). The production, storage and release of the neurotrophins nerve growth factor, brain-derived neurotrophic factor and neurotrophin-3 by human peripheral eosinophils in allergics and non-allergics. *Clinical and Experimental Allergy*, 33: 649–654.

Nograles KE, Zaba LC, Shemer A, et al. (2009). IL-22-producing 'T22' T cells account for upregulated IL-22 in atopic dermatitis despite reduced IL-17-producing TH17 T cells.

Journal of Allergy and Clinical Immunology, 123: 1244–52.e2.

Novak N, Bieber T (2005). The role of dendritic cell subtypes in the pathophysiology of atopic dermatitis. *Journal of the American Academy of Dermatology*, 53(2 suppl 2): S171–176.

Novak N, Valenta R, Bohle B, et al. (2004). FcepsilonRI engagement of Langerhans cell-like dendritic cells and inflammatory dendritic epidermal cell-like dendritic cells induces chemotactic signals and different T-cell phenotypes in vitro. *Journal of Allergy and Clinical Immunology*, 113: 949–957.

Novak N, Peng W, Yu C (2007). Network of myeloid and plasmacytoid dendritic cells in atopic dermatitis. *Advances in Experimental Medicine and Biology*, 601: 97–104.

Novak N, Baurecht H, Schäfer T, et al. (2008). Loss-of-function mutations in the filaggrin gene and allergic contact sensitization to nickel. *Journal of Investigative Dermatology*, 128: 1430–1435.

O'Riain S (1973). New and simple test of nerve function in hand. *British Medical Journal*, 3: 615–616.

Obara W, Kawa Y, Ra C, Nishioka K, Soma Y, Mizoguchi M (2002). T cells and mast cells as a major source of interleukin-13 in atopic dermatitis. *Dermatology*, 205: 11–17.

Ogawa H, Yoshiike T (1993). A speculative view of atopic dermatitis: barrier dysfunction in pathogenesis. *Journal of Dermatological Science*, 5: 197–204.

Ohmen JD, Hanifin JM, Nickoloff BJ, et al. (1995). Overexpression of IL-10 in atopic dermatitis. Contrasting cytokine patterns with delayed-type hypersensitivity reactions. *Journal of Immunology*, 154: 1956–1963.

Ohnishi Y, Okino N, Ito M, Imayama S (1999). Ceramidase activity in bacterial skin flora as a possible cause of ceramide deficiency in atopic dermatitis. *Clinical and Diagnostic Laboratory Immunology*, 6: 101–104.

Ohtani T, Memezawa A, Okuyama R, et al. (2009). Increased hyaluronan production and decreased E-cadherin expression by cytokine-stimulated keratinocytes lead to spongiosis formation. *Journal of Investigative Dermatology*, 129: 1412–1420.

Okamoto R, Arikawa J, Ishibashi M, Kawashima M, Takagi Y, Imokawa G (2003). Sphingosylphosphorylcholine is upregulated in the stratum corneum of patients with atopic dermatitis. *Journal of Lipid Research*, 44: 93–102.

Oldhoff JM, Bihari IC, Knol EF, Bruijnzeel-Koomen CA, de Bruin-Weller MS (2004). Atopy patch test in patients with atopic eczema/dermatitis syndrome: comparison of petrolatum and aqueous solution as a vehicle. *Allergy*, 59: 451–456.

Olesen AB, Andersen G, Jeppesen DL, Benn CS, Juul S, Thestrup-Pedersen K (2005). Thymus is enlarged in children with current atopic dermatitis. A cross-sectional study. *Acta DermatoVenereologica*, 85: 240–24.

Omoto Y, Tokime K, Yamanaka K, et al. (2006). Human mast cell chymase cleaves pro-IL-18 and generates a novel and biologically active IL-18 fragment. *Journal of Immunology*, 177: 8315–8319.

Ong PY, Ohtake T, Brandt C, et al. (2002). Endogenous antimicrobial peptides and skin infections in atopic dermatitis. *New England Journal of Medicine*, 347: 1151–1160.

Oppel T, Schuller E, Günther S, et al. (2000). Phenotyping of epidermal dendritic cells allows the differentiation between extrinsic and intrinsic forms of atopic dermatitis. *British Journal of Dermatology*, 143: 1193–1198.

Orihara K, Narita M, Tobe T, et al. (2007) Circulating Foxp3+CD4+ cell numbers in atopic patients and healthy control subjects. *Journal of Allergy and Clinical Immunology*, 120: 960–962.

Otsuka A, Tanioka M, Nakagawa Y, et al. (2011). Effects of cyclosporine on pruritus and serum IL-31 levels in patients with atopic dermatitis. *European Journal of Dermatology*, 21: 816–817.

Ou LS, Goleva E, Hall C, Leung DY (2004). T regulatory cells in atopic dermatitis and subversion of their activity by superantigens. *Journal of Allergy and Clinical Immunology*, 113: 756–763.

Palmer CN, Irvine AD, Terron-Kwiatkowski A, et al. (2006). Common loss-of-function variants of the epidermal barrier protein filaggrin are a major predisposing factor for atopic dermatitis. *Nature Genetics*, 38: 441–446.

Park CO, Lee HJ, Lee JH, et al. (2008). Increased expression of CC chemokine ligand 18 in extrinsic atopic dermatitis patients. Experimental Dermatology, 17: 24–29.

Park do S, Youn YH (2007). Clinical significance of serum interleukin-18 concentration in the patients with atopic dermatitis]. Korean Journal of Laboratory Medicine, 27: 128–132.

Park JH, Choi YL, Namkung JH, et al. (2006). Characteristics of extrinsic vs. intrinsic atopic dermatitis in infancy: correlations with laboratory variables. British Journal of Dermatology, 155: 778–783.

Parkkinen MU, Kiistala R, Kiistala U (1991). Baseline water loss and cholinergic sweat stimulation in atopic dermatitis: a gravimetric measurement of local skin water loss. Archives of Dermatological Research, 283: 382–386.

Parkkinen MU, Kiistala R, Kiistala U (1992). Sweating response to moderate thermal stress in atopic dermatitis. British Journal of Dermatology, 126: 346–350.

Parwez Q, Stemmler S, Epplen JT, Hoffjan S (2008). Variation in genes encoding eosinophil granule proteins in atopic dermatitis patients from Germany. Journal of Negative Results in BioMedicine, 13(7): 9.

Pastore S, Fanales-Belasio E, Albanesi C, Chinni LM, Giannetti A, Girolomoni G (1997). Granulocyte macrophage colony-stimulating factor is overproduced by keratinocytes in atopic dermatitis. Implications for sustained dendritic cell activation in the skin. Journal of Clinical Investigation, 99: 3009–3017.

Pastore S, Corinti S, La Placa M, Didona B, Girolomoni G (1998). Interferon-gamma promotes exaggerated cytokine production in keratinocytes cultured from patients with atopic dermatitis. Journal of Allergy and Clinical Immunology, 101(4 Pt 1): 538–544.

Piletta PA, Wirth S, Hommel L, Saurat JH, Hauser C (1996). Circulating skin-homing T cells in atopic dermatitis. Selective up-regulation of HLA-DR, interleukin-2R, and CD30 and decrease after combined UV-A and UV-B phototherapy. Archives of Dermatology, 132: 1171–1176.

Pincelli C, Fantini F, Massimi P, Giannetti A (1990). Neuropeptide Y-like immunoreactivity in Langerhans cells from patients with atopic dermatitis. International Journal of Neuroscience, 51: 219–220.

Proksch E, Fölster-Holst R, Jensen JM (2006). Skin barrier function, epidermal proliferation and differentiation in eczema. Journal of Dermatological Science, 43: 159–169.

Prose PH, Sedlis E (1960). Morphologic and histochemical studies of atopic eczema in infants and children. Journal of Investigative Dermatology, 34: 149–165.

Raap U, Goltz C, Deneka N, et al. (2005). Brain-derived neurotrophic factor is increased in atopic dermatitis and modulates eosinophil functions compared with that seen in nonatopic subjects. Journal of Allergy and Clinical Immunology, 115: 1268–1275.

Raap U, Wichmann K, Bruder M, et al. (2008a). Correlation of IL-31 serum levels with severity of atopic dermatitis. Journal of Allergy and Clinical Immunology, 122: 421–423.

Raap U, Deneka N, Bruder M, Kapp A, Wedi B (2008b). Differential up-regulation of neurotrophin receptors and functional activity of neurotrophins on peripheral blood eosinophils of patients with allergic rhinitis, atopic dermatitis and nonatopic subjects. Clinical and Experimental Allergy, 38: 1493–1498.

Raap U, Weißmantel S, Gehring M, Eisenberg AM, Kapp A, Fölster-Holst R (2012). IL-31 significantly correlates with disease activity and Th2 cytokine levels in children with atopic dermatitis. Pediatric Allergy and Immunology, 23: 285–288.

Rajka G (1989). Essential Aspects of Atopic Dermatitis, Springer-Verlag, Berlin, p. 29.

Reefer AJ, Satinover SM, Solga MD, et al. (2008). Analysis of CD25hiCD4+ 'regulatory' T-cell subtypes in atopic dermatitis reveals a novel T(H)2-like population. Journal of Allergy and Clinical Immunology, 121: 415–422.

Rieg S, Steffen H, Seeber S, et al. (2005). Deficiency of dermcidin-derived antimicrobial peptides in sweat of patients with atopic dermatitis correlates with an impaired innate defense of human skin in vivo. Journal of Immunology, 174: 8003–8010.

Riley G, Siebers R, Rains N, Crane J, Fitzharris P (1998). House-dust mite antigen on skin and sheets. Lancet, 351: 649–650.

Ring J, Thomas P (1989). Histamine and atopic eczema. Acta Dermato-Venereologica Supplementum (Stockholm), 144: 70–77.

Rippke F, Schreiner V, Schwanitz HJ (2002). The acidic milieu of the horny layer: new findings on the physiology and pathophysiology of skin pH. American Journal of Clinical Dermatology, 3: 261–272.

Rochman I, Watanabe N, Arima K, Liu YJ, Leonard WJ (2007). Cutting edge: direct action of thymic stromal lymphopoietin on activated human CD4+ T cells. Journal of Immunology, 178: 6720–6724.

Rossbach K, Wendorff S, Sander K, et al. (2009). Histamine H_4 receptor antagonism reduces hapten-induced scratching behaviour but not inflammation. Experimental Dermatology, 18: 57–63.

Sakurai K, Sugiura H, Matsumoto M, Uehara M (2002). Occurrence of patchy parakeratosis in normal-appearing skin in patients with active atopic dermatitis and in patients with healed atopic dermatitis: a cause of impaired barrier function of the atopic skin. Journal of Dermatological Science, 30: 37–42.

Saloga J, Renz H, Larsen GL, Gelfand EW (1994). Increased airways responsiveness in mice depends on local challenge with antigen. American Journal of Respiratory and Critical Care Medicine, 149: 65–70.

Sampson HA, Jolie PL (1984). Increased plasma histamine concentrations after food challenges in children with atopic dermatitis. New England Journal of Medicine, 311: 372–376.

Sandilands A, O'Regan GM, Liao H, et al. (2006). Prevalent and rare mutations in the gene encoding filaggrin cause ichthyosis vulgaris and predispose individuals to atopic dermatitis. Journal of Investigative Dermatology, 126: 1770–1775.

Sandilands A, Sutherland C, Irvine AD, McLean WH (2009). Filaggrin in the frontline: role in skin barrier function and disease. Journal of Cell Science, 122(Pt 9): 1285–1294.

Sandoval-Lopez G, Teran LM (2001). TARC: novel mediator of allergic inflammation. Clinical and Experimental Allergy, 31: 1809–1812.

Schlüter H, Wepf R, Moll I, Franke WW (2004). Sealing the live part of the skin: the integrated meshwork of desmosomes, tight junctions and curvilinear ridge structures in the cells of the uppermost granular layer of the human epidermis. *European Journal of Cell Biology*, **83**: 655–665.

Schmid-Wendtner MH, Korting HC (2006). The pH of the skin surface and its impact on the barrier function. *Skin Pharmacology and Physiology*, **19**: 296–302.

Seneviratne SL, Jones L, Bailey AS, Black AP, Ogg GS (2006). Severe atopic dermatitis is associated with a reduced frequency of IL-10 producing allergen-specific CD4+ T cells. *Clinical and Experimental Dermatology*, **31**: 689–694.

Shaker OG, El-Komy M, Tawfic SO, Zeidan N, Tomairek RH (2009). Possible role of nerve growth factor and interleukin-18 in pathogenesis of eczematous lesions of atopic dermatitis. *Journal of Dermatological Science*, **53**: 153–154.

Shelley WB and Crissey JT (2003). *Classics in Clinical Dermatology with Biographical Sketches, 50th Anniversary.* CRC Press, pp. 243–246.

Shimizu T, Abe R, Ohkawara A, Mizue Y, Nishihira J (1997). Macrophage migration inhibitory factor is an essential immunoregulatory cytokine in atopic dermatitis. *Biochemical and Biophysical Research Communications*, **240**: 173–8.

Sillevis Smitt JH, Bos JD, Hulsebosch HJ, Krieg SR (1986). *In situ* immunophenotyping of antigen presenting cells and T cell subsets in atopic dermatitis. *Clinical and Experimental Dermatology*, **11**: 159–168.

Simon D, Lindberg RL, Kozlowski E, Braathen LR, Simon HU (2006). Epidermal caspase-3 cleavage associated with interferon-gamma-expressing lymphocytes in acute atopic dermatitis lesions. *Experimental Dermatology*, **15**: 441–446.

Smith TP, Bailey CJ (1986). Epidermolytic toxin from *Staphylococcus aureus* binds to filaggrins. *FEBS Letters*, **194**: 309–312.

Sohn MH, Song JS, Kim KW, *et al.* (2007). Association of interleukin-10 gene promoter polymorphism in children with atopic dermatitis. *Journal of Pediatrics*, **150**: 106–108.

Sondell B, Jonsson M, Dyberg P, Egelrud T (1997). *In situ* evidence that the population of Langerhans cells in normal human epidermis may be heterogeneous. *British Journal of Dermatology*, **136**: 687–693.

Sonkoly E, Muller A, Lauerma AI, *et al.* (2006). IL-31: a new link between T cells and pruritus in atopic skin inflammation. *Journal of Allergy and Clinical Immunology*, **117**: 411–417.

Soumelis V, Reche PA, Kanzler H, *et al.* (2002). Human epithelial cells trigger dendritic cell mediated allergic inflammation by producing TSLP. *Nature Immunology*, **3**: 673–680.

Souwer Y, Szegedi K, Kapsenberg ML, de Jong EC (2010). L-17 and IL-22 in atopic allergic disease. *Current Opinion in Immunology*, **22**: 821–6.

Spergel JM (2005). Atopic march: link to upper airways. *Current Opinion in Allergy and Clinical Immunology*, **5**: 17–21.

Steinhoff M, Neisius U, Ikoma A, *et al.* (2003). Proteinase-activated receptor-2 mediates itch: a novel pathway for pruritus in human skin. *Journal of Neuroscience*, **23**: 6176–6180.

Suárez JDA (1901). *Etiologia del eczema por el estafilococus aureus*, Ricardo Rojas, Madrid.

Sugimoto Y, Iba Y, Nakamura Y, Kayasuga R, Kamei C (2004). Pruritus-associated response mediated by cutaneous histamine H_3 receptors. *Clinical and Experimental Allergy*, **34**: 456–459.

Sugiura H, Omoto M, Hirota Y, Danno K, Uehara M (1997). Density and fine structure of peripheral nerves in various skin lesions of atopic dermatitis. *Archives of Dermatological Research*, **289**: 125–131.

Suh KY (2010). Food allergy and atopic dermatitis: separating fact from fiction. *Seminars in Cutaneous Medicine and Surgery*, **29**: 72–8.

Sulzberger MB (1955). Atopic dermatitis: its clinical and histological picture. In: Baer RL (ed.), *Atopic Dermatitis*. New York University Press, New York, p. 11.

Sybert VP, Dale BA, Holbrook KA (1985). Ichthyosis vulgaris: identification of a defect in synthesis of filaggrin correlated with an absence of keratohyaline granules. *Journal of Investigative Dermatology*, **84**: 191–194.

Syed S, Weibel L, Kennedy H, Harper JI (2008). A pilot study showing pulsed-dye laser treatment improves localized areas of chronic atopic dermatitis. *Clinical and Experimental Dermatology*, **33**: 243–248.

Taha RA, Leung DY, Ghaffar O, Boguniewicz M, Hamid Q (1998). *In vivo* expression of cytokine receptor mRNA in atopic dermatitis. *Journal of Allergy and Clinical Immunology*, **102**: 245–250.

Takaoka A, Arai I, Sugimoto M, Yamaguchi A, Tanaka M, Nakaike S (2005). Expression of IL-31 gene transcripts in NC/Nga mice with atopic dermatitis. *European Journal of Pharmacology*, **516**: 180–181.

Takehashi M, Izekawa Z (2000). Dry skin in atopic dermatitis and patients on hemodialysis. In: Lodén M, Maibach HI (eds), *Dry Skin and Moisturizers: Chemistry and Function*. CRC Press, Boca Raton.

Tanaka A, Tanaka T, Suzuki H, Ishii K, Kameyoshi Y, Hide M (2006). Semi-purification of the immunoglobulin E-sweat antigen acting on mast cells and basophils in atopic dermatitis. *Experimental Dermatology*, **15**: 283–290.

Tanaka Y, Anan S, Yoshida H (1990). Immunohistochemical studies in mite antigen-induced patch test sites in atopic dermatitis. *Journal of Dermatological Science*, **1**: 361–368.

Taylor RS, Baadsgaard O, Hammerberg C, Cooper KD (1991). Hyperstimulatory CD1a+CD1b+CD36+ Langerhans cells are responsible for increased autologous T lymphocyte reactivity to lesional epidermal cells of patients with atopic dermatitis. *Journal of Immunology*, **147**: 3794–3802.

Tazawa T, Sugiura H, Sugiura Y, Uehara M (2004). Relative importance of IL-4 and IL-13 in lesional skin of atopic dermatitis. *Archives of Dermatological Research*, **295**: 459–464.

Thepen T, Langeveld-Wildschut EG, Bihari IC, *et al.* (1996). Biphasic response against aeroallergen in atopic dermatitis showing a switch from an initial TH2 response to a TH1 response *in situ*: an immunocytochemical study. *Journal of Allergy and Clinical Immunology*, **97**: 828–837.

Thomsen SF, Ulrik CS, Kyvik KO, *et al.* (2007). Importance of genetic factors in the etiology of atopic dermatitis:

a twin study. *Allergy and Asthma Proceedings*, 28: 535–539.

Thurmond RL, Gelfand EW, Dunford PJ (2008). The role of histamine H1 and H4 receptors in allergic inflammation: the search for new antihistamines. *Nature Reviews Drug Discovery*, 7: 41–53.

Toda M, Leung DY, Molet S, *et al.* (2003). Polarized *in vivo* expression of IL-11 and IL-17 between acute and chronic skin lesions. *Journal of Allergy and Clinical Immunology*, 111: 875–881.

Tokura Y (2010). Extrinsic and intrinsic types of atopic dermatitis. *Journal of Dermatological Science*, 58: 1–7.

Toma T, Mizuno K, Okamoto H, *et al.* (2005). Expansion of activated eosinophils in infants with severe atopic dermatitis. *Pediatrics International*, 47: 32–38.

Tominaga M, Ozawa S, Ogawa H, Takamori K (2007). A hypothetical mechanism of intraepidermal neurite formation in NC/Nga mice with atopic dermatitis. *Journal of Dermatological Science*, 46: 199–210.

Toyoda M, Morohashi M (1998). Morphological assessment of the effects of cyclosporin A on mast cell–nerve relationship in atopic dermatitis. *Acta Dermato-Venereologica*, 78: 321–325.

Trautmann A, Akdis M, Kleemann D, *et al.* (2000). T cell-mediated Fas-induced keratinocyte apoptosis plays a key pathogenetic role in eczematous dermatitis. *Journal of Clinical Investigation*, 106: 25–35.

Trautmann A, Akdis M, Bröcker EB, *et al.* (2001). New insights into the role of T cells in atopic dermatitis and allergic contact dermatitis. *Trends in Immunology*, 22: 530–532.

Troilius A, Moller H (1989). Unilateral eruption of endogenous eczema after hemiparesis. *Acta Dermato-Venereologica*, 69: 256–258.

Uno H, Hanifin JM (1980). Langerhans cells in acute and chronic epidermal lesions of atopic dermatitis, observed by L-dopa histofluorescence, glycol methacrylate thin secretion, and electron microscopy. *Journal of Investigative Dermatology*, 75: 52–60.

Urashima R, Mihara M (1998). Cutaneous nerves in atopic dermatitis. A histological, immunohistochemical and electron microscopic study. *Virchows Archiv*, 432: 363–370.

Valenta R, Maurer D, Steiner R, *et al.* (1996). Immunoglobulin E response to human proteins in atopic patients. *Journal of Investigative Dermatology*, 107: 203–208.

Van der Heijden FL, Wierenga EA, Bos JD, Kapsenberg ML (1991). Allergen-specific CD4+ T lymphocytes in atopic dermatitis lesional skin. In: Czernielewski J (ed.), *Pharmacology of the Skin*, Vol 4, Karger, Basel, pp. 149–154.

van Reijsen FC, Bruijnzeel-Koomen CA, Kalthoff FS, *et al.* (1992). Skin-derived aeroallergen-specific T-cell clones of Th2 phenotype in patients with atopic dermatitis. *Journal of Allergy and Clinical Immunology*, 90: 184–193.

Vasilopoulos Y, Cork MJ, Teare D, *et al.* (2007). A nonsynonymous substitution of cystatin A, a cysteine protease inhibitor of house dust mite protease, leads to decreased mRNA stability and shows a significant association with atopic dermatitis. *Allergy*, 62: 514–519.

Verhagen J, Akdis M, Traidl-Hoffmann C, *et al.* (2006). Absence of T-regulatory cell expression and function in atopic dermatitis skin. *Journal of Allergy and Clinical Immunology*, 117: 176–183.

Voegeli R, Rawlings AV, Breternitz M, Doppler S, Schreier T, Fluhr JW (2009). Increased stratum corneum serine protease activity in acute eczematous atopic skin. *British Journal of Dermatology*, 161: 70–77.

Vyas H, Krishnaswamy G (2006). Paul Ehrlich's 'Mastzellen' – from aniline dyes to DNA chip arrays: a historical review of developments in mast cell research. *Methods in Molecular Biology*, 315: 3–11.

Wang LF, Lin JY, Hsieh KH, Lin RH (1996). Epicutaneous exposure of protein antigen induces a predominant Th2-like response with high IgE production in mice. *Journal of Immunology*, 156: 4077–4082.

Wassom DL, Loegering DA, Solley GO, *et al.* (1981). Elevated serum levels of the eosinophil granule major basic protein in patients with eosinophilia. *Journal of Clinical Investigation*, 67: 651–661.

Watanabe N, Wang YH, Lee HK, *et al.* (2005). Hassall's corpuscles instruct dendritic cells to induce CD4+CD25+ regulatory T cells in human thymus. *Nature*, 436: 1181–1185.

Wedi B, Raap U, Lewrick H, Kapp A (1997). Delayed eosinophil programmed cell death *in vitro*: a common feature of inhalant allergy and extrinsic and intrinsic atopic dermatitis. *Journal of Allergy and Clinical Immunology*, 100: 536–543.

Wedi B, Raap U, Kapp A (1999). Significant delay of apoptosis and Fas resistance in eosinophils of subjects with intrinsic and extrinsic type of atopic dermatitis. *International Archives of Allergy and Immunology*, 118: 234–235.

Weidenthaler B, Hausser I, Anton-Lamprecht I (1993). Is filaggrin really a filament-aggregating protein *in vivo*? *Archives of Dermatological Research*, 285: 111–120.

Weidinger S, Illig T, Baurecht H, *et al.* (2006). Loss-of-function variations within the filaggrin gene predispose for atopic dermatitis with allergic sensitizations. *Journal of Allergy and Clinical Immunology*, 118: 214–219.

Weiss E, Mamelak AJ, La Morgia S, *et al.* (2004). The role of interleukin 10 in the pathogenesis and potential treatment of skin diseases. *Journal of the American Academy of Dermatology*, 50: 657–675.

Werfel T (2009). The role of leukocytes, keratinocytes, and allergen-specific IgE in the development of atopic dermatitis. *Journal of Investigative Dermatology*, 129: 1878–1891.

Werfel T, Morita A, Grewe M, *et al.* (1996). Allergen specificity of skin-infiltrating T cells is not restricted to a type-2 cytokine pattern in chronic skin lesions of atopic dermatitis. *Journal of Investigative Dermatology*, 107: 871–876.

Werner Y, Lindberg M, Forslind B (1982). The water-binding capacity of stratum corneum in dry non-eczematous skin of atopic eczema. *Acta DermatoVenereologica*, 62: 334–337.

Wiesner-Menzel L, Schulz B, Vakilzadeh F, Czarnetzki BM (1981). Electron microscopical evidence for a direct contact between nerve fibres and mast cells. *Acta Dermato-Venereologica*, 61: 465–469.

Williams DH (1938). Skin temperature reaction to histamine in atopic dermatitis (disseminated neurodermatitis). *Journal of Investigative Dermatology*, 1: 119–129.

Williams HC, Johansson SG (2005). Two types of eczema – or are there? *Journal of Allergy and Clinical Immunology*, **116**: 1064–1066.

Wollenberg A, Kraft S, Hanau D, Bieber T (1996). Immunomorphological and ultrastructural characterization of Langerhans cells and a novel, inflammatory dendritic epidermal cell (IDEC) population in lesional skin of atopic eczema. *Journal of Investigative Dermatology*, **106**: 446–453.

Wollenberg A, Räwer HC, Schauber J (2010). Innate immunity in atopic dermatitis. *Clinical Reviews in Allergy and Immunology*, **41**: 272–281.

Wollina U (2008). Botulinum toxin: Non-cosmetic indications and possible mechanisms of action. *Journal of Cutaneous and Aesthetic Surgery*, **1**: 3–6.

Wollina U, Karamfilov T (2002). Adjuvant botulinum toxin A in dyshidrotic hand eczema: A controlled prospective pilot study with left-right comparison. *Journal of the European Academy of Dermatology and Venereology*, **16**: 40–42.

Wood LC, Elias PM, Calhoun C, Tsai JC, Grunfeld C, Feingold KR (1996). Barrier disruption stimulates interleukin-1 alpha expression and release from a pre-formed pool in murine epidermis. *Journal of Investigative Dermatology*, **106**: 397–403.

Yamamoto T, Yodogawa K, Wakita S, *et al.* (2007). Recurrent prosthetic valve endocarditis caused by *Staphylococcus aureus* colonizing skin lesions in severe atopic dermatitis. *International Medicine*, **46**: 571–573.

Yoshihisa Y, Makino T, Matsunaga K (2010). Macrophage migration inhibitory factor is essential for eosinophil recruitment in allergen-induced skin inflammation. *Journal of Investigative Dermatology*, **131**: 925–931.

Yu B, Shao Y, Zhang J, *et al.* (2010). Polymorphisms in human histamine receptor H4 gene are associated with atopic dermatitis. *British Journal of Dermatology*, **162**: 1038–1043.

Yuki T, Haratake A, Koishikawa H, Morita K, Miyachi Y, Inoue S (2007). Tight junction proteins in keratinocytes: localization and contribution to barrier function.

Experimental Dermatology, **16**: 324–330.

Zeller S, Rhyner C, Meyer N, Schmid-Grendelmeier P, Akdis CA, Crameri R (2009). Exploring the repertoire of IgE-binding self-antigens associated with atopic eczema. *Journal of Allergy and Clinical Immunology*, **124**: 278–85, .

Ziegler SF, Liu YJ (2006). Thymic stromal lymphopoietin in normal and pathogenic T cell development and function. *Nature Immunology*, **7**: 709–714.

CHAPTER 7

Adkinson NF, Middleton E (2003). *Middleton's Allergy: Principles and Practice*, Mosby, Philadelphia.

Akdis CA, Akdis M, Bieber T, *et al.* (2006). Diagnosis and treatment of atopic dermatitis in children and adults: European Academy of Allergology and Clinical Immunology/American Academy of Allergy, Asthma and Immunology/PRACTALL Consensus Report. *Allergy*, **61**: 969–987.

Baker BS (2006). The role of microorganisms in atopic dermatitis. *Clinical and Experimental Immunology*, **144**: 1–9.

Ball TM, Castro-Rodriguez JA, Griffith KA, Holberg CJ, Martinez FD, Wright AL (2000). Siblings, day-care attendance, and the risk of asthma and wheezing during childhood. *New England Journal of Medicine*, **343**: 538–543.

Balloch A, Kemp A, Shelton M, Hill D (1996). Breastmilk specific antibodies and infant sensitization. *Allergy and Asthma Proceedings*, **17**: 126.

Bardana EJ Jr (2004). Immunoglobulin E- (IgE) and non-IgE-mediated reactions in the pathogenesis of atopic eczema/dermatitis syndrome (AEDS). *Allergy*, **59**(suppl)78: 25–29.

Beck LA, Leung DY (2000). Allergen sensitization through the skin induces systemic allergic responses. *Journal of Allergy and Clinical Immunology*, **106**(5 Suppl): S258-S263.

Bergmann RL, Bergmann KE, Lau-Schadensdorf S, *et al.* (1994). Atopic diseases in infancy. The German multicenter atopy study (MAS-90). *Pediatric Allergy and Immunology*, **5**(suppl 6): 19–25.

Bergmann RL, Edenharter G, Bergmann KE, *et al.* (1998). Atopic dermatitis in early infancy predicts

allergic airway disease at 5 years. *Clinical and Experimental Allergy*, **28**: 965–970.

Bernstein IL, Storms WW (1995). Practice parameters for allergy diagnostic testing. Joint Task Force on Practice Parameters for the Diagnosis and Treatment of Asthma. The American Academy of Allergy, Asthma and Immunology and the American College of Allergy, Asthma and Immunology. *Annals of Allergy and Asthma Immunology*, **75**: 543–625.

Björkstén B, Naaber P, Sepp E, Mikelsaar M (1999). The intestinal microflora in allergic Estonian and Swedish 2-year-old children. *Clinical and Experimental Allergy*, **29**: 342–346. [Erratum in: *Clinical and Experimental Allergy*, 2000; **30**: 1047.]

Boguniewicz M, Leung DY (2006). Atopic dermatitis. *Journal of Allergy and Clinical Immunology*, **117** (suppl); S475–480.

Bråbäck L, Breborowicz A, Julge K, *et al.* (1995). Risk factors for respiratory symptoms and atopic sensitisation in the Baltic area. *Archives of Disease in Childhood*, **72**: 487–493.

Broide DH (2001). Molecular and cellular mechanisms of allergic disease. *Journal of Allergy and Clinical Immunology*, **108**(suppl 2): S65–S71.

Burks AW, James JM, Hiegel A, *et al.* (1998). Atopic dermatitis and food hypersensitivity reactions. *Journal of Pediatrics*, **132**: 132–136.

Carvalho NF, Kenney RD, Carrington PH, Hall DE (2001). Severe nutritional deficiencies in toddlers resulting from health food milk alternatives. *Pediatrics*, **107**: E46.

Celedon JC, Litonjua AA, Weiss ST, Gold DR (1999). Day care attendance in the first year of life and illnesses of the upper and lower respiratory tract in children with a familial history of atopy. *Pediatrics*, **104**: 495–500.

Darsow U, Lübbe J, Taïeb A, *et al.* (2005). Position paper on diagnosis and treatment of atopic dermatitis. *Journal of the European Academy of Dermatology and Venereology*, **19**: 286–295.

Di Prisco DE, Fuenmayor MC, Champion RH (1979). Specific hyposensitization in atopic dermatitis. *British Journal of Dermatology*, **101**: 697–700.

Diepgen TL (2001). Atopic dermatitis: the role of environmental and social factors, the European experience. *Journal of the American Academy of Dermatology*, **45**(suppl 1): S44–S48.

Early Treatment of the Atopic Child (1998). Allergic factors associated with the development of asthma and the influence of cetirizine in a double-blind, randomised, placebo-controlled trial: first results of ETAC. *Pediatric Allergy and Immunology*, **9**: 116–124.

Echechipía S, Gómez B, Lasa E, et al. (2003). Epicutaneous test with inhalers in the study of atopic dermatitis [in Spanish]. *Anales del Sistema Sanitario de Navarra*, **26**(suppl 2): 31–37.

Eder W, Klimecki W, Yu L, et al. (2004). Toll-like receptor 2 as a major gene for asthma in children of European farmers. *Journal of Allergy and Clinical Immunology*, **113**: 482–488.

Eichenfield LF, Hanifin JM, Beck LA, et al. (2003). Atopic dermatitis and asthma: parallels in the evolution of treatment. *Pediatrics*, **111**: 608–616.

Eigenmann PA, Sicherer SH, Borkowski TA, et al. (1998). Prevalence of IgE-mediated food allergy among children with atopic dermatitis. *Pediatrics*, **101**: E8.

Eyerich K, Pennino D, Scarpor C, et al. (2009). Il-17 in atopic dermatitis. Linking allergen-specific adoptive and microbial-triggered innate immune response. *Journal of Allergy and Clinical Immunology*, **123**: 59–66.

Fergusson DM, Horwood LJ, Shannon FT (1990). Early solid feeding and recurrent childhood eczema: a 10-year longitudinal study. *Pediatrics*, **86**: 541–546.

Friedmann PS, Tan BB (1998). Mite elimination – clinical effect on eczema. *Allergy*, **53** (suppl 48): 97–100.

Fuiano N, Incorvaia C (2004). Value of skin prick test and atopy patch test in mite-induced respiratory allergy and/or atopic eczema/dermatitis syndrome [in Italian]. *Minerva Pediatrica*, **56**: 537–540.

Genentech (2008). Xolair (Omalizumab) for subcutaneous use. Available at: www.gene.com/gene/products/information/pdf/xolair-prescribing.pdf (accessed February 12, 2011).

Gern JE, Weiss ST (2000). Protection against atopic diseases by measles – a rash conclusion? *Journal of the American Medical Association*, **283**: 394–395.

Glover MT, Atherton DJ (1992). A double-blind controlled trial of hyposensitization to *Dermatophagoides pteronyssinus* in children with atopic eczema. *Clinical and Experimental Allergy*, **22**: 440–446.

Greenhawt M (2010). The role of food allergy in atopic dermatitis. *Allergy and Asthma Proceedings*, **31**: 392–397.

Grulee C, Sanford H (1936). The influence of breast and artificial feeding on infantile eczema. *Journal of Pediatrics*, **9**: 223–225.

Halken S, Høst A, Hansen LG, Osterballe O (1992). Effect of an allergy prevention programme on incidence of atopic symptoms in infancy. A prospective study of 159 'high-risk' infants. *Allergy*, **47**: 545–553.

Hamid Q, Boguniewicz M, Leung DY (1994). Differential in situ cytokine gene expression in acute versus chronic atopic dermatitis. *Journal of Clinical Investigation*, **94**: 870–876.

Hanifin JM, Cooper KD, Ho VC, et al. (2004). Administrative regulations for evidence-based clinical practice guidelines. *Journal of the American Academy of Dermatology*, **50**: 391–404. [Erratum in: *Journal of the American Academy of Dermatology*, 2005; **52**: 156.]

Henderson J, Northstone K, Lee SP, et al. (2008). The burden of disease associated with filaggrin mutations: a population-based, longitudinal birth cohort study. *Journal of Allergy and Clinical Immunology*, **121**: 872–877.

Herz U, Bunikowski R, Renz H (1998). Role of T cells in atopic dermatitis. New aspects on the dynamics of cytokine production and the contribution of bacterial superantigens. *International Archives of Allergy and Immunology*, **115**: 179–190.

Humbert M, Menz G, Ying S, et al. (1999). The immunopathology of extrinsic (atopic) and intrinsic (non-atopic) asthma: more similarities than differences. *Immunology Today*, **20**: 528–533.

Illi S, von Mutius E, Lau S, et al. (2001). Early childhood infectious diseases and the development of asthma up to school age: a birth

cohort study. *British Medical Journal*, **322**: 390–395.

International Study of Asthma and Allergies in Childhood (ISAAC) Steering Committee (1998). Worldwide variation in prevalence of symptoms of asthma, allergic rhinoconjunctivitis, and atopic eczema: ISAAC. *Lancet*, **351**: 1225–1232.

Irvine AD, McLean WH (2006). Breaking the (un)sound barrier: filaggrin is a major gene for atopic dermatitis. *Journal of Investigative Dermatology*, **126**: 1200–1202.

Johansson SG, Hourihane JO, Bousquet J, et al. (2001). A revised nomenclature for allergy. An EAACI position statement from the EAACI nomenclature task force. *Allergy*, **56**: 813–824 Review. [Erratum in: *Allergy*, 2001; **56**: 1229.]

Johansson SG, Bieber T, Dahl R, et al. (2004). Revised nomenclature for allergy for global use: Report of the Nomenclature Review Committee of the World Allergy Organization, October 2003. *Journal of Allergy and Clinical Immunology*, **113**: 832–836.

Kaufman HS, Roth HL (1974). Hyposensitization with alum precipitated extracts in atopic dermatitis: a placebo-controlled study. *Annals of Allergy*, **32**: 321–330.

Kleinman RE, Walker WA (1984). Antigen processing and uptake from the intestinal tract. *Clinical Reviews in Allergy*, **2**: 25–37.

Koga C, Kabashima K, Shirassishi N, et al. (2008). Possible pathogenic role of Th17 cells for atopic dermatitis. *Journal of Investigative Dermatology*, **128**: 2625–2630.

Kramer MS, Moroz B (1981). Do breastfeeding and delayed introduction of solid foods protect against subsequent atopic eczema? *Journal of Pediatrics*, **98**: 546–550.

Ladoyanni E, Cheung ST, North J, Tan CY (2007). Pellagra occurring in a patient with atopic dermatitis and food allergy. *Journal of the European Academy of Dermatology and Venereology*, **21**: 394–396.

Leung DY, Bieber T (2003). Atopic dermatitis. *Lancet*, **361**: 151–160.

Leung DY, Boguniewicz M, Howell MD, Nomura I, Hamid QA (2004a). New insights into atopic dermatitis. *Journal of Clinical Investigation*, **113**: 651–657.

Leung DY, Nicklas RA, Li JT, *et al.* (2004b). Disease management of atopic dermatitis: an updated practice parameter. Joint Task Force on Practice Parameters. *Annals of Allergy Asthma and Immunology,* 93(3 suppl 2): S1-S21.

Lever R (2001). The role of food in atopic eczema. *Journal of the American Academy of Dermatology,* 45(suppl 1): S57-S60.

Lewin Group I (2005). *The Burden of Skin Diseases.* Executive summary prepared by The Society for Investigative Dermatology and the American Academy of Dermatology Association, Falls Chuch, pp. 40–44.

Lilja G, Dannaeus A, Foucard T, Graff-Lonnevig V, Johansson SG, Oman H (1991). Effects of maternal diet during late pregnancy and lactation on the development of IgE and egg- and milk-specific IgE and IgG antibodies in infants. *Clinical and Experimental Allergy,* 21: 195–202.

Lipozencić J, Wolf R (2007). Atopic dermatitis: an update and review of the literature. *Dermatologic Clinics,* 25: 605–612.

Lugović L, Lipozencić J, Jakić-Razumović J (2005). Prominent involvement of activated Th1-subset of T-cells and increased expression of receptor for IFN-gamma on keratinocytes in atopic dermatitis acute skin lesions. *International Archives of Allergy and Immunology,* 137: 125–133.

Lugović L, Cupić H, Lipozencić J, Jakić-Razumović J (2006). The role of adhesion molecules in atopic dermatitis. *Acta Dermato-Venereologica Croatia,* 14: 2–7.

McFadden JP, White JM, Basketter DA, Kimber I (2009). Does hapten exposure predispose to atopic disease? The hapten–atopy hypothesis. *Trends in Immunology,* 30: 67–74.

McFadden JP, Dearman RJ, White JM, Basketter DA, Kimber I (2011). The hapten–atopy hypothesis II: the 'cutaneous hapten paradox'. *Clinical and Experimental Allergy,* 41: 327–337.

Machtinger S, Moss R (1986). Cow's milk allergy in breastfed infants: the role of allergen and maternal secretory IgA antibody. *Journal of Allergy and Clinical Immunology,* 77: 341–347.

Majamaa H, Isolauri E (1997). Probiotics: a novel approach in the management of food allergy. *Journal of Allergy and Clinical Immunology,* 99: 179–185.

Naleway AL (2004). Asthma and atopy in rural children: is farming protective? *Clinical and Medical Research,* 2: 5–12.

Nassif A, Chan SC, Storrs FJ, Hanifin JM (1994). Abnormal skin irritancy in atopic dermatitis and in atopy without dermatitis. *Archives of Dermatology,* 130: 1402–1407.

Nguyen J, Cazassus F, Atallah A, Baba N, Sibille G, Coriatt D (2001). Kwashiorkor after an exclusion diet for eczema. *La Presse Médicale,* 30: 1496–1497.

Niggemann B (2004). Role of oral food challenges in the diagnostic work-up of food allergy in atopic eczema dermatitis syndrome. *Allergy,* 59(suppl 78): 32–34.

Nowak D, Heinrich J, Jörres R, *et al.* (1996). Prevalence of respiratory symptoms, bronchial hyper-responsiveness and atopy among adults: west and east Germany. *European Respiratory Journal,* 9: 2541–2552.

Oyoshi M, Murphy GF, Geha RS (2009). Filaggrin-deficient mice exhibit Th17 dominated skin inflammation and permissiveness to epicutaneous sensitization with protein antigen. *Journal of Allergy and Clinical Immunology,* 124: 485–493.

Parslow TG, Stites DP, Terr AI, Imboden JB, eds (2001). *Medical Immunology,* 10th edn, McGraw Hill, New York.

Patki A (2007). Eat dirt and avoid atopy: the hygiene hypothesis revisited. *Indian Journal of Dermatology, Venereology and Leprology,* 73: 2–4.

Pesonen M, Kallio MJ, Ranki A, Siimes MA (2006). Prolonged exclusive breastfeeding is associated with increased atopic dermatitis: a prospective follow-up study of unselected healthy newborns from birth to age 20 years. *Clinical and Experimental Allergy,* 36: 1011–1018.

Roberts G, Lack G (2005). Diagnosing peanut allergy with skin prick and specific IgE testing. *Journal of Allergy and Clinical Immunology,* 115: 1291–1296.

Robinson DS, Larche M, Durham SR (2004). Tregs and allergic disease. *Journal of Clinical Investigation,* 114: 1389–97.

Romagnani S (1992a). Human TH1 and TH2 subsets: regulation of differentiation and role in protection and immunopathology. *International Archives of Allergy and Immunology,* 98: 279–285.

Romagnani S (1992b). Induction of TH1 and TH2 responses: a key role for the 'natural' immune response? *Immunology Today,* 13: 379–381.

Rosenthal E, Schlesinger Y, Birnbaum Y, Goldstein R, Benderly A, Freier S (1991). Intolerance to casein hydrolysate formula. Clinical aspects. *Acta Paediatrica Scandinavica,* 80: 958–960.

Rowlands D, Tofte SJ, Hanifin JM (2006). Does food allergy cause atopic dermatitis? Food challenge testing to dissociate eczematous from immediate reactions. *Dermatologic Therapy,* 19: 97–103.

Sampson HA (1999). Food allergy. Part 1: immunopathogenesis and clinical disorders. *Journal of Allergy and Clinical Immunology,* 103: 717–728.

Sampson HA (2001). Utility of food-specific IgE concentrations in predicting symptomatic food allergy. *Journal of Allergy and Clinical Immunology,* 107: 891–896.

Sampson HA, Albergo R (1984). Comparison of results of skin tests, RAST, and double-blind, placebo-controlled food challenges in children with atopic dermatitis. *Journal of Allergy and Clinical Immunology,* 74: 26–33.

Savilahti E, Järvenpää AL, Räihä NC (1983). Serum immunoglobulins in preterm infants: comparison of human milk and formula feeding. *Pediatrics,* 72: 312–316.

Scheinfeld N (2005). Omalizumab: a recombinant humanized monoclonal IgE-blocking antibody. *Dermatology Online Journal,* 11: 2.

Schmid-Grendelmeier P, Simon D, Simon HU, Akdis CA, Wüthrich B (2001). Epidemiology, clinical features, and immunology of the 'intrinsic' (non-IgE-mediated) type of atopic dermatitis (constitutional dermatitis). *Allergy,* 56: 841–849.

Schultz Larsen F, Hanifin J (2002). Epidemiology of atopic dermatitis. *Immunology and Allergy Clinics of North America,* 22: 1–24.

Sepp E, Julge K, Vasar M, Naaber P, Björksten B, Mikelsaar M (1997). Intestinal microflora of Estonian and Swedish infants. *Acta Paediatrica,* 86: 956–961.

Sicherer SH, Morrow EH, Sampson HA (2000). Dose-response in double-blind, placebo-controlled oral food challenges in children with atopic dermatitis. *Journal of Allergy and Clinical Immunology*, **105**: 582–586.

Spergel JM, Mizoguchi E, Brewer JP, Martin TR, Bhan AK, Geha RS (1998). Epicutaneous sensitization with protein antigen induces localized allergic dermatitis and hyper-responsiveness to methacholine after single exposure to aerosolized antigen in mice. *Journal of Clinical Investigation*, **101**: 1614–1622.

Stein RT, Sherrill D, Morgan WJ, *et al.* (1999). Respiratory syncytial virus in early life and risk of wheeze and allergy by age 13 years. *Lancet*, **354**: 541–545.

Strachan DP (1989). Hay fever, hygiene, and household size. *British Medical Journal*, **299**: 1259–1260.

Tan BB, Weald D, Strickland I, Friedmann PS (1996). Double-blind controlled trial of effect of house dust mite allergen avoidance on atopic dermatitis. *Lancet*, **347**: 15–18.

van den Oord RA, Sheikh A (2009). Filaggrin gene defects and risk of developing allergic sensitization and allergic disorders: systematic review and meta-analysis. *British Medical Journal*, **339**: b2433.

von Bubnoff D, Geiger E, Bieber T (2001). Antigen-presenting cells in allergy. *Journal of Allergy and Clinical Immunology*, **108**: 329–339.

von Mutius E (1998). The influence of birth order on the expression of atopy in families: a gene–environment interaction? *Clinical and Experimental Allergy*, **28**: 1454–1456.

von Mutius E (2000). The environmental predictors of allergic disease. *Journal of Allergy and Clinical Immunology*, **105**: 9–19.

von Mutius E (2001). Infection: friend or foe in the development of atopy and asthma? The epidemiological evidence. *European Respiratory Journal*, **18**: 872–881.

von Mutius E, Nicolai T (1996). Familial aggregation of asthma in a South Bavarian population. *American Journal of Respiratory and Critical Care Medicine*, **153**: 1266–1272.

von Mutius E, Martinez FD, Fritzsch C, Nicolai T, Roell G, Thiemann HH (1994). Prevalence of asthma and atopy in two areas of West and East Germany. *American Journal of Respiratory and Critical Care Medicine*, **149**: 358–364.

Wahn U, von Mutius E (2001). Childhood risk factors for atopy and the importance of early intervention. *Journal of Allergy and Clinical Immunology*, **107**: 567–574.

Weidinger S, O'Sullivan M, Illig T, *et al.* (2008). Filaggrin mutations, atopic eczema, hay fever, and asthma in children. *Journal of Allergy and Clinical Immunology*, **121**: 1203–1210.

Werfel T (2009). The role of leukocytes, keratinocytes, and allergen-specific IgE in the development of atopic dermatitis. *Journal of Investigative Dermatology*, **129**: 1878–1891.

Werfel T, Ballmer-Weber B, Eigenmann PA, *et al.* (2007). Eczematous reactions to food in atopic eczema: position paper of the EAACI and GA2LEN. *Allergy*, **62**: 723–728.

Williams HC (2005). Clinical practice. Atopic dermatitis. *New England Journal of Medicine*, **352**: 2314–2324.

Wüthrich B (1999). Clinical aspects, epidemiology, and prognosis of atopic dermatitis. *Annals of Allergy Asthma and Immunology*, **83**: 464–470.

Zachariae H, Cramers M, Herlin T, *et al.* (1985). Non-specific immunotherapy and specific hyposensitization in severe atopic dermatitis. *Acta Dermato-Venereologica Supplementum (Stockholm)*, **114**: 48–54.

Zeiger RS, Heller S (1995). The development and prediction of atopy in high-risk children: follow-up at age 7 years in a prospective randomized study of combined maternal and infant food allergen avoidance. *Journal of Allergy and Clinical Immunology*, **95**: 1179–1190.

Zeiger RS, Heller S, Mellon MH, *et al.* (1989). Effect of combined maternal and infant food-allergen avoidance on development of atopy in early infancy: a randomized study. *Journal of Allergy and Clinical Immunology*, **84**: 72–89. [Erratum in: *Journal of Allergy and Clinical Immunology*, **84**: 677.]

CHAPTER 8

Abbas S, Goldberg JW, Massaro M (2004). Personal cleanser technology and clinical performance. *Dermatologic Therapy*, **17**(suppl 1): 35–42.

Abramovits W, Gover MD, Gupta AK (2005). Atopiclair nonsteroidal cream. *Skinmed*, **4**: 369.

Abramovits W, Perlmutter A (2006a). MimyX cream. *Skinmed*, **5**: 29–30.

Abramovits W, Perlmutter A (2006b). Steroids versus other immune modulators in the management of allergic dermatoses. *Current Opinion in Allergy and Clinical Immunology*, **6**: 345–354.

Ananthapadmanabhan KP, Moore DJ, Subramanyan K, *et al.* (2004). Cleansing without compromise: the impact of cleansers on the skin barrier and the technology of mild cleansing. *Dermatologic Therapy*, **17**(suppl 1): 16–25.

Bergstrand N (2003). Liposomes for drug delivery: from physico-chemical studies to applications. *Acta Universitatis Upsaliensis*, 1–71.

Bettzuege-Pfaff BI, Melzer A (2005). Treating dry skin and pruritus with a bath oil containing soya oil and lauromacrogols. *Current Medical Research Opinion*, **21**: 1735–1739.

Bikle DD, Chang S, Crumrine D, *et al.* (2004). 25 Hydroxyvitamin D 1 alpha-hydroxylase is required for optimal epidermal differentiation and permeability barrier homeostasis. *Journal of Investigative Dermatology*, **122**: 984–992.

Borrek S, Hildebrandt A, Forster J (1997). Gamma-linolenic-acid-rich borage seed oil capsules in children with atopic dermatitis. A placebo-controlled double-blind study. *Klinische Pädiatrie*, **209**: 100–104.

Braff M H, Gallo RL (2006). Antimicrobial peptides: an essential component of the skin defensive barrier. *Current topics in Microbiology and Immunology*, **306**: 91–110.

Buraczewska I, Berne B, Lindberg M, *et al.* (2007). Changes in skin barrier function following long-term treatment with moisturizers, a randomized controlled trial. *British Journal of Dermatology*, **156**: 492–498.

Candi E, Schmidt R, Melino G (2005). The cornified envelope: a model of cell death in the skin. *Nature Reviews in Molecular and Cellular Biology*, **6**: 328–340.

Cao C, Sun Y, Healey S, *et al.* (2006). EGFR-mediated expression of aquaporin-3 is involved in human skin fibroblast migration. *Biochemical Journal*, **400**: 225–234.

Cardona ID, Cho SH, Leung DY (2006). Role of bacterial superantigens in atopic dermatitis: implications for future therapeutic strategies. *American Journal of Clinical Dermatology*, **7**: 273–279.

Chamlin SL, Kao J, Frieden IJ, *et al.* (2002). Ceramide-dominant barrier repair lipids alleviate childhood atopic dermatitis: changes in barrier function provide a sensitive indicator of disease activity. *Journal of the American Academy of Dermatology*, **47**: 198–208.

Choi EH, Brown BE, Crumrine D, *et al.* (2005). Mechanisms by which psychologic stress alters cutaneous permeability barrier homeostasis and stratum corneum integrity. *Journal of Investigative Dermatology*, **124**: 587–595.

Cork MJ, Robinson DA, Vasilopoulos Y, *et al.* (2006). New perspectives on epidermal barrier dysfunction in atopic dermatitis: gene–environment interactions. *Journal of Allergy and Clinical Immunology*, **118**: 3–21.

Denda M, Sokabe T, Fukumi-Tominaga T, *et al.* (2007). Effects of skin surface temperature on epidermal permeability barrier homeostasis. *Journal of Investigative Dermatology*, **127**: 654–659.

Draelos ZD (2000). Therapeutic moisturizers. *Dermatologic Clinics*, **18**: 597–607.

Draelos ZD (2005). Concepts in skin care maintenance. *Cutis*, **76**(6 suppl): 19–25.

Dumas M, Sadick NS, Noblesse E, *et al.* (2007). Hydrating skin by stimulating biosynthesis of aquaporins. *Journal of Drugs in Dermatology*, **6**(6 suppl): s20–24.

Eichenfield LF, Fowler JF Jr, Rigel DS, *et al.* (2007). Natural advances in eczema care. *Cutis*, **80**(6 suppl): 2–16.

Elias PM (1983). Epidermal lipids, barrier function, and desquamation. *Journal of Investigative Dermatology*, **80**(suppl): 44s–49s.

Elias PM (2005). Physiological lipids for barrier repair in dermatology. In: Draelos Z (ed.), *Cosmeceuticals*, Elsevier, Philadelphia, pp. 63–70.

Elias PM, Hatano Y, Williams ML (2008). Basis for the barrier abnormality in atopic dermatitis: Outside-inside-outside pathogenic mechanisms. *Journal of Allergy and Clinical Immunology*, **121**: 1337–1343.

Engel K, Reuter J, Seiler C, *et al.* (2008). Anti-inflammatory effect of pimecrolimus in the sodium lauryl sulphate test. *Journal of the European Academy of Dermatology and Venereology*, **22**: 447–450.

Faurschou A, Wiegell SR, Wulf HC (2007). Transepidermal water loss after photodynamic therapy, UVB radiation and topical corticosteroid is independent of inflammation. *Skin Research and Technology*, **13**: 202–206.

Fluhr JW, Kao J, Jain M, *et al.* (2001). Generation of free fatty acids from phospholipids regulates stratum corneum acidification and integrity. *Journal of Investigative Dermatology*, **117**: 44–51.

Gfatter R, Hackl P, Braun F (1997). Effects of soap and detergents on skin surface pH, stratum corneum hydration and fat content in infants. *Dermatology*, **195**: 258–262.

Ginger RS, Blachford S, Rowland J, *et al.* (2005). Filaggrin repeat number polymorphism is associated with a dry skin phenotype. *Archives of Dermatological Research*, **297**: 235–241.

Hanson KM, Behne MJ, Barry NP, *et al.* (2002).Two-photon fluorescence lifetime imaging of the skin stratum corneum pH gradient. *Biophysical Journal*, **83**: 1682–1690.

Hara-Chikuma M, Verkman AS (2006). Physiological roles of glycerol-transporting aquaporins: the aquaglyceroporins. *Cellular and Molecular Life Sciences*, **63**: 1386–1392.

Harding CR (2004). The stratum corneum: structure and function in health and disease. *Dermatologic Therapy*, **17**(suppl 1): 6–15.

Irvine AD, McLean WH (2006). Breaking the (un)sound barrier: filaggrin is a major gene for atopic dermatitis. *Journal of Investigative Dermatology*, **126**: 1200–1202.

Ishibashi M, Arikawa J, Okamoto R, *et al.* (2003). Abnormal expression of the novel epidermal enzyme, glucosylceramide deacylase, and the accumulation of its enzymatic reaction product, glucosylsphingosine, in the skin of patients with atopic dermatitis. *Laboratory Investigation*, **83**: 397–408.

Kim DW, Park JY, Na GY, *et al.* (2006). Correlation of clinical features and skin barrier function in adolescent and adult patients with atopic dermatitis. *International Journal of Dermatology*, **45**: 698–701.

Kircik L, Del Rosso J (2007). A novel hydrogel vehicle formulated for the treatment of atopic dermatitis. *Journal of Drugs in Dermatology*, **6**: 718–722.

Kircik LH, Del Rosso JQ (2011). Evaluating clinical use of a ceramide-dominant, physiologic lipid-based topical emulsion for atopic dermatitis. *Journal of Clinical and Aesthetic Dermatology*, **4**: 25–31.

Kisich KO, Howell MD, Boguniewicz M, *et al.* (2007). The constitutive capacity of human keratinocytes to kill *Staphylococcus aureus* is dependent on beta-defensin 3. *Journal of Investigative Dermatology*, **127**: 2368–2380.

Lebwohl M, Herrmann LG (2005). Impaired skin barrier function in dermatologic disease and repair with moisturization. *Cutis*, **76**(6 suppl): 7–12.

Leung DY, Boguniewicz M, Howell MD, *et al.* (2004). New insights into atopic dermatitis. *Journal of Clinical Investigation*, **113**: 651–657.

Levin CY, Maibach HI (2001). Do cool water or physiologic saline compresses enhance resolution of experimentally-induced irritant contact dermatitis? *Contact Dermatitis*, **45**: 146–150.

Leyvraz C, Charles RP, Rubera I, *et al.* (2005). The epidermal barrier function is dependent on the serine protease CAP1/Prss8. *Journal of Cell Biology*, **170**: 487–496.

Loden M (2003). Role of topical emollients and moisturizers in the treatment of dry skin barrier disorders. *American Journal of Clinical Dermatology*, **4**: 771–788.

Madison KC (2003). Barrier function of the skin: 'la raison d'être' of the epidermis. *Journal of Investigative Dermatology*, **121**: 231–241.

Man MQ M, Feingold KR, Thornfeldt CR, *et al.* (1996). Optimization of physiological lipid mixtures for barrier repair. *Journal of Investigative Dermatology*, **106**: 1096–1101.

Martens-Lobenhoffer J, Meyer FP (1998). Pharmacokinetic data of gamma-linolenic acid in healthy volunteers after the administration of evening primrose oil (Epogam). *International Journal of Clinical Pharmacology and Therapeutics*, **36**: 363–366.

Maytin EV, Chung HH, Seetharaman VM (2004). Hyaluronan participates in the epidermal response to disruption of the permeability barrier *in vivo*. *American Journal of Pathology*, **165**: 1331–1341.

Miller DW, Koch SB, Yentzer BA, *et al.* (2011). An over-the-counter moisturizer is as clinically effective as, and more cost-effective than, prescription barrier creams in the treatment of children with mild-to-moderate atopic dermatitis: a randomized, controlled trial. *Journal of Drugs in Dermatology*, **10**: 531–537.

Morar N, Cookson WO, Harper JI, *et al.* (2007). Filaggrin mutations in children with severe atopic dermatitis. *Journal of Investigative Dermatology*, **127**: 1667–1672.

Olsson M, Broberg A, Jernås M, *et al.* (2006).ê Increased expression of aquaporin 3 in atopic eczema. *Allergy*, **61**: 1132–1137.

Ong PY, Boguniewicz M (2008). Atopic dermatitis. *Primary Care*, **35**: 105–117.

Palmer CN, Irvine AD, Terron-Kwiatkowski A, *et al.* (2006). Common loss-of-function variants of the epidermal barrier protein filaggrin are a major predisposing factor for atopic dermatitis. *Nature Genetics*, **38**: 441–446.

Park CW, Lee BH, Lee CH (2005). Tacrolimus reduces staphylococcal colonization on the skin in Korean atopic dermatitis patients. *Drugs under Experimental and Clinical Research*, **31**: 77–87.

Parneix-Spake A, Goustas P, Green R (2001). Eumovate (clobetasone butyrate) 0.05% cream with its moisturizing emollient base has better healing properties than hydrocortisone 1% cream: a study in nickel-induced contact dermatitis. *Journal of Dermatologic Treatment*, **12**: 191–197.

Pasonen-Seppänen S, Karvinen S, Törrönen K, *et al.* (2003). EGF upregulates, whereas TGF-beta downregulates, the hyaluronan synthases Has2 and Has3 in organotypic keratinocyte cultures: correlations with epidermal proliferation and differentiation. *Journal of Investigative Dermatology*, **120**: 1038–1044.

Puig A, Bonilla A, Cebrian J, *et al.* (2004). *New Delivery Systems for Hair and Fabric Care*, Business Briefing, Global Cosmetics Manufacturing. Lipotec, Barcelona, pp. 1–7.

Rawlings AV, Harding CR (2004). Moisturization and skin barrier function. *Dermatologic Therapy*, **17**(suppl 1): 43–48.

Rawlings AV, Matts PJ (2005). Stratum corneum moisturization at the molecular level: an update in relation to the dry skin cycle. *Journal of Investigative Dermatology*, **124**: 1099–1110.

Rawlings AV, Canestrari DA, Dobkowski B (2004). Moisturizer technology versus clinical performance. *Dermatologic Therapy*, **17**(suppl 1): 49–56.

Rosen MR (2005). *Delivery System Handbook for Personal Care and Cosmetic Products: Technology, Applications, and Formulations*, William Andrew, Norwich.

Sandilands AF, Smith FJ, Irvine AD, *et al.* (2007). Filaggrin's fuller figure: a glimpse into the genetic architecture of atopic dermatitis. *Journal of Investigative Dermatology*, **127**: 1282–1284.

Schmid MH, Korting HC (1995). The concept of the acid mantle of the skin: its relevance for the choice of skin cleansers. *Dermatology*, **191**: 276–280.

Schmid-Wendtner MH, Korting HC (2006). The pH of the skin surface and its impact on the barrier function. *Skin Pharmacology and Physiology*, **19**: 296–302.

Segre JA (2006). Epidermal differentiation complex yields a secret: mutations in the cornification protein filaggrin underlie ichthyosis vulgaris. *Journal of Investigative Dermatology*, **118**: 1202–1204.

Sheu HM, Lee JY, Chai Cy, *et al.* (1997). Depletion of stratum corneum intercellular lipid lamellae and barrier function abnormalities after long-term topical corticosteroids. *British Journal of Dermatology*, **136**: 884–890.

Simpson E, Dutronc Y (2011). A new body moisturizer increases skin hydration and improves atopic dermatitis symptoms among children and adults. *Journal of Drugs in Dermatology*, **10**: 744–749.

Strobel CT, Byrne WJ, Abramovits W, *et al.* (1978). A zinc-deficiency dermatitis in patients on total parenteral nutrition. *International Journal of Dermatology*, **17**: 575–581.

Sugarman JL, Parish LC (2009). Efficacy of a lipid-based barrier repair formulation in moderate-to-severe pediatric atopic dermatitis. *Journal of Drugs and Dermatology*, **8**: 1106–1111.

Tagami H, Kobayashi H, O'goshi K, *et al.* (2006). Atopic xerosis: employment of noninvasive biophysical instrumentation for the functional analyses of the mildly abnormal stratum corneum and for the efficacy assessment of skin care products. *Journal of Cosmetic Dermatology*, **5**: 140–149.

Takwale A, Tan E, Agarwal S, *et al.* (2003). Efficacy and tolerability of borage oil in adults and children with atopic eczema: randomised, double blind, placebo controlled, parallel group trial. *British Medical Journal*, **327**: 1385.

Umeda-Sawada R, Fujiwara Y, Ushiyama I, *et al.* (2006). Distribution and metabolism of dihomo-gamma-linolenic acid (DGLA, 20:3n-6) by oral supplementation in rats. *Bioscience, Biotechnology, and Biochemistry*, **70**: 2121–2130.

Warner RR, Stone KJ, Boissy YL (2003). Hydration disrupts human stratum corneum ultrastructure. *Journal of Investigative Dermatology*, **120**: 275–284.

Weidinger S, Illig T, Baurecht H (2006). Loss-of-function variations within the filaggrin gene predispose for atopic dermatitis with allergic sensitizations. *Journal of Allergy and Clinical Immunology*, **118**: 214–219.

Xhauflaire-Uhoda E, Thirion L, Piérard-Franchimont C, *et al.* (2007). Comparative effect of tacrolimus and betamethasone valerate on the passive sustainable hydration of the stratum corneum in atopic dermatitis. *Dermatology*, **214**: 328–332.

Zettersten EM, Ghadially R, Feingold KR, *et al.* (1997). Optimal ratios of topical stratum corneum lipids improve barrier recovery in chronologically aged skin. *Journal of the American Academy of Dermatology*, **37**(3 Pt 1): 403–408.

CHAPTER 9

Abeck D, Mempel M (1998). *Staphylococcus aureus* colonization in atopic dermatitis and its therapeutic implications. *British Journal of Dermatology*, **139**(suppl 53): 13–16.

Adachi J, Endo K, Fukuzumi T, Tanigawa N, Aoki T (1998). Increasing incidence of streptococcal impetigo in atopic dermatitis. *Journal of Dermatological Science*, **17**: 45–53.

Akiyama H, Yamasaki O, Kanzaki H, Tada J, Arata J (1999). Streptococci isolated from various skin lesions: the interaction with *Staphylococcus aureus* strains. *Journal of Dermatological Science*, **19**: 17–22.

Asano S, Ichikawa Y, Kumagai T, Kawashima M, Imokawa G (2008). Microanalysis of an antimicrobial peptide, beta-defensin-2, in the stratum corneum from patients with atopic dermatitis. *British Journal of Dermatology*, **159**: 97–104.

Bäck O, Bartosik J (2001). Systemic ketoconazole for yeast allergic patients with atopic dermatitis. *Journal of the European Academy of Dermatology and Venereology*, **15**: 34–38.

Bäck O, Scheynius A, Johansson SG (1995). Ketoconazole in atopic dermatitis: therapeutic response is correlated with decrease in serum IgE. *Archives of Dermatological Research*, **287**: 448–451.

Bath-Hextall FJ, Birnie AJ, Ravenscroft JC, Williams HC (2010). Interventions to reduce *Staphylococcus aureus* in the management of atopic eczema: an updated Cochrane review. *British Journal of Dermatology*, **163**: 12–26.

Beck LA, Boguniewicz M, Hata T, *et al.* (2009). Phenotype of atopic dermatitis subjects with a history of eczema herpeticum. *Journal of Allergy and Clinical Immunology*, **124**: 260–269, 269.

Bieber T (2008). Atopic dermatitis. *New England Journal of Medicine*, **358**: 1483–1494.

Binkley GW, Deoreo GA, Johnson HH Jr (1956). An eczematous reaction associated with molluscum contagiosum. *American Medical Association Archives of Dermatology*, **74**: 344–348.

Boguniewicz M, Schmid-Grendelmeier P, Leung DY (2006). Atopic dermatitis. *Journal of Allergy and Clinical Immunology*, **118**: 40–43.

Bork K, Bräuninger W (1988). Increasing incidence of eczema herpeticum: analysis of 75 cases. *Journal of the American Academy of Dermatology*, **19**: 1024–1029.

Broberg A, Faergemann J, Johansson S, Johansson SG, Strannegård IL, Svejgaard E (1992). *Pityrosporum ovale* and atopic dermatitis in children and young adults. *Acta Dermato-Venereologica*, **72**: 187–192.

Brook I, Frazier EH, Yeager JK (1996). Microbiology of infected atopic dermatitis. *International Journal of Dermatology*, **35**: 791–793.

Bunikowski R, Mielke M, Skarabis H, *et al.* (1999). Prevalence and role of serum IgE antibodies to the *Staphylococcus aureus*-derived superantigens SEA and SEB in children with atopic dermatitis. *Journal of Allergy and Clinical Immunology*, **103**: 119–124.

Bussmann C, Peng WM, Bieber T, Novak N (2008). Molecular pathogenesis and clinical implications of eczema herpeticum. *Expert Review of Molecular Diagnostics*, **14**: e21.

Cardona ID, Cho SH, Leung DY (2006). Role of bacterial superantigens in atopic dermatitis: implications for future therapeutic strategies. *American Journal of Clinical Dermatology*, **7**: 273–279.

Cho SH, Strickland I, Boguniewicz M, Leung DY (2001). Fibronectin and fibrinogen contribute to the enhanced binding of *Staphylococcus aureus* to atopic skin. *Journal of Allergy and Clinical Immunology*, **108**: 269–274.

Chung HJ, Jeon HS, Sung H, Kim MN, Hong SJ (2008). Epidemiological characteristics of methicillin-resistant *Staphylococcus aureus* isolates from children with eczematous atopic dermatitis lesions. *Journal of Clinical Microbiology*, **46**: 991–995.

Cono J, Casey CG, Bell DM (2003). Smallpox vaccination and adverse events: guidelines for clinicians. Centers for Disease Control and Prevention. *Morbidity and Mortality Weekly Report Recommendations and Reports*, **52**: 1–28.

Copeman PW, Wallace HJ (1964). Eczema vaccinatum. *British Medical Journal*, ii: 906–908.

Craig FE, Smith EV, Williams HC (2010). Bleach baths to reduce severity of atopic dermatitis colonized by *Staphylococcus*. *Archives of Dermatology*, **146**: 541–543.

Darabi K, Hostetler SG, Bechtel MA, *et al.* (2009). The role of *Malassezia* in atopic dermatitis affecting the head and neck of adults. *Journal of the American Academy of Dermatology*, **60**(1): 125–136.

David TJ (1989). Infection and prevention: current controversies in childhood atopic eczema: a review. *Journal of the Royal Society of Medicine*, **82**: 420–422.

David TJ, Cambridge GC (1986). Bacterial infection and atopic eczema. *Archives of Disease in Childhood*, **61**: 20–23.

David TJ, Longson M (1985). Herpes simplex infections in atopic eczema. *Archives of Disease in Childhood*, **60**: 338–343.

Dohil MA, Lin P, Lee J, Lucky AW, Paller AS, Eichenfield LF (2006). The epidemiology of molluscum contagiosum in children. *Journal of the American Academy of Dermatology*, **54**: 47–54.

Engler RJ, Kenner J, Leung DY (2002). Smallpox vaccination: Risk considerations for patients with atopic dermatitis. *Journal of Allergy and Clinical Immunology*, **110**: 357–365.

Faergemann J (1999). *Pityrosporum* species as a cause of allergy and infection. *Allergy*, **54**: 413–419.

Faergemann J (2002). Atopic dermatitis and fungi. *Clinical Microbiology Reviews*, **15**: 545–563.

Faergemann J, Aly R, Maibach HI (1983). Quantitative variations in distribution of *Pityrosporum orbiculare* on clinically normal skin. *Acta Dermato-Venereologica*, **63**: 346–348.

Falanga V, Campbell DE, Leyden JJ, Douglas SD (1985). Nasal carriage of *Staphylococcus aureus* and antistaphylococcal immunoglobulin E antibodies in atopic dermatitis. *Journal of Clinical Microbiology*, **22**: 452–454.

Fery-Blanco C, Pelletier F, Humbert P, Aubin F (2007). Disseminated molluscum contagiosum during topical treatment of atopic dermatitis with tacrolimus: efficacy of cidofovir [in French]. *Annales de Dermatologie et de Venereologie*, **134**: 457–459.

Friedman SJ, Schroeter AL, Homburger HA (1985). IgE antibodies to *Staphylococcus aureus*. Prevalence in patients with atopic dermatitis. *Archives of Dermatology*, **121**: 869–872.

Gao PS, Rafaels NM, Hand T, *et al.* (2009). Filaggrin mutations that confer risk of atopic dermatitis confer greater risk for eczema herpeticum. *Journal of Allergy and Clinical Immunology*, **124**: 507–513.

Gauger A, Fischer S, Mempel M, *et al.* (2006). Efficacy and functionality of silver-coated textiles in patients with atopic eczema. *Journal of the European Academy of Dermatology and Venereology*, **20**: 534–541. [Erratum in: *Journal of the European Academy of Dermatology and Venereology*, **20**: 771.]

Gong JQ, Lin L, Lin T, *et al.* (2006). Skin colonization by *Staphylococcus aureus* in patients with eczema and atopic dermatitis and relevant combined topical therapy: a double-blind multicentre randomized controlled trial. *British Journal of Dermatology*, **155**: 680–687.

Goo J, Ji JH, Jeon H, *et al.* (2010). Expression of antimicrobial peptides such as LL-37 and hBD-2 in nonlesional skin of atopic individuals. *Pediatric Dermatology*, **27**: 341–348.

Guého E, Boekhout T, Ashbee HR, Guillot J, Van Belkum A, Faergemann J (1998). The role of *Malassezia* species in the ecology of human skin and as pathogens. *Medical Mycology*, **36**(suppl 1): 220–229.

Haim M, Gdalevich M, Mimouni D, Ashkenazi I, Shemer J (2000). Adverse reactions to smallpox vaccine: the Israel Defense Force experience, (1991) to 1996. A comparison with previous surveys. *Military Medicine*, **165**: 287–289.

Hanifin JM, Rogge JL (1977). Staphylococcal infections in patients with atopic dermatitis. *Archives of Dermatology*, **113**: 1383–1386.

Hata TR, Kotol P, Boguniewicz M, *et al.* (2010). History of eczema herpeticum is associated with the inability to induce human β-defensin (HBD)-2, HBD-3 and cathelicidin in the skin of patients with atopic dermatitis. *British Journal of Dermatology*, **163**: 659–661.

Higaki S, Inoue Y, Yoshida A, *et al.* (2008). Case of bilateral multiple herpetic epithelial keratitis manifested as dendriform epithelial edema during primary Kaposi's varicelliform eruption. *Japanese Journal of Ophthalmology*, **52**: 127–129.

Hill SE, Yung A, Rademaker M (2011). Prevalence of *Staphylococcus aureus* and antibiotic resistance in children with atopic dermatitis: a New Zealand experience. *Australasian Journal of Dermatology*, **52**: 27–31.

Hinz T, Zaccaro D, Byron M, *et al.* (2011). Atopic dermo-respiratory syndrome is a correlate of eczema herpeticum. *Allergy*, **66**: 925–33.

Hoeger PH (2004). Antimicrobial susceptibility of skin-colonizing *S. aureus* strains in children with atopic dermatitis. *Pediatric Allergy and Immunology*, **15**: 474–477.

Hon KL, Leung AK, Kong AY, Leung TF, Ip M (2008). Atopic dermatitis complicated by methicillin-resistant *Staphylococcus aureus* infection. *Journal of the National Medical Association*, **100**: 797–800.

Howell MD, Novak N, Bieber T, *et al.* (2005). Interleukin-10 downregulates anti-microbial peptide expression in atopic dermatitis. *Journal of Investigative Dermatology*, **125**: 738–745 Erratum in: *Journal of Investigative Dermatology*, **125**: 1320.

Howell MD, Boguniewicz M, Pastore S, *et al.* (2006). Mechanism of HBD-3 deficiency in atopic dermatitis. *Clinical Immunology*, **121**: 332–338.

Howell MD, Streib JE, Kim BE, *et al.* (2009). Ceragenins: a class of antiviral compounds to treat orthopox infections. *Journal of Investigative Dermatology*, **129**: 2668–2675.

Huang JT, Abrams M, Tlougan B, Rademaker A, Paller AS (2009). Treatment of *Staphylococcus aureus* colonization in atopic dermatitis decreases disease severity. *Pediatrics*, **123**: e808–814.

Huang JT, Rademaker A, Paller AS (2011). Dilute bleach baths for *Staphylococcus aureus* colonization in atopic dermatitis to decrease disease severity. *Archives of Dermatology*, **147**: 246–247.

Ikezawa Z, Kondo M, Okajima M, Nishimura Y, Kono M (2004). Clinical usefulness of oral itraconazole, an antimycotic drug, for refractory atopic dermatitis. *European Journal of Dermatology*, **14**: 400–406.

Inoue Y, Aihara M, Kirino M, *et al.* (2010). Interleukin-18 is elevated in the horny layer in atopic dermatitis patients and associated with *Staphylococcus aureus* colonisation. *British Journal of Dermatology*, **164**: 560–567.

Jekler J, Bergbrant IM, Faergemann J, Larkö O (1992). The *in vivo* effect of UVB radiation on skin bacteria in patients with atopic dermatitis. *Acta Dermato-Venereologica*, **72**: 33–36.

Jen M, Chang MW (2010). Eczema herpeticum and eczema vaccinatum

in children. *Pediatric Annals*, **39**: 658–664.

Johansson C, Eshaghi H, Linder MT, Jakobson E, Scheynius A (2002). Positive atopy patch test reaction to *Malassezia furfur* in atopic dermatitis correlates with a T helper 2-like peripheral blood mononuclear cells response. *Journal of Investigative Dermatology*, **118**: 1044–1051.

Johansson C, Sandström MH, Bartosik J, *et al.* (2003). Atopy patch test reactions to *Malassezia* allergens differentiate subgroups of atopic dermatitis patients. *British Journal of Dermatology*, **148**: 479–488.

Jones HE, Reinhardt JH, Rinaldi MG (1973). A clinical, mycological, and immunological survey for dermatophytosis. *Archives of Dermatology*, **108**: 61–65.

Jones HE, Reinhardt JH, Rinaldi MG (1974). Immunologic susceptibility to chronic dermatophytosis. *Archives of Dermatology*, **110**: 213–220.

Kanda N (2004). Antimycotics suppress interleukin-4 and interleukin-5 production in anti-CD3 plus anti-CD28-stimulated T cells from patients with atopic dermatitis [in Japanese]. *Nippon Ishinkin Gakkai Zasshi*, **45**: 137–142.

Kempe CH (1960). Studies of smallpox and complications of smallpox vaccination. *Pediatrics*, **26**: 176–189.

Kisich KO, Carspecken CW, Fiéve S, Boguniewicz M, Leung DY (2008). Defective killing of *Staphylococcus aureus* in atopic dermatitis is associated with reduced mobilization of human beta-defensin-3. *Journal of Allergy and Clinical Immunology*, **122**: 62–68.

Klein PA, Clark RA, Nicol NH (1999). Acute infection with *Trichophyton rubrum* associated with flares of atopic dermatitis. *Cutis*, **63**: 171–172.

Krakowski AC, Eichenfield LF, Dohil MA (2008). Management of atopic dermatitis in the pediatric population. *Pediatrics*, **122**: 812–824.

Krutmann J (2000). Phototherapy for atopic dermatitis. *Clinical and Experimental Dermatology*, **25**: 552–558.

Lane JM, Millar JD (1971). Risks of smallpox vaccination complications in the United States. *American Journal of Epidemiology*, **93**: 238–240.

Leclercq R, Bismuth R, Casin I, *et al.* (2000). *In vitro* activity of fusidic acid against *streptococci* isolated from skin and soft tissue infections. *Journal of Antimicrobial Chemotherapy*, **45**: 27–29.

Leung DY (2003). Infection in atopic dermatitis. *Current Opinions in Pediatrics*, **15**: 399–404.

Leung DY, Harbeck R, Bina P, *et al.* (1993). Presence of IgE antibodies to staphylococcal exotoxins on the skin of patients with atopic dermatitis. Evidence for a new group of allergens. *Journal of Clinical Investigation*, **92**: 1374–1380.

Lever R (1996). Infection in atopic dermatitis. *Dermatologic Therapy*, **1**: 32–37.

Lever R, Hadley K, Downey D, Mackie R (1988). Staphylococcal colonization in atopic dermatitis and the effect of topical mupirocin therapy. *British Journal of Dermatology*, **119**: 189–198.

Leyden JJ, Kligman AM (1977). The case for steroid–antibiotic combinations. *British Journal of Dermatology*, **96**: 179–187.

Lübbe J (2003). Secondary infections in patients with atopic dermatitis. *American Journal of Clinical Dermatology*, **4**: 641–654.

Matiz C, Tom WL, Eichenfield LF, *et al.* (2010). Children with atopic dermatitis appear less likely to be infected with community acquired methicillin-resistant *Staphylococcus aureus*: the San Diego experience. *Pediatric Dermatology*, **28**: 6–11.

Metry D, Browning J, *et al.* (2007). Sodium hypochlorite (bleach) baths: a potential measure to reduce the incidence of recurrent, cutaneous *Staphylococcus aureus* superinfection among susceptible populations. Poster presented at the Society for Pediatric Dermatology, annual meeting. Chicago.

Miajlovic H, Fallon PG, Irvine AD, Foster TJ (2010). Effect of filaggrin breakdown products on growth of and protein expression by *Staphylococcus aureus*. *Journal of Allergy and Clinical Immunology*, **126**: 1184–1190.

Motala C, Potter PC, Weinberg EG, Malherbe D, Hughes J (1986). Anti-*Staphylococcus aureus*-specific IgE in atopic dermatitis. *Journal of Allergy and Clinical Immunology*, **78**: 583–589.

Niebuhr M, Mai U, Kapp A, Werfel T (2008). Antibiotic treatment of cutaneous infections with *Staphylococcus aureus* in patients with atopic dermatitis: current antimicrobial resistances

and susceptibilities. *Experimental Dermatology*, **17**: 953–957.

Nomura I, Tanaka K, Tomita H, *et al.* (1999). Evaluation of the staphylococcal exotoxins and their specific IgE in childhood atopic dermatitis. *Journal of Allergy and Clinical Immunology*, **104**: 441–446.

Nomura I, Goleva E, Howell MD, *et al.* (2003). Cytokine milieu of atopic dermatitis, as compared to psoriasis, skin prevents induction of innate immune response genes. *Journal of Immunology*, **171**: 3262–3269.

Ong PY, Ohtake T, Brandt C, *et al.* (2002). Endogenous antimicrobial peptides and skin infections in atopic dermatitis. *New England Journal of Medicine*, **347**: 1151–1160.

Osawa K, Etoh T, Ariyoshi N, *et al.* (2007). Relationship between Kaposi's varicelliform eruption in Japanese patients with atopic dermatitis treated with tacrolimus ointment and genetic polymorphisms in the IL-18 gene promoter region. *Journal of Dermatology*, **34**: 531–536.

Rajka G (1989). *Essential Aspects of Atopic Dermatitis*, Springer-Verlag, Berlin, p. 30.

Ramirez de Knott HM, McCormick TS, Kalka K, *et al.* (2006). Cutaneous hypersensitivity to *Malassezia sympodialis* and dust mite in adult atopic dermatitis with a textile pattern. *Contact Dermatitis*, **54**: 92–99.

Reginald K, Westritschnig K, Linhart B, *et al.* (2011). *Staphylococcus aureus* fibronectin-binding protein specifically binds IgE from patients with atopic dermatitis and requires antigen presentation for cellular immune responses. *Journal of Allergy and Clinical Immunology*, **128**: 82–91.

Ricci G, Patrizi A, Mandrioli P, *et al.* (2006). Evaluation of the antibacterial activity of a special silk textile in the treatment of atopic dermatitis. *Dermatology*, **213**: 224–227.

Rico T, Green J, Kirsner RS (2009). Novel antiviral therapy based on innate immunity. *Journal of Investigative Dermatology*, **129**: 2540.

Rieg S, Steffen H, Seeber S, *et al.* (2005). Deficiency of dermcidin-derived antimicrobial peptides in sweat of patients with atopic dermatitis correlates with an impaired innate defense of human

skin *in vivo*. *Journal of Immunology*, **174**: 8003–8010.

Ring J, Brockow K, Abeck D (1996). The therapeutic concept of 'patient management' in atopic eczema. *Allergy*, **51**: 206–215.

Sais G, Jucglà A, Curcó N, Peyrí J (1994). Kaposi's varicelliform eruption with ocular involvement. *Archives of Dermatology*, **130**: 1209–1210.

Sanderson IR, Brueton LA, Savage MO, Harper JI (1987). Eczema herpeticum: a potentially fatal disease. *British Medical Journal (Clinical Research Edition)*, **294**: 693–694.

Savolainen J, Lintu P, Kosonen J, *et al.* (2001). *Pityrosporum* and *Candida* specific and non-specific humoral, cellular and cytokine responses in atopic dermatitis patients. *Clinical and Experimental Allergy*, **31**: 125–134.

Schempp CM, Effinger T, Czech W, Krutmann J, Simon JC, Schöpf E (1997). Characterization of nonresponders in high dosage UVA1 therapy of acute exacerbated atopic dermatitis [in German]. *Hautarzt*, **48**: 94–99.

Schnopp C, Ring J, Mempel M (2010). The role of antibacterial therapy in atopic eczema. *Expert Opinion in Pharmacotherapy*, **11**: 929–936.

Schopfer K, Baerlocher K, Price P, Krech U, Quie PG, Douglas SD (1979). Staphylococcal IgE antibodies, hyperimmunoglobulinemia E and *Staphylococcus aureus* infections. *New England Journal of Medicine*, **12**: 835–838.

Silva SH, Guedes AC, Gontijo B, *et al.* (2006). Influence of narrow-band UVB phototherapy on cutaneous microbiota of children with atopic dermatitis. *Journal of the European Academy of Dermatology and Venereology*, **20**: 1114–1120.

Solomon LM, Telner P (1966). Eruptive molluscum contagiosum in atopic dermatitis. *Canadian Medical Association Journal*, **95**: 978–979.

Suh L, Coffin S, Leckerman KH, Gelfand JM, Honig PJ, Yan AC (2008). Methicillin-resistant *Staphylococcus aureus* colonization in children with atopic dermatitis. *Pediatric Dermatology*, **25**: 528–534.

Svejgaard E, Faergeman J, Jemec G, Kieffer M, Ottevanger V (1989). Recent investigations on the relationship between fungal skin diseases and atopic dermatitis.

Acta Dermato-Venereologica Supplementum (Stockholm), **144**: 140–142.

Svejgaard E, Larsen PØ, Deleuran M, Ternowitz T, Roed-Petersen J, Nilsson J (2004). Treatment of head and neck dermatitis comparing itraconazole 200 mg and 400 mg daily for 1 week with placebo. *Journal of the European Academy of Dermatology and Venereology*, **18**: 445–449.

Takechi M (2005). Minimum effective dosage in the treatment of chronic atopic dermatitis with itraconazole. *Journal of International Medical Research*, **33**: 273–283.

Tomimori Y, Kawakami Y, McCausland MM, et al. (2011). Protective murine and human monoclonal antibodies against eczema vaccinatum. *Antiviral Therapy*, **16**: 67–75.

Verbist L (1990). The antimicrobial activity of fusidic acid. *Journal of Antimicrobial Chemotherapy*, (suppl B): 1–5.

Voorhees T, Chang J, Yao Y, et al. (2011). Dendritic cells produce inflammatory cytokines in response to bacterial products from *Staphylococcus aureus*-infected atopic dermatitis lesions. *Cellular Immunology*, **267**: 17–22.

Vora S, Damon I, Bulginiti V et al. (2008). Severe eczema vaccinatum in a household contact of smallpox vaccinee. *Clinical Infectious Diseases*, **46**: 1555–1561.

Vu AT, Baba T, Chen X, Le TA, et al. (2010). *Staphylococcus aureus* membrane and diacylated lipopeptide induce thymic stromal lymphopoietin in keratinocytes through the Toll-like receptor 2-Toll-like receptor 6 pathway. *Journal of Allergy and Clinical Immunology*, **126**: 985–993.

Wachs GN, Maibach HI (1976). Cooperative double-blind trial of an antibiotic/corticoid combination in impetiginized atopic dermatitis. *British Journal of Dermatology*, **95**: 323–328.

Wahn U, Bos JD, Goodfield M, et al. (2002). Efficacy and safety of pimecrolimus cream in the long-term management of atopic dermatitis in children. *Pediatrics*, **110**: e2.

Walsh GA, Richards KL, Douglas SD, Blumenthal MN (1981). Immunoglobulin E anti-*Staphylococcus aureus* antibodies in atopic patients. *Journal of Clinical Microbiology*, **13**: 1046–1048.

Wann ER, Gurusiddappa S, Hook M (2000). The fibronectin-binding MSCRAMM FnbpA of *Staphylococcus aureus* is a bifunctional protein that also binds to fibrinogen. *Journal of Biological Chemistry*, **275**: 13863–13871.

Wetzel S, Wollenberg A (2004). Eczema molluscatum in tacrolimus treated atopic dermatitis. European *Journal of Dermatology*, **14**: 73–74.

Wheeler CE Jr, Abele DC (1966). Eczema herpeticum, primary and recurrent. *Archives of Dermatology*, **93**: 162–173.

White MI, Noble WC (1985). The cutaneous reaction to staphylococcal protein A in normal subjects and patients with atopic dermatitis or psoriasis. *British Journal of Dermatology*, **113**: 179–183.

Williams RE, Gibson AG, Aitchison TC, Lever R, Mackie RM (1990). Assessment of a contact-plate sampling technique and subsequent quantitative bacterial studies in atopic dermatitis. *British Journal of Dermatology*, **123**: 493–501.

Wilson BB, Deuell B, Mills TA (1993). Atopic dermatitis associated with dermatophyte infection and Trichophyton hypersensitivity. *Cutis*, **51**: 191–192.

Wollenberg A, Wagner M, Günther S, et al. (2002). Plasmacytoid dendritic cells: a new cutaneous dendritic cell subset with distinct role in inflammatory skin diseases. *Journal of Investigative Dermatology*, **119**: 1096–1102.

Wollenberg A, Zoch C, Wetzel S, Plewig G, Przybilla B (2003a). Predisposing factors and clinical features of eczema herpeticum: a retrospective analysis of 100 cases. *Journal of the American Academy of Dermatology*, **49**: 198–205.

Wollenberg A, Wetzel S, Burgdorf WH, Haas J (2003b). Viral infections in atopic dermatitis: pathogenic aspects and clinical management. *Journal of Allergy and Clinical Immunology*, **112**: 667–674.

Yoshimura M, Namura S, Akamatsu H, Horio T (1996). Antimicrobial effects of phototherapy and photochemotherapy *in vivo* and *in vitro*. *British Journal of Dermatology*, **135**: 528–532.

Yoshimura-Mishima M, Akamatsu H, Namura S, Horio T (1999). Suppressive effect of ultraviolet (UVB and PUVA) radiation on superantigen production by *Staphylococcus*

aureus. *Journal of Dermatological Science*, **19**: 31–36.

Zargari A, Eshaghi H, Bäck O, Johansson S, Scheynius A (2001). Serum IgE reactivity to *Malassezia furfur* extract and recombinant *M. furfur* allergens in patients with atopic dermatitis. *Acta Dermato-Venereologica*, **81**: 418–422.

CHAPTER 10

Abramovits W (2005). A clinician's paradigm in the treatment of atopic dermatitis. *Journal of the American Academy of Dermatology*, **53**(1 suppl 1): S70–77.

Abramovits W, Boguniewicz M (2006). A multicenter, randomized, vehicle-controlled clinical study to examine the efficacy and safety of MAS063DP (Atopiclair) in the management of mild to moderate atopic dermatitis in adults. *Journal of Drugs in Dermatology*, **5**: 236–244.

Abramovits W, Perlmutter A (2006). MimyX cream. *Skinmed*, **5**: 29–30.

Abramovits W, Perlmutter A (2007). Atopiclair™: its position within a topical paradigm for the treatment of atopic dermatitis. *Expert Reviews in Dermatology*, **2**: 115–119.

Abramovits W, Goldstein AM, Stevenson LC (2003). Changing paradigms in dermatology: topical immunomodulators within a permutational paradigm for the treatment of atopic and eczematous dermatitis. *Clinics in Dermatology*, **21**: 383–391.

Abramovits W, Boguniewicz M, Paller AS, et al. (2005). The economics of topical immunomodulators for the treatment of atopic dermatitis. *Pharmacoeconomics*, **23**: 543–566.

Alomar A, Berth-Jones J, Bos JD, et al. (2004). The role of topical calcineurin inhibitors in atopic dermatitis. *British Journal of Dermatology*, **151**(suppl 70): 3–27.

Ashcroft DM, Dimmock P, Garside R, Stein K, Williams HC (2005). Efficacy and tolerability of topical pimecrolimus and tacrolimus in the treatment of atopic dermatitis: meta-analysis of randomised controlled trials. *British Medical Journal*, **330**: 516.

Callen J, Chamlin S, Eichenfield LF, et al. (2007). A systematic review of the safety of topical therapies for atopic dermatitis. *British Journal of Dermatology*, **156**: 203–221.

Del Rosso J, Friedlander SF (2005). Corticosteroids: options in the era of steroid-sparing therapy. *Journal of the American Academy of Dermatology*, 53(1 suppl 1): S50–58.

Finlay AY, Edwards PH, Harding KG (1989). 'Fingertip unit' in dermatology. *Lancet*, ii: 155.

Fleischer AB Jr (2006). Black box warning for topical calcineurin inhibitors and the death of common sense. *Dermatology Online Journal*, 12: 2.

Fleischer AB Jr, Abramovits W, Breneman D, Jaracz E (2007). Tacrolimus ointment is more effective than pimecrolimus cream in adult patients with moderate to very severe atopic dermatitis. *Journal of Dermatological Treatment*, 18: 151–157.

Kaufmann R, Bieber T, Helgesen AL, *et al.* (2006). Onset of pruritus relief with pimecrolimus cream 1% in adult patients with atopic dermatitis: a randomized trial. *Allergy*, 61: 375–381.

Kempers S, Boguniewicz M, Carter E, *et al.* (2004). A randomized investigator-blinded study comparing pimecrolimus cream 1% with tacrolimus ointment 0.03% in the treatment of pediatric patients with moderate atopic dermatitis. *Journal of the American Academy of Dermatology*, 51: 515–525.

Koo JY, Fleischer AB Jr, Abramovits W, *et al.* (2005). Tacrolimus ointment is safe and effective in the treatment of atopic dermatitis: results in 8000 patients. *Journal of the American Academy of Dermatology*, 53(2 suppl 2): S195-S205.

Langeveld-Wildschut EG, Riedl H, Thepen T, Bihari IC, Bruijnzeel PL, Bruijnzeel-Koomen CA (2000). Modulation of the atopy patch test reaction by topical corticosteroids and tar. *Journal of Allergy and Clinical Immunology*, 106: 737–743.

Leung DY, Hanifin JM, Pariser DM, *et al.* (2009). Effects of pimecrolimus cream 1% in the treatment of patients with atopic dermatitis who demonstrate a clinical insensitivity to topical corticosteroids: a randomized, multicentre vehicle-controlled trial. *British Journal of Dermatology*, 161: 435–443.

Long CC, Finlay AY, Averill RW (1998). A practical guide to topical therapy in children. *British Journal of Dermatology*, 138: 293–296.

Margolis DJ, Hoffstad O, Bilker W (2007). Lack of association between exposure to topical calcineurin inhibitors and skin cancer in adults. *Dermatology*, 214: 289–295.

Meingassner JG, Aschauer H, Stuetz A, Billich A (2005). Pimecrolimus permeates less than tacrolimus through normal, inflamed, or corticosteroid-pretreated skin. *Experimental Dermatology*, 14: 752–757.

Munkvad M (1989). A comparative trial of Clinitar versus hydrocortisone cream in the treatment of atopic eczema. *British Journal of Dermatology*, 121: 763–766.

National Psoriasis Foundation (1998). *Steroids*, National Psoriasis Foundation, Portland.

Paller AS, Lebwohl M, Fleischer AB Jr, *et al.* (2005). Tacrolimus ointment is more effective than pimecrolimus cream with a similar safety profile in the treatment of atopic dermatitis: results from 3 randomized, comparative studies. *Journal of the American Academy of Dermatology*, 52: 810–822.

Park CW, Lee BH, Lee CH (2005). Tacrolimus reduces staphylococcal colonization on the skin in Korean atopic dermatitis patients. *Drugs under Experimental and Clinical Research*, 31: 77–87.

Rigopoulos D, Ioannides D, Kalogeromitros D, Gregoriou S, Katsambas A (2004). Pimecrolimus cream 1% vs. betamethasone 17-valerate 0.1% cream in the treatment of seborrhoeic dermatitis. A randomized open-label clinical trial. *British Journal of Dermatology*, 151: 1071–1075.

Sabroe RA, Kennedy CT, Archer CB (1997). The effects of topical doxepin on responses to histamine, substance P and prostaglandin E2 in human skin. *British Journal of Dermatology*, 137: 386–390.

Simpson D, Noble S (2005). Tacrolimus ointment: a review of its use in atopic dermatitis and its clinical potential in other inflammatory skin conditions. *Drugs*, 65: 827–858.

Taylor JS, Praditsuwan P, Handel D, Kuffner G (1996). Allergic contact dermatitis from doxepin cream. One-year patch test clinic experience. *Archives of Dermatology*, 132: 515–518.

Thaci D, Salgo R (2010). Malignancy concerns of topical calcineurin inhibitors for atopic dermatitis: facts and controversies. *Clinics in Dermatology*, 28: 52–56.

Thomas KS, Armstrong S, Avery A, *et al.* (2002). Randomised controlled trial of short bursts of a potent topical corticosteroid versus prolonged use of a mild preparation for children with mild or moderate atopic eczema. *British Medical Journal*, 324: 768.

Winiski A, Wang S, Schwendinger B, Stuetz A (2007). Inhibition of T-cell activation *in vitro* in human peripheral blood mononuclear cells by pimecrolimus and glucocorticosteroids and combinations thereof. *Experimental Dermatology*, 16: 699–704.

CHAPTER 11

Akdis CA, Akdis M, Bieber T, *et al.* (2006). Diagnosis and treatment of atopic dermatitis in children and adults: European Academy of Allergology and Clinical Immunology/American Academy of Allergy, Asthma and Immunology/PRACTALL Consensus Report. *Allergy*, 61: 969–987.

Akhavan A, Rudikoff D (2003). The treatment of atopic dermatitis with systemic immunosuppressive agents. *Clinics in Dermatology*, 21: 225–240.

Almawi WY, Melemedjian OK, Rieder MJ (1999). An alternate mechanism of glucocorticoid anti-proliferative effect: promotion of a Th2 cytokine-secreting profile. *Clinical Transplantation*, 13: 365–374.

Alves C, Robazzi TC, Mendonca M (2008). Withdrawal from glucocorticosteroid therapy: clinical practice recommendations. *Jornal de Pediatria (Rio de Janeiro)*, 84: 192–202.

Andres C, Belloni B, Mempel M, Ring J (2008). Omalizumab for patients with severe and therapy-refractory atopic eczema? *Current Allergy and Asthma Reports*, 8: 179–180.

Ballester I, Silvestre JF, Pérez-Crespo M, Lucas A (2009). Severe adult atopic dermatitis: treatment with mycophenolate mofetil in 8 patients. *Actas Dermosifiliograficas*, 100: 883–887.

Beck LA, Saini S (2006). Wanted: a study with omalizumab to determine the role of IgE-mediated pathways in atopic dermatitis. *Journal of the*

American Academy of Dermatology, 55: 540–541; author reply 541–542.

Berth-Jones J, Finlay AY, Zaki I, *et al.* (1996). Cyclosporine in severe childhood atopic dermatitis: a multicenter study. *Journal of the American Academy of Dermatology*, 34: 1016–1021.

Berth-Jones J, Graham-Brown RA, Marks R, *et al.* (1997). Long-term efficacy and safety of cyclosporin in severe adult atopic dermatitis. *British Journal of Dermatology*, 136: 76–81.

Berth-Jones J, Takwale A, Tan E, Barclay G, *et al.* (2002). Azathioprine in severe adult atopic dermatitis: a double-blind, placebo-controlled, crossover trial. *British Journal of Dermatology*, 147: 324–330.

Borchard KL, Orchard D (2008). Systemic therapy of paediatric atopic dermatitis: an update. *Australasian Journal of Dermatology*, 49: 123–134.

Brandt C, Pavlovic V, Radbruch A, Worm M, Baumgrass R (2009). Low-dose cyclosporine A therapy increases the regulatory T cell population in patients with atopic dermatitis. *Allergy*, 64: 1588–1596.

Brinkmann V, Kristofic C (1995). Regulation by corticosteroids of Th1 and Th2 cytokine production in human CD4+ effector T cells generated from CD45RO- and CD45RO+ subsets. *Journal of Immunology*, 155: 3322–3328.

Buys LM (2007). Treatment options for atopic dermatitis. *American Family Physician*, 75: 523–528.

Caruso C, Gaeta F, Valluzzi RL, *et al.* (2010). Omalizumab efficacy in a girl with atopic eczema. *Allergy*, 65: 278–279.

Chacko M, Weinberg JM (2007). Efalizumab. *Dermatologic Therapy*, 20: 265–269.

Cronstein BN, Kimmel SC, Levin RI, Martiniuk F, Weissmann G (1992). A mechanism for the anti-inflammatory effects of corticosteroids: the glucocorticoid receptor regulates leukocyte adhesion to endothelial cells and expression of endothelial-leukocyte adhesion molecule 1 and intercellular adhesion molecule 1. *Proceedings of the National Academy of Science of the United States of America*, 89: 9991–9995.

Dasgupta N, Gelber AC, Racke F, Fine DM (2005). Central nervous system lymphoma associated with mycophenolate mofetil in lupus nephritis. *Lupus*, 14: 910–913.

Denby KS, Beck LA (2012). Update on systemic therapies for atopic dermatitis. *Current Opinion in Allergy and Clinical Immunology*, 12: 421.

Dicarlo JB, McCall CO (2001). Pharmacologic alternatives for severe atopic dermatitis. *International Journal of Dermatology*, 40: 82–88.

Egan CA, Rallis TM, Meadows KP, Krueger GG (1999). Low-dose oral methotrexate treatment for recalcitrant palmoplantar pompholyx. *Journal of the American Academy of Dermatology*, 40: 612–614.

el-Azhary RA, Farmer SA, Drage LA, *et al.* (2009). Thioguanine nucleotides and thiopurine methyltransferase in immunobullous diseases. *Archives of Dermatology*, 145: 644–652.

Fauci AS, Dale DC, Balow JE (1976). Glucocorticosteroid therapy: mechanisms of action and clinical considerations. *Annals of Internal Medicine*, 84: 304–315.

Finotto S, Mekori YA, Metcalfe DD (1997). Glucocorticoids decrease tissue mast cell number by reducing the production of the c-kit ligand, stem cell factor, by resident cells: *in vitro* and *in vivo* evidence in murine systems. *Journal of Clinical Investigation*, 99: 1721–1728.

Forman SB, Garrett AB (2007). Success of omalizumab as monotherapy in adult atopic dermatitis: case report and discussion of the high-affinity immunoglobulin E receptor, FcepsilonRI. *Cutis*, 80: 38–40.

Forte WC, Sumita JM, Rodrigues AG, Liuson D, Tanaka E (2005). Rebound phenomenon to systemic corticosteroid in atopic dermatitis. *Allergologia et immunopathologia (Madrid)*, 33: 307–311.

Ghosh K, Ghosh K (2007). Strongyloides stercoralis septicaemia following steroid therapy for eosinophilia: report of three cases. *Transactions of the Royal Society of Tropical Medicine and Hygiene*, 101: 1163–1165.

Goldsmith P, McGarity B, Walls AF, Church MK, Millward-Sadler GH, Robertson DA (1990). Corticosteroid treatment reduces mast cell numbers in inflammatory bowel disease. *Digestive Disease Science*, 35: 1409–1413.

Goujon C, Berard F, Dahel K, *et al.* (2006). Methotrexate for the treatment of adult atopic dermatitis.

European Journal of Dermatology, 16: 155–158.

Griffiths CE, Dubertret L, Ellis CN, *et al.* (2004). Ciclosporin in psoriasis clinical practice: an international consensus statement. *British Journal of Dermatology*, 150 (suppl 67): 11–23.

Grundmann-Kollmann M, Podda M, Ochsendorf F, *et al.* (2001). Mycophenolate mofetil is effective in the treatment of atopic dermatitis. *Archives of Dermatology*, 137: 870–873.

Haeck IM, Knol MJ, Ten Berge O, van Velsen SG, de Bruin-Weller MS, Bruijnzeel-Koomen CA (2011). Enteric-coated mycophenolate sodium versus cyclosporin A as long-term treatment in adult patients with severe atopic dermatitis: a randomized controlled trial. *Journal of the American Academy of Dermatology*, 64: 1074–1084.

Hanifin JM, Schneider LC, Leung DY, *et al.* (1993). Recombinant interferon gamma therapy for atopic dermatitis. *Journal of the American Academy of Dermatology*, 28(2 Pt 1): 189–197.

Harper JI, Ahmed I, Barclay G, *et al.* (2000). Cyclosporin for severe childhood atopic dermatitis: short course versus continuous therapy. *British Journal of Dermatology*, 142: 52–58.

Heddle RJ, Soothill JF, Bulpitt CJ, *et al.* (1984). Combined oral and nasal beclomethasone diproprionate in children with atopic eczema: a randomised controlled trial. *British Medical Journal (Clinical Research Edition)*, 289: 651–654.

Heil PM, Maurer D, Klein B, *et al.* (2010). Omalizumab therapy in atopic dermatitis: depletion of IgE does not improve the clinical course – a randomized, placebo-controlled and double blind pilot study. *Journal der Deutschen Dermatologischen Gesellschaft*, 8: 990–998.

Heller M, Shin HT, Orlow SJ, *et al.* (2007). Mycophenolate mofetil for severe childhood atopic dermatitis: experience in 14 patients. *British Journal of Dermatology*, 157: 127–132.

Hijnen D, Haeck I, van Kraats AA, *et al.* (2009). Cyclosporin A reduces CD4(+)CD25(+) regulatory T-cell numbers in patients with atopic dermatitis. *Journal of Allergy and Clinical Immunology*, 124: 856–858.

Hong J, Koo B, Koo J (2008). The psychosocial and occupational impact of chronic skin disease. *Dermatologic Therapy*, **21**: 54–59.

Jacobi A, Antoni C, Manger B, *et al.* (2005). Infliximab in the treatment of moderate to severe atopic dermatitis. *Journal of the American Academy of Dermatology*, **52**(3 Pt 1): 522–526.

Jang IG, Yang JK, Lee HJ, *et al.* (2000). Clinical improvement and immunohistochemical findings in severe atopic dermatitis treated with interferon gamma. *Journal of the American Academy of Dermatology*, **42**: 1033–1040.

Kalb RE, Strober B, Weinstein G, *et al.* (2009). Methotrexate and psoriasis: (2009). National Psoriasis Foundation Consensus Conference. *Journal of the American Academy of Dermatology*, **60**: 824–837.

Kazlow Stern D, Tripp JM, Ho VC, *et al.* (2005). The use of systemic immune moderators in dermatology: an update. *Dermatologic Clinics*, **23**: 259–300.

Khan S, Subedi D, Chowdhury MM (2006). Use of amino terminal type III procollagen peptide (P3NP) assay in methotrexate therapy for psoriasis. *Postgraduate Medical Journal*, **82**: 353–354.

Knowles SR, Gupta AK, Shear NH, Sauder D (1995). Azathioprine hypersensitivity-like reactions – a case report and a review of the literature. *Clinical and Experimental Dermatology*, **20**: 353–356.

Krathen RA, Hsu S (2005). Failure of omalizumab for treatment of severe adult atopic dermatitis. *Journal of the American Academy of Dermatology*, **53**: 338–340.

Krynetski EY, Evans WE (2000). Genetic polymorphism of thiopurine *S*-methyltransferase: molecular mechanisms and clinical importance. *Pharmacology*, **61**: 136–146.

Kuanprasert N, Herbert O, Barnetson RS (2002). Clinical improvement and significant reduction of total serum IgE in patients suffering from severe atopic dermatitis treated with oral azathioprine. *Australasian Journal of Dermatology*, **43**: 125–127.

La Rosaa M, Musarraa I, Rannoa C, *et al.* (1995). A randomized, double-blind, placebo-controlled, crossover trial of systemic flunisolide in the treatment of children with severe atopic dermatitis. *Current Therapeutic Research*, **56**: 720–726.

Lear JT, English JS, Jones P, *et al.* (1996). Retrospective review of the use of azathioprine in severe atopic dermatitis. *Journal of the American Academy of Dermatology*, **35**: 642–643.

Liu HN, Wong CK (1997). *In vitro* immunosuppressive effects of methotrexate and azathioprine on Langerhans cells. *Archives of Dermatological Research*, **289**: 94–97.

Lucky AW (1984). Principles of the use of glucocorticosteroids in the growing child. *Pediatric Dermatology*, **1**: 226–235.

Lyakhovitsky A, Barzilai A, Heyman R, *et al.* (2010). Low-dose methotrexate treatment for moderate-to-severe atopic dermatitis in adults. *Journal of the European Academy of Dermatology and Venereology*, **24**: 43–49.

Meggitt SJ, Reynolds NJ (2001). Azathioprine for atopic dermatitis. *Clinical and Experimental Dermatology*, **26**: 369–375.

Miyaura H, Iwata M (2002). Direct and indirect inhibition of Th1 development by progesterone and glucocorticoids. *Journal of Immunology*, **168**: 1087–1094.

Murphy LA, Atherton DJ (2003). Azathioprine as a treatment for severe atopic eczema in children with a partial thiopurine methyl transferase (TPMT) deficiency. *Pediatric Dermatology*, **20**: 531–534.

Murray ML, Cohen JB (2007). Mycophenolate mofetil therapy for moderate to severe atopic dermatitis. *Clinical and Experimental Dermatology*, **32**: 23–27.

Musial J, Milewski M, Undas A, *et al.* (1995). Interferon-gamma in the treatment of atopic dermatitis: influence on T cell activation. *Allergy*, **50**: 520–523.

Nakamura S, Takeda K, Hashimoto Y, *et al.* (2011). Favorable clinical response by pre-prandial administration of low-dose ciclosporin to severe adult atopic dermatitis. *Journal of Dermatological Treatment*, [Epub ahead of print].

Nakano T, Ohara O, Teraoka H, *et al.* (1990). Glucocorticoids suppress group II phospholipase A2 production by blocking mRNA synthesis and post-transcriptional expression. *Journal of Biological Chemistry*, **265**: 12745–12748.

Neuber K, Schwartz I, Itschert G, *et al.* (2000). Treatment of atopic eczema with oral mycophenolate mofetil.

British Journal of Dermatology, **143**: 385–391.

Porter CM, Clipstone NA (2002). Sustained NFAT signaling promotes a Th1-like pattern of gene expression in primary murine CD4+ T cells. *Journal of Immunology*, **168**: 4936–4945.

Qureshi A, Scheinfeld N (2008). Myfortic (mycophenolate sodium) delayed-release tablets. *Dermatology Online Journal*, **14**: 4.

Rouse C, Siegfried E (2008). Methotrexate for atopic dermatitis in children. *Journal of the American Academy of Dermatology*, **58**(suppl 2): AB7.

Sabbagh F, El Tawil Z, Lecerf F, *et al.* (2008). Impact of cyclosporine A on magnesium homeostasis: clinical observation in lung transplant recipients and experimental study in mice. *Transplantation*, **86**: 436–444.

Santini MP, Talora C, Seki T, Bolgan L, Dotto GP (2001). Cross talk among calcineurin, Sp1/Sp3, and NFAT in control of p21(WAF1/CIP1) expression in keratinocyte differentiation. *Proceedings of the National Academy of Sciences of the USA*, **98**: 9575–9580.

Schreiber SL, Crabtree GR (1992). The mechanism of action of cyclosporin A and FK506. *Immunology Today*, **13**: 136–142.

Sediva A, Kayserova J, Vernerova E, *et al.* (2008). Anti-CD20 (rituximab) treatment for atopic eczema. *Journal of Allergy and Clinical Immunology*, **121**: 1515–1516; author reply 1516–1517.

Shaffrali FC, Colver GB, Messenger AG, *et al.* (2003). Experience with low-dose methotrexate for the treatment of eczema in the elderly. *Journal of the American Academy of Dermatology*, **48**: 417–419.

Shaw MG, Burkhart CN, Morrell DS (2009). Systemic therapies for pediatric atopic dermatitis: a review for the primary care physician. *Pediatric Annals*, **38**: 380–387.

Sheinkopf LE, Rafi AW, Do LT, *et al.* (2008). Efficacy of omalizumab in the treatment of atopic dermatitis: a pilot study. *Allergy and Asthma Proceedings*, **29**: 530–537.

Shulman DI, Palmert MR, Kemp SF (2007). Adrenal insufficiency: still a cause of morbidity and death in childhood. *Pediatrics*, **119**: e484–494.

Simon D, Hösli S, Kostylina G, Yawalkar N, Simon HU (2008). Anti-CD20 (rituximab) treatment improves atopic eczema. *Journal of Allergy and Clinical Immunology*, **121**: 122–128.

Sonenthal KR, Grammer LC, Patterson R (1993). Do some patients with atopic dermatitis require long-term oral steroid therapy? *Journal of Allergy and Clinical Immunology*, **91**: 971–973.

Truhan AP, Ahmed AR (1989). Corticosteroids: a review with emphasis on complications of prolonged systemic therapy. *Annals of Allergy*, **62**: 375–391.

Tsang HH, Trendell-Smith NJ, Wu AK, Mok MY (2010). Diffuse large B-cell lymphoma of the central nervous system in mycophenolate mofetil-treated patients with systemic lupus erythematosus. *Lupus*, **19**: 330–3.

van Velsen SG, Haeck IM, Bruijnzeel-Koomen CA, de Bruin-Weller MS (2009). First experience with enteric-coated mycophenolate sodium (Myfortic) in severe recalcitrant adult atopic dermatitis: an open label study. *British Journal of Dermatology*, **160**: 687–691.

Vane J, Botting R (1987). Inflammation and the mechanism of action of anti-inflammatory drugs. *Faseb Journal*, **1**: 89–96.

Vernino S, Salomao DR, Habermann TM, O'Neill BP (2005). Primary CNS lymphoma complicating treatment of myasthenia gravis with mycophenolate mofetil. *Neurology*, **65**: 639–641.

Weatherhead SC, Wahie S, Reynolds NJ, Meggitt SJ (2007). An open-label, dose-ranging study of methotrexate for moderate-to-severe adult atopic eczema. *British Journal of Dermatology*, **156**: 346–351.

Wee JS, Marinaki A, Smith CH (2011). Life threatening myelotoxicity secondary to azathioprine in a patient with atopic eczema and normal thiopurine methyltransferase activity. *British Medical Journal*, **342**: d1417.

Wolverton SE (2009). Optimizing clinical use of azathioprine with newer pharmacogenetic data. *Archives of Dermatology*, **145**: 707–710.

Woolley KL, Gibson PG, Carty K, Wilson AJ, Twaddell SH, Woolley MJ (1996). Eosinophil apoptosis and the resolution of airway inflammation in asthma. *American Journal of Respiratory and Critical Care Medicine*, **154**: 237–243.

Zaki I, Emerson R, Allen BR (1996). Treatment of severe atopic dermatitis in childhood with cyclosporin. *British Journal of Dermatology*, **135**(suppl 48): 21–24.

Zonneveld IM, De Rie MA, Beljaards RC, et al. (1996). The long-term safety and efficacy of cyclosporin in severe refractory atopic dermatitis: a comparison of two dosage regimens. *British Journal of Dermatology*, **135**(suppl 48): 15–20.

CHAPTER 12

Abeck D, Schmidt T, Fesq H, et al. (2000). Long-term efficacy of medium-dose UVA1 phototherapy in atopic dermatitis. *Journal of the American Academy of Dermatology*, **42**: 254–257.

Atherton DJ, Carabott F, Glover MT, et al. (1988). The role of psoralen photochemotherapy (PUVA) in the treatment of severe atopic eczema in adolescents. *British Journal of Dermatology*, **118**: 791–795.

Autio P, Komulainen P, Larni HM (2002). Heliotherapy in atopic dermatitis: a prospective study on climatotherapy using the SCORAD index. *Acta Dermato-Venereologica*, **82**: 436–40.

Baltás E, Csoma Z, Bodai L, Ignácz F, Dobozy A, Kemény L (2006). Treatment of atopic dermatitis with the xenon chloride excimer laser. *Journal of the European Academy of Dermatology and Venereology*, **20**: 657–660.

Breuckmann F, von Kobyletzki G, Avermaete A, et al. (2002a). Mononuclear cells in atopic dermatitis *in vivo*: immunomodulation of the cutaneous infiltrate by medium-dose UVA1 phototherapy. *European Journal of Medical Research*, 7(7): 315–22.

Breuckmann F, von Kobyletzki G, Avermaete A, et al. (2002b). Modulation of cathepsin G expression in severe atopic dermatitis following medium-dose UVA1 phototherapy. *BMC Dermatology*, **2**: 12.

Bulkley LD (1881). *Eczema and Its Management*, 2nd edn, G.P. Putnam's Sons, New York, p. 318.

Calzavara-Pinton P, Monari P, Manganoni AM, et al. (2010). Merkel cell carcinoma arising in immunosuppressed patients treated with high-dose ultraviolet A1 (320–400 nm) phototherapy: a report of two cases. *Photodermatology, Photoimmunology and Photomedicine*, **26**: 263–265.

Clayton TH, Clark SM, Turner D, Goulden V (2007). The treatment of severe atopic dermatitis in childhood with narrowband ultraviolet B phototherapy. *Clinical and Experimental Dermatology*, **32**: 28–33.

Collins P, Ferguson J (1995). Narrowband (TL-01) UVB air-conditioned phototherapy for atopic eczema in children. *British Journal of Dermatology*, **133**: 653–667.

Darsow U, Wollenberg A, Simon D et al. (2010). ETFAD/EADV eczema task force (2009) position paper on diagnosis and treatment of atopic dermatitis. *Journal of the European Academy of Dermatology and Venereology*, **24**: 317–28.

Dawe RS (2003). Ultraviolet A1 phototherapy. *British Journal of Dermatology*, **148**: 626–637.

de Kort WJ, van Weelden H (2000). Bath psoralen-ultraviolet A therapy in atopic eczema. *Journal of the European Academy of Dermatology and Venereology*, **14**: 172–174.

Der-Petrossian M, Seeber A, Hönigsmann H, et al. (2000). Half-side comparison study on the efficacy of 8-methoxypsoralen bath-PUVA versus narrowband ultraviolet B phototherapy in patients with severe chronic atopic dermatitis. *British Journal of Dermatology*, **142**: 39–43.

Dittmar HC, Pflieger D, Schempp CM, et al. (1999). Comparison of balneophototherapy and UVA/B monophototherapy in patients with subacute atopic dermatitis. *Hautarzt*, **50**: 649–653.

Dogra S, De D (2010). Phototherapy and photochemotherapy in childhood dermatoses. *Indian Journal of Dermatology, Venereology and Leprology*, **76**: 521–526.

Gambichler T (2007). Balneophototherapy for psoriasis using saltwater baths and UVB irradiation, revisited. *Archives of Dermatology*, **143**: 647–649.

Gambichler T (2009). Management of atopic dermatitis using photo(chemo) therapy. *Archives of Dermatological Research*, **301**: 197–203.

Gambichler T, Küster W, Kreuter A, et al. (2000). Balneophototherapy – combined treatment of psoriasis vulgaris and atopic dermatitis with saltwater baths and artificial ultraviolet radiation. *Journal of the European Academy of Dermatology and Venereology*, **14**: 425–428.

Gambichler T, Breuckmann F, Boms S, et al. (2005). Narrowband UVB phototherapy in skin conditions beyond psoriasis. *Journal of the American Academy of Dermatology*, **52**: 660–670.

Gambichler T, Kreuter A, Tomi NS, Othlinghaus N, Altmeyer P, Skrygan M (2008). Gene expression of cytokines in atopic eczema before and after ultraviolet A1 phototherapy. *British Journal of Dermatology*, **158**: 1117–1120.

George SA, Bilsland DJ, Johnson BE, et al. (1993). Narrowband (TL-01) UVB airconditioned phototherapy for chronic severe adult atopic dermatitis. *British Journal of Dermatology*, **128**: 49–56.

Green C, Ferguson J, Lakshmipathi T, Johnson BE (1988). 311 nm UVB phototherapy – an effective treatment for psoriasis. *British Journal of Dermatology*, **119**: 691–696.

Grundmann-Kollmann M, Behrens S, Podda M, Peter RU, Kaufmann R, Kerscher M (1999). Phototherapy for atopic eczema with narrowband UVB. *Journal of the American Academy of Dermatology*, **40**(6 Pt 1): 995–997.

Hannuksela M, Karvonen J, Husa M, et al. (1985). Ultraviolet light therapy in atopic dermatitis. *Acta Dermato-Venereologica*, **114**(suppl): 137–139.

Harari M, Shani J, Seidl V, et al. (2000). Climatotherapy of atopic dermatitis at the Dead Sea: demographic evaluation and cost-effectiveness. *International Journal of Dermatology*, **39**: 59–69.

Heinlin J, Schiffner-Rohe J, Schiffner R, et al. (2011). A first prospective randomized controlled trial on the efficacy and safety of synchronous balneophototherapy vs. narrowband UVB monotherapy for atopic dermatitis. *Journal of the European Academy of Dermatology and Venereology*, **25**: 765–773.

Hjerppe M, Hasan T, Saksala I, et al. (2001). Narrowband UVB treatment in atopic dermatitis. *Acta Dermato-Venereologica*, **81**: 439–440.

Horio T (1998). Skin disorders that improve by exposure to sunlight. *Clinics in Dermatology*, **16**: 59–65.

Hudson-Peacock MJ, Diffey BL, Farr PM (1996). Narrowband UVB phototherapy for severe atopic dermatitis. *British Journal of Dermatology*, **135**: 332.

Jekler J, Larkö O (1990a). The effect of ultraviolet radiation with peaks at 300 nm and 350 nm in the treatment of atopic dermatitis. *Photodermatology, Photoimmunology and Photomedicine*, **7**: 169–172.

Jekler J, Larkö O (1990b). Combined UVA-UVB versus UVB phototherapy for atopic dermatitis: a paired-comparison study. *Journal of the American Academy of Dermatology*, **22**: 49–53.

Jekler J, Larkö O (1991). Phototherapy for atopic dermatitis with ultraviolet A (UVA), low-dose UVB and combined UVA and UVB: two paired-comparison studies. *Photodermatology, Photoimmunology and Photomedicine*, **8**: 151–156.

Jury CS, McHenry P, Burden AD, Lever R, Bilsland D (2006). Narrowband ultraviolet B (UVB) phototherapy in children. *Clinical and Experimental Dermatology*, **31**: 196–199.

Kowalzick L, Kleinheinz A, Weichenthal M, et al. (1995). Low dose versus medium dose UV-A1 treatment in severe atopic eczema. *Acta Dermato-Venereologica*, **75**: 43–45.

Krutmann J (2000). Phototherapy for atopic dermatitis. *Clinical and Experimental Dermatology*, **25**: 552–558.

Krutmann J, Czech W, Diepgen T, et al. (1992). High-dose UVA1 therapy in the treatment of patients with atopic dermatitis. *Journal of the American Academy of Dermatology*, **26**: 225–230.

Krutmann J, Diepgen TL, Luger TA, et al. (1998). High-dose UVA1 therapy for atopic dermatitis: results of a multicenter trial. *Journal of the American Academy of Dermatology*, **38**: 589–593.

Larkö O (1996). Phototherapy of eczema. *Photodermatology, Photoimmunology and Photomedicine*, **12**: 91–94.

Lee E, Koo J, Berger T (2005). UVB phototherapy and skin cancer risk: a review of the literature. *International Journal of Dermatology*, **44**: 355–360.

Legat FJ, Hofer A, Brabek E, et al. (2003). Narrowband UV-B vs medium-dose UV-A1 phototherapy in chronic atopic dermatitis. *Archives of Dermatology*, **139**: 223–224.

Meduri NB, Vandergriff T, Rasmussen H, et al. (2007). Phototherapy in the management of atopic dermatitis: a systematic review. *Photodermatology, Photoimmunology and Photomedicine*, **23**: 106–112.

Midelfart K, Stenvold SE, Volden G (1985). Combined UVB and UVA phototherapy of atopic eczema. *Dermatologica*, **171**: 95–98.

Morita A, Krutmann J (2000). Ultraviolet A radiation-induced apoptosis. *Methods in Enzymology*, **319**: 302–309.

Morita A, Werfel T, Stege H, et al. (1997). Evidence that singlet oxygen-induced human T helper cell apoptosis is the basic mechanism of ultraviolet-A radiation phototherapy. *Journal of Experimental Medicine*, **186**: 1763–1768.

Mutzhas MF, Hölzle E, Hofmann C, Plewig G (1981). A new apparatus with high radiation energy between 320-460 nm: physical description and dermatological applications. *Journal of Investigative Dermatology*, **76**: 42–47.

Nexmand PH (1948). *Clinical Studies of Besnier's Prurigo*, Rosenkilde & Bagger, Copenhagen, pp. 132–148.

Nisticò SP, Saraceno R, Capriotti E, Felice CD, Chimenti S (2008). Efficacy of monochromatic excimer light (308 nm) in the treatment of atopic dermatitis in adults and children. *Photomedicine and Laser Surgery*, **26**(1): 14–18.

Pavlovsky M, Baum S, Shpiro D, Pavlovsky L, Pavlotsky F (2011). Narrowband UVB: is it effective andsafe for pediatric psoriasis and atopic dermatitis? *Journal of the European Academy of Dermatology and Venereology*, **25**: 727–729.

Polderman MCA, Wintzen M, le Cessie S, et al. (2005). UVA-1 cold light therapy in the treatment of atopic dermatitis: 61 patients treated in the Leiden University Medical Center. *Photodermatology, Photoimmunology and Photomedicine*, **21**: 93–96.

Prinz B, Michelsen S, Pfeiffer C, et al. (1999). Long-term application of extracorporeal photochemotherapy in severe atopic dermatitis. *Journal of the American Academy of Dermatology*, **40**: 577–582.

Pugashetti R, Lim HW, Koo J (2010). Broadband UVB revisited: is the narrowband UVB fad limiting our therapeutic options? *Journal of Dermatologic Treatment*, **21**: 326–330.

Radenhausen M, Michelsen S, Plewig G, *et al.* (2004). Bicentre experience in the treatment of severe generalised atopic dermatitis with extracorporeal photochemotherapy. *Journal of Dermatology*, **31**: 961–9670.

Reynolds NJ, Franklin V, Gray JC, *et al.* (2001). Narrowband ultraviolet B and broadband ultraviolet A phototherapy in adult atopic eczema: a randomized controlled trial. *Lancet*, **357**: 2012–2016.

Richter HI, Billmann-Eberwein C, Grewe M, *et al.* (1998). Successful monotherapy of severe and intractable atopic dermatitis by photopheresis. *Journal of the American Academy of Dermatology*, **38**: 585–588.

Sand M, Bechara FG, Sand D, *et al.* (2007). Extracorporeal photopheresis as a treatment for patients with severe, refractory atopic dermatitis. *Dermatology*, **215**: 134–138.

Scheinfeld NS, Tutrone WD, Weinberg JM, *et al.* (2003). Phototherapy of atopic dermatitis. *Clinics in Dermatology*, **21**: 241–248.

Schiffner R, Schiffner-Rohe J, Gerstenhauer M, *et al.* (2002). Dead Sea treatment – principle for outpatient use in atopic dermatitis: safety and efficacy of synchronous balneophototherapy using narrowband UVB and bathing in Dead Sea salt solution. *European Journal of Dermatology*, **12**: 543–548.

Sheehan MP, Atherton DJ, Norris P, *et al.* (1993). Oral psoralen photochemotherapy in severe childhood atopic eczema: an update. *British Journal of Dermatology*, **129**: 431–436.

Stern RS (2001). PUVA Follow up Study. The risk of melanoma in association with long-term exposure to PUVA. *Journal of the American Academy of Dermatology*, **44**: 755–761.

Tintle S, Shemer A, Suárez-Fariñas M, *et al.* (2011). Reversal of atopic dermatitis with narrowband UVB phototherapy and biomarkers for therapeutic response. *Journal of Allergy and Clinical Immunology*, **128**: 583–593.

Turner MA, Devlin J, David TJ (1991). Holidays and atopic eczema. *Archives of Disease in Childhood*, **66**: 212–215.

Tzaneva S, Seeber A, Schwaiger M, *et al.* (2001). High-dose versus medium-dose UVA1 phototherapy for patients with severe generalized atopic dermatitis. *Journal of the American Academy of Dermatology*, **45**: 503–507.

Tzaneva S, Kittler H, Holzer G, *et al.* (2010). Methoxypsoralen plus ultraviolet (UV) A is superior to medium-dose UVA1 in the treatment of severe atopic dermatitis: a randomized crossover trial. *British Journal of Dermatology*, **162**: 655–60.

Uetsu N, Horio T (2003). Treatment of persistent severe atopic dermatitis in 113 Japanese patients with oral psoralen photochemotherapy. *Journal of Dermatology*, **30**: 450–457.

Valkova S, Velkova A (2004). UVA/UVB phototherapy for atopic dermatitis revisited. *Journal of Dermatological Treatment*, **15**: 239–244.

von Kobyletzki G, Pieck C, Hoffmann K, *et al.* (1999). Medium-dose UVA1 cold-light phototherapy in the treatment of severe atopic dermatitis. *Journal of the American Academy of Dermatology*, **41**: 931–937.

Weischer M, Blum A, Eberhard F, *et al.* (2004). No evidence for increased skin cancer risk in psoriasis patients treated with broadband or narrowband UVB phototherapy: a first retrospective study. *Acta Dermato-Venereologica*, **84**: 370–374.

Wollenschläger I, Hermann J, Ockenfels HM (2009). Targeted UVB-308 nm (NUVB) therapy with excimer laser in the treatment of atopic dermatitis and other inflammatory dermatoses. *Hautarzt*, **60**: 898–906.

Yoshiike T, Aikawa Y, Sindhvananda J, *et al.* (1993). A proposed guideline for psoralen photochemotherapy (PUVA) with atopic dermatitis: successful therapeutic effect on severe and intractable cases. *Journal of Dermatological Science*, **5**: 50–53.

Zimmermann J, Utermann S (1994). Photobrine therapy in patients with psoriasis and neurodermatitis atopica [in German]. *Hautarzt*, **45**: 849–853.

CHAPTER 13

Aggarwal R, Potamitis T, Chong N, Guarro M, Shah P, Kheterpal S (1993). Extensive visual loss with topical facial steroids. *Eye*, **7**: 664–666.

Akova Y, Jabbur N, Neumann R, Foster C (1993). Atypical ocular atopy. *Ophthalmology*, **100**: 1367–1371.

Amemiya T, Matsuda H, Uehara M (1980). Ocular findings in atopic dermatitis with special reference to the clinical features of atopic cataract. *Ophthalmologica*, **180**: 129–132.

Amer R, Bamonte G, Forrester J (2007). Uveitis associated with immunoglobulin E-mediated allergic diseases. *Clinical Experimental Ophthalmology*, **35**: 677–678.

Amin K, Belsito D (2006). The etiology of eyelid dermatitis: a 10-year retrospective analysis. *Contact Dermatitis*, **55**: 280–285.

Anderson K, Broesby-Olsen S (2006). Allergic contact dermatitis from oleyl alcohol in Elidel cream. *Contact Dermatitis*, **55**: 354–356.

Anonymous (2007). Topical tacrolimus plus oral alcohol: skin irritation. *Prescribe International* **16**(92): 249.

Armaly M (1965). Statistical attributes of the steroid hypertensive response in the clinically normal eye. *Investigative Ophthalmology*, **4**: 187–197.

Asano-Kato N, Fukagawa K, Tsubota K, Urayama K, Takahashi S, Fujishima H (2001). Quantitative evaluation of atopic blepharitis by scoring of eyelid conditions and measuring the water content of the skin and evaporation from the eyelid surface. *Cornea*, **20**: 255–259.

Asano-Kato N, Fukagawa K, Takano Y, *et al.* (2003). Treatment of atopic blepharitis by controlling eyelid skin water retention ability with ceramide gel application. *British Journal of Ophthalmology*, **87**: 362–363.

Assiri A, Yousuf B, Quantock A, Murphy P (2005). Incidence and severity of keratoconus in Asir province, Saudi Arabia. *British Journal of Ophthalmology*, **89**: 1403–1406.

Ayaki M, Ohoguro N, Azuma N, *et al.* (2002). Detection of cytotoxic anti-lens epithelium-derived growth factor autoantibodies in atopic dermatitis. *Autoimmunity* **35**: 319–327.

Bawazeer A, Hodge W, Lorimer B (2000). Atopy and keratoconus: a multivariate analysis. *British Journal of Ophthalmology*, 84: 834–836.

Brandonisio T, Bachman J, Sears J (2001). Atopic dermatitis: a case report and current clinical review of systemic and ocular manifestations. *Optometry*, 72: 94–102.

Carmi E, Defossez-Tribout C, Ganry O, *et al.* (2006). Ocular complications of atopic dermatitis in children. *Acta Dermato-Venereologica*, 86: 515–517.

Carnahan M, Goldstein D (2000). Ocular complications of topical, periocular, and systemic corticosteroids. *Current Opinion in Ophthalmology*, 11: 478–483.

Castrow F (1981). Atopic cataracts versus steroid cataracts. *Journal of the American Academy of Dermatology*, 5: 64–66.

Chang P, Yang C, Yang C, *et al.* (2005). Clinical characteristics and surgical outcomes of pediatric rhegmatogenous retinal detachment in Taiwan. *American Journal of Ophthalmology*, 139: 1067–1072.

Chen C, Huang J, Yang K, Chen H (2000). Atopic cataracts in a child with atopic dermatitis: a case report and review of the literature. *Asian Pacific Journal of Allergy and Immunology*, 18: 69–71.

Chen S, Jiunn-Feng H, Te-Cheng Y (2006). Pediatric rhegmatogenous retinal detachment in Taiwan. *Retina*, 26: 410–414.

Chin MS, Caruso R, Detrick B, Hooks J (2006). Autoantibodies to p75/lens epithelium-derived growth factor, a cell survival factor, found in patients with atypical retinal degeneration. *Journal of Autoimmunity*, 27: 17–27.

Clark A, Brotchie D, Read A, *et al.* (2005). Dexamethasone alters F-actin architecture and promotes cross-linked actin network formation in human trabecular meshwork tissue. *Cell Motility and the Cytoskeleton*, 60: 83–95.

Cornish KS, Gregory ME, Ramaesh K (2010). Systemic cyclosporin A in severe atopic keratoconjunctivitis. *European Journal of Ophthalmology*, 20: 844–851.

Cubey R (1976). Glaucoma following the application of corticosteroid to the skin of the eyelids. *British Journal of Dermatology*, 95: 207–208.

David M, el-Azhary R, Farmer S (2007). Results of patch testing to a corticosteroid series: a retrospective review of 1188 patients during 6 years at Mayo Clinic. *Journal of the American Academy of Dermatology*, 56: 921–927.

Dogru M, Nakagawa N, Tetsumoto K, Katakami C, Yamamoto M (1999). Ocular surface disease in atopic dermatitis. *Japanese Journal of Ophthalmology*, 43: 53–57.

Dogru M, Asano-Kato N, Tanaka M, *et al.* (2005a). Ocular surface and MUC5AC alterations in atopic patients with corneal shield ulcers. *Current Eye Research*, 30: 897–908.

Dogru M, Okada N, Asano-Kato N, *et al.* (2005b). Atopic ocular surface disease: implications on tear function and ocular surface mucins. *Cornea*, 24(8 suppl): S18–S23.

Dogru M, Okada N, Asano-Kato A, *et al.* (2006). Alterations of the ocular surface epithelial mucins 1, 2, 4 and the tear functions in patients with atopic keratoconjunctivitis. *Clinical and Experimental Allergy*, 36: 1556–1565.

Donshik P, Cavanaugh H, Boruchoff S, Dohlman C (1981). Posterior subcapsular cataracts induced by topical corticosteroids following keratoplasty for keratoconus. *Annals of Ophthalmology*, 13: 29–32.

Ehst B, Warshaw E (2004). Alcohol-induced application site erythema after topical immunomodulator use and its inhibition by aspirin. *Archives of Dermatology*, 140: 1014–1015.

Eisenlohr J (1983). Glaucoma following the prolonged use of topical steroid medication to the eyelids. *Journal of the American Academy of Dermatology*, 8: 878–881.

Fisher A (1986). The role of patch testing. In: *Contact Dermatitis*, Lea & Febiger, Philadelphia.

Francois J (1984). Corticosteroid glaucoma. *Ophthalmologica*, 188: 76–81.

Freeman A, Serle J, Van Veldhuisen P, *et al.* (2004). Tacrolimus ointment in the treatment of eyelid dermatitis. *Cutis*, 73: 267–271.

Ganapathy V, Casiano C (2004). Autoimmunity to the nuclear autoantigen DFS70 (LEDGF): What exactly are the autoantibodies trying to tell us? *Arthritis and Rheumatism*, 50: 684–688.

Garrity J, Liesegang (1984). Ocular complications of atopic dermatitis. *Canadian Journal of Ophthalmology*, 19: 21–24.

Garrott H, Walland M (2004). Glaucoma from topical corticosteroids to the eyelids. *Clinical Experimental Ophthalmology*, 32: 224–226.

Guglielmetti S, Dart JK, Calder V (2010). Atopic keratoconjunctivitis and atopic dermatitis. *Current Opinion in Allergy and Clinical Immunology*, 10: 478–485.

Guin J (2002). Eyelid dermatitis: experience in 203 cases. *Journal of the American Academy of Dermatology*, 47: 755–765.

Haeck IM, Rouwen TJ, Mik LT, *et al.* (2011). Topical corticosteroids in atopic dermatitis and the risk of glaucoma and cataracts. *Journal of the American Academy of Dermatology*, 64: 275–81.

Hida T, Tano Y, Okinami S, Ogino N, Inoue M (2000). Multicenter retrospective study of retinal detachment associated with atopic dermatitis. *Japanese Journal of Ophthalmology*, 44: 407–418.

Hoang-Xuan T, Prisant O, Hannouche D, Robin H (1997). Systemic cyclosporine A in severe atopic keratoconjunctivitis. *Ophthalmology*, 104: 1300–1305.

Hutnik C, Nichols B (1999). Cataracts in systemic diseases and syndromes. *Current Opinion in Ophthalmology*, 10: 22–28.

Ibarra-Duran M, Mena-Cedillos C, Rodriguez-Almaraz M (1992). Cataracts and atopic dermatitis in children. A study of 68 patients. *Boletin Medico del Hospital Infantil de Mexico*, 49: 851–855.

Inomata M, Hayashi M, Shumiya S, Kawashima S, Ito Y (2001). Involvement of inducible nitric oxide synthase in cataract formation in Shumiya cataract rat (SCR). *Current Eye Research*, 23: 307–311.

Inoue M, Shinoda K, Ishida S, *et al.* (2005). Intraocular lens implantation after atopic cataract surgery decreases incidence of postoperative retinal detachment. *Ophthalmology*, 112: 1719–1724.

Ito Y, Nabekura T, Takeda M, *et al.* (2001). Nitric oxide participates in cataract development in selenite-treated rats. *Current Eye Research*, 22: 215–220.

Jobling A, Augusteyn R (2002). What causes steroid cataracts? A review of steroid-induced posterior subcapsular cataracts. *Clinical Experimental Optometry*, 85: 61–75.

Jones R, Rhee D (2006). Corticosteroid-induced ocular hypertension and glaucoma: a brief review and update of the literature. *Current Opinion in Ophthalmology*, 17: 163–167.

Kallen C, Reinhard T, Schilgen G, *et al.* (2003). Atopic keratoconjunctivitis: probably a risk factor for the development of conjunctival carcinoma. *Ophthalmology*, 100: 808–814.

Katshushima H, Miyazaki I, Sekina N, Nishio C, Matsuda M (1994). Incidence of cataract and retinal detachment associated with atopic dermatitis. *Nippon Ganka Gakkai Zasshi*, 98: 495–500.

Katsura H, Hida T (1984). Retinal detachment associated with atopic dermatitis. *Retina*, 4: 148–151.

Katsura H, Oda H, Utsumi Y (1994). Breaks in the pars plicata following surgery for atopic cataract. *Ophthalmic Surgery*, 25: 514–515.

Kaufman P, Alm A (2003). *Adler's Physiology of the Eye: Clinical application*, Mosby, St Louis.

Kenney C, Brown D (2003). The cascade hypothesis of keratoconus. *Contact Lens and the Anterior Eye*, 26: 139–146.

Kersey J, Broadway D (2006). Corticosteroid-induced glaucoma: review of the literature. *Eye*, 20: 407–416.

Knight A, Boxer M, Chandler J (2005). Alcohol-induced rash caused by topical tacrolimus. *Annals of Allergy, Asthma, and Immunology*, 95: 291–292.

Kobatashi S, Roy D, Spector A (1982). Sodium/potassium ATPase in normal and cataractous human lenses. *Current Eye Research*, 11: 327–334.

Kubo E, Singh D, Fatma N, *et al.* (2003). Cellular distribution of lens epithelium-derived growth factor (LEDGF) in the rat eye: loss of LEDGF from nuclei of differentiating cells. *Histochemistry and Cell Biology*, 119: 289–299.

Kymionis G, Tsilimbaris M, Iliaki O, Christodoulakis E, Siganos C, Pallikaris I (2004). Treatment of atopic eyelid disease using topical tacrolimus following corticosteroid discontinuation in a patient with open-angle glaucoma. *Cornea*, 23: 828–830.

Lens A, Langley T, Nemeth S, *et al.* (2008). *Ocular Anatomy and Physiology*, second edition, John H Bond, Thorofare, p. 76.

Lim W, Chee S (2004). Retinal detachment in atopic dermatitis can masquerade as acute panuveitis with rapidly progressive cataract. *Retina*, 24: 953–956.

Loewenstein J, Lee S (2004). *Ophthalmology – Just the Facts*, McGraw-Hill, New York, 158–159.

McGhee C, Dean S, Danesh-Meyer H (2002). Locally administered ocular corticosteroids: benefits and risks. *Drug Safety*, 25: 33–55.

Margolin L, Hershko K, Garcia-Rojas M, Ingber A (2003). Andogsky syndrome variant: atopic dermatitis associated with bilateral cataracts and retinal degeneration with left retinal detachment. *Pediatric Dermatology*, 20: 419–420.

Marsh P, Pflugfelder S (1999). Topical nonpreserved methylprednisolone therapy for keratoconjunctivitis sicca in Sjögren syndrome. *Ophthalmology*, 106: 811–816.

Matsuda A, Ebihara N, Kumagai N, *et al.* (2007). Genetic polymorphisms in the promoter of the interferon gamma receptor 1 gene are associated with atopic cataracts. *Investigative Ophthalmology, and Visual Science*, 48: 583–589.

Matsui H, Lin L, Singh D, Shinohara T, Reddy V (2001). Lens epithelium-derived growth factor: increased survival and decreased DNA breakage of human RPE cells induced by oxidative stress. *Investigative Ophthalmology, and Visual Science*, 42: 2935–2941.

Matsuo T, Saito H, Matsuo N (1997). Cataract and aqueous flare levels in patients with atopic dermatitis. *American Journal of Ophthalmology*, 124: 36–39.

Mayer K, Reinhard T, Reis A, Bohringer D, Sundmacher R (2001). FK406 ointment 0.1% – a new therapeutic option for atopic blepharitis. Clinical trial with 14 patients. *Klinische Monatsblatter fur Augenheilkunde*, 218: 733–736.

Mayman C, Miller D, Tijerina M (1979). *In vitro* production of steroid cataract in bovine lens. Part II: measurement of sodium-potassium adenosine triphosphate activity. *Acta Ophthalmologica (Copenhagen)*, 57: 1107–1116.

Mihara E, Miyata H, Nagata M, Ohama E (2000). Lens epithelial cell damage and apoptosis in atopic cataract – histopathological and immunohistochemical studies.

Nippon Ganka Gakkai Zasshi, 104: 409–416.

Miyake-Kashima M, Fukagawa K, Tanaka M (2004). Kaposi varicelliform eruption associated with 0.1% tacrolimus ointment treatment in atopic blepharitis. *Cornea*, 23: 190–193.

Mohan R, Muralidharan A (1989). Steroid-induced glaucoma and cataract. *Indian Journal of Ophthalmology*, 37: 13–16.

Munjal V, Dhir S, Jain I (1982). Steroid-induced glaucoma. *Indian Journal of Ophthalmology*, 30: 379–382.

Munjal V, Dhir S, Jain I, Gangwar D, D'Souza M (1984). Topical corticosteroids and cataract. *Indian Journal of Ophthalmology*, 32: 478–480.

Nagai N, Liu Y, Fukuhata T, Ito Y (2006). Inhibitors of inducible nitric oxide synthase prevent damage to human lens epithelial cells induced by interferon-gamma and lipopolysaccharide. *Biological and Pharmaceutical Bulletin*, 29: 2077–2081.

Nagaki Y, Hayasaka S, Kadoi C (1999). Cataract progression in patients with atopic dermatitis. *Journal of Cataract and Refractive Surgery*, 25: 96–99.

Nakano E, Iwasaki T, Osanai T, Yamamoto K, Miyauchi M (1997). Ocular complications of atopic dermatitis. *Nippon Ganka Gakkai Zasshi*, 101: 64–48.

Namazi M, Handjani F (2006). Increased oxidative activity from hydrogen peroxide may be the cause of the predisposition to cataracts among patients with atopic dermatitis. *Medical Hypotheses*, 66: 863–864.

National Surveillance of Infectious Keratitis in Japan (2006). National surveillance of infectious keratitis in Japan – current status of isolates, patient background, and treatment. *Nippon Ganka Gakkai Zasshi*, 110: 961–972.

Nguyen D, Sidebottom R, Bates A (2007). Microbial keratitis in keratoglobus-associated vernal keratoconjunctivitis and atopic dermatitis. *Eye and Contact Lens*, 33: 109–110.

Nivenius E, Van der Ploeg I, Jung K, Chryssanthou E, van Hage M, Montan P (2007). Tacrolimus ointment vs steroid ointment for eyelid dermatitis in patients with atopic keratoconjunctivitis. *Eye*, 21: 968–975.

Ohmachi N, Sasabe T, Kojima M, *et al.* (1994). Eye complications in atopic dermatitis. *Areruga*, 43: 796–799.

Oka C, Ideta H, Nagasaki H, Watanabe K, Shinagawa K (1994). Retinal detachment with atopic dermatitis similar to traumatic retinal detachment. *Ophthalmology*, 101: 1050–1054.

Oshita M, Goto H, Yamakawa N, Usui M, Uga S (2005). Experimental cataract models produced by repeated blunt mechanical stimulation and elucidation of the pathogenetic mechanism. *Nippon Ganka Gakkai Zasshi*, 109: 197–204.

Rahi A, Davies P, Ruben M, Lobascher D, Menon J (1977). Keratoconus and coexisting atopic disease. *British Journal of Ophthalmology*, 61: 761–764.

Rapaport M, Rapaport V (1999). Eyelid dermatitis to red face syndrome to cure: clinical experience in 100 cases. *Journal of the American Academy of Dermatology*, 41: 435–442.

Reinhard T, Sundmacher R (1992). Perforating keratoplasty in endogenous eczema. An indication for systemic cyclosporine A – a retrospective study of 18 patients. *Klinische Monatsblatter Augenheilkunde*, 201: 159–63.

Reinhard T, Moller M, Sundmacher R (1999). Penetrating keratoplasty in patients with atopic dermatitis with and without systemic cyclosporine A. *Cornea*, 18: 645–651.

Rikkers S, Holland G, Drayton G, Michel F, Torres M, Takahashi S (2003). Topical tacrolimus treatment of atopic eyelid disease. *American Journal of Ophthalmology*, 135: 297–302.

Romero-Jiménez M, Santodomingo-Rubido J, Wolffsohn JS (2010). Keratoconus: a review. *Contact Lens and Anterior Eye*, 33: 157–166.

Ross J, Jacob A, Batterbury M (2004). Facial eczema and sight-threatening glaucoma. *Journal of the Royal Society of Medicine*, 97: 485–486.

Rozsa FW, Reed DM, Scott KM, *et al.* (2006). Gene expression profile of human trabecular meshwork cells in response to long-term dexamethasone exposure. *Molecular Vision*, 12: 125–141.

Sahni D, Darley C, Hawk J (2004). Glaucoma induced by periorbital topical steroid use –

a rare complication. *Clinical and Experimental Dermatology*, 29: 617–619.

Sasabe T, Suwa Y, Kawamura T, Aoiki T (1997). Cataracts occur in patients with atopic dermatitis when the serum IgE increases. *Nippon Ganka Gakkai Zasshi*, 101: 389–392.

Sasaki K, Kojima M, Nakaizumi H, Kitagawa K, Yamada Y, Ishizaki H (1998). Early lens changes seen in patients with atopic dermatitis applying image analysis processing of Scheimpflug and specular microscopic images. *Ophthalmologica*, 212: 88–94.

Shaw D, Eichenfield L, Shainhouse T, Maibach H (2004). Allergic contact dermatitis from tacrolimus. *Journal of the American Academy of Dermatology*, 50: 962–965.

Shinohara T, Singh D, Fatma N (2002). LEDGF, a survival factor, activates stress-related genes. *Progress in Retinal and Eye Research*, 21: 341–358.

Sim D, Chen R, Hove M, Verma S (2009). Acute irreversible cortical cataracts in prolonged topical corticosteroid overuse for chronic eczema. *Eye (London)*, 23: 984.

Singh D, Ohguru N, Chylack L, Shinohara T (1999). Lens epithelium-derived growth factor: increased resistance to thermal and oxidative stress. *Investigative Ophthalmology, and Visual Science*, 40: 1444–1451.

Singh D, Ohguro N, Kikuchi T, *et al.* (2000). Lens epithelium-derived growth factor: effects on growth and survival of lens epithelial cells, keratinocytes, and fibroblasts. *Biochemical and Biophysical Research Communications*, 267: 373–381.

Singh G, Mathur J (1968). Atopic erythroderma with bilateral cataract, unilateral keratoconus and iridocyclitis and undescended testes. *British Journal of Ophthalmology*, 52: 61–63.

Spaeth G, Rodrigues M, Weinreb S (1977). Steroid-induced glaucoma: A. Persistent elevation of intraocular pressure. B. Histopathological aspects. *Transactions of the American Ophthalmological Society*, 75: 353–381.

Sugiura K, Muro Y, Nishizawa Y, *et al.* (2007). LEDGF/DFS70, a major autoantigen of atopic dermatitis, is a component of keratohyalin granules. *Journal of Investigative Dermatology*, 127: 75–80.

Takano Y, Fukagawa K, Dogru M, *et al.* (2004). Inflammatory cells in brush cytology samples correlate with the severity of corneal lesions in atopic keratoconjunctivitis. *British Journal of Ophthalmology*, 88: 1504–1505.

Tan M, Lebwohl M, Esser A, Wei H (2001). The penetration of 0.005% fluticasone propionate ointment in eyelid skin. *Journal of the American Academy of Dermatology*, 45: 392–396.

Tane N, Dhar S, Roy S, Pinheiro A, Ohira A, Roy S (2007). Effect of excess synthesis of extracellular matrix components by trabecular meshwork cells: possible consequence of aqueous outflow. *Experimental Eye Research*, 84: 832–842.

Tao Q, Hollenburg N, Graves S (1999). Sodium pump inhibition and regional expression of sodium pump α-isoforms in lens. *Hypertension*, 34: 1168–1174.

Tuft S, Kemeny D, Dart J, Buckley R (1991). Clinical features of atopic keratoconjunctivitis. *Ophthalmology*, 98: 150–158.

Uchio E, Miyakawa K, Ikezawa Z, Ohno S (1998). Systemic and local immunological features of atopic dermatitis patients with ocular complications. *British Journal of Ophthalmology*, 82: 82–87.

Uehara M, Sato T (1986). Atopic cataract induced by severe allergic contact dermatitis on the face. *Dermatologica*, 172: 54–57.

Uehara M, Amemiya T, Arai M (1985). Atopic cataracts in a Japanese population. With special reference to factors possibly relevant to cataract formation. *Dermatologica*, 170: 180–184.

Van Boxtel L, Hardus P, Al Hassan W, Van Voorst Vader P, Jansonium N (2005). Corticosteroids and the risk of glaucoma. *Nederlands Tijdschrift voor Geneesekunde*, 149: 2485–2489.

Vie R (1980). Glaucoma and amaurosis associated with long-term application of topical corticosteroids to the eyelids. *Acta Dermato-Venereologica*, 60: 541–542.

Virganen H, Reitamo S, Kari M, Kari O (2006). Effect of 0.03% tacrolimus ointment on conjunctival cytology in patients with severe atopic blepharoconjunctivitis: a retrospective study. *Acta Ophthalmologica Scandinavica*, 84: 693–695.

Wang N, Tsai C, Chen Y, et al. (2005). Pediatric rhegmatogenous retinal detachment in East Asians. *Ophthalmology*, 112: 1890–1895.

Watanabe A, Kodera M, Sugiura K, et al. (2004). Anti-DFS70 antibodies in 597 healthy hospital workers. *Arthritis and Rheumatism*, 50: 892–900.

Williamson J, Jasani M (1967). Examination for posterior subcapsular cataracts in patients treated with topical steroids. *British Journal of Ophthalmology*, 51: 554–556.

Yablonski M, Burde R, Kolker A, Becker B (1978). Cataracts induced by topical dexamethasone in diabetics. *Archives of Ophthalmology*, 96: 474–476.

Yamada K, Senju S, Shinohara, et al. (2001). Humoral immune response directed against lens epithelium-derived growth factor in patients with VKH. *Immunology Letters*, 78: 161–168.

Yokoi K, Yokoi N, Kinoshita S (1998). Impairment of ocular surface epithelium barrier function in patients with atopic dermatitis. *British Journal of Ophthalmology*, 82: 979–800.

Zhang X, Ognibene C, Clark A, Yorio T (2007). Dexamethasone inhibition of trabecular meshwork cell phagocytosis and its modulation by glucocorticoid receptor beta. *Experimental Eye Research*, 84: 275–284.

Zugerman C, Saunders D, Levit F (1976). Glaucoma from topically applied steroids. *Archives of Dermatology*, 112: 1326.

CHAPTER 14

Adachi A, Horikawa T (2007). Pompholyx of the infant possibly induced by systemic metal allergy to chromium in mother's milk [in Japanese]. *Arerugi*, 56: 703–708.

Ahmed AR, Moy R (1981). Azathioprine. *International Journal of Dermatology*, 20: 461–467.

Astner S, Burnett N, Rius-Díaz F, Doukas AG, González S, Gonzalez E (2006). Irritant contact dermatitis induced by a common household irritant: a noninvasive evaluation of ethnic variability in skin response. *Journal of the American Academy of Dermatology*, 54: 458–465.

Beissert S, Luger TA (1999). Future developments of antipsoriatic therapy. *Dermatologic Therapy*, 11: 104–117.

Belsito DV (2000). The diagnostic evaluation, treatment, and prevention of allergic contact dermatitis in the new millennium. *Journal of Allergy and Clinical Immunology*, 105: 409–420.

Belsito DV, Fowler JF, Marks JG, et al. (2004). Pimecrolimus cream 1%: a potential new treatment for chronic hand dermatitis. *Cutis*, 73: 31–38.

Berardesca E, Maibach HI (1988). Racial differences in sodium lauryl sulphate induced cutaneous irritation: black and white. *Contact Dermatitis*, 18: 65–70.

Berth-Jones J, Takwale A, Tan E, et al. (2002). Azathioprine in severe adult atopic dermatitis: a double-blind, placebo-controlled, crossover trial. *British Journal of Dermatology*, 147: 324–330.

Boffa MJ, Chalmers RJ (1996). Methotrexate for psoriasis. *Clinical and Experimental Dermatology*, 21: 399–408.

Bollag W, Ott F (1999). Successful treatment of chronic hand eczema with oral 9-cis-retinoic acid. *Dermatology*, 199: 308–312.

Bryld LE, Agner T, Menné T (2003). Relation between vesicular eruptions on the hands and tinea pedis, atopic dermatitis and nickel allergy. *Acta Dermato-Venereologica*, 83: 186–188.

Bureau of Labor Statistics (BLS) (1999). *Occupational injuries and illnesses in the United States*, US Department of Labor.

Burnett CA, Lushniak BD, McCarthy W, Kaufman J (1998). Occupational dermatitis causing days away from work in U.S. private industry, 1993. *American Journal of Industrial Medicine*, 34: 568–573.

Buxton PK (1987). ABC of dermatology. Treatment of eczema and inflammatory dermatoses. *British Medical Journal (Clinical Research Edition)*, 295: 1112–1114.

Cartwright PH, Rowell NR (1987). Comparison of Grenz rays versus placebo in the treatment of chronic hand eczema. *British Journal of Dermatology*, 117: 73–76.

Centers for Disease Control (1986). Leading work-related diseases and injuries. *MMWR Morbidity and Mortality Weekly Report*, 35: 561–563.

Chen JJ, Liang YH, Zhou FS, et al. (2006). The gene for a rare autosomal dominant form of pompholyx maps to chromosome 18q22.1–18q22.3. *Journal of Investigative Dermatology*, 126: 300–304.

Cipollaro VA (1991). Grenz rays. *International Journal of Dermatology*, 30: 225–226.

Coenraads PJ, Nater JP, van der Lende R (1983). Prevalence of eczema and other dermatoses of the hands and arms in the Netherlands. Association with age and occupation. *Clinical and Experimental Dermatology*, 8: 495–503.

Coenraads PJ, Ruzicka T, Lynde C, et al. (2008). Alitretinoin re-induces response in relapsed CHE patients. 9th Biennial Congress of the European Society of Contact Dermatitis, Lisbon, Portugal, Poster 49.

Colebunders R, Zolfo M, Lynen L (2005). Severe dyshidrosis in two patients with HIV infection shortly after starting highly active antiretroviral treatment. *Dermatology Online Journal*, 11: 31.

Cvetkovski RS, Jensen H, Olsen J, Johansen JD, Agner T (2005). Relation between patients' and physicians' severity assessment of occupational hand eczema. *British Journal of Dermatology*, 153: 596–600.

Cvetkovski RS, Zachariae R, Jensen H, Olsen J, Johansen JD, Agner T (2006a). Quality of life and depression in a population of occupational hand eczema patients. *Contact Dermatitis*, 54: 106–111.

Cvetkovski RS, Zachariae R, Jensen H, Olsen J, Johansen JD, Agner T (2006b). Prognosis of occupational hand eczema: a follow-up study. *Archives of Dermatology*, 142: 305–311.

de Jongh CM, Khrenova L, Verberk MM, et al. (2008). Loss-of-function polymorphisms in the filaggrin gene are associated with an increased susceptibility to chronic irritant contact dermatitis: a case-control study. *British Journal of Dermatology*, 159: 621–627.

De Rie MA, Meinardi MM, Bos JD (1991). Lack of efficacy of topical cyclosporin A in atopic dermatitis and allergic contact dermatitis. *Acta Dermato-Venereologica*, 71: 452–454.

De Rie MA, Van Eendenburg JP, Versnick AC, Stolk LM, Bos JD,

Westerhof W (1995). A new psoralen-containing gel for topical PUVA therapy: development, and treatment results in patients with palmoplantar and plaque-type psoriasis, and hyperkeratotic eczema. *British Journal of Dermatology*, 132: 964–969.

Deleo VA, Taylor SC, Belsito DV, *et al.* (2002). The effect of race and ethnicity on patch test results. *Journal of the American Academy of Dermatology*, 46(suppl 2): S107–112.

Diepgen TL, Fartasch M (1994). General aspects of risk factors in hand eczema. In: Menne T, Maibach HI (eds), *Hand Eczema*, CRC Press, Boca Raton, pp. 142–156.

Drake LA, Dorner W, Goltz RW *et al.* (1995). Guidelines of care for contact dermatitis. Committee on Guidelines of Care. *Journal of the American Academy of Dermatology*, 32: 109–113.

Duarte I, Nakano JT, Lazzarini R (1998). Hand eczema: evaluation of 250 patients. *American Journal of Contact Dermatitis*, 9: 216–223.

Duff M, Cruchfield CE 3rd, Moore J, Farniok K, Potish RA, Gallego H (2006). Radiation therapy for chronic vesicular hand dermatitis. *Dermatitis*, 17: 128–132.

Edman B (2000). Statistical relations between hand eczema and contact allergens. In: Menne T, Maibach HI (eds), *Hand Eczema*, CRC Press, Boca Raton, pp. 75–83.

Edwards EK Jr, Edwards EK Sr (1990). Grenz ray therapy. *International Journal of Dermatology*, 29: 17–18 Erratum in: *International Journal of Dermatology*, 29: 257.

Egan CA, Rallis TM, Meadows KP, Krueger GG (1999). Low-dose oral methotrexate treatment for recalcitrant palmoplantar pompholyx. *Journal of the American Academy of Dermatology*, 40: 612–614.

Egawa K (2005). Topical vitamin D3 derivatives in treating hyperkeratotic palmoplantar eczema: a report of 5 patients. *Journal of Dermatology*, 32: 381–386.

Elston DM, Ahmed DD, Watsky KL, Schwarzenberger K (2002). Hand dermatitis. *Journal of the American Academy of Dermatology*, 47: 291–299.

Epling C, Duncan J, Archibong E, Østbye T, Pompeii LA, Dement J (2011). Latex allergy symptoms among health care workers: results from a university health and safety surveillance system. *International Journal of Occupational and Environmental Health*, 17: 17–23.

Epstein E (1984). Hand dermatitis: practical management and current concepts. *Journal of the American Academy of Dermatology*, 10: 395–424.

Fairris GM, Mack DP, Rowell NR (1984). Superficial X-ray therapy in the treatment of constitutional eczema of the hands. *British Journal of Dermatology*, 111: 445–449.

Fairris GM, Jones DH, Mack DP, Rowell NR (1985). Conventional superficial X-ray versus Grenz ray therapy in the treatment of constitutional eczema of the hands. *British Journal of Dermatology*, 112: 339–341.

Färm G (1996). Contact allergy to colophony and hand eczema. A follow-up study of patients with previously diagnosed contact allergy to colophony. *Contact Dermatitis*, 34: 93–100.

Flyvholm MA, Lindberg M; OEESC-2005 organizing committee. (2006). OEESC-2005 – summing up on the theme irritants and wet work. *Contact Dermatitis*, 55: 317–321.

Forrester BG, Roth VS (1998). Hand dermatitis in intensive care units. *Journal of Occupational and Environmental Medicine*, 40: 881–885.

Fowler JF, Ghosh A, Sung J, *et al.* (2006). Impact of chronic hand dermatitis on quality of life, work productivity, activity impairment, and medical costs. *Journal of the American Academy of Dermatology*, 54: 448–457.

Funke U, Diepgen TL, Fartasch M (1996). Risk-group-related prevention of hand eczema at the workplace. *Current Problems in Dermatology*, 25: 123–132.

Ghadially R, Brown BE, Sequeira-Martin SM, Feingold KR, Elias PM (1995). The aged epidermal permeability barrier. Structural, functional, and lipid biochemical abnormalities in humans and a senescent marine model. *Journal of Clinical Investigation*, 95: 2281–2290.

Goh CL (1989). An epidemiological comparison between occupational and non-occupational hand eczema. *British Journal of Dermatology*, 120: 77–82.

Goujon C, Bérard F, Dahel K, *et al.* (2006). Methotrexate for the treatment of adult atopic dermatitis. *European Journal of Dermatology*, 16: 155–158.

Gould WM (1991). Friction dermatitis of the thumbs caused by pantyhose. *Archives of Dermatology*, 127: 1740.

Granlund H, Erkko P, Eriksson E, Reitamo S (1996). Comparison of cyclosporine and topical betamethasone-17, 21-dipropionate in the treatment of severe chronic hand eczema. *Acta Dermato-Venereologica*, 76: 371–376.

Granlund H, Erkko P, Reitamo S (1998). Long-term follow-up of eczema patients treated with cyclosporine. *Acta Dermato-Venereologica*, 78: 40–43.

Grassberger M, Baumruker T, Enz A, *et al.* (1999). A novel anti-inflammatory drug, SDZ ASM 981, for the treatment of skin diseases: *in vitro* pharmacology. *British Journal of Dermatology*, 141: 264–273.

Grattan CE, Carmichael AJ, Shuttleworth GJ, Foulds IS (1991). Comparison of topical PUVA with UVA for chronic vesicular hand eczema. *Acta Dermato-Venereologica*, 71: 118–122.

Gritiyarangsan P, Sukhum A, Tresukosol P, Kullavanijaya P (1998). Topical PUVA therapy for chronic hand eczema. *Journal of Dermatology*, 25: 299–301.

Grundmann-Kollmann M, Behrens S, Peter RU, Krescher M (1999). Treatment of severe recalcitrant dermatoses of the palms and soles with PUVA-bath versus PUVA-cream therapy. *Photodermatology Photoimmunology, and Photomedicine*, 15: 87–89.

Halbert AR, Gebauer KA, Wall LM (1992). Prognosis of occupational chromate dermatitis. *Contact Dermatitis*, 27: 214–219.

Hantash B, Fiorentino D (2006). Liver enzyme abnormalities in patients with atopic dermatitis treated with mycophenolate mofetil. *Archives of Dermatology*, 142: 109–110.

Hartmann M, Enk A (2005). Mycophenolate mofetil and skin diseases. *Lupus*, 14(suppl 1): s58–63.

Heine G, Schnuch A, Uter W, *et al.* (2006). Type IV sensitization profile of individuals with atopic eczema: results from the Information Network of Departments of Dermatology (IVDK) and the German Contact Dermatitis, Research Group (DKG). *Allergy*, 61: 611–616.

Heller M, Shin HT, Orlow SJ, Schaffer JV (2007). mofetil for severe childhood atopic dermatitis: experience in 14 patients. *British Journal of Dermatology*, 157: 127–132.

Hersle K, Mobacken H (1982). Hyperkeratotic dermatitis of the palms. *British Journal of Dermatology*, 107: 195–201.

Holness DL (2001). Results of a quality of life questionnaire in a patch test clinic population. *Contact Dermatitis*, 44: 80–84.

Holness DL (2004). Health care services use by workers with work-related contact dermatitis. *Dermatitis*, 15: 18–24.

Ingram JR, Batchelor JM, Williams HC (2009). Alitretinoin as a potential advance in the management of severe chronic hand eczema. *Archives of Dermatology*, 145: 314–315.

Inui S, Itami S, Katayama I (2004). Frictional dermatitis due to paper tissues. *Contact Dermatitis*, 50: 374–375.

Itschner L, Hinnen U, Elsner P (1996). Prevention of hand eczema in the metal-working industry: risk awareness and behavior of metal worker apprentices. *Dermatology*, 193: 226–229.

Jain VK, Aggarwal K, Passi S, Gupta S (2004). Role of contact allergens in pompholyx. *Journal of Dermatology*, 31: 188–181.

Jolivet J, Cowan KH, Curt GA, Clendeninn NJ, Chabner BA (1983). The pharmacology and clinical use of methotrexate. *New England Journal of Medicine*, 309: 1094–1104.

Jordan WP Jr (1974). Allergic contact dermatitis in hand eczema. *Archives of Dermatology*, 110: 567–569.

Jordan WP Jr, King SE (1979). Nickel feeding in nickel-sensitive patients with hand eczema. *Journal of the American Academy of Dermatology*, 1: 506–508.

Josefson A, Färm G, Stymne B, Meding B (2006). Nickel allergy and hand eczema – a 20-year follow up. *Contact Dermatitis*, 55: 286–290.

Kaaber K, Veien NK, Tjell JC (1978). Low nickel diet in the treatment of patients with chronic nickel dermatitis. *British Journal of Dermatology*, 98: 197–201.

Kaaber K, Menné T, Tjell JC, Veien N (1979). Antabuse treatment of nickel dermatitis. Chelation – a new principle in the treatment of nickel dermatitis. *Contact Dermatitis*, 5: 221–228.

Kaaber K, Menné T, Veien N, Hougaard P (1983). Treatment of nickel dermatitis with Antabuse; a double-blind study. *Contact Dermatitis*, 9: 297–300.

Kadyk DL, McCarter K, Achen F, Belsito DV (2003). Quality of life in patients with allergic contact dermatitis. *Journal of the American Academy of Dermatology*, 49: 1037–1048.

Kedrowski DA, Warshaw EM (2008). Hand dermatitis: a review of clinical features, diagnosis, and management. *Dermatology Nursing*, 20: 17–25.

Keil JE, Shmunes E (1983). The epidemiology of work-related skin disease in South Carolina. *Archives of Dermatology*, 119: 650–654.

Kelly KJ, Kurup V, Zacharisen M, Resnick A, Fink JN (1993). Skin and serologic testing in the diagnosis of latex allergy. *Journal of Allergy and Clinical Immunology*, 91: 1140–1145.

King CM, Chalmers RJ (1984). A double-blind study of superficial radiotherapy in chronic palmar eczema. *British Journal of Dermatology*, 111: 451–454.

Kissling S, Wüthrich B (1994). Sites, types of manifestations and micromanifestations of atopic dermatitis in young adults. A personal follow-up 20 years after diagnosis in childhood [in German]. *Hautarzt*, 45: 368–371.

Klein AW (2004). Treatment of dyshidrotic hand dermatitis with intradermal botulinum toxin. *Journal of the American Academy of Dermatology*, 50: 153–154; author reply 154.

Klein LR, Fowler JF Jr (1992). Nickel dermatitis recall during disulfiram therapy for alcohol abuse. *Journal of the American Academy of Dermatology*, 26: 645–646.

Laing ME, Powell FC, O'Sullivan D, Nagle CM, Keane FM (2006). The influence of contact dermatitis on career change in hairdressers. *Contact Dermatitis*, 54: 218–219.

Lampel HP, Patel N, Boyse K, O'Brien SH, Zirwas MJ (2007). Prevalence of hand dermatitis in inpatient nurses at a United States hospital. *Dermatitis*, 18: 140–142.

Lerbaek A, Kyvik KO, Ravn H, Menné T, Agner T (2007a). Incidence of hand eczema in a population-based twin cohort: genetic and environmental risk factors. *British Journal of Dermatology*, 157: 552–557.

Lerbaek A, Kyvik K, Mortensen J, Bryld LE, Menné T, Agner T (2007b). Heritability of hand eczema is not explained by comorbidity with atopic dermatitis. *Journal of Investigative Dermatology*, 127: 1632–1640.

Lerbaek A, Bisgaard H, Agner T, Ohm Kyvik K, Palmer CN, Menné T (2007c). Filaggrin null alleles are not associated with hand eczema or contact allergy. *British Journal of Dermatology*, 157: 1199–1204.

Lillis JV, Guo CS, Lee JJ, Blauvelt A (2010). Increased IL-23 expression in palmoplantar psoriasis and hyperkeratotic hand dermatitis. *Archives of Dermatology*, 146: 918–919.

Lindelof B, Beitner H (1990). The effect of Grenz ray therapy on pustulosis palmoplantaris, a double-blind bilateral trial. *Acta Dermato-Venereologica Supplementum*, 70: 529–531.

Lindelof B, Wrangsjo K, Liden S (1987). A double-blind study of Grenz ray therapy in chronic eczema of the hands. *British Journal of Dermatology*, 117: 77–80.

Llombart M, García-Abujeta JL, Sánchez-Pérez RM (2007). Pompholyx induced by intravenous immunoglobulin therapy. *Journal of Investigational Allergology and Clinical Immunology*, 14: 277–285.

Löffler H, Bruckner T, Diepgen T, Effendy I (2006). Primary prevention in health care employees: a prospective intervention study with a 3-year training period. *Contact Dermatitis*, 54: 202–209.

Lushniak BD (1995). The epidemiology of occupational contact dermatitis. *Dermatologic Clinics*, 13: 671–680.

MacConnachie AA, Smith CC (2007). Pompholyx eczema as a manifestation of HIV infection, response to antiviral therapy. *Acta Dermato-Venereologica*, 84: 378–379.

McDonald JC, Beck MH, Chen Y, Cherry NM (2006). Incidence by occupation and industry of work-related skin diseases in the United Kingdom, 1996–2001. *Occupational Medicine (London)*, 56: 398–405.

McMullen E, Gawkrodger DJ (2006). Physical friction is under-recognized as an irritant that can cause or contribute to contact dermatitis.

British Journal of Dermatology, **154**: 154–156.

Magina S, Barros MA, Ferreira JA, Mesquita-Guimarães J (2003). Atopy, nickel sensitivity, occupation, and clinical patterns in different types of hand dermatitis. *American Journal of Contact Dermatitis*, **14**: 63–68.

Maibach H (1976). Immediate hypersensitivity in hand dermatitis. Role of food-contact dermatitis. *Archives of Dermatology*, **112**: 1289–1291.

Mäkelä L, Lammintausta K, Kalimo K (2007). Contact sensitivity and atopic dermatitis: association with prognosis, a follow-up study in 801 atopic patients. *Contact Dermatitis*, **56**: 76–80.

Malten KE (1981). Thoughts on irritant contact dermatitis. *Contact Dermatitis*, **7**: 238–247.

Man I, Ibbotson SH, Ferguson J (2004). Photoinduced pompholyx: a report of 5 cases. *Journal of the American Academy of Dermatology*, **50**: 55–60.

Mathias CG (1985). The cost of occupational skin disease. *Archives of Dermatology*, **121**: 332–334.

Meding B (1994). Epidemiology of hand eczema. In: Menné T, Maibach HI (eds), *Hand Eczema*, CRC Press, Boca Raton, pp. 157–164.

Meding B (1996). Prevention of hand eczema in atopics. *Current Problems in Dermatology*, **25**: 116–122.

Meding B, Järvholm B (2004). Incidence of hand eczema – a population-based retrospective study. *Journal of Investigational Dermatology*, **122**: 873–877.

Meding B, Swanbeck G (1989). Epidemiology of different types of hand eczema in an industrial city. *Acta Dermato-Venereologica*, **69**: 227–233.

Meding B, Swanbeck G (1990a). Predictive factors for hand eczema. *Contact Dermatitis*, **23**: 154–161.

Meding B, Swanbeck G (1990b). Consequences of having hand eczema. *Contact Dermatitis*, **23**: 6–14.

Meding B, Lantto R, Lindahl G, Wrangsjö K, Bengtsson B (2005a). Occupational skin disease in Sweden – a 12-year follow-up. *Contact Dermatitis*, **53**: 308–313.

Meding B, Wrangsjö K, Järvholm B (2005b). Fifteen-year follow-up of hand eczema: predictive

factors. *Journal of Investigational Dermatology*, **124**: 893–897.

Meding B, Wrangsjö K, Järvholm B (2007). Hand eczema extent and morphology – association and influence on long-term prognosis. *Journal of Investigational Dermatology*, **127**: 2147–2151.

Meggitt SJ, Gray JC, Reynolds NJ (2006). Azathioprine dosed by thiopurine methyltransferase activity for moderate-to-severe atopic eczema: a double-blind, randomized controlled trial. *Lancet*, **367**: 839–846.

Menné T (1985). Flare-up of cobalt dermatitis from Antabuse treatment. *Contact Dermatitis*, **12**: 53.

Menné T, Hjorth N (1985). Frictional contact dermatitis. *American Journal of Industrial Medicine*, **8**: 401–402.

Menné T, Kaaber K (1978). Treatment of pompolyx due to nickel allergy with chelating agents. *Contact Dermatitis*, **4**: 289–290.

Menné T, Borgan O, Green A (1982). Nickel allergy and hand dermatitis in a stratified sample of the Danish female population: an epidemiological study including a statistic appendix. *Acta Dermato-Venereologica*, **62**: 35–41.

Moller H (2000). Atopic hand eczema. In: Menné T, Maibach HI (eds), *Hand Eczema*, CRC Press, Boca Raton, pp. 141–146.

Montnémery P, Nihlén U, Löfdahl CG, Nyberg P, Svensson A (2005). Prevalence of hand eczema in an adult Swedish population and the relationship to risk occupation and smoking. *Acta Dermato-Venereologica*, **85**: 429–432.

Morison WL, Parrish JA, Fitzpatrick TB (1978). Oral methoxsalen photochemotherapy of recalcitrant dermatoses of the palms and soles. *British Journal of Dermatology*, **99**: 293–302.

Morren MA, Przybilla B, Bamelis M, Heykants B, Reynaers A, Degreef H (1994). Atopic dermatitis: triggering factors. *Journal of the American Academy of Dermatology*, **31**: 467–473.

Mygind K, Sell L, Flyvholm MA, Jepsen KF (2006). High-fat petrolatum-based moisturizers and prevention of work-related skin problems in wet-work occupations. *Contact Dermatitis*, **54**: 35–41.

Nassif A, Chan SC, Storrs FJ, Hanifin JM (1994). Abnormal skin irritancy in atopic dermatitis

and in atopy without dermatitis. *Archives of Dermatology*, **130**: 1402–1407 [Erratum in: *Archives of Dermatology*, 1995; **131**: 464.]

Nesbitt LT Jr (1995). Minimizing complications from systemic glucocorticosteroid use. *Dermatologic Clinics*, **13**: 925–939.

Nicholson PJ, Llewellyn D, English JS, Guidelines Development Group (2010). Evidence-based guidelines for the prevention, identification and management of occupational contact dermatitis and urticaria. *Contact Dermatitis*, **63**: 177–186.

Niinai H, Kawamoto M, Yuge O (2004). Severe pompholyx following endoscopic thoracic sympathectomy for palmar hyperhidrosis. *Interactive and Cardiovascular Thoracic Surgery*, **3**: 593–595.

Nilsson E (1994). Individual and environmental risk factors for hand eczema in hospital workers. In: Menné T, Maibach HI (eds), *Hand Eczema*, CRC Press, Boca Raton, pp. 115–130.

Nilsson EJ, Knutsson A (1995). Atopic dermatitis, nickel sensitivity and xerosis as risk factors for hand eczema in women. *Contact Dermatitis*, **33**: 401–406.

Nilsson E, Mikaelsson B, Andersson S (1985). Atopy, occupation and domestic work as risk factors for hand eczema in hospital workers. *Contact Dermatitis*, **13**: 216–223.

Nousari HC, Sragovich A, Kimyai-Asadi A, Orlinsky D, Anhalt GJ (1999a). Mycophenolate mofetil in autoimmune and inflammatory skin disorders. *Journal of the American Academy of Dermatology*, **40**: 265–268.

Nousari HC, Anhalt GJ, Morison WL (1999b). Mycophenolate in psoralen-UVA desensitization therapy for chronic actinic dermatitis. *Archives of Dermatology*, **135**: 1128–1129.

Nyrén M, Lindberg M, Stenberg B, Svensson M, Svensson A, Meding B (2005). Influence of childhood atopic dermatitis on future worklife. *Scandinavian Journal of Work and Environmental Health*, **31**: 474–378.

Odia S, Vocks E, Rakoski J, Ring J (1996). Successful treatment of dyshidrotic hand eczema using tap water iontophoresis with pulsed direct current. *Acta Dermato-Venereologica*, **76**: 472–474.

Ogden S, Clayton TH, Goodfield MJ (2006). Recalcitrant hand pompholyx: variable response to etanercept. *Clinical and Experimental Dermatology*, **31**: 145–146.

Patil S, Maibach HI (1994). Effect of age and sex on the elicitation of irritant contact dermatitis. *Contact Dermatitis*, 30: 257–264.

Paul MA, Fleischer AB, Sherertz EF (1995). Patients' benefit from contact dermatitis evaluation: results of a follow-up study. *American Journal of Contact Dermatitis*, 6: 63–66.

Paulsen E, Andersen KE (1991). Irritant contact dermatitis of a gardener's hands caused by handling of fur-covered plant ornaments. *American Journal of Contact Dermatitis*, 2: 113–116.

Petering H, Breuer C, Herbst R, Kapp A, Werfel T (2004). Comparison of localized high-dose UVA1 irradiation versus topical cream psoralen-UVA for treatment of chronic vesicular dyshidrotic eczema. *Journal of the American Academy of Dermatology*, 50: 68–72.

Petersen CS, Menné T (1992). Cyclosporin A responsive chronic severe vesicular hand eczema. *Acta Dermato-Venereologica*, **72**: 436–437.

Pickenäcker A, Luger TA, Schwarz T (1998). Dyshidrotic eczema treated with mycophenolate mofetil. *Archives of Dermatology*, **134**: 378–379.

Pigatto PD, Legori A, Bigardi AS (1992). Occupational dermatitis from physical causes. *Clinical Dermatology*, 10: 231–243.

Pitché P, Boukari M, Tchangai-Walla K (2006). Factors associated with palmoplantar or plantar pompholyx: a case-control study. *Annales de dermatologie et de vénéréologie*, 133: 139–143.

Polderman MC, Govaert JC, le Cessie S, Pavel S (2003). A double-blind placebo-controlled trial of UVA-1 in the treatment of dyshidrotic eczema. *Clinical and Experimental Dermatology*, **28**: 584–587.

Pryce DW, Irvine D, English JS, Rycroft RJ (1989). Soluble oil dermatitis: a follow-up study. *Contact Dermatitis*, 21: 28–35.

Queille-Roussel C, Paul C, Duteil L, et al. (2001). The new topical ascomycin derivative SDZ ASM 981 does not induce skin atrophy when applied to normal skin for 4 weeks: a randomized, double-blind controlled study. *British*

Journal of Dermatology, 144: 507–513.

Rajka G (1989). *Essential Aspects of Atopic Dermatitis*, Springer-Verlag, Berlin.

Ramsing DW, Agner T (1996). Effect of glove occlusion on human skin (II). Long-term experimental exposure. *Contact Dermatitis*, 34: 258–262.

Reilly MC, Lavin PT, Kahler KH, Pariser DM (2003). Validation of the Dermatology Life Quality Index and the Work Productivity and Activity Impairment–Chronic Hand Dermatitis questionnaire in chronic hand dermatitis. *Journal of the American Academy of Dermatology*, 48: 128–130.

Reitamo S, Rissanen J, Remitz A, et al. (1998). Tacrolimus ointment does not affect collagen synthesis: results of a single-center randomized trial. *Journal of Investigative Dermatology*, 111: 396–398.

Rietschel RL, Nethercott JR, Emmett EA, et al. (1990). Methylchloroisothiazolinone-methylisothiazolinone reactions in patients screened for vehicle and preservative hypersensitivity. *Journal of the American Academy of Dermatology*, 22: 734–738.

Rosén K, Mobacken H, Swanbeck G (1987). Chronic eczematous dermatitis of the hands: a comparison of PUVA and UVB treatment. *Acta Dermato-Venereologica*, 67: 48–54.

Rowell N (1978). Adverse effects of superficial X-ray therapy and recommendations for safe use in benign dermatoses. *Journal of Dermatology, Surgical Oncology*, 4: 630–634.

Rustemeyer T, van Hoogstraten IMW, von Blomberg BME, et al. (2011). Mechanisms of irritant and allergic contact dermatitis. In: Johansen JD, Frosch PJ, Lepoitteven J-P (eds), *Contact Dermatitis*, 5th edn, Springer, Heidelberg, p. 47.

Ruzicka T, Larsen FG, Galewicz D, et al. (2004). Oral alitretinoin (9-*cis*-retinoic acid) therapy for chronic hand dermatitis in patients refractory to standard therapy: results of a randomized, double-blind, placebo-controlled, multicenter trial. *Archives of Dermatology*, 140: 1453–1459.

Ruzicka T, Lynde CW, Jemec GB, et al. (2008). Efficacy and safety of oral alitretinoin (9-cis retinoic acid) in patients with severe

chronic hand eczema refractory to topical corticosteroids: results of a randomized, double-blind, placebo-controlled, multicentre trial. *British Journal of Dermatology*, 158: 808–817.

Rystedt I (1985). Work-related hand eczema in atopics. *Contact Dermatitis*, 12: 164–171.

Scerri L (1999). Azathioprine in dermatological practice: an overview with special emphasis on its use in non-bullous inflammatory dermatoses. *Advances in Experimental Medicine and Biology*, 455: 343–348.

Schempp CM, Müller H, Czech W, Schöpf E, Simon JC (1997). Treatment of chronic palmoplantar eczema with local bath-PUVA therapy. *Journal of the American Academy of Dermatology*, 36: 733–737.

Schiener R, Gottlöber P, Müller B, et al. (2005). PUVA-gel vs. PUVA-bath therapy for severe recalcitrant palmoplantar dermatoses. A randomized, single-blinded prospective study. *Photodermatology, Photoimmunology and Photomedicine*, 21: 62–67.

Schliemann S, Kelterer D, Bauer A, et al. (2008). Tacrolimus ointment in the treatment of occupationally induced chronic hand dermatitis. *Contact Dermatitis*, 58: 299–306.

Schmidt M, Raghavan B, Müller V, et al. (2010). Crucial role for human Toll-like receptor 4 in the development of contact allergy to nickel. *Nature Immunology*, 11: 814–819.

Schmidt T, Abeck D, Boeck K, Mempel M, Ring J (1998). UVA1 irradiation is effective in treatment of chronic vesicular dyshidrotic hand eczema. *Acta Dermato-Venereologica Supplementum*, 78: 318–319.

Schmitt J, Schmitt N, Meurer M (2007). Cyclosporin in the treatment of patients with atopic eczema- a systematic review and meta-analysis. *Journal of the European Academy of Dermatology and Venereology*, 21: 606–619.

Semhoun-Ducloux S, Ducloux D, Miguet JP (2000). Mycophenolate mofetil-induced dyshidrotic eczema. *Annals of Internal Medicine*, 132: 417.

Seyfarth F, Schliemann S, Antonov D, Elsner P (2011). Dry skin, barrier function, and irritant contact dermatitis in the elderly. *Clinics in Dermatology*, 29: 31–36.

Sezer E, Etikan I (2007). Local narrowband UVB phototherapy vs. local PUVA in the treatment of chronic hand eczema. *Photodermatology, Photoimmunology and Photomedicine*, 23: 10–4.

Sheehan-Dare RA, Goodfield MJ, Rowell NR (1989). Topical psoralen photochemotherapy (PUVA) and superficial radiotherapy in the treatment of chronic hand eczema. *British Journal of Dermatology*, 121: 65–69.

Sherertz EF (1999). Allergic contact dermatitis. In: Adams RM (ed.), *Occupational Skin Disease*, WB Saunders, Philadelphia, p. 23–27.

Sherertz EF (2000). The role of dermatologists in the delivery of occupational dermatologic care. *Dermatologic Clinics*, 18: 235–240.

Simons JR, Bohnen IJ, van der Valk PG (1997). A left–right comparison of UVB phototherapy and topical photochemotherapy in bilateral chronic hand dermatitis after 6 weeks treatment. *Clinical and Experimental Dermatology*, 22: 7–10.

Simpson EL, Thompson MM, Hanifin JM (2006). Prevalence and morphology of hand eczema in patients with atopic dermatitis. *Dermatitis*, 17: 123–127.

Skoet R, Olsen J, Mathiesen B, Iversen L, Johansen JD, Agner T (2004). A survey of occupational hand eczema in Denmark. *Contact Dermatitis*, 51: 159–166.

Skudlik C, Schwanitz HJ (2004). Tertiary prevention of occupational skin diseases. *Journal der Deutschen Dermatologischen Gesellschaft*, 2: 424–433.

Smit HA, Burdorf A, Coenraads PJ (1993). Prevalence of hand dermatitis in different occupations. *International Journal of Epidemiology*, 22: 288–293.

Smith HR, Armstrong DK, Wakelin SH, Rycroft RJ, White IR, McFadden JP (2000). Descriptive epidemiology of hand dermatitis at the St John's contact dermatitis clinic 1983–97. *British Journal of Dermatology*, 142: 284–287.

Smith TA (2004). Incidence of occupational skin conditions in a food manufacturing company: results of a health surveillance programme.

Occupational Medicine (London), 54: 227–230.

Sollinger HW (1995). US renal transplant mycophenolate mofetil study group. Mycophenolate mofetil for the prevention of acute rejection in primary cadaveric renal allograft recipients. *Transplantation*, 60: 225–232.

Soni BP, Sherertz EF (1997). Evaluation of previously patch-tested patients referred to a contact dermatitis clinic. *American Journal of Contact Dermatitis*, 8: 10–14.

Stingeni L, Lapomarda V, Lisi P (1995). Occupational hand dermatitis in hospital environments. *Contact Dermatitis*, 33: 172–176.

Storrs FJ (1979). Use and abuse of systemic corticosteroid therapy. *Journal of the American Academy of Dermatology*, 1: 95–106.

Suli C, Lorini M, Mistrello G, Tedeschi A (2006). Diagnosis of latex hypersensitivity: comparison of different methods. *European Annals of Allergy and Clinical Immunology*, 38: 24–30.

Sun CC, Guo YL, Lin RS (1995). Occupational hand dermatitis in a tertiary referral dermatology clinic in Taipei. *Contact Dermatitis*, 33: 414–418.

Sutton RL Jr, Ayres S Jr (1953). Dermatitis of the hands; etiology and principles of treatment with observations concerning a hyperkeratotic dermatitis of the volar skin. *AMA Archives of Dermatology, and Syphilology*, 68: 266–285.

Swartling C, Naver H, Lindberg M, Anveden I (2002). Treatment of dyshidrotic hand dermatitis with intradermal botulinum toxin. *Journal of the American Academy of Dermatology*, 47: 667–671.

Szepietowski J, Salomon J (2005). Hand dermatitis: a problem commonly affecting nurses. *Roczniki Akademii Medycznej w Bialymstoku*, 50(suppl 1): 46–48.

Templet JT, Hall S, Belsito DV (2004). Etiology of hand dermatitis among patients referred for patch testing. *Dermatitis*, 15: 25–32.

Turjanmaa K (1987). Incidence of immediate allergy to latex gloves in hospital personnel. *Contact Dermatitis*, 17: 270–275.

Uter W, Pfahlberg A, Gefeller O, Schwanitz HJ (1999). Hand dermatitis in a prospectively-followed cohort of hairdressing apprentices: final results of the POSH study. Prevention of occupational

skin disease in hairdressers. *Contact Dermatitis*, 41: 280–286.

Van der Walle HB (2000). Irritant contact dermatitis. In: Menné T, Maibach HI (eds), *Hand Eczema*, CRC Press, Boca Raton, pp. 133–139.

Veien NK, Menné T (1990). Nickel contact allergy and a nickel-restricted diet. *Seminars in Dermatology*, 9: 197–205.

Veien NK, Hattel T, Justesen O, Nørholm A (1983). Oral challenge with metal salts. (II). Various types of eczema. *Contact Dermatitis*, 9: 407–410.

Vestey JP, Gawkrodger DJ, Wong WK, Buxton PK (1986). An analysis of 501 consecutive contact clinic consultations. *Contact Dermatitis*, 15: 119–125.

Wahlberg JE (1985). Occupational hyperkeratosis in carpet installers. *American Journal of Industrial Medicine*, 8: 351–353.

Wallenhammar LM, Nyfjäll M, Lindberg M, Meding B (2004). Health-related quality of life and hand eczema – a comparison of two instruments, including factor analysis. *Journal of Investigational Dermatology*, 122: 1381–1389.

Walling HW, Swick BL, Storrs FJ, Boddicker ME (2008). Frictional hyperkeratotic hand dermatitis responding to Grenz ray therapy. *Contact Dermatitis*, 58: 49–55.

Warshaw EM (1998). Latex allergy. *Journal of the American Academy of Dermatology*, 39: 1–24.

Warshaw EM (2004). Therapeutic options for chronic hand dermatitis. *Dermatologic Therapy*, 17: 240–250.

Warshaw E, Lee G, Storrs FJ (2003). Hand dermatitis: a review of clinical features, therapeutic options, and long-term outcomes. *American Journal of Contact Dermatitis*, 14: 119–137.

Warshaw EM, Ahmed RL, Belsito DV, et al. (2007). Contact dermatitis of the hands: cross-sectional analyses of North American *Contact Dermatitis*, Group Data, 1994–2004. *Journal of the American Academy of Dermatology*, 57: 301–314.

Weatherhead SC, Wahie S, Reynolds NJ, Meggitt SJ (2007). An open-label, dose-ranging study of methotrexate for moderate-to-severe adult atopic eczema. *British Journal of Dermatology*, 156: 346–351.

Weisshaar E, Radulescu M, Bock M, Albrecht U, Zimmermann E,

Diepgen TL (2005). Skin protection and skin disease prevention courses for secondary prevention in healthcare workers: first results after two years of implementation. *Journal der Deutschen Dermatologischen Gesellschaft*, 3: 33–338.

Wigger-Alberti W, Iliev D, Elsner P (1999). Contact dermatitis due to irritation. In: Adams RM (ed.), *Occupational Skin Disease*, WB Saunders, Philadelphia, pp. 1–21.

Wilkinson SM, Heagerty AH, English JS (1992). A prospective study into the value of patch and intradermal tests in identifying topical corticosteroid allergy. *British Journal of Dermatology*, 127: 22–25.

Williams JD, Lee AY, Matheson MC, Frowen KE, Noonan AM, Nixon RL (2008). Occupational contact urticaria: Australian data. *British Journal of Dermatology*, 159: 125–131.

Wollina U, Karamfilov T (2002). Adjuvant botulinum toxin A in dyshidrotic hand eczema: a controlled prospective pilot study with left-right comparison. *Journal of the European Academy of Dermatology and Venereology*, 16: 40–42.

Woolner D, Soltani K (1994). Management of hand dermatitis. *Comprehensive Therapy*, 20: 422–426.

Zemtsov A (1998). Treatment of palmoplantar eczema with bath-PUVA therapy. *Journal of the American Academy of Dermatology*, 38: 505–506.

Zimmerman SW, Esch J (1978). Skin lesions treated with azathioprine and prednisone. Comparison of nontransplant patients and renal transplant recipients. *Archives of Internal Medicine*, 138: 912–914.

CHAPTER 15

Agner T (1991a). Skin susceptibility in uninvolved skin of hand eczema patients and healthy controls. *British Journal of Dermatology*, 125: 140–146.

Agner T (1991b). Susceptibility of atopic dermatitis patients to irritant dermatitis caused by sodium lauryl sulphate. *Acta Dermato-Venereologica*, 71: 296–300.

Ale IS, Maibach HA (2010). Diagnostic approach in allergic and irritant contact dermatitis. *Expert Reviews in Clinical Immunology*, 6: 291–310.

Alomar A, Berth-Jones J, Bos JD, et al. (2007). The role of topical calcineurin inhibitors in atopic dermatitis. *British Journal of Dermatology*, 151: 3-27.

Basketter DA, Miettinen J, Lahti A (1998). Acute irritant reactivity to sodium lauryl sulfate in atopics and nonatopics. *Contact Dermatitis*, 38: 253–257.

Belsito D, Wilson DC, Warshaw E, et al. (2006). A prospective randomized clinical trial of 0.1% tacrolimus ointment in a model of chronic allergic contact dermatitis. *Journal of the American Academy of Dermatology*, 55: 40-46.

Brasch J, Burgard J, Sterry W (1992). Common pathogenetic pathways in allergic and irritant contact dermatitis. *Journal of Investigative Dermatology*, 98: 166–170.

Bruynzeel-Koomen C, van Wichen DF, Toonstra J, et al. (1986). The presence of IgE molecules on epidermal Langerhans cells in patients with atopic dermatitis. *Archives of Dermatologic Research*, 278: 199–205.

Bursch LS, Wang L, Igyarto B, et al. (2007). Identification of a novel population of langerin+ dendritic cells. *Journal of Experimental Medicine*, 204: 3147–3156.

Carlsen BC, Johansen JD, Menné T, et al. (2010). Filaggrin null mutations and association with contact allergy and allergic contact dermatitis: results from a tertiary dermatology clinic. *Contact Dermatitis*, 63(2): 89–95.

Coenraads PJ, Diepgen TL (1998). Risk for hand eczema in employees with past or present atopic dermatitis. *International Archives of Occupational and Environmental Health*, 71: 7–13.

Cohen PR, Cardullo AC, Ruszkowski AM, et al. (1990). Allergic contact dermatitis to nickel in children with atopic dermatitis. *Annals of Allergy*, 65: 73–79.

Cohen SR (1996). Contact dermatitis: an overview. *Cross Section in Dermatology: A Primary Care Perspective*, 2: 1–12.

Compalati E, Rogkakou A, Passalacqua G, Canonica GW (2012). Evidences of efficacy of allergen immunotherapy in atopic dermatitis: an updated review. *Current Opinion in Allergy and Clinical Immunology*, 12: 427–433.

Cronin E, Bandmann HJ, Calnan CD, et al. (1970). Contact dermatitis in the atopic. *Acta Dermato-Venereologica (Stockholm)*, 50: 183–187.

Cronin E, McFadden JP (1993). Patients with atopic eczema do become sensitized to contact allergens. *Contact Dermatitis*, 28: 225–228.

Dahl MV (1990). Flare factors and atopic dermatitis: the role of allergy. *Journal of Dermatological Science*, 1: 311–318.

Davis JA, Visscher MO, Wickett RR, et al. (2010). Influence of tumour necrosis factor-α polymorphism-308 and atopy on irritant contact dermatitis in healthcare workers. *Contact Dermatitis*, 63: 320-332.

de Groot AC (1990). The frequency of contact allergy in atopic patients with dermatitis. *Contact Dermatitis*, 22: 273–277.

de Jongh CM, John SM, Bruynzeel DP, et al. (2008). Cytokine gene polymorphisms and susceptibility to chronic irritant contact dermatitis. *Contact Dermatitis*, 58: 269–277.

Dearman RJ, Kimber I (2000). Role of CD4+ T helper 2-type cells in cutaneous inflammatory responses induced by fluorescein isothiocyanate. *Immunology*, 101: 442–451.

Di Nardo A, Braff MH, Taylor KR, et al. (2007). Cathelicidin antimicrobial peptides block dendritic cell TLR4 activation and allergic contact sensitization. *Journal of Immunology*, 178: 1829-1834.

Dilulio NA, Xu H, Fairchild RL (1996). Diversion of CD4+ T cell development from regulatory T helper to effector T helper cells alters the contact hypersensitivity response. *European Journal of Immunology*, 26: 2606–2612.

Enk AH, Knop J (2000). T-cell receptor mimic peptides and their potential application in T-cell-mediated disease. *International Archives of Allergy and Immunology*, 123: 275–281.

Friedmann PS (1998). Allergy and the skin. II. Contact and atopic eczema. *British Medical Journal*, 316: 1226–1229.

Ginhoux F, Collin MP, Bogunovic M, et al. (2007). Blood-derived dermal langerin+ dendritic cells survey the skin in the steady state. *Journal of Experimental Medicine*, 204: 3133–3146.

Giordano-Labadie F, Rance F, Pellegrin F, et al. (1999). Frequency of contact allergy in children with atopic dermatitis: results of a prospective study of 137 cases. *Contact Dermatitis*, 40: 192–195.

Göllner GP, Müller G, Alt R, et al. (2000). Therapeutic application of T-cell receptor mimic peptides or cDNA in the treatment of T-cell-mediated skin diseases. *Gene Therapy*, 7: 1000–1004.

Grewe M, Gyufko K, Schopf E, et al. (1994). Lesional expression of interferon-γ in atopic eczema. *Lancet*, 343: 25–26.

Grewe M, Walther S, Gyufko K, et al. (1995). Analysis of the cytokine pattern expressed *in situ* in inhalant allergen patch test reactions of atopic dermatitis patients. *Journal of Investigative Dermatology*, 105: 407–410.

Grewe M, Bruijnzeel-Koomen CA, Schopf E, et al. (1998). A role for Th1 and Th2 cells in the immunopathogenesis of atopic dermatitis. *Immunology Today*, 19: 359–361.

Hanifin JM, Chan S (1999). Biochemical and immunologic mechanisms in atopic dermatitis: new targets for emerging therapies. *Journal of the American Academy of Dermatology*, 41: 72–77.

Hanifin JM, Rajka G (1980). Diagnostic features of atopic dermatitis. *Acta Dermato-Venereologica Supplementum (Stockholm)*, 92: 44–47.

Ingordo V, D'Andria G, D'Andria C, et al. (2001). Clinical relevance of contact sensitization in atopic dermatitis. *Contact Dermatitis*, 45: 239–240.

Izadpanah A, Gallo RL (2005). Antimicrobial peptides. *Journal of the American Academy of Dermatology*, 52: 381–390.

Jenkinson HA (1997). Contact dermatitis in a chimney sweep. *Contact Dermatitis*, 37: 35.

Johnson EE, Irons JS, Patterson R, et al. (1974). Serum IgE concentration in atopic dermatitis. Relationship to severity of disease and presence of atopic respiratory disease. *Journal of Allergy and Clinical Immunology*, 54: 94–99.

Kapsenberg ML, Wierenga EA, Stiekema FE, et al. (1992). Th1 lymphokine production profiles of nickel-specific CD4+ T lymphocyte clones from nickel contact allergic and nonallergic individuals. *Journal*

of *Investigative Dermatology*, 98: 59–63.

Klas PA, Corey G, Storrs FJ, et al. (1996). Allergic and irritant patch test reactions and atopic disease. *Contact Dermatitis*, 34: 121–124.

Lammintausta K, Kalimo K, Fagerlund VL (1992). Patch test reactions in atopic patients. *Contact Dermatitis*, 26: 234–240.

Larsen JM, Bonefeld CM, Poulsen SS, et al. (2009). IL-23 and T(H)17-mediated inflammation in human allergic contact dermatitis. *Journal of Allergy and Clinical Immunology*, 123: 486–492.

Lever R, Forsyth A (1992). Allergic contact dermatitis in atopic dermatitis. *Acta Dermato-Venereologica Supplementum (Stockholm)*, 176: 95–98.

Loffler H, Effendy I (1999). Skin susceptibility of atopic individuals. *Contact Dermatitis*, 40: 239–242.

Lugovic L, Lipozencic J (1997). Contact hypersensitivity in atopic dermatitis. *Arhiv za Higijenu Rada i Toksikologiju (Archives of Industrial Hygiene and Toxicology)*, 48: 287–296.

Magnusson B, Fregert S, Hjorth N, et al. (1969). Routine patch testing V. Correlations of reactions to the site of dermatitis and the history of the patient. *Acta Dermato-Venereologica*, 49: 556–563.

Mäkelä L, Lammintausta K, Kalimo K (2007). Contact sensitivity and atopic dermatitis: association with prognosis, a follow-up study in 801 atopic patients. *Contact Dermatitis*, 56: 76-80.

Marghescu S (1985). Patch test reactions in atopic patients. *Acta Dermato-Venereologica Supplementum (Stockholm)*, 114: 113–116.

Mark B, Slavin R (2006). Allergic contact dermatitis. *Medical Clinics of North America*, 90: 169–185.

Medi BM, Singh J (2006). Prospects for vaccines for allergic and other immunologic skin disorders. *American Journal of Clinical Dermatology*, 7: 146–153.

Mohammad AH, Cohen S, Hadi S (2005). Patch testing: a retrospective analysis of 103 patients with emphasis on practical aspects for the clinician. *Skinmed*, 4: 340–344.

Nettis E, Colanardi MC, Soccio AL, et al. (2002). Occupational irritant and allergic contact dermatitis

among healthcare workers. *Contact Dermatitis*, 46: 101–107.

Novak N, Baurecht H, Schäfer T, et al. (2008). Loss-of-function mutations in the filaggrin gene and allergic contact sensitization to nickel. *Journal of Investigative Dermatology*, 128(6):1430–1435.

Ouwehand K, Oosterhoff D, Breetveld M, et al. (2010). Irritant-induced migration of Langerhans cells coincides with an IL-10 dependent switch to a macrophage-like phenotype. *Journal of Investigative Dermatology*, 131: 418–425.

Pennino D, Eyerich K, Scarponi C, et al. (2010). IL-17 amplifies human contact hypersensitivity by licensing hapten nonspecific Th1 cells to kill autologous keratinocytes. *Journal of Immunology*, 184: 4880–4888.

Poulin LF, Henri S, de Bovis B, et al. (2007). The dermis contains langerin+ dendritic cells that develop and function independently of epidermal Langerhans cells. *Journal of Experimental Medicine*, 204: 3119–3131.

Probst P, Kuntzlin D, Fleischer B (1995). TH2-type infiltrating T cells in nickel-induced contact dermatitis. *Cellular Immunology*, 165: 134–140.

Romani N, Clausen BE, Stoitzner P (2010). Langerhans cells and more: langerin-expressing dendritic cell subsets in the skin. *Immunological Reviews*, 234: 120–141.

Rothenberg ME (2010). Innate sensing of nickel. *Nature Immunology*, 11: 781–782.

Rudikoff D, Lebwohl M (1998). Atopic dermatitis. *Lancet*, 351: 1715–1721.

Rustemeyer T, van Hoogstraten IMW, von Blomberg BME, et al. (2011). Mechanisms of irritant and allergic contact dermatitis. In: Johansen JD, Frosch PJ, Lepoitteven J-P (eds), *Contact Dermatitis*, 5th edn, Springer, Heidelberg, p. 47.

Schmidt M, Raghavan B, Müller V, et al. (2010). Crucial role for human Toll-like receptor 4 in the development of contact allergy to nickel. *Nature Immunology*, 11: 814-819.

Schmunes E (1986). The role of atopy in occupational skin diseases. *Occupational Medicine*, 1: 219-228.

Schöpf E, Baumgärtner A (1989). Patch testing in atopic dermatitis. *Journal of the American Academy of Dermatology*, 21(4 Pt 2): 860–862.

Schwarz A, Grabbe S, Riemann H, et al. (1994). *In vivo* effects of interleukin-10 on contact hypersensitivity and delayed-type hypersensitivity reactions. *Journal of Investigative Dermatology*, **103**: 211–216.

Seidenari S (1994). Reactivity to nickel sulfate at sodium lauryl sulfate pretreated skin sites is higher in atopics: an echographic evaluation by means of image analysis performed on 20 MHz B-scan recordings. *Acta Dermato-Venereologica*, **74**: 245–249.

Stolz R, Hinnen U, Elsner P (1997). An evaluation of the relationship between 'atopic skin' and skin irritability in metalworker trainees. *Contact Dermatitis*, **36**: 281–284.

Stuetz A, Baumann K, Grassberger M, et al. (2006). Discovery of topical calcineurin inhibitors and pharmacological profile of pimecrolimus. *International Archives of Allergy and Immunology*, **141**: 199–212.

Szepietowski JC, McKenzie RC, Keohane SG, et al. (1997). Atopic and nonatopic individuals react to nickel challenge in a similar way. A study of the cytokine profile in nickel-induced contact dermatitis. *British Journal of Dermatology*, **137**: 195–200.

Thepen T, Langeveld–Wildschut EG, Bihari IC, et al. (1996). Biphasic response against aeroallergen in atopic dermatitis showing a switch from an initial TH2 response to a TH1 response *in situ*: an immunocytochemical study. *Journal of Allergy and Clinical Immunology*, **97**: 828–837.

Thyssen JP, Johansen JD, Linneberg A, et al. (2010). The association between null mutations in the filaggrin gene and contact sensitization to nickel and other chemicals in the general population. *British Journal of Dermatology*, **162(6)**: 1278–1285.

Tupker RA, Pinnagoda J, Coenraads PJ, et al. (1990). Susceptibility to irritants: role of barrier function, skin dryness and history of atopic dermatitis. *British Journal of Dermatology*, **123**: 199–205.

Uehara M, Sawai T (1989). A longitudinal study of contact sensitivity in patients with atopic dermatitis. *Archives of Dermatology*, **125**: 366–368.

Uehara M, Izukura R, Sawai T (1990). Blood eosinophilia in atopic dermatitis. *Clinical and Experimental Dermatology*, **15**: 264–266.

Uno H, Hanifin JM (1980). Langerhans cells in acute and chronic epidermal lesions of atopic dermatitis, observed by L-dopa histofluorescence, glycol methacrylate thin secretion, and electron microscopy. *Journal of Investigative Dermatology*, **75**: 52–60.

van der Valk PG, Kruis-de Vries MH, Nater JP et al. (1985). Eczematous (irritant and allergic) reactions of the skin and barrier function as determined by water vapour loss. *Clinical and Experimental Dermatology*, **10**: 185–193.

Wang B, Fujisawa H, Zhuang L, et al. (2000). CD4+ Th1 and CD8+ type 1 cytotoxic T cells both play a crucial role in the full development of contact hypersensitivity. *Journal of Immunology*, **165**: 6783–6790.

Young E, Bruijnzeel-Koomen C, Berrens L (1985). Delayed type hypersensitivity in atopic dermatitis. *Acta Dermato-Venereologica Supplementum (Stockholm)*, **114**: 77–81.

CHAPTER 16

Ackerman AB (1978). *Histologic Diagnosis of Inflammatory Skin Diseases*, Lea & Febiger, Philadelphia, p. 499.

Adachi A, Horikawa T, Takashima T, Ichihashi M (2000). Mercury-induced nummular dermatitis. *Journal of the American Academy of Dermatology*, **43(2 Pt 2)**: 383–385.

Aoyama H, Tanaka M, Hara M, Tabata N, Tagami H (1999). Nummular eczema: an addition of senile xerosis and unique cutaneous reactivities to environmental aeroallergens. *Dermatology*, **199**: 135–139.

Bazin E (1862). Des espèces d'eczéma. In: *Lecons theoriques et cliniques sur les affections generiques de la peau*, Volume 1, Adrien Delahaye, Paris, pp. 191–193.

Belsito DV (1987). Contact dermatitis to ethyl-cyanoacrylate-containing glue. *Contact Dermatitis*, **17**: 234–236.

Bendl BJ (1979). Nummular eczema of statis origin. The backbone of a morphologic pattern of diverse etiology. *International Journal of Dermatology*, **18**: 129–135.

Bettoli V, Tosti A, Varotti C (1987). Nummular eczema during isotretinoin treatment. *Journal of the American Academy of Dermatology*, **16(3 Pt 1)**: 617.

Bos JD, van Garderen ID, Krieg SR, Poulter LW (1986). Different *in situ* distribution patterns of dendritic cells having Langerhans (T6+) and interdigitating (RFD1+) cell immunophenotype in psoriasis, atopic dermatitis, and other inflammatory dermatoses. *Journal of Investigative Dermatology*, **87**: 358–361.

Bos JD, Hagenaars C, Das PK, Krieg SR, Voorn WJ, Kapsenberg ML (1989). Predominance of 'memory' T cells (CD4+, CDw29+) over 'naive' T cells (CD4+, CD45R+) in both normal and diseased human skin. *Archives of Dermatological Research*, **281**: 24–30.

Calnan CD, Meara RH (1956). Discoid eczema – dry type. *Transactions of the St John's Hospital Dermatological Society*, **37**: 26–28.

Caraffini S, Lisi P (1987). Nummular dermatitis-like eruption from ethylenediamine hydrochloride in 2 children. *Contact Dermatitis*, **17**: 313–314.

Carr RD, Berke M, Becker SW (1964). Incidence of atopy in patients with various neurodermatoses. *Archives of Dermatology*, **89**: 20–26.

Chipman ED (1934). Nummular eczema. *California and Western Medicine*, **41**: 316–318.

Cowan MA (1961). Nummular eczema. A review, follow-up and analysis of a series of 325 cases. *Acta Dermato-Venereologica*, **41**: 453–460.

Flendrie M, Vissers WH, Creemers MC, de Jong EM, van de Kerkhof PC, van Riel PL (2005). Dermatological conditions during TNF–alpha-blocking therapy in patients with rheumatoid arthritis: a prospective study. *Arthritis Research and Therapy*, **7(3)**: R666–676.

Fowle LP, Rice JW (1953). Etiology of nummular eczema. *AMA Archives of Dermatology and Syphilology*, **68**: 69–79.

Gordon S (1954). Eczematous eruptions with special features. In: Loewenthal LJA (ed.), *The Eczemas*, Livingstone, Edinburgh.

Gutman AB, Kligman AM, Sciacca J, James WD (2005). Soak and smear: a standard technique revisited. *Archives of Dermatology*, **141**: 1556–1559.

Hellgren L, Mobacken H (1969). Nummular eczema – clinical and statistical data. *Acta Dermato-Venereologica*, **49**: 189–196.

Hill LW (1956). *The Treatment of Eczema in Infants and Children*, Mosby, St Louis.

Jansen T, Küppers U, Plewig G (1992). Sulzberger-Garbe exudative discoid and lichenoid chronic dermatosis ('Oid-Oid disease') – reality or fiction?. *Hautarzt*, **43**: 426–431.

Järvikallio A, Naukkarinen A, Harvima IT, Aalto ML, Horsmanheimo M (1997). Quantitative analysis of tryptase- and chymase-containing mast cells in atopic dermatitis and nummular eczema. *British Journal of Dermatology*, **136**: 871–877.

Järvikallio A, Harvima IT, Naukkarinen A (2003). Mast cells, nerves and neuropeptides in atopic dermatitis and nummular eczema. *Archives of Dermatological Research*, **295**: 2–7.

Johnson M-LT, Roberts J (1978). *Prevalence of Dermatological Disease among Persons 1–74 Years of Age*, Washington DC: US Department of Health Education, National Center for Health Statistics, 1978, DHEW Publication number PHS 79-1660. Data from the national health survey. Vital and Health Statistics Series 11, number 212.

Kaminska R, Mortenhumer M (2003). Nummular allergic contact dermatitis after scabies treatment. *Contact Dermatitis*, **48**: 337.

Krogh HK (1960). Nummular eczema. Its relationship to internal foci of infection. A survey of 84 case records. *Acta Dermato-Venereologica*, **40**: 114–126.

Krupa Shankar DS, Shrestha S (2005). Relevance of patch testing in patients with nummular dermatitis. *Indian Journal of Dermatology, Venereology and Leprology*, **71**: 406–408.

Le Coz CJ (2002). Contact nummular (discoid) eczema from depilating cream. *Contact Dermatitis*, **46**: 111–112.

Moore MM, Elpern DJ, Carter DJ (2004). Severe, generalized nummular eczema secondary to interferon alfa-2b plus ribavirin combination therapy in a patient with chronic hepatitis C virus infection. *Archives of Dermatology*, **140**: 215–217.

Patrizi A, Rizzoli L, Vincenzi C, Trevisi P, Tosti A (1999). Sensitization to thimerosal in atopic children. *Contact Dermatitis*, **40**: 94–97.

Pavithran K (1990). Non-pruritic eczemas as presenting manifestation of leprosy. *Indian Journal of Leprology*, **62**: 202–207.

Pietrzak A, Chodorowska G, Urban J, Bogucka V, Dybiec E (2005). Cutaneous manifestation of giardiasis – case report. *Annals of Agricultural and Environmental Medicine*, **12**: 299–303.

Pollitzer S (1912). A recurrent eczematoid affection of the hands. *Journal of Cutaneous Diseases*, **30**: 716–721.

Reed WB, Pidgeon J, Becker SW (1961). Patients with spinal cord injury. Clinical cutaneous studies. *Archives of Dermatology*, **83**: 379–385.

Roberts H, Orchard D (2010). Methotrexate is a safe and effective treatment for paediatric discoid (nummular) eczema: a case series of 25 children. *Australasian Journal of Dermatology*, **51**: 128–130.

Rollins TG (1968). From xerosis to nummular dermatitis. The dehydration dermatosis. *Journal of the American Medical Association*, **206**: 637.

Rosen R, Paver K, Kossard S (1990). Halo eczema surrounding seborrhoeic keratoses: an example of perilesional nummular dermatitis. *Australasian Journal of Dermatology*, **31**: 73–76.

Sakurane M, Shiotani A, Furukawa F (2002). Therapeutic effects of antibacterial treatment for intractable skin diseases in *Helicobacter pylori*-positive Japanese patients. *Journal of Dermatology*, **29**: 23–27.

Satoh T, Takayama K, Sawada Y, Yokozeki H, Nishioka K (2003). Chronic nodular prurigo associated with nummular eczema: possible involvement of odontogenic infection. *Acta Dermato-Venereologica*, **83**: 376–377.

Shelley WB, Crissey JT (2003). *Classics in Clinical Dermatology: With biographical sketches*, Parthenon, Boca Raton, p. 75.

Sulzberger MB (1979). Distinctive exudative discoid and lichenoid chronic dermatosis (Sulzberger and Garbe) re-examined – 1978. *British Journal of Dermatology*, **100**:13–20.

Sulzberger MD, Garbe W (1937). Nine cases of a distinctive exudative discoid and lichenoid chronic dermatosis. *Archives of Dermatology*, **36**: 247.

Tanaka T, Satoh T, Yokozeki H (2009). Dental infection associated with nummular eczema as an overlooked focal infection. *Journal of Dermatology*, **36**: 462–465.

Wilkinson DS (1979). Discoid eczema as a consequence of contact with irritants. *Contact Dermatitis*, **5**: 118–119.

Wilkinson SM, Smith AG, Davis MJ, Mattey D, Dawes PT (1992). Pityriasis rosea and discoid eczema: dose-related reactions to treatment with gold. *Annals of Rheumatic Diseases*, **51**: 881–884.

CHAPTER 17

Beauregard S, Gilchrest BA (1987). A survey of skin problems and skincare regimens in the elderly. *Archives of Dermatology*, **123**: 1638–1643.

Browse NL, Burnand KG (1982). The cause of venous ulceration. *Lancet*, ii: 243–245.

Charles CA, Romanelli P, Martinez ZB, Ma F, Roberts B, Kirsner RS (2009). Tumor necrosis factor-α in nonhealing venous leg ulcers. *Journal of the American Academy of Dermatology*, **60**: 951–955.

Cheatle TR, McMullin GM, Farrah J, Smith PD, Scurr JH (1990). Skin damage in chronic venous insufficiency: does an oxygen diffusion barrier really exist? *Journal of the Royal Society of Medicine*, **83**: 493–494.

Cheatle TR, Scott HJ, Scurr JH, Coleridge Smith PD (1991a). White cells, skin blood flow and venous ulcers. *British Journal of Dermatology*, **125**: 288–290.

Cheatle TR, Scurr JH, Smith PD (1991b). Drug treatment of chronic venous insufficiency and venous ulceration: a review. *Journal of the Royal Society of Medicine*, **84**: 354–358.

Coleridge Smith PD, Thomas P, Scurr JH, Dormandy JA (1988). Causes of venous ulceration: a new hypothesis. British Medical Journal. *Clinical Research Edition*, **296**: 1726–1727.

Cowin AJ, Hatzirodos N, Rigden J, Fitridge R, Belford DA (2006). Etanercept decreases tumor necrosis factor-α activity in chronic wound fluid. *Wound Repair and Regeneration*, **14**: 421–426.

Deguchi E, Imafuku S, Nakayama J (2010). Ulcerating stasis dermatitis of the forearm due to arteriovenous fistula: a case report and review of the published work. *Journal of Dermatology*, 37: 550–3.

Dillon RS (1986). Treatment of resistant venous stasis ulcers and dermatitis with the end-diastolic pneumatic compression boot. *Angiology*, 37: 47–56.

Dissemond J, Knab J, Lehnen M, Franckson T, Goos M (2004). Successful treatment of stasis dermatitis with topical tacrolimus. *VASA*, 33: 260–262.

Dodd HJ, Gaylarde PM, Sarkany I (1985). Skin oxygen tension in venous insufficiency of the lower leg. *Journal of the Royal Society of Medicine*, 78: 373–376.

Dooms-Goossens A, Degreef H, Parijs M, Maertens M (1979). A retrospective study of patch test results from 163 patients with stasis dermatitis or leg ulcers. II. Retesting of 50 patients. *Dermatologica*, 159: 231–238.

Droller H (1955). Dermatologic findings in a random sample of old persons. *Geriatrics*, 10: 421–424.

Falanga V, Moosa HH, Nemeth AJ, Alstadt SP, Eaglstein WH (1987). Dermal pericapillary fibrin in venous disease and venous ulceration. *Archives of Dermatology*, 123: 620–623.

Farber EM, Barnes VR (1956). The stasis syndrome. *AMA Archives of Dermatology*, 73: 277–282.

Gooptu C, Powell SM (1999). The problems of rubber hypersensitivity (Types I and IV) in chronic leg ulcer and stasis eczema patients. *Contact Dermatitis*, 41: 89–93.

Herouy Y, Mellios P, Bandemir E, *et al.* (2001). Inflammation in stasis dermatitis upregulates MMP-1, MMP-2 and MMP-13 expression. *Journal of Dermatological Science*, 25: 198–205.

Isoda H, Shimauchi T, Ogaki T, *et al.* (2006). Stasis ulcer and dermatitis caused by artificial arteriovenous fistula created 33 years previously for the treatment of poliomyelitis. *Clinical and Experimental Dermatology*, 31: 470–472.

Jappe U, Schnuch A, Uter W (2003). Frequency of sensitization to antimicrobials in patients with atopic eczema compared with nonatopic individuals: analysis of multicentre surveillance data, 1995–1999.

British Journal of Dermatology, 149:87–93.

Kasteler JS, Petersen MJ, Vance JE, Zone JJ (1992). Circulating activated T lymphocytes in autoeczematization. *Archives of Dermatology*, 128: 795–798.

Kirsner RS, Pardes JB, Eaglstein WH, Falanga V (1993). The clinical spectrum of lipodermatosclerosis. *Journal of the American Academy of Dermatology*, 28: 623–627.

Lever WF, Schaumburg-Lever G (1990). *Histopathology of the Skin*, 7th edn, Lippincott-Raven, Philadelphia, p. 690.

Lotti T, Fabbri P, Panconesi E (1987). The pathogenesis of venous ulcers. *Journal of the American Academy of Dermatology*, 16: 877–879.

Morris SD, Rycroft RJ, White IR, Wakelin SH, McFadden JP (2002). Comparative frequency of patch test reactions to topical antibiotics. *British Journal of Dermatology*, 146: 1047–1051.

Pappas PJ, You R, Rameshwar P, *et al.* (1999). Dermal tissue fibrosis in patients with chronic venous insufficiency is associated with increased transforming growth factor-beta1 gene expression and protein production. *Journal of Vascular Surgery*, 30: 1129–1145.

Pardes JB, Nemeth AJ (1993). Adverse sequelae of venous hypertension. *Seminars in Dermatology*, 12: 66–71.

Pascarella L, Schonbein GW, Bergan JJ (2005). Microcirculation and venous ulcers: a review. *Annals of Vascular Surgery*, 19: 921–927.

Peschen M, Lahaye T, Hennig B, Weyl A, Simon JC, Vanscheidt W (1999). Expression of the adhesion molecules ICAM-1, VCAM-1, LFA-1 and VLA-4 in the skin is modulated in progressing stages of chronic venous insufficiency. *Acta Dermato-Venereologica*, 79: 27–32.

Pimentel CL, Rodriguez-Salido MJ (2008). Pigmentation due to stasis dermatitis treated successfully with a noncoherent intense pulsed light source. *Dermatologic Surgery*, 34: 950–951.

Purwins S, Herberger K, Debus ES, *et al.* (2010). Cost-of-illness of chronic leg ulcers in Germany. *International Wound Journal*, 7: 97–102.

Raju, S, Hollis, K, Neglen P (2007). Use of compression stockings in chronic venous disease: patient compliance and efficacy. *Annals of Vascular Surgery*, 21: 790–795.

Reich-Schupke S, Kreuter A, Altmeyer P, Stücker M (2009). Wrong diagnosis erysipelas: hypodermitis – case series and review of literature. *Journal der Deutschen Dermatologischen Gesellschaft*, 7: 222–225.

Weaver J, Billings SD (2009). Initial presentation of stasis dermatitis mimicking solitary lesions: a previously unrecognized clinical scenario. *Journal of the American Academy of Dermatology*, 61: 1028–1032.

Weismann K, Krakauer R, Wanscher B (1980). Prevalence of skin diseases in old age. *Acta Dermato-Venereologica*, 60: 352–353.

Wilkinson SM (1994). Hypersensitivity to topical corticosteroids. *Clinical and Experimental Dermatology*, 19: 1–11.

Wilkinson SM, English JS (1992). Hydrocortisone sensitivity: clinical features of 59 cases. *Journal of the American Academy of Dermatology*, 27: 683–687.

CHAPTER 18

Ackerman AB (1977). Histopathologic differentiation of eczematous dermatitides from psoriasis and seborrheic dermatitis. *Cutis*, 20: 619–623.

Alessi E, Cusini M, Zerboni R (1988). Mucocutaneous manifestations in patients infected with human immunodeficiency virus. *Journal of the American Academy of Dermatology*, 19: 290–297.

Aly R, Katz HI, Kempers SE, *et al.* (2003). Ciclopirox gel for seborrheic dermatitis of the scalp. *Journal of the American Academy of Dermatology*, 42(suppl 1): 19–22.

Andersen SL, Thomsen K (1971). Psoriasiform napkin dermatitis. *British Journal of Dermatology*, l84: 316–319.

Barba A, Piubello W, Vantini I, *et al.* (1982). Skin lesions in chronic alcoholic pancreatitis. *Dermatologica*, 164: 322–326.

Barr RJ, Young EM Jr (1985). Psoriasiform and related papulosquamous disorders. *Journal of Cutaneous Pathology*, 12: 412–425.

Bergbrant IM, Faergemann J (1989). Seborrheic dermatitis and *Pityrosporum ovale*: a cultural and immunological study. *Acta Dermato-Venereologica*, l69: 332–335.

Bergbrant IM, Johansson S, Robbins D, Scheynius A, Faergemann J, Söderström T (1991). An immunological study in patients with seborrheic dermatitis. *Clinical and Experimental Dermatology*, 16: 331–338.

Berger RS, Stoner MF, Hobbs ER, Hayes TJ, Boswell RN (1988). Cutaneous manifestations of early human immunodeficiency virus exposure. *Journal of the American Academy of Dermatology*, 19: 298–303.

Brenner S, Horwitz C (1988). Possible nutrient mediators in psoriasis and seborrheic dermatitis. II. Nutrient mediators: essential fatty acids; vitamins A, E and D; vitamins B_1, B_2, B_6, niacin and biotin; vitamin C selenium; zinc; iron. *World Review of Nutrition and Dietetics*, 55: 165–182.

Burton JL, Pye RJ (1983). Seborrhea is not a feature of seborrheic dermatitis. *British Medical Journal (Clinical Research Edition)*, 286: 1169–1170.

Burton JL, Cunliffe WJ, Saunders IG, Shuster S (1971). The effect of facial nerve paresis on sebum excretion. *British Journal of Dermatology*, 84: 135–138.

Burton JL, Cartlidge M, Cartlidge NE, Shuster S (1973a). Sebum excretion in Parkinsonism. *British Journal of Dermatology*, 88: 263–266.

Burton JL, Cartlidge M, Shuster S (1973b). Effect of L-dopa on the seborrhea of Parkinsonism. *British Journal of Dermatology*, 88: 475–479.

Caputo R, Gelmetti C (2002). *Pediatric Dermatology and Dermatopathology: A Concise Atlas*, Martin Dunitz, London.

Carr MM, Pryce DM, Ive FA (1987). Treatment of seborrhoeic dermatitis with ketoconazole: I. Response of seborrheic dermatitis of the scalp to topical ketoconazole. *British Journal of Dermatology*, 116: 213–216.

Cassano N, Amoruso A, Loconsole F, Vena GA (2002). Oral terbinafine for the treatment of seborrheic dermatitis in adults. *Journal of the American Academy of Dermatology*, 41: 821–822.

Christodoulou GN, Vareltzides AG (1978). Positive side effects of lithium? *American Journal of Psychiatry*, 135: 1249.

Christodoulou GN, Georgala S, Vareltzides A, Catsarou A (1983). Lithium in seborrheic dermatitis. *Psychiatric Journal of the University of Ottawa*, 8: 27–29.

Clift DC, Dodd HJ, Kirby JD, Midgley G, Noble WC (1988). Seborrheic dermatitis and malignancy. An investigation of the skin flora. *Acta Dermato-Venereologica*, 68: 48–52.

Cowley NC, Farr PM, Shuster S (1990). The permissive effect of sebum in seborrheic dermatitis: an explanation of the rash in neurological disorders. *British Journal of Dermatology*, 122: 71–76.

Cribier B, Samain F, Vetter D, Heid E, Grosshans E (1998). Systematic cutaneous examination in hepatitis C virus-infected patients. *Acta Dermato-Venereologica*, 78: 355–357.

Dawson TL Jr (2007). *Malassezia globosa* and *restricta*: breakthrough understanding of the etiology and treatment of dandruff and seborrheic dermatitis through whole-genome analysis. *Journal of Investigative Dermatology Symposium Proceedings*, 12: 15–19.

DeAngelis YM, Gemmer CM, Kaczvinsky JR, Kenneally DC, Schwartz JR, Dawson TL Jr (2005). Three etiologic facets of dandruff and seborrheic dermatitis: Malassezia fungi, sebaceous lipids, and individual sensitivity. *Journal of Investigative Dermatology Symposium Proceedings*, 10: 295–297.

DeAngelis YM, Saunders CW, Johnstone KR, *et al.* (2007). Isolation and expression of a *Malassezia globosa* lipase gene, LIP1. *Journal of Investigative Dermatology*, 127: 2138–2146.

DHEW (1978). *Skin conditions and related need for medical care among persons 1–74 years, United States, 1971–1974*, National Center for Health Statistics, Hyattsville, DHEW publication no. 79-1660.

Eisenstat BA, Wormser GP (1984). Seborrheic dermatitis and butterfly rash in AIDS. *New England Journal of Medicine*, 311: 189.

Ercis M, Balci S, Atakan N (1996). Dermatological manifestations of 71 Down syndrome children admitted to a clinical genetics unit. *Clinical Genetics*, 317–320.

Eyre RW, Burton CS, Callaway JL (1984). Dandruff and seborrheic dermatitis. *North Carolina Medical Journal*, 45: 789–790.

Faergemann J (1999). *Pityrosporum* species as a cause of allergy and infection. *Allergy*, 54: 413–419.

Faergemann J, Johansson S, Bäck O, Scheynius A (1986). An immunologic and cultural study of *Pityrosporum* folliculitis. *Journal of the American Academy of Dermatology*, 14: 429–433.

Ford GP, Farr PM, Ive FA, Shuster S (1984). The response of seborrhoeic dermatitis to ketoconazole. *British Journal of Dermatology*, 111: 603–607.

Fredriksson T (1985). Controlled comparison of Clinitar Shampoo and Selsun Shampoo in the treatment of seborrheic dermatitis of the scalp. *British Journal of Clinical Practice*, 39: 25–28.

Gaitanis G, Magiatis P, Stathopoulou K, *et al.* (2008). AhR ligands, malassezin, and indolo[3,2-b]carbazole are selectively produced by *Malassezia furfur* strains isolated from seborrheic dermatitis. *Journal of Investigative Dermatology*, 128: 1620–1625.

Garcia RL, Miller JD, Miller WN (1978). Occlusive tar extract therapy for recalcitrant psoriasis and seborrheic dermatitis of the scalp. *Cutis*, 22: 90–91.

Gross-Tsur V, Gross-Kieselstein E, Amir N (1990). Cardio-facio cutaneous syndrome: neurological manifestations. *Clinical Genetics*, 38: 382–386.

Guého E, Faergemann J, Lyman C, Anaissie EJ (1994). *Malassezia* and *Trichosporon*: two emerging pathogenic basidiomycetous yeast-like fungi. *Journal of Medical and Veterinary Mycology*, 32(suppl 1): 367–378.

Gupta AK (2001). A random survey concerning aspects of acne rosacea [abstract]. *Journal of Cutaneous Medicine and Surgery*, 5(suppl): 38.

Gupta AK, Bluhm R (2004). Seborrheic dermatitis. *Journal of the European Academy of Dermatology and Venereology*, 18: 13–26.

Gupta AK, Batra R, Bluhm R, Boekhout T, Dawson TL Jr (2004a). Skin diseases associated with *Malassezia* species. *Journal of the American Academy of Dermatology*, 51: 785–798.

Gupta AK, Madzia SE, Batra R (2004b). Etiology and management of seborrheic dermatitis. *Dermatology*, 208: 89–93.

Honig PJ, Frieden IJ, Kim HJ, Yan AC (2003). Streptococcal intertrigo:

an underrecognized condition in children. *Pediatrics*, **112**(6 Pt 1): 1427–1429.

Ilchyshyn A, Meldelsohn SS, Macfarlane A, Verbov J (1987). *Candida albicans* and infantile seborrheic dermatitis. *British Journal of Clinical Practice*, 41: 557–559.

Jacobs JC, Miller ME (1972). Fatal familial Leiner's disease: a deficiency of the opsonic activity of serum complement. *Pediatrics*, 49: 225–232.

Janniger CK (1993). Infantile seborrheic dermatitis: an approach to cradle cap. *Cutis*, 51: 233–235.

Janniger CK, Schwartz RA (1995). Seborrheic dermatitis. *American Family Physician*, **52**: 149–55, 159–160. Review. Erratum in: *American Family Physician*, 1995; 52: 782.

Janniger CK, Schwartz RA, Musumeci ML, Tedeschi A, Mirona B, Micali G (2005). Infantile psoriasis. *Cutis*, **76**: 173–177.

Kaplan MH, Sadick N, McNutt NS, Meltzer M, Sarngadharan MG, Pahwa S (1987). Dermatologic findings and manifestations of acquired immunodeficiency syndrome (AIDS). *Journal of the American Academy of Dermatology*, **16**: 485–506.

Kasteler JS, Callen JP (1994). Scalp involvement in dermatomyositis. Often overlooked or misdiagnosed. *Journal of the American Medical Association*, **272**: 1939–1941.

Keipert JA (1990). Rashes commonly starting in the first few months: various forms of dermatitis. In: Keipert JA (ed.), *Essential Pediatric Dermatology*, Harwood, London.

Kerr K, Darcy T, Henry J, *et al.* (2011). Epidermal changes associated with symptomatic resolution of dandruff: biomarkers of scalp health. *International Journal of Dermatology*, 50: 102–113.

Kligman AM (1979). Perspectives and problems in cutaneous gerontology. *Journal of Investigative Dermatology*, 73: 39–46.

Kligman AM, McGinley KJ, Leyden JJ (1976). The nature of dandruff. *Journal of the Society of Cosmetic Chemists*, 27: 111–139.

Krfstin D (1927). The seborrheic facies as a manifestation of postencephalitic Parkinsonism and allied disorders. *Quarterly Journal of Medicine*, 21: 177.

Ljubojevic S, Lipozencic J, Basta-Juzbasic A (2010). Contact allergy to corticosteroids and *Malassezia furfur* in seborrheic dermatitis patients. *Journal of the European Academy of Dermatology and Venereology*, 25: 647–651.

Lynch PJ (1982). Dermatologic problems of the head and neck in the aged. *Otolaryngologic Clinics of North America*, **15**: 271–285.

McCulley JP, Dougherty JM (1985). Blepharitis associated with acne rosacea and seborrheic dermatitis. *International Ophthalmology Clinics*, **25**: 159–172.

McGinley KJ, Leyden JJ, Marples RR, Kligman AM (1975). Quantitative microbiology of the scalp in nondandruff, dandruff, and seborrheic dermatitis. *Journal of Investigative Dermatology*, **64**: 401–405.

Mahé A, Boulais C, Blanc L, Kéita S, Bobin P (1994). Seborrheic dermatitis as a revealing feature of HIV infection in Bamako, Mali. *Journal of the American Academy of Dermatology*, **33**: 601–602.

Mahé A, Simon F, Coulibaly S, Tounkara A, Bobin P (1996). Predictive value of seborrheic dermatitis and other common dermatoses for HIV infection in Bamako, Mali. *Journal of the American Academy of Dermatology*, **34**: 1084–1086.

Maietta G, Fornaro P, Rongioletti F, Rebora A (1990). Patients with mood depression have a high prevalence of seborrheic dermatitis. *Acta Dermato-Venereologica*, 70: 432–434.

Marino CT, McDonald E, Romano JF (1991). Seborrheic dermatitis in acquired immunodeficiency syndrome. *Cutis*, **48**: 217–218.

Marks R, Pearse AD, Walker AP (1985). The effects of a shampoo containing zinc pyrithione on the control of dandruff. *British Journal of Dermatology*, **112**: 415–422.

Mathes BM, Douglass MC (1985). Seborrheic dermatitis in patients with acquired immunodeficiency syndrome. *Journal of the American Academy of Dermatology*, **13**: 947–951.

Matis WL, Triana A, Shapiro R, Eldred L, Polk BF, Hood AF (1987). Dermatologic findings associated with human immunodeficiency virus infection. *Journal of the American Academy of Dermatology*, **17**: 746–751.

Mayser P, Gross A (2000). IgE antibodies to *Malassezia furfur*, *M. sympodialis* and *Pityrosporum orbiculare* in patients with atopic dermatitis, seborrheic eczema or pityriasis versicolor, and identification of respective allergens. *Acta Dermato-Venereologica*, **80**: 357–361.

Menni S, Piccinno R, Baietta S, Ciuffreda A, Scotti L (1989). Infantile seborrheic dermatitis: 7-year follow-up and some prognostic criteria. *Pediatric Dermatology*, **6**: 13–15.

Meshkinpour A, Sun J, Weinstein G (2003). An open pilot study using tacrolimus ointment in the treatment of seborrheic dermatitis. *Journal of the American Academy of Dermatology*, **49**: 145–147.

Mills KJ, Hu P, Henry J, Tamura M, Tiesman JP, Xu J (2012). Dandruff/seborrheic dermatitis is characterized by an inflammatory genomic signature and possible immune dysfunction: transcriptional analysis of the condition and treatment effects of zinc pyrithione. *British Journal of Dermatology*, **166**(suppl 2): 33–40.

Mimouni K, Mukamel M, Zeharia A, Mimouni M (1995). Prognosis of infantile seborrheic dermatitis. *Journal of Pediatrics*, **127**: 744–746.

Moises-Alfaro CB, Caceres-Rios HW, Rueda M, Velazquez-Acosta A, Ruiz-Maldonado R (2002). Are infantile seborrheic and atopic dermatitis clinical variants of the same disease? *Journal of the American Academy of Dermatology*, **41**: 349–351.

Moore M, Kile RL (1935). *Pityrosporum ovalis* as a causative agent of seborrheic dermatitis. *Science*, **81**: 277–278.

Nakabayashi A, Sei Y, Guillot J (2000). Identification of *Malassezia* species isolated from patients with seborrheic dermatitis, atopic dermatitis, pityriasis versicolor and normal subjects. *Medical Mycology*, **38**: 337–341.

Neville EA, Finn OA (1975). Psoriasiform napkin dermatitis – a follow-up study. *British Journal of Dermatology*, **92**: 279–285.

Olansky S (1980). Whole coal tar shampoo: a therapeutic hair repair system. *Cutis*, **25**: 99–104.

Opdyke DL, Burnett CM, Brauer EW (1967). Anti-seborrheic qualities of zinc pyrithione in a cream vehicle. II. Safety evaluation. *Food Cosmetics Toxicology*, **5**: 321–326.

Ostlere LS, Taylor CR, Harris DW, Rustin MH, Wright S, Johnson M (1996). Skin surface lipids in HIV-positive patients with and without seborrheic dermatitis. *Journal of the American Academy of Dermatology*, 35: 276–279.

Passi S, Morrone A, De Luca C, Picardo M, Ippolito F (1991). Blood levels of vitamin E, polyunsaturated fatty acids of phospholipids, lipoperoxides and glutathione peroxidase in patients affected with seborrheic dermatitis. *Journal of Dermatological Science*, 2: 171–178.

Peter RU, Richarz-Barthauer U (1995). Successful treatment and prophylaxis of scalp seborrheic dermatitis and dandruff with 2% ketoconazole shampoo: results of a multicentre, double-blind, placebo-controlled trial. *British Journal of Dermatology*, 132: 441–445.

Pierard GE, Arrese JE, Pierard-Franchimont C, *et al.* (1997). Prolonged effects of antidandruff shampoos – time to recurrence of *Malassezia ovalis* colonization of skin. *International Journal of Cosmetic Science*, 19: 111–117.

Piérard-Franchimont C, Hermanns JF, Degreef H, Piérard GE (2000). From axioms to new insights into dandruff. *Dermatology*, 200: 93–98.

Podmore P, Burrows D, Eedy DJ, Stanford CF (1986). Seborrheic eczema – a disease entity or a clinical variant of atopic eczema? *British Journal of Dermatology*, 115: 341–350.

Priestley GC, Savin JA (1976). The microbiology of dandruff. *British Journal of Dermatology*, 94: 469–471.

Prohic A (2010). Distribution of *Malassezia* species in seborrheic dermatitis: correlation with patients' cellular immune status. *Mycoses*, 53: 344–349.

Rigopoulos D, Ioannides D, Kalogeromitros D, Gregoriou S, Katsambas A (2004). Pimecrolimus cream 1% vs. betamethasone 17-valerate 0.1% cream in the treatment of seborrheic dermatitis. A randomized open-label clinical trial. *British Journal of Dermatology*, 151: 1071–1075.

Ro BI, Dawson TL (2005). The role of sebaceous gland activity and scalp microfloral metabolism in the etiology of seborrheic dermatitis and dandruff. *Journal of Investigative Dermatology Symposium Proceedings*, 10: 194–197.

Rook A, Wilkinson DS, Ebling FJG, eds (1998). *Textbook of Dermatology*, Blackwell Science, Oxford.

Ruiz-Maldonado R, López-Matínez R, Pérez Chavarría EL, Rocio Castañón L, Tamayo L (1989a). *Pityrosporum ovale* in infantile seborrheic dermatitis. *Pediatric Dermatology*, 6: 16–20.

Ruiz-Maldonado R, Parish LC, Beare JM, (eds) (1989b). *Textbook of Pediatric Dermatology*, Grune & Stratton, Philadelphia.

Sandyk R, Kay SR (1990). The relationship of negative schizophrenia to parkinsonism. *International Journal of Neuroscience*, 55: 1–59.

Scaparro E, Quadri G, Virno G, Orifici C, Milani M (2001). Evaluation of the efficacy and tolerability of oral terbinafine (Daskil) in patients with seborrheic dermatitis. A multicentre, randomized, investigator-blinded, placebo-controlled trial. *British Journal of Dermatology*, 144: 854–857.

Schachner LA, Hansen RC (1988). *Pediatric Dermatology*, Churchill Livingstone, New York, p. 659.

Schwartz JR, Shah R, Krigbaum H, Sacha J, Vogt A, Blume-Peytavi U (2011). New insights on dandruff/seborrheic dermatitis: the role of the scalp follicular infundibulum in effective treatment strategies. *British Journal of Dermatology*, 165(suppl 2): 18–23.

Schwartz RA, Janusz CA, Janniger CK (2006). Seborrheic dermatitis: an overview. *American Family Physician*, 74: 125–30.

Senaldi G, Di Perri G, Di Silverio A, Minoli L (1987). Seborrheic dermatitis: an early manifestation in AIDS. *Clinical and Experimental Dermatology*, 12: 72–73.

Shemer A, Kaplan B, Nathanson N, Grunwald MH, Amichai B, Trau H (2008). Treatment of moderate to severe facial seborrheic dermatitis with itraconazole: an open non-comparative study. *Israel Medical Association Journal*, 10: 417–418.

Shuster S (1984). The etiology of dandruff and the mode of action of therapeutic agents. *British Journal of Dermatology*, 111: 235–242.

Soeprono FF, Schinella RA, Cockerell CJ, Comite SL (1986). Seborrheic-like dermatitis of acquired immunodeficiency syndrome. A clinicopathologic study. *Journal of the American Academy of Dermatology*, 14: 242–248.

Sonea MJ, Moroz BE, Reece ER (1987). Leiner's disease associated with diminished third component of complement. *Pediatric Dermatology*, 4: 105–107.

Stratigos JD, Antoniou C, Katsambas A, *et al.* (1988). Ketoconazole 2% cream versus hydrocortisone 1% cream in the treatment of seborrheic dermatitis. A double-blind comparative study. *Journal of the American Academy of Dermatology*, 19: 850–853.

Tajima M, Sugita T, Nishikawa A, Tsuboi R (2008). Molecular analysis of *Malassezia* microflora in seborrheic dermatitis patients: comparison with other diseases and healthy subjects. *Journal of Investigative Dermatology*, 128: 345–351.

Tilstra JS, Prevost N, Khera P, English JC 3rd (2009). Scalp dermatomyositis revisited. *Archives of Dermatology*, 145: 1062–1063.

Tollesson A, Frithz A (1993). Borage oil, an effective new treatment for infantile seborrheic dermatitis. *British Journal of Dermatology*, 129: 95.

Tollesson A, Frithz A, Berg A, Karlman G (1993). Essential fatty acids in infantile seborrheic dermatitis. *Journal of the American Academy of Dermatology*, 28: 957–961.

Tollesson A, Frithz A, Stenlund K (1997). *Malassezia furfur* in infantile seborrheic dermatitis. *Pediatric Dermatology*, 14: 423–425.

Turner JD, Schwartz RA (2006). Atopic dermatitis. A clinical challenge. *Acta Dermato Venereologica Alpina, Panonica, et Adriatica*, 15(2): 59–68.

Valia RG (2006). Etiopathogenesis of seborrheic dermatitis. *Indian Journal of Dermatology, Venereology and Leprology*, 72: 253–255.

Veien NK, Pilgaard CE, Gade M (1980). Seborrheic dermatitis of the scalp treated with a tar/zinc pyrithione shampoo. *Clinical and Experimental Dermatology*, 5: 53–56.

Vickers CFH (1980). The natural history of atopic eczema. *Acta Dermato-Venereologica*, 92(suppl): 113–115.

Vidal C, Girard PM, Dompmartin D, et al. (1990). Seborrheic dermatitis and HIV infection. Qualitative analysis of skin surface lipids in men seropositive and seronegative for HIV. Journal of the American Academy of Dermatology, 23: 1106–1110.

Wananukul S, Chatproedprai S, Charutragulchai W (2011). Randomized, double-blind, split-side comparison study of moisturizer containing licochalcone vs. 1% hydrocortisone in the treatment of infantile seborrheic dermatitis. Journal of the European Academy of Dermatology and Venereology, 26: 894–897.

Yates VM, Kerr RE, MacKie RM (1983). Early diagnosis of infantile seborrheic dermatitis and atopic dermatitis – clinical features. British Journal of Dermatology, 108: 633–638.

Zug KA, Palay DA, Rock B (1996). Dermatologic diagnosis and treatment of itchy red eyelids. Survey of Ophthalmology, 40: 293–306.

CHAPTER 19

Alcalay J, Wolf JE Jr (1988). Pruritic urticarial papules and plaques of pregnancy: the enigma and the confusion. Journal of the American Academy of Dermatology, 19: 1115–1116.

Aronson IK, Bond S, Fiedler VC, Vomvouras S, Gruber D, Ruiz C (1998). Pruritic urticarial papules and plaques of pregnancy: clinical and immunopathologic observations in 57 patients. Journal of the American Academy of Dermatology, 39: 933–939. (Erratum in: Journal of the American Academy of Dermatology, 1999; 40: 611.)

Arpey CJ, Nagashima-Whalen LS, Chren MM, Zaim MT (1992). Congenital miliaria crystallina: case report and literature review. Pediatric Dermatology, 9: 283–287.

Bassukas ID (1992). Is erythema toxicum neonatorum a mild self-limited acute cutaneous graft-versus-host reaction from maternal-to-fetal lymphocyte transfer? Medical Hypotheses, 38: 334–338.

Borrego L (2000). Follicular lesions in polymorphic eruption of pregnancy. Journal of the American Academy of Dermatology, 42: 146.

Borrego L, Peterson EA, Diez LI, et al. (1999). Polymorphic eruption of

pregnancy and herpes gestationis: comparison of granulated cell proteins in tissue and serum. Clinical and Experimental Dermatology, 24: 213–225.

Brand CU, Hunziker T, Schaffner T, Limat A, Gerber HA, Braathen LR (1995). Activated immunocompetent cells in human skin lymph derived from irritant contact dermatitis: an immunomorphological study. British Journal of Dermatology, 132: 39–45.

Cambiaghi S, Scarabelli G, Pistritto G, Gelmetti C (1995). Gianotti–Crosti syndrome in an adult after influenza virus vaccination. Dermatology, 191: 340–341.

Chen JJ, Liang YH, Zhou FS, et al. (2006). The gene for a rare autosomal dominant form of pompholyx maps to chromosome 18q22.1-18q22.3. Journal of Investigative Dermatology, 126: 300–304.

Chien YH, Hwu WL, Chiang BL (2007). The genetics of atopic dermatitis. Clinical Reviews in Allergy and Immunology, 33: 178–190.

Choudhri SH, Magro CM, Crowson AN, Nicolle LE (1994). An Id reaction to Mycobacterium leprae: first documented case. Cutis, 54: 282–286.

Chuh A, Lee A, Zawar V, Sciallis G, Kempf W (2005). Pityriasis rosea – an update. Indian Journal of Dermatology Venereology and Leprology, 71: 311–315.

Elling SV, McKenna P, Powell FC (2000). Pruritic urticarial papules and plaques of pregnancy in twin and triplet pregnancies. Journal of the European Academy of Dermatology and Venereology, 14: 378–381.

Enomoto H, Noguchi E, Iijima S, et al. (2007). Single nucleotide polymorphism-based genome-wide linkage analysis in Japanese atopic dermatitis families. BMC Dermatology, 7: 5.

Erkek E, Senturk GB, Ozkaya O, Bükülmez G (2001). Gianotti–Crosti syndrome preceded by oral polio vaccine and followed by varicella infection. Pediatric Dermatology, 18: 516–518.

Fierro MT, Novelli M, Quaglino P, et al. (2008). Heterogeneity of circulating CD4+ memory T-cell subsets in erythrodermic patients: CD27 analysis can help to distinguish cutaneous T-cell lymphomas from inflammatory

erythroderma. Dermatology, 216: 213–221.

Fyhrquist-Vanni N, Alenius H, Lauerma A (2007). Contact dermatitis. Dermatologic Clinics, 25: 613–623.

Goepel J (1959). The Sulzberger–Garbe syndrome [in German]. Dermatologische Wochenschrift, 140: 1338–1341.

Gourdin FW, Smith JG Jr (1993). Etiology of venous ulceration. Southern Medical Journal, 86: 1142–1146.

Guillet MH, Wierzbicka E, Guillet S, Dagregorio G, Guillet G (2007). A 3-year causative study of pompholyx in 120 patients. Archives of Dermatology, 143: 1504–1508.

Hon KL, Lam MC, Leung TF, et al. (2007). Are age-specific high serum IgE levels associated with worse symptomatology in children with atopic dermatitis? International Journal of Dermatology, 46: 1258–1262.

Jain VK, Aggarwal K, Passi S, Gupta S (2004). Role of contact allergens in pompholyx. Journal of Dermatology, 31: 188–193.

Kanda N, Watanabe S (2007). Leukotriene B (4) enhances tumor necrosis factor-alpha-induced CCL27 production in human keratinocytes. Clinical and Experimental Allergy, 37: 1074–1082.

Kang NG, Oh CW (2003). Gianotti-Crosti syndrome following Japanese encephalitis vaccination. Journal of Korean Medical Science, 18: 459–461.

Karakaş M, Durdu M, Tuncer I, Cevlik F (2007). Gianotti–Crosti syndrome in a child following hepatitis B virus vaccination. Journal of Dermatology, 34: 117–120.

Karvonen J (2001). Nummular eczema [in Finnish]. Duodecim, 117: 1140–1146.

Kirk JF, Wilson BB, Chun W, Cooper PH (1996). Miliaria profunda. Journal of the American Academy of Dermatology, 35: 854–856.

Kwan T (2004). Spongiotic dermatitis. In: Barnhill RL, Crowson AN (eds), Textbook of Dermatopathology, McGraw-Hill, New York, pp. 17–34.

Lin RL, Janniger CK (2005). Pityriasis alba. Cutis, 76: 21–24.

Lipozencić J, Wolf R (2007). Atopic dermatitis: an update and review of the literature. Dermatologic Clinics, 25: 605–612.

Lisby S, Müller KM, Jongeneel CV, et al. (1995). Nickel and skin irritants upregulate tumor necrosis factor-alpha mRNA in keratinocytes by different but potentially synergistic mechanisms. *International Immunology*, 7: 343–352.

Llombart M, García-Abujeta JL, Sánchez-Pérez RM, et al. (2007). Pompholyx induced by intravenous immunoglobulin therapy. *Journal of Investigative Allergology and Clinical Immunology*, 17: 277–278.

Magro CM, Crowson AN (2000). Necrotizing eosinophilic folliculitis as a manifestation of the atopic diathesis. *International Journal of Dermatology*, 39: 672–677.

Magro C, Crowson AN, Kovatich A, et al. (2002). Pityriasis lichenoides: a clonal T-cell lymphoproliferative disorder. *Human Pathology*, 33: 788–795.

Magro CM, Nuovo GJ, Crowson AN (2003). The utility of the *in situ* detection of T-cell receptor beta rearrangements in cutaneous T-cell-dominant infiltrates. *Diagnostic and Molecular Pathology*, 12: 133–141.

Magro CM, Dyrsen ME, Crowson AN (2008). Acute infectious id panniculitis/panniculitic bacterid: a distinctive form of neutrophilic lobular panniculitis. *Journal of Cutaneous Pathology*, 35: 941–946.

Mikulowska A, Falck B (1994). Distributional changes of Langerhans cells in human skin during irritant contact dermatitis. *Archives of Dermatology Research*, 286: 429–433.

Monastirli A, Varvarigou A, Pasmatzi E, et al. (2007). Gianotti–Crosti syndrome after hepatitis A vaccination. *Acta Dermato-Venereologica*, 87: 174–175.

Mowad CM, McGinley KJ, Foglia A, et al. (1995). The role of extracellular polysaccharide substance produced by *Staphylococcus epidermidis* in miliaria. *Journal of the American Academy of Dermatology*, 33: 729–733.

Murphy LA, Buckley C (2000). Gianotti–Crosti syndrome in an infant following immunization. *Pediatric Dermatology*, 17: 225–226.

Murray JC (1990). Pregnancy and the skin. *Dermatologic Clinics*, 8: 327–334.

Niinai H, Kawamoto M, Yuge O (2004). Severe pompholyx following endoscopic thoracic sympathectomy for palmar hyperhidrosis. *Interactive Cardiovascular Thoracic Surgery*, 3: 593–595.

Ortonne N, Le Gouvello S, Mansour H, et al. (2008). CD158K/KIR3DL2 transcript detection in lesional skin of patients with erythroderma is a tool for the diagnosis of Sézary syndrome. *Journal of Investigative Dermatology*, 128: 465–472.

Park do S, Youn YH (2007). Clinical significance of serum interleukin-18 concentration in the patients with atopic dermatitis [in Korean]. *Korean Journal of Laboratory Medicine*, 27: 128–132.

Parsons JM (1996). Transient acantholytic dermatosis (Grover's disease): a global perspective. *Journal of the American Academy of Dermatology*, 35: 653–666. [Erratum in: *Journal of the American Academy of Dermatology*, 1997; 36: 370.]

Raby BA, Klanderman B, Murphy A, et al. (2007). A common mitochondrial haplogroup is associated with elevated total serum IgE levels. *Journal of Allergy and Clinical Immunology*, 120: 351–358.

Razzaque Ahmed A (1984). Diagnosis of bullous disease and studies in the pathogenesis of blister formation using immunopathological techniques. *Journal of Cutaneous Pathology*, 11: 237–248.

Rudolph CM, Al-Fares S, Vaughan-Jones SA, et al. (2006). Polymorphic eruption of pregnancy: clinicopathology and potential trigger factors in 181 patients. *British Journal of Dermatology*, 154: 54–60.

Schwartz RA, Janniger CK (1996). Erythema toxicum neonatorum. *Cutis*, 58: 153–155.

Schwartz RA, Janusz CA, Janniger CK (2006). Seborrheic dermatitis: an overview. *American Family Physician*, 74: 125–130.

Sehgal VN, Srivastava G, Aggarwal AK (2007). Parapsoriasis: a complex issue. *Skinmed*, 6: 280–286.

Sherard GB 3rd, Atkinson SM Jr. (2001). Focus on primary care: pruritic dermatological conditions in pregnancy. *Obstetrical and Gynecological Survey*, 56: 427–432.

Snijders BE, Thijs C, Kummeling I, et al. (2007). Breastfeeding and infant eczema in the first year of life in the KOALA birth cohort study: a risk period-specific analysis. *Pediatrics*, 119: e137–e141.

Söderhäll C, Marenholz I, Kerscher T, et al. (2007). Variants in a novel epidermal collagen gene (COL29A1) are associated with atopic dermatitis. *PLoS Biology*, 5: e242.

Stone OJ (1990). High viscosity of newborn extracellular matrix is the etiology of erythema toxicum neonatorum: neonatal jaundice?: hyaline membrane disease? *Medical Hypotheses*, 33: 15–17.

Straka BF, Cooper PH, Greer KE (1991). Congenital miliaria crystallina. *Cutis*, 47: 103–106.

Szepietowski J, Walker C, Hunter JA, et al. (2001). Elevated leukaemia inhibitory factor (LIF) expression in lesional psoriatic skin: correlation with interleukin (IL)-8 expression. *Journal of Dermatology*, 28: 115–122.

Vasconcellos C, Domingues PP, Aoki V, et al. (1995). Erythroderma: analysis of 247 cases. *Revista de Saúde Pública*, 29: 177–182.

Vaughan Jones SA, Hern S, Nelson-Piercy C, et al. (1999). A prospective study of 200 women with dermatoses of pregnancy correlating clinical findings with hormonal and immunopathological profiles. *British Journal of Dermatology*, 141: 71–81.

Velangi SS, Tidman MJ (1998). Gianotti–Crosti syndrome after measles, mumps and rubella vaccination. *British Journal of Dermatology*, 139: 1122–1123.

Vidimos AT, Camisa C (1992). Tongue and cheek: oral lesions in pityriasis rosea. *Cutis*, 50: 276–280.

Walsh NM, Prokopetz R, Tron VA, et al. (1994). Histopathology in erythroderma: review of a series of cases by multiple observers. *Journal of Cutaneous Pathology*, 21: 419–423.

Zurn A, Celebi CR, Bernard P, et al. (1992). A prospective immunofluorescence study of 111 cases of pruritic dermatoses of pregnancy: IgM anti-basement membrane zone antibodies as a novel finding. *British Journal of Dermatology*, 126: 474–478.

CHAPTER 20

Adams AE, Zwicker J, Curiel C, et al. (2004). Aggressive cutaneous T-cell lymphomas after TNFalpha blockade. *Journal of the American Academy of Dermatology*, 51: 660–662.

Al-Dhalimi MA (2007). Neonatal and infantile erythroderma: a clinical and follow-up study of 42 cases. *Journal of Dermatology*, 34: 302–307.

Anderson PC, Loeffel ED (1970). Erythrodermatitis. A review of 40 cases. *Missouri Medicine*, 67: 252–255.

Axelrod JH, Herbold DR, Freel JH, Palmer SM (1988). Exfoliative dermatitis: presenting sign of fallopian tube carcinoma. *Obstetrics and Gynecology*, 71(6 Pt 2): 1045–1047.

Berth-Jones J (2002). Erythroderma. In: Lebwohl M, Heymann WR, Berth-Jones J, Coulson I (eds), *Treatment of Skin Disease: Comprehensive Therapeutic Strategies*, Mosby, London, pp. 205–208.

Bi MY, Curry JL, Christiano AM, *et al.* (2011). The spectrum of hair loss in patients with mycosis fungoides and Sézary syndrome. *Journal of the American Academy of Dermatology*, 64: 53–63.

Byer RL, Bachur RG (2006). Clinical deterioration among patients with fever and erythroderma. *Pediatrics*, 118: 2450–2460.

Campbell JJ, Clark RA, Watanabe R, Kupper TS (2010). Sézary syndrome and mycosis fungoides arise from distinct T-cell subsets: a biologic rationale for their distinct clinical behaviors. *Blood*, 116: 767–771.

Dahten A, Mergemeier, S *et al.* (2007). PPAR gamma expression profile and its cytokine driven regulation in atopic dermatitis. *Allergy*, 62: 926–933.

Deffer TA, Overton-Keary PP, Goette DK (1985). Erythroderma secondary to esophageal carcinoma. *Journal of the American Academy of Dermatology*, 13(2 Pt 1): 311–313.

Ekmekci TR, Koslu A (2006). Erythroderma in a young healthy man. *Dermatology Online Journal*, 12(6): 23.

Faure M, Bertrand C, Mauduit G, Souteyrand P, Thivolet J (1985). Paraneoplastic erythroderma: apropos of a case. *Dermatologica*, 170: 147–151.

Flugman SL, McClain SA, Clark RA (2001). Transient eruptive seborrheic keratoses associated with erythrodermic psoriasis and erythrodermic drug eruption: report of two cases. *Journal of the American Academy of Dermatology*, 45(6 suppl): S212–214.

Glassman BD, Muglia JJ (1993). Widespread erythroderma and desquamation in a neonate. Congenital cutaneous candidiasis (CCC). *Archives of Dermatology*, 129: 899, 902.

Grant-Kels JM, Bernstein M, *et al.* (2007). Exfoliative dermatitis. In: Wolff K, Goldsmith LA, Katz SI, *et al.* (eds), *Fitzpatrick's Text book of Dermatology in General Medicine*, 7th edn, McGraw-Hill, New York, pp. 225–232.

Harmon CB, Witzig TE, Katzmann JA, Pittelkow MR (1996). Detection of circulating T cells with CD4+CD7- immunophenotype in patients with benign and malignant lymphoproliferative dermatoses. *Journal of the American Academy of Dermatology*, 35(3 Pt 1): 404–410.

Heikkilä H, Ranki A, Cajanus S, Karvonen SL (2005). Infliximab combined with methotrexate as long-term treatment for erythrodermic psoriasis. *Archives of Dermatology*, 141: 1607–1610.

Kokturk A, Ikizoglu G, Kaya TI, Baz K, Ulubas B, Apa DD (2004). Seborrheic dermatitis-like manifestation of lung cancer evolving into erythrodermia. *Journal of the European Academy of Dermatology and Venereology*, 18: 381–382.

Kotz EA, Anderson D, Thiers BH (2003). Cutaneous T-cell lymphoma. *Journal of the European Academy of Dermatology and Venereology*, 17: 131–137.

Lafaille P, Bouffard D, Provost N (2009). Exacerbation of undiagnosed mycosis fungoides during treatment with etanercept. *Archives of Dermatology*, 145: 94–95.

Lewis TG, Tuchinda C, Lim HW, Wong HK (2006). Life-threatening pustular and erythrodermic psoriasis responding to infliximab. *Journal of Drugs in Dermatology*, 5: 546–548.

Matutes E (2007). Adult T-cell leukaemia/lymphoma. *Journal of Clinical Pathology*, 60: 1373–1377.

Momm F, Pflieger D, Lutterbach J (2002). Paraneoplastic erythroderma in a prostate cancer patient. *Strahlentherapie und Onkologie*, 178: 393–395.

Morar N, Dlova N, Gupta AK, Naidoo DK, Aboobaker J, Ramdial PK (1999). Erythroderma: a comparison between HIV positive and negative patients. *International Journal of Dermatology*, 38: 895–900.

Müller H, Gattringer C, Zelger B, Höpfl R, Eisendle K (2008).

Infliximab monotherapy as first-line treatment for adult-onset pityriasis rubra pilaris: case report and review of the literature on biologic therapy. *Journal of the American Academy of Dermatology*, 59(5 suppl): S65–70.

Munyao TM, Abinya NA, Ndele JK, *et al.* (2007). Exfoliative erythroderma at Kenyatta National Hospital, Nairobi. *East African Medical Journal*, 84: 566–570.

Nassem S, Kashyap R, Awasthi NP, *et al.* (2009). Sézary syndrome presenting with 'leonine facies'. *Australasian Journal of Dermatology*, 50: 285–288.

Nicolis GD, Helwig EB (1973). Exfoliative dermatitis. A clinicopathologic study of 135 cases. *Archives of Dermatology*, 108: 788–797.

Oranje AP, Devillers AC, Kunz B (2006). Treatment of patients with atopic dermatitis using wet-wrap dressings with diluted steroids and/or emollients. An expert panel's opinion and review of the literature. *Journal of the European Academy of Dermatology and Venereology*, 20: 1277–1286.

Parving HH, Worm AM, Rossing N (1976). Plasma volume, intravascular albumin and its transcapillary escape rate in patients with extensive skin disease. *British Journal of Dermatology*, 95: 519–524.

Patrizi A, Pileri S, Rivano MT, Di Lernia V (1990). Malignant histiocytosis presenting as erythroderma. *International Journal of Dermatology*, 29: 214–216.

Pruszkowski A, Bodemer C, Fraitag S, Teillac-Hamel D, Amoric JC, de Prost Y (2000). Neonatal and infantile erythrodermas: a retrospective study of 51 patients. *Archives of Dermatology*, 136: 875–880.

Quéreux G, Renaut JJ, Peuvrel L, Knol AC, Brocard A, Dréno B (2010). Sudden onset of an aggressive cutaneous lymphoma in a young patient with psoriasis: role of immunosuppressants. *Acta Dermato-Venereologica*, 90: 616–620.

Querfeld C, Guitart J, Kuzel TM, Rosen S (2004). Successful treatment of recalcitrant, erythroderma-associated pruritus with etanercept. *Archives of Dermatology*, 140: 1539–1540.

Rongioletti F, Borenstein M, Kirsner R, Kerdel F (2003). Erythrodermic, recalcitrant psoriasis: clinical resolution with infliximab. *Journal of Dermatological Treatment*, 14: 222–225.

Rosen T, Chappell R, Drucker C (1979). Exfoliative dermatitis: presenting sign of internal malignancy. *Southern Medical Journal*, 72: 652–653.

Rosenbach M, Hsu S, Korman NJ, et al. (2010). Treatment of erythrodermic psoriasis: from the medical board of the National Psoriasis Foundation. *Journal of the American Academy of Dermatology*, 62: 655–662.

Rothe MJ, Bialy TL, Grant-Kels JM (2000). Erythroderma. *Dermatologic Clinics*, 18: 405–415.

Rothe MJ, Bernstein ML, Grant-Kels JM (2005). Life-threatening erythroderma: diagnosing and treating the 'red man'. *Clinics in Dermatology*, 23: 206–217.

Russell-Jones R, Whittaker S (2000). Sézary syndrome: diagnostic criteria and therapeutic options. *Seminars in Cutaneous Medicine and Surgery*, 19: 100–108.

Sahin MT, Oztürkcan S, Ermertcan AT, Saçar T, Türkdogan P (2004). Transient eruptive seborrheic keratoses associated with erythrodermic pityriasis rubra pilaris. *Clinical and Experimental Dermatology*, 29: 554–555.

Santos-Juanes J, Coto-Segura P, Mas-Vidal A, Galache Osuna C (2010). Ustekinumab induces rapid clearing of erythrodermic psoriasis after failure of antitumor necrosis factor therapies. *British Journal of Dermatology*, 162: 1144–1146.

Sarkar R, Sharma RC, Koranne RV, Sardana K (1999). Erythroderma in children: a clinico-etiological study. *Journal of Dermatology*, 26: 507–511.

Sehgal VN, Srivastava G (2006). Erythroderma/generalized exfoliative dermatitis in pediatric practice: an overview. *International Journal of Dermatology*, 45: 831–839.

Sehgal VN, Srivastava G, Sardana K (2004). Erythroderma/ exfoliative dermatitis: a synopsis. *International Journal of Dermatology*, 43: 39–47.

Shelley WB, Shelley ED (1985). Shoreline nails: sign of drug-induced erythroderma. *Cutis*, 35: 220–222, 224.

Shuster S (1963). High-output cardiac failure from skin disease. *Lancet*, i: 1338–1340.

Sigurdsson V, de Vries IJ, Toonstra J, et al. (2000). Expression of VCAM-1, ICAM-1, E-selectin, and P-selectin on endothelium *in situ* in patients with erythroderma, mycosis fungoides and atopic dermatitis. *Journal of Cutaneous Pathology*, 27: 436–440. .

Tebbe B, Schlippert U, Garbe C, Orfanos CE (1991). Erythroderma 'en nappes claires' as a marker of metastatic kidney cancer. Lasting, successful treatment with rIFN-alpha-2a. *Hautarzt*, 42: 324–327.

Thestrup-Pedersen K, Halkier-Sørensen L, Søgaard H, Zachariae H (1988). The red man syndrome. Exfoliative dermatitis of unknown etiology: a description and follow-up of 38 patients. *Journal of the American Academy of Dermatology*, 18: 1307–1312.

Thomson M, Berth Jones J (2009). Erythroderma and exfoliative dermatitis. In: Revuz J, Roujeau JC, Kerdel FA, Valeyrie-Allanore L (eds), *Life-Threatening Dermatoses and Emergencies in Dermatology*, Springer, Berlin, pp. 79–87.

Walsh NM, Prokopetz R, Tron VA, et al. (1994). Histopathology in erythroderma: review of a series of cases by multiple observers. *Journal of Cutaneous Pathology*, 21: 419–423.

CHAPTER 21

Albert MH, Notarangelo LD, Ochs HD (2011). Clinical spectrum, pathophysiology and treatment of the Wiskott–Aldrich syndrome. *Current Opinion in Hematology*, 18: 42–48.

Aleman K, Noordzij JG, de Groot R, van Dongen JJ, Hartwig NG (2001). Reviewing Omenn syndrome. *European Journal of Pediatrics*, 160: 718–725.

Andreu N, Pujol-Moix N, Martinez-Lostao L, et al. (2003). Wiskott–Aldrich syndrome in a female with skewed X-chromosome inactivation. *Blood, Cells, Molecules and Disease*, 31: 332–337.

Bacchetta R, Passerini L, Gambineri E, et al. (2006). Defective regulatory and effector T cell functions in patients with FOXP3 mutations. *Journal of Clinical Investigation*, 116: 1713–1722.

Bard S, Paravisini A, Avilés-Izquierdo JA, Fernandez-Cruz E, Sánchez-Ramón S (2008).

Eczematous dermatitis in the setting of hyper-IgE syndrome successfully treated with omalizumab. *Archives of Dermatology*, 144: 1662–1663.

Barth RF, Vergara GG, Khurana SK, Lowman JT, Beckwith JB (1972). Rapidly fatal familial histiocytosis associated with eosinophilia and primary immunological deficiency. *Lancet*, ii: 503–506.

Bennett CL, Christie J, Ramsdell F, et al. (2001). The immune dysregulation, polyendocrinopathy, enteropathy, X-linked syndrome (IPEX) is caused by mutations of FOXP3. *Nature Genetics*, 27: 20–21.

Berron-Ruiz A, Berron-Perez R, Ruiz-Maldonado R (2000). Cutaneous markers of primary immunodeficiency diseases in children. *Pediatric Dermatology*, 17: 91–96.

Bienemann K, Gudowius S, Niehues T (2007). Topical tacrolimus is effective against eczema in Wiskott–Aldrich syndrome (WAS). *Acta Paediatrica*, 96: 312–314.

Bindl L, Torgerson T, Perroni L, et al. (2005). Successful use of the new immune-suppressor sirolimus in IPEX (immune dysregulation, polyendocrinopathy, enteropathy, X-linked syndrome). *Journal of Pediatrics*, 147: 256–259.

Bittner TC, Pannicke U, Renner ED, et al. (2010). Successful long-term correction of autosomal recessive hyper-IgE syndrome due to DOCK8 deficiency by hematopoietic stem cell transplantation. *Klinische Padiatrie*, 222: 351–355.

Boraz RA (1989). Dental considerations in the treatment of Wiskott–Aldrich syndrome: report of case. *ASDC Journal of Dentistry for Children*, 56: 225–227.

Borges WG, Hensley T, Carey JC, Petrak BA, Hill HR (1998). The face of Job. *Journal of Pediatrics*, 133: 303–305.

Borges WG, Augustine NH, Hill HR (2000). Defective interleukin-12/interferon-gamma pathway in patients with hyperimmunoglobulinemia E syndrome. *Journal of Pediatrics*, 136: 176–180.

Bos JD (2002). Atopiform dermatitis. *British Journal of Dermatology*, 147: 426–429.

Boztug K, Schmidt M, Schwarzer A, et al. (2010). Stem-cell gene therapy for the Wiskott–Aldrich syndrome. *New England Journal of Medicine*, 363: 1918–1927.

Buckley RH, Fiscus SA (1975). Serum IgD and IgE concentrations in immunodeficiency diseases. *Journal of Clinical Investigation*, 55: 157–165.

Buckley RH, Wray BB, Belmaker EZ (1972). Extreme hyperimmunoglobulinemia E and undue susceptibility to infection. *Pediatrics*, 49: 59–70.

Burroughs LM, Torgerson TR, Storb R, et al. (2010). Stable hematopoietic cell engraftment after low-intensity nonmyeloablative conditioning in patients with immune dysregulation, polyendocrinopathy, enteropathy, X-linked syndrome. *Journal of Allergy and Clinical Immunology*, 126: 1000–1005.

Caudy AA, Reddy ST, Chatila T, Atkinson JP, Verbsky JW (2007). CD25 deficiency causes an immune dysregulation, polyendocrinopathy, enteropathy, X-linked-like syndrome, and defective IL-10 expression from CD4 lymphocytes. *Journal of Allergy and Clinical Immunology*, 119: 482–487.

Cavadini P, Vermi W, Facchetti F (2005). AIRE deficiency in thymus of 2 patients with Omenn syndrome. *Journal of Clinical Investigation*, 115: 728–732.

Chamlin SL, McCalmont TH, Cunningham BB, et al. (2002). Cutaneous manifestations of hyper-IgE syndrome in infants and children. *Journal of Pediatrics*, 141: 572–575.

Chehimi J, Elder M, Greene J, et al. (2001). Cytokine and chemokine dysregulation in hyper-IgE syndrome. *Clinical Immunology*, 100: 49–56.

Cho JS, Pietras EM, Garcia NC, et al. (2010). IL-17 is essential for host defense against cutaneous *Staphylococcus aureus* infection in mice. *Journal of Clinical Investigation*, 120: 1762–1773.

Conley ME, Notarangelo LD, Etzioni A (1999). Diagnostic criteria for primary immunodeficiencies. Representing PAGID (Pan-American Group for Immunodeficiency) and ESID (European Society for Immunodeficiencies). *Clinical Immunology*, 93: 190–197.

Conley ME, Saragoussi D, Notarangelo L, Etzioni A, Casanova JL (2003). An international study examining therapeutic options used in treatment of Wiskott–Aldrich syndrome. *Clinical Immunology*, 109: 272–277.

Conti HR, Shen F, Nayyar N, et al. (2009). Th17 cells and IL-17 receptor signaling are essential for mucosal host defense against oral candidiasis. *Journal of Experimental Medicine*, 206: 299–311.

Corneo B, Moshous D, Güngör T, et al. (2001). Identical mutations in *RAG1* or *RAG2* genes leading to defective V (D)J recombinase activity can cause either T–B-severe combined immune deficiency or Omenn syndrome. *Blood*, 97: 2772–2776.

Cotelingam JD, Witebsky FG, Hsu SM, Blaese RM, Jaffe ES (1985). Malignant lymphoma in patients with the Wiskott–Aldrich syndrome. *Cancer Investigation*, 3: 515–522.

d'Hennezel E, Ben-Shoshan M, Ochs HD (2009). FOXP3 forkhead domain mutation and regulatory T cells in the IPEX syndrome. *New England Journal of Medicine*, 361: 1710–1713.

Davis SD, Schaller J, Wedgwood RJ (1966). Job's syndrome. Recurrent, 'cold', staphylococcal abscesses. *Lancet* i: 1013–1015.

Davutoglu M, Guler E, Karabiber H, Arican O (2009). Eczematous skin lesions in an infant. *American Family Physician*, 80(2):191.

De Meester J, Calvez R, Valitutti S, Dupré L (2010). The Wiskott–Aldrich syndrome protein regulates CTL cytotoxicity and is required for efficient killing of B cell lymphoma targets. *Journal of Leukocyte Biology*, 88: 1031–1040.

de Saint-Basile G, Le Deist F, de Villartay JP, et al. (1991). Restricted heterogeneity of T lymphocytes in combined immunodeficiency with hypereosinophilia (Omenn's syndrome). *Journal of Clinical Investigation*, 87: 1352–1359.

DeWitt CA, Bishop AB, Buescher LS, Stone SP (2006). Hyperimmunoglobulin E syndrome: two cases and a review of the literature. *Journal of the American Academy of Dermatology*, 54: 855–865.

Eberting CL, Davis J, Puck JM, Holland SM, Turner ML (2004). Dermatitis and the newborn rash of hyper-IgE syndrome. *Archives of Dermatology*, 140: 1119–1125.

Ege M, Ma Y, Manfras B, et al. (2005). Omenn syndrome due to ARTEMIS mutations. *Blood*, 105: 4179–4186.

Engelhardt KR, McGhee S, Winkler S, et al. (2009). Large deletions and point mutations involving the dedicator of cytokinesis 8 (DOCK8)

in the autosomal-recessive form of hyper-IgE syndrome. *Journal of Allergy and Clinical Immunology*, 124: 1289–1302.

Erlewyn-Lajeunesse MD (2000). Hyperimmunoglobulin-E syndrome with recurrent infection: a review of current opinion and treatment. *Pediatric Allergy and Immunology*, 11: 133–141.

Faaij CM, Annels NE, Ruigrok G et al. (2010). Decrease of skin infiltrating and circulating CCR10+ T cells coincides with clinical improvement after topical tacrolimus in Omenn syndrome. *Journal of Investigative Dermatology*, 130: 308–311.

Filipovich AH, Stone JV, Tomany SC, et al. (2001). Impact of donor type on outcome of bone marrow transplantation for Wiskott–Aldrich syndrome: collaborative study of the International Bone Marrow Transplant Registry and the National Marrow Donor Program. *Blood*, 97: 1598–1603.

Fontenot JD, Gavin MA, Rudensky AY (2003). Foxp3 programs the development and function of CD4+CD25+ regulatory T cells. *Nature Immunology*, 4: 330–336.

Freeman AF, Holland SM (2010). Clinical manifestations of hyper IgE syndromes. *Disease Markers*, 29: 123–130.

Freeman AF, Collura-Burke CJ, Patronas NJ, et al. (2007). Brain abnormalities in patients with hyperimmunoglobulin E syndrome. *Pediatrics*, 119: e1121–e1125.

Freeman AF, Avila EM, Shaw PA, et al. (2011). Coronary artery abnormalities in hyper-IgE syndrome. *Journal of Clinical Immunology*, 31: 338–345.

Garraud O, Mollis SN, Holland SM, et al. (1999). Regulation of immunoglobulin production in hyper-IgE (Job's) syndrome. *Journal of Allergy and Clinical Immunology*, 103(2 Pt 1): 333–340.

Gatz SA, Benninghoff U, Schütz C, et al. (2011). Curative treatment of autosomal-recessive hyper-IgE syndrome by hematopoietic cell transplantation. *Bone Marrow Transplantation*, 46: 552–556.

Gelfand EW, McCurdy D, Rao CP, Cohen A (1984). Absence of lymphocyte ecto-5'-nucleotidase in infants with reticuloendotheliosis and eosinophilia (Omenn's syndrome). *Blood*, 63: 1475–1480.

Gomez L, Le Deist F, Blanche S, Cavazzana-Calvo M, Griscelli

C, Fischer A (1995). Treatment of Omenn syndrome by bone marrow transplantation. *Journal of Pediatrics*, **127**: 76–81.

Goussetis E, Peristeri I, Kitra V, *et al.* (2010). Successful long-term immunologic reconstitution by allogeneic hematopoietic stem cell transplantation cures patients with autosomal dominant hyper-IgE syndrome. *Journal of Allergy and Clinical Immunology*, **126**: 392–394.

Grimbacher B, Holland SM, Gallin JI, *et al.* (1999). Hyper-IgE syndrome with recurrent infections – an autosomal dominant multisystem disorder. *New England Journal of Medicine*, **340**: 692–702.

Grimbacher B, Holland SM, Puck JM (2005). Hyper-IgE syndromes. *Immunological Reviews*, **203**: 244–250.

Grunebaum E, Bates A, Roifman CM (2008). Omenn syndrome is associated with mutations in DNA ligase IV. *Journal of Allergy and Clinical Immunology*, **122**: 1219–1220.

Gudmundsson KO, Sigurjonsson OE, Gudmundsson S, Goldblatt D, Weemaes CM, Haraldsson A (2002). Increased expression of interleukin-13 but not interleukin-4 in CD4+ cells from patients with the hyper-IgE syndrome. *Clinical and Experimental Immunology*, **128**: 532–537.

Halabi-Tawil M, Ruemmele FM, Fraitag S (2009). Cutaneous manifestations of immune dysregulation, polyendocrinopathy, enteropathy, X-linked (IPEX) syndrome. *British Journal of Dermatology*, **160**: 645–651.

Heimall J, Freeman A, Holland SM (2010). Pathogenesis of hyper IgE syndrome. *Clinical Reviews in Allergy and Immunology*, **38**: 32–38.

Heltzer ML, Choi JK, Ochs HD, Sullivan KE, Torgerson TR, Ernst LM (2007). A potential screening tool for IPEX syndrome. *Pediatric and Developmental Pathology*, **10**: 98–105.

Hill HR, Ochs HD, Quie PG, *et al.* (1974). Defect in neutrophil granulocyte chemotaxis in Job's syndrome of recurrent 'cold' staphylococcal abscesses. *Lancet*, **ii**: 617–619.

Hoeger PH, Harper JI (1998). Neonatal erythroderma: differential diagnosis and management of the 'red baby'. *Archives of Diseases in Childhood*, **79**: 186–191.

Imai K, Morio T, Zhu Y, *et al.* (2004). Clinical course of patients with WASP gene mutations. *Blood*, **103**: 456–464.

Jang E, Cho WS, Cho ML, *et al.* (2011). Foxp3+ regulatory T cells control humoral autoimmunity by suppressing the development of long-lived plasma cells. *Journal of Immunology*, **186**: 1546–1553.

Jouan H, Le Deist F, Nezelof C (1987). Omenn's syndrome – pathologic arguments in favor of a graft versus host pathogenesis: a report of nine cases. *Human Pathology*, **18**: 1101–1108.

Kato M, Kimura H, Seki M, *et al.* (2006). Omenn syndrome – review of several phenotypes of Omenn syndrome and *RAG1/RAG2* mutations in Japan. *Allergology International*, **55**: 115–119.

Krivit W, Good RA (1959). Aldrich's syndrome (thrombocytopenia, eczema, and infection in infants) studies of the defense mechanisms. *AMA Journal of Diseases of Children*, **97**: 137–153.

Leonardo SM, Josephson JA, Hartog NL, Gauld SB (2010). Altered B cell development and anergy in the absence of Foxp3. *Journal of Immunology*, **185**: 2147–2156.

Litzman J, Jones A, Hann I, Chapel H, Strobel S, Morgan G (1996). Intravenous immunoglobulin, splenectomy, and antibiotic prophylaxis in Wiskott–Aldrich syndrome. *Archives of Diseases in Childhood*, **75**: 436–439.

Ma CS, Chew GY, Simpson N, *et al.* (2008). Deficiency of Th17 cells in hyper IgE syndrome due to mutations in *STAT3*. *Journal of Experimental Medicine*, **205**: 1551–1557.

Mancebo E, Recio MJ, Martínez-Busto E, *et al.* (2011). Possible role of Artemis c.512C>G polymorphic variant in Omenn syndrome. *DNA Repair (Amsterdam)*, **10**: 3–4.

Mazzolari E, Moshous D, Forino C, *et al.* (2005). Hematopoietic stem cell transplantation in Omenn syndrome: a single-center experience. *Bone Marrow Transplantation*, **36**: 107–114.

Milner JD, Brenchley JM, Laurence A, *et al.* (2008). Impaired T(H)17 cell differentiation in subjects with autosomal dominant hyper-IgE syndrome. *Nature*, **452**: 773–776.

Minegishi Y, Karasuyama H (2008). Genetic origins of hyper-IgE syndrome. *Current Allergy and Asthma Reports*, **8**: 386–391.

Minegishi Y, Saito M, Morio T, *et al.* (2006). Human tyrosine kinase 2 deficiency reveals its requisite roles in multiple cytokine signals involved in innate and acquired immunity. *Immunity*, **25**: 745–755.

Minegishi Y, Saito M, Tsuchiya S, *et al.* (2007). Dominant-negative mutations in the DNA-binding domain of STAT3 cause hyper-IgE syndrome. *Nature*, **448**: 1058–1062.

Minegishi Y, Saito M, Nagasawa M, *et al.* (2009). Molecular explanation for the contradiction between systemic Th17 defect and localized bacterial infection in hyper-IgE syndrome. *Journal of Experimental Medicine*, **206**: 1291–1301.

Mintz R, Garty BZ, Meshel T, *et al.* (2010). Reduced expression of chemoattractant receptors by polymorphonuclear leukocytes in hyper IgE syndrome patients. *Immunology Letters*, **130**: 97–106.

Moore MM, Hurst EB, Chastain S, Barnes CJ (2007). A child with multiple petechiae and eczematous plaques. *Pediatric Dermatology*, **24**: 417–418.

Morales-Tirado V, Sojka DK, Katzman SD, *et al.* (2010). Critical requirement for the Wiskott–Aldrich syndrome protein in Th2 effector function. *Blood*, **115**: 3498–3507.

Netea MG, Kullberg BJ, van der Meer JW (2005). Severely impaired IL-12/IL-18/IFNgamma axis in patients with hyper IgE syndrome. *European Journal of Clinical Investigation*, **35**: 718–721.

Nieves DS, Phipps RP, Pollock SJ, *et al.* (2004). Dermatologic and immunologic findings in the immune dysregulation, polyendocrinopathy, enteropathy, X-linked syndrome. *Archives of Dermatology*, **140**: 466–472.

Notarangelo LD (2010). Primary immunodeficiencies. *Journal of Allergy and Clinical Immunology*, **125**(2 suppl 2): S182–194.

O'Connell AC, Puck JM, Grimbacher B, *et al.* (2000). Delayed eruption of permanent teeth in hyperimmunoglobulinemia E recurrent infection syndrome. *Oral Surgery, Oral Medicine, Oral Pathology, Oral Radiology and Endodontics*, **89**: 177–185.

Ochs HD, Thrasher AJ (2006). The Wiskott–Aldrich syndrome. *Journal* of Allergy and Clinical Immunology, 117: 725–738.

Ochs HD, Filipovich AH, Veys P, Cowan MJ, Kapoor N (2009). Wiskott–Aldrich syndrome: diagnosis, clinical and laboratory manifestations, and treatment. Biology of Blood and Marrow Transplantation, 15(1 suppl): 84–90.

Omenn GS (1965). Familial reticuloendotheliosis with eosinophilia. New England Journal of Medicine, 273: 427–432.

Orange JS, Stone KD, Turvey SE, Krzewski K (2004). The Wiskott–Aldrich syndrome. Cellular and Molecular Life Sciences, 61: 2361–2385.

Paller A (2003). Genetic disorders of the immune system: Wiskott–Aldrich syndrome. In: Schachner LA, Hansen RC (eds), Pediatric Dermatology, 3rd edn, Mosby, St Louis, pp. 314–316.

Paller AS (2005). Genetic immunodeficiency disorders. Clinics in Dermatology, 23: 68–77.

Passerini L, Di Nunzio S, Gregori S, et al. (2011). Functional type 1 regulatory T cells develop regardless of FOXP3 mutations in patients with IPEX syndrome. European Journal of Immunology, 41: 1120–1131.

Peacocke M, Siminovitch KA (1992). Wiskott–Aldrich syndrome: new molecular and biochemical insights. Journal of the American Academy of Dermatology, 27: 507–519.

Powell BR, Buist NR, Stenzel P (1982). An X-linked syndrome of diarrhea, polyendocrinopathy, and fatal infection in infancy. Journal of Pediatrics, 100: 731–737.

Presotto F, Trentin L, Agostini C (1999). Hyper-IgE syndrome. New England Journal of Medicine, 341: 375–376.

Pruszkowski A, Bodemer C, Fraitag S, Teillac-Hamel D, Amoric JC, de Prost Y (2000). Neonatal and infantile erythrodermas: a retrospective study of 51 patients. Archives of Dermatology, 136: 875–880.

Puck JM, Candotti F (2006). Lessons from the Wiskott–Aldrich syndrome. New England Journal of Medicine, 355: 1759–1761.

Puzenat E, Rohrlich P, Thierry P, et al. (2007). Omenn syndrome: a rare case of neonatal erythroderma. European Journal of Dermatology, 17: 137–139.

Rescigno R, Dinowitz M (2001). Ophthalmic manifestations of immunodeficiency states. Clinical Reviews in Allergy and Immunology, 20: 163–181.

Rodríguez MF, Patiño PJ, Montoya F, Montoya CJ, Sorensen RU, García de Olarte D (1998). Interleukin 4 and interferon-gamma secretion by antigen and mitogen-stimulated mononuclear cells in the hyper-IgE syndrome: no TH-2 cytokine pattern. Annals of Allergy, Asthma and Immunology, 81(5 Pt 1): 443–447.

Roifman CM, Gu Y, Cohen A (2006). Mutations in the RNA component of RNase mitochondrial RNA processing might cause Omenn syndrome. Journal of Allergy and Clinical Immunology, 117: 897–903.

Roifman CM, Zhang J, Atkinson A, et al. (2008). Adenosine deaminase deficiency can present with features of Omenn syndrome. Journal of Allergy and Clinical Immunology, 121: 1056–1058.

Rubio-Cabezas O, Minton JA, Caswell R (2009). Clinical heterogeneity in patients with FOXP3 mutations presenting with permanent neonatal diabetes. Diabetes Care, 32: 111–116.

Saijo M, Suzutani T, Murono K, Hirano Y, Itoh K (1998). Recurrent aciclovir-resistant herpes simplex in a child with Wiskott–Aldrich syndrome. British Journal of Dermatology, 139: 311–314.

St Geme JW Jr, Prince JT, Burke BA, Krivit W (1962). Studies of persistent herpes virus infection in children with the Aldrich syndrome. Journal of Pediatrics, 61: 302–303.

Saurat JH (1985). Eczema in primary immune-deficiencies. Clues to the pathogenesis of atopic dermatitis with special reference to the Wiskott–Aldrich syndrome. Acta Dermato-Venereologica Supplementum (Stockholm), 114: 125–128.

Saurat JH, Woodley D, Helfer N (1985). Cutaneous symptoms in primary immunodeficiencies. Current Problems in Dermatology, 13: 50–91.

Scheimberg I, Hoeger PH, Harper JI, Lake B, Malone M (2001). Omenn syndrome: differential diagnosis in infants with erythroderma and immunodeficiency. Pediatric and Developmental Pathology, 4: 237–245.

Schimke LF, Sawalle-Belohradsky J, Roesler J, et al. (2010). Diagnostic approach to the hyper-IgE syndromes: immunologic and clinical key findings to differentiate hyper-IgE syndromes from atopic dermatitis. Journal of Allergy and Clinical Immunology, 126: 611–617.

Schwarz K, Notarangelo LD, Spanopoulou E, Vezzoni P, Villa A (1999). Recombination defects. In: Ochs HD, Smith CIE, Puck JM (eds), Primary Immunodeficiency Diseases. A Molecular and Genetic Approach, Oxford University Press, New York, pp. 155–166.

Shcherbina A, Candotti F, Rosen FS, Remold-O'Donnell E (2003). High incidence of lymphomas in a subgroup of Wiskott–Aldrich syndrome patients. British Journal of Haematology, 121: 529–530.

Sillevis Smitt JH, Wulffraat NM, Kuijpers TW (2005). The skin in primary immunodeficiency disorders. European Journal of Dermatology, 15: 425–432.

Sullivan KE, Mullen CA, Blaese RM, Winkelstein JA (1994). A multi-institutional survey of the Wiskott–Aldrich syndrome. Journal of Pediatrics, 125(6 Pt 1): 876–885.

Takeda K, Noguchi K, Shi W, et al. (1997). Targeted disruption of the mouse STAT3 gene leads to early embryonic lethality. Proceedings of the National Academy of Science of the United States of America, 94: 3801–3804.

Tangye SG, Cook MC, Fulcher DA (2009). Insights into the role of STAT3 in human lymphocyte differentiation as revealed by the hyper-IgE syndrome. Journal of Immunology, 182: 21–28.

Tatli MM, Sarraoglu S, Shermatov K, Gurel MS, Karadag A (2007). Exfoliative erythroderma, recurrent infections, generalized lymphadenopathy and hepatosplenomegaly in a newborn: Omenn syndrome. Australasian Journal of Dermatolou, 48: 133–134.

Taylor MD, Sadhukhan S, Kottangada P, et al. (2010). Nuclear role of WASP in the pathogenesis of dysregulated TH1 immunity in human Wiskott–Aldrich syndrome. Science Translational Medicine, 2(37): 37–44.

Thampakkul S, Ballow M (2001). Replacement intravenous immune serum globulin therapy in patients with antibody immune deficiency. Immunology and Allergy Clinics of North America, 21: 165–184.

Thrasher (2009). New Insights into the Biology of Wiskott–Aldrich

Syndrome (WAS), Hematology American Society of Hematology Education Program, 2009: 132–138.

Torgerson TR, Ochs HD (2007). Immune dysregulation, polyendocrinopathy, enteropathy, X-linked: forkhead box protein 3 mutations and lack of regulatory T cells. *Journal of Allergy and Clinical Immunology*, 120: 744–750.

Torgerson TR, Linane A, Moes N, *et al.* (2007). Severe food allergy as a variant of IPEX syndrome caused by a deletion in a noncoding region of the FOXP3 gene. *Gastroenterology*, 132: 1705–1717.

Van Eendenburg JP, Smitt JH, Weening RS (1991). Hyperimmunoglobulin E recurrent infection (Job) syndrome. *British Journal of Dermatology*, 125: 397.

Villa A, Santagata S, Bozzi F, *et al.* (1998). Partial V (D)J recombination activity leads to Omenn syndrome. *Cell*, 93: 885–896.

Villa A, Notarangelo LD, Roifman CM (2008). Omenn syndrome: inflammation in leaky severe combined immunodeficiency. *Journal of Allergy and Clinical Immunology*, 122: 1082–1086.

Wada T, Candotti F (2008). Somatic mosaicism in primary immune deficiencies. *Current Opinion in Allergy and Clinical Immunology*, 8: 510–514.

Wildin RS, Freitas A (2005). IPEX and FOXP3: clinical and research perspectives. *Journal of Autoimmunity*, 25(suppl): 56–62.

Wildin RS, Ramsdell F, Peake J, *et al.* (2001). X-linked neonatal diabetes mellitus, enteropathy and endocrinopathy syndrome is the human equivalent of mouse scurfy. *Nature Genetics*, 27: 18–20.

Woellner C, Schäffer AA, Puck JM, *et al.* (2007). The hyper IgE syndrome and mutations in TYK2. *Immunity*, 26: 535; author reply 536.

Yarmohammadi H, Cunningham-Rundles C (2008). Treatment of primary immunodeficiency diseases. In: Rezaei N, Aghamohammadi A, Notarangelo LD (eds), *Primary Immunodeficiency Diseases*, Springer-Verlag, Berlin, pp. 315–334.

Yong PL, Russo P, Sullivan KE (2008). Use of sirolimus in IPEX and IPEX-like children. *Journal of Clinical Immunology*, 28: 581–587.

Zhang Q, Davis JC, Lamborn IT, *et al.* (2009). Combined immunodeficiency associated with *DOCK8* mutations.
New England Journal of Medicine, 361: 2046–2055.

CHAPTER 22

Bacot BK, Paul ME, Navarro M, *et al.* (1997). Objective measures of allergic disease in children with human immunodeficiency virus infection. *Journal of Allergy and Clinical Immunology*, 100: 707–711.

Ball LM, Harper JI (1987). Atopic eczema in HIV-seropositive haemophiliacs. *Lancet*, ii: 627–628.

Bannister MJ , Freeman S (2000). Adult-onset atopic dermatitis. *Australasian Journal of Dermatology*, 41: 225–228.

Becker Y (2004). HIV-1 induced AIDS is an allergy and the allergen is the Shed gp120 – a review, hypothesis, and implications. *Virus Genes*, 28: 319–331.

Bowser CS, Kaye J, Joks RO, Charlot CA, Moallem HJ (2007). IgE and atopy in perinatally HIV-infected children. *Pediatric Allergy and Immunology*, 18: 298–303.

Chen H, Hayashi G, Lai OY, *et al.* (2012). Psoriasis patients are enriched for genetic variants that protect against HIV-1 disease. *PloS Genetics*, 8: e100251.

Chen TM, Cockerell CJ (2003). Cutaneous manifestations of HIV infection and HIV-related disorders. In: Bolognia JL, Jorizzo JL, Rapini RP (eds), *Dermatology*, Mosby, St Louis, pp. 1206–1208.

Corominas M, Garcia JF, Mestre M, Fernández-Viladrich P, Buendia E (2000). Predictors of atopy in HIV-infected patients. *Annals of Allergy, Asthma and Immunology*, 84: 607–611.

de Moraes AP, de Arruda EA, Vitoriano MA, *et al.* (2007). An open-label efficacy pilot study with pimecrolimus cream 1% in adults with facial seborrheic dermatitis infected with HIV. *Journal of the European Academy of Dermatology and Venereology*, 21: 596–601.

Elias PM, Steinhoff M (2008). 'Outside-to-inside' (and now back to 'outside') pathogenic mechanisms in atopic dermatitis. *Journal of Investigative Dermatology*, 128: 1067–1070.

Elias PM, Hatano Y, Williams ML (2008). Basis for the barrier abnormality in atopic dermatitis: outside-inside-outside pathogenic mechanisms. *Journal of Allergy and*
Clinical Immunology, 121: 1337–1343.

Ellaurie M, Rubinstein A, Rosenstreich DL (1995). IgE levels in pediatric HIV-1 infection. *Annals of Allergy, Asthma and Immunology*, 75: 332–336.

Gunathilake R, Schmuth M, Scharschmidt TC, *et al.* (2010). Epidermal barrier dysfunction in non-atopic HIV: evidence for an 'inside-to-outside' pathogenesis. *Journal of Investigative Dermatology*, 130: 1185–1188.

Hatano Y, Terashi H, Arakawa S, Katagiri K (2005). Interleukin-4 suppresses the enhancement of ceramide synthesis and cutaneous permeability barrier functions induced by tumor necrosis factor-alpha and interferon-gamma in human epidermis. *Journal of Investigative Dermatology*, 124: 786–792.

Hawk JLM, Magnus IA (1979). Chronic actinic dermatitis: An idiopathic photosensitivity syndrome including actinic reticuloid and photosensitive eczema. *British Journal of Dermatology*, 101(suppl 17): 24.

Hoare C, Li Wan Po A, Williams H (2000). Systematic review of treatments for atopic eczema. *Health Technology Assessment*, 4(37): 1–191.

Howell MD, Kim BE, Gao P, *et al.* (2007). Cytokine modulation of atopic dermatitis filaggrin skin expression. *Journal of Allergy and Clinical Immunology*, 120: 150–155.

Huang JT, Rademaker A, Paller AS (2009). Dilute bleach baths for *Staphylococcus aureus* colonization in atopic dermatitis to decrease disease severity. *Archives of Dermatology*, 147: 246–247.

Israël-Biet D, Labrousse F, Tourani JM, Sors H, Andrieu JM, Even P (1992). Elevation of IgE in HIV-infected subjects: a marker of poor prognosis. *Journal of Allergy and Clinical Immunology*, 89(1 Pt 1): 68–75.

Junqueira Magalhães Afonso JP, Tomimori J, Michalany NS, Nonogaki S, Porro AM (2012). Pruritic papular eruption and eosinophilic folliculitis associated with human immunodeficiency virus (HIV) infection: A histopathological and immunohistochemical comparative study. *Journal of the American Academy of Dermatology*, 67: 269–275.

Klein SA, Dobmeyer JM, Dobmeyer TS, *et al.* (1997). Demonstration of the Th1 to Th2 cytokine shift during the course of HIV-1 infection using cytoplasmic cytokine detection on single cell level by flow cytometry. *Aids*, 11: 1111–1118.

Koutsonikolis A, Nelson RP Jr, Fernandez-Caldas E, *et al.* (1996). Serum total and specific IgE levels in children infected with human immunodeficiency virus. *Journal of Allergy and Clinical Immunology*, 97: 692–697.

Kurahashi R, Hatano Y, Katagiri K (2008). IL-4 suppresses the recovery of cutaneous permeability barrier functions *in vivo*. *Journal of Investigative Dermatology*, 128: 1329–1331.

Lin RY, Lazarus TS (1995). Asthma and related atopic disorders in outpatients attending an urban HIV clinic. *Annals of Allergy Asthma and Immunology*, 74: 510–515.

Marone G, Florio G, Triggiani M, Petraroli A, de Paulis A (2000). Mechanisms of IgE elevation in HIV-1 infection. *Critical Reviews in Immunology*, 20: 477–496.

Ozkaya E (2005). Adult-onset atopic dermatitis. *Journal of the American Academy of Dermatology*, 52: 579–582.

Paganelli R, Fanales-Belasio E, Scala E, *et al.* (1991). Serum eosinophil cationic protein (ECP) in human immunodeficiency virus (HIV) infection. *Journal of Allergy and Clinical Immunology*, 88: 416–418.

Rodwell GE, Berger TG (2000). Pruritus and cutaneous inflammatory conditions in HIV disease. *Clinics in Dermatology*, 18: 479–484.

Sample S, Chernoff DN, Lenahan GA, *et al.* (1990). Elevated concentration of IgE antibodies to environmental antigens in HIV-seropositive homosexuals. *Journal of Allergy and Clinical Immunology*, 86(6 Pt 1): 876–880.

Sanchez-Borges M, Orozco A, Di Biagio E, Tami I, Suarez-Chacon R (1993). Eosinophilia in early-stage human immunodeficiency virus infection. *Journal of Allergy and Clinical Immunology*, 92: 494–495.

Skiest DJ, Keiser P (1997). Clinical significance of eosinophilia in HIV-infected individuals. *American Journal of Medicine*, 102: 449–453.

Supanaranond W, Desakorn V, Sitakalin C, Naing N, Chirachankul P (2001). Cutaneous manifestations in HIV positive patients. *Southeast Asian Journal of Tropical Medicine and Public Health*, 32: 171–176.

Tay YK, Khoo BP, Goh CL (1999). The profile of atopic dermatitis in a tertiary dermatology outpatient clinic in Singapore. *International Journal of Dermatology*, 38: 689–692.

Toutous-Trellu L, Abraham S, Pechère M, *et al.* (2005). Topical tacrolimus for effective treatment of eosinophilic folliculitis associated with human immunodeficiency virus infection. *Archives of Dermatology*, 141: 1203–1208.

Tubiolo VC, Vazzo LA, Beall GN (1997). Food allergy in human immunodeficiency virus (HIV) infection. *Annals of Allergy, Asthma and Immunology*, 78: 209–212.

Vigano A, Principi N, Crupi L, Onorato J, Vincenzo ZG, Salvaggio A (1995). Elevation of IgE in HIV-infected children and its correlation with the progression of disease. *Journal of Allergy and Clinical Immunology*, 95: 627–632.

Wilkins K, Turner R, Dolev JC, LeBoit PE, Berger TG, Maurer TA (2006). Cutaneous malignancy and human immunodeficiency virus disease. *Journal of the American Academy of Dermatology*, 54: 189–206.

CHAPTER 23

Akiyama M (2010). FLG mutations in ichthyosis vulgaris and atopic eczema: spectrum of mutations and population genetics. *British Journal of Dermatology*, 162: 472–477.

Anton-Lamprecht I, Hofbauer M (1972). Ultrastructural distinction of autosomal dominant ichthyosis vulgaris and X-linked recessive ichthyosis. *Humangenetik*, 15: 261–264.

Bellew S, Del Rosso JQ (2010). Overcoming the barrier treatment of ichthyosis: a combination-therapy approach. *Journal of Clinical and Aesthetic Dermatology*, 3: 49–53.

Compton JG, DiGiovanna J, Johnston KA, Fleckman P, Bale SJ (2002). Mapping of the associated phenotype of an absent granular layer in ichthyosis vulgaris to the epidermal differentiation complex on chromosome 1. *Experimental Dermatology*, 11: 518–526.

Elsayed-Ali H, Barton S, Marks R (1992). Stereological studies of desmosomes in ichthyosis vulgaris. *British Journal of Dermatology*, 126: 24–28.

Feinstein A, Ackerman AB, Ziprkowski L (1970). Histology of autosomal dominant ichthyosis vulgaris and X-linked ichthyosis. *Archives of Dermatology*, 101: 524–527.

Fleckman P, Holbrook KA, Dale BA, Sybert VP (1993). Keratinocytes cultured from subjects with ichthyosis vulgaris are phenotypically abnormal. *Journal of Investigative Dermatology*, 88: 640–645.

Liu P, Yang Q, Wang X, *et al.* (2008). Identification of a genetic locus for ichthyosis vulgaris on chromosome 10q22.3-q24.2. *Journal of Investigative Dermatology*, 128: 1418–1422.

Nirunsuksiri W, Zhang SH, Fleckman P (1998). Reduced stability and bi-allelic, coequal expression of profilaggrin mRNA in keratinocytes cultured from subjects with ichthyosis vulgaris. *Journal of Investigative Dermatology*, 110: 854–861.

Oji V, Traupe H (2009). Ichthyosis: clinical manifestations and practical treatment options. *American Journal of Clinical Dermatology*, 10: 351–364.

Okulicz JF, Schwartz RA (2003). Hereditary and acquired ichthyosis vulgaris. *International Journal of Dermatology*, 42: 95–98.

Patel N, Spencer LA, English JC 3rd, Zirwas MJ (2006). Acquired ichthyosis. *Journal of the American Academy of Dermatology*, 55: 647–56.

Rabinowitz LG, Esterly NB (1994). Atopic dermatitis and ichthyosis vulgaris. *Pediatrics in Review*, 15: 220–226.

Rubeiz N, Kibbi AG (2003). Management of ichthyosis in infants and children. *Clinics in Dermatology*, 21: 325–328.

Sandilands A, O'Regan GM, Liao H, *et al.* (2006). Prevalent and rare mutations in the gene encoding filaggrin cause ichthyosis vulgaris and predispose individuals to atopic dermatitis. *Journal of Investigative Dermatology*, 126: 1770–1775.

Sandilands A, Terron-Kwiatkowski A, Hull PR, *et al.* (2007). Comprehensive analysis of the gene encoding filaggrin uncovers prevalent and rare mutations in ichthyosis vulgaris and atopic eczema. *Nature Genetics*, **39**: 650–654.

Shwayder T, Ott F (1991). All about ichthyosis. *Pediatric Clinics of North America*, **38**: 835–857.

Smith FJ, Irvine AD, Terron-Kwiakowski A (2006). Loss-of-function mutations in the gene encoding filaggrin cause ichthyosis vulgaris. *Nature Genetics*, **38**: 337–342.

Sybert VP, Dale BA, Holbrook KA (1985). Ichthyosis vulgaris: identification of a defect in synthesis of filaggrin correlated with an absence of keratohyaline granules. *Journal of Investigative Dermatology*, **84**: 191–194.

Ziprkowski L, Feinstein A (1972). A survey of ichthyosis vulgaris in Israel. *British Journal of Dermatology*, **86**: 1–8.

CHAPTER 24

Aaronson DW (2006). The 'black box' warning and allergy drugs. *Journal of Allergy and Clinical Immunology*, **117**: 40–44.

Ault A (2005). Adrenal suppression from topical corticosteroids surprisingly high. Medical Page Today: March 25 2005. Available at: www.medpagetoday.com/Dermatology/Steroids/tb/777 (accessed November 5, 2011).

Fleischer AB Jr (2006). Black box warning for topical calcineurin inhibitors and the death of common sense. *Dermatology Online Journal*, **12**: 2.

Glusac EJ (2003). Under the microscope: doctors, lawyers, and melanocytic neoplasms. *Journal of Cutaneous Pathology*, **30**: 287–293.

Goldberg DJ (2007). Legal issues in dermatology: informed consent, complications and medical malpractice. *Seminars in Cutaneous Medicine and Surgery*, **26**: 2–5.

Kubetin SK (2003). FDA panel: docs don't consider adrenal suppression in kids on topical steroids. *Skin & Allergy News*, **34**(12): 19.

Lydiatt DD (2004). Medical malpractice and cancer of the skin. *American Journal of Surgery*, **187**: 688–694.

Maccaro (1993). The treating physician rule and the adjudication of claims for social security disability benefits. *Social Security Report Service*, **833**: 833–834.

Marks JG, Elsner P, DeLeo VA (2002). *Contact and Occupational Dermatology*, 3rd edn, Mosby, St Louis.

Mathias CG (1989). Contact dermatitis and workers' compensation: criteria for establishing occupational causation and aggravation. *Journal of the American Academy of Dermatology*, **20**: 842–848.

Read S, Hill HF 3rd (2005). Dermatology's malpractice experience: clinical settings for risk management. Journal of the American *Academy of Dermatology*, **53**: 134–137.

Ruzicka T, Ring J, Przybilla B (1991). *Handbook of Atopic Eczema*, Springer-Verlag, Berlin.

Skin-Cap (2008). Overview. Injury Board. Available at: www.injuryboard.com/topic/skin-cap-overview.aspx (accessed November 5, 2011).

Williams HC (2000). *Atopic Dermatitis: The Epidemiology, Causes, and Prevention of Atopic Eczema*. Cambridge University Press, Cambridge.

INDEX

Note: Page numbers in *italic* refer to tables, boxes or figures in the text

abscesses, staphylococcal 'cold' 330, 331
acantholytic dermatosis, transient (Grover disease) 307
acanthosis 283, 290, 293
acetylcholine 96, 98–9
acid ceramidase 136
acid mantle 136–7, 162
aclometasone dipropionate *182*
acne vulgaris 280
acroangiodermatitis 272
acrodermatitis enteropathica 71, 282
actinic dermatitis 348
acupuncture 105
acute eczema 40, 122–4
acyclovir (aciclovir) 85, 175
ADAM10 123
Adamson, Horatio George 14
adolescent AD 42, 43, 54–6
adrenal insufficiency 188, 361
adult AD, differential diagnosis 74–6
adult T-cell leukemia/lymphoma 312
adult-onset atopic dermatitis 39, 341
aeroallergens 112, 127, 137–8, 147, 152
    avoidance 154
    skin penetration 138
Aetius of Amila 13
African patients 298
African–Americans 46, 57, 104, 234
age 32, 234
airway reactivity 147
albumin, loss 317
alitretinoin 241
allergens 34–7
    allergic contact dermatitis 247–8
    contact 247–8, 273
    dietary 37, 91, 112
    dust mite 34–5, 36–7, 108, 112, 127, 137, 152
    identification 150–2
    maternal exposure 34–5
    skin penetration 138
    types 112
    See also aeroallergens; food allergies
allergic contact dermatitis (ACD) 247
    adults 74
    association with AD 251
    children 65–6
    diagnosis 252
    hands 224

histopathology 296–7
    misdiagnosis 362–3
    pathogenesis 248–51
    treatment 252–4
allergic rhinitis 78, 127, 147, 342
allergy
    factors in 145
    role in AD 23
alloknesis ('itchy skin') 96
alopecia
    chronic erythroderma 313
    Omenn syndrome 334, 335
amcinonide *181*
American Academy of Dermatology, diagnostic criteria *77*
Americans with Disabilities Act 360
ammonium lactate 273, 356
AMPs, *See* antimicrobial peptides
anaphylaxis 228
annular lesions
    nummular dermatitis 258
    seborrheic dermatitis 278–9
antecubital fossa 52, 53
anterior uveitis 216
antibiotics
    bacterial skin infections 90–1, 168, *177*
    and gut flora 35
    infants 35, 90–1, 92
    primary immunodeficiency diseases 337
    routine use 169
antidepressants *103*, 104
antifungal agents 170, 171, 285, 286
antigen presentation 137
antihistamines 94, 143, 155
    contact dermatitis 253
    oral 90, 102, *103*, 264
    topical 90, 101
antimicrobial peptides (AMPs) 130, 132, 160, 165–6, 174, 250
antioxidants 37
apoptosis, keratinocytes 122–3, 160
APT, *See* atopy patch test
aquaporins 125, 160
aqueous humor 212, 220
arachidonic acid 163, 283
Artemis mutations 335, 336
'arthritic eczema' 255
artistic representations of AD 15
Asian patients 212, 298
Aspergillus spp. 333
aspirin, topical *101*, 102
associations, atopic dermatitis 34

asteatotic eczema 259, 290
asthma 78, 127, 146–7, 149
    association with AD 20, 34
    HIV/AIDS 342
atopic dermatitis (AD), introduction of term 39, 107
atopic march 77–8, 127–8, 146–7
    and antihistamines 90
'atopic salute' 57
'atopic shiners' 50, 57
atopic skin care 86–8
atopic 'volcano' 110
atopiform dermatitis 108, 125, 128–9, 341, *346*
atoporrheic dermatitis 83
atopy
    first use of term 20
    in HIV/AIDS 342
atopy patch test (APT) 117, 137–8, 151
Augustus 12
Australia *29, 31*
autoeczematization 259, 263, 274, 330
autonomic nervous system 98–9
avenanthramides 162–3
azathioprine 190, 241, 320
    adverse effects *196*, 241
    interactions *196*
    mechanism of action *196*
    monitoring guidelines *197*
    pruritus of AD *103*, 104
azole antifungal agents 170, 286

β-hemolytic streptococci 168
BACH study 241
bacitracin 273
bacterial infections
    infantile AD 84, 85, 90–1
    S. aureus 130, 132, 139–40, 165–6
    stasis dermatitis 268–9
bacterid reactions 290
Baer, Rudolph L 11, 21
balneotherapy *202*, 207
balsam of Peru 226
bamboo hair 68–9
barrier repair agents 90, 163–4, 356
Bateman, Thomas 13, 14
bathing 155, 162–3
    dilute bleach 168, *169, 177*, 334, 350
    frequent 36
    infants 86–7, 92
    salt-water 207
Bazin, Ernest 17, 255
benefits law 358–9
Besnier, Ernest 20, 108
betamethasone dipropionate *181–2*
betamethasone valerate *182*
biblical references 12
Biett, Laurent-Theodore 13
bifonazole 286
bioflavonoid antioxidants 184
biologic therapies 193–4, 237, 319
biphasic model 118
birthweight 81
bleach baths 168, *169, 177*, 334, 350
blepharitis 216–18, 280
Bloch, Dr Bruno 21

blood urea nitrogen (BUN) *198*
Blount disease 332
bone marrow transplant 336
borage oil 283
botulinum toxin 124, 242
bradykinin 96
brain, processing of pruritus 94–5
brain-derived neurotropic factor 144
Brazil *29*
breast involvement 58–60
breast milk 35, 79, 154
'bricks-and-mortar' model 159–60, 351
Brocq, Louis-Anne-Jean 19
Bulkley, Lucius Duncan 20
bullous dermatoses 290
Bureau of Labor Statistics 228
Burow solution 253
butorphanol *103*, 104

C-nerve fibers 94
Caillault, Charles 16
calcineurin inhibitors 89–90, 100
    adverse effects/cautions 100–1, 174–5, 183, 221,
        237, 319
    contact dermatitis 253
    in glaucoma 221
    hand dermatitis 237
    HIV/AIDS patient 350
    legal issues 362
    skin barrier function 163, 164
    stasis dermatitis 273
calcipotriol 237
calcitonin gene-related peptide (CGRP) 124, 144, 264
calcium channel blockers 260, 262
candidiasis 268–9, 334
    congenital 314
cannabinoids 163, 184
Canterbury Tales 12
canthelicidins 130, 132, 165, 174
carba mix 226
cardiac failure 315, 317
cataracts 214–15
    corticosteroid-induced 218–21
cathelicidins 160, 250–1
cathepsins 97
CCL17/CCL18 chemokines *116*
CD20 antigen 193
CD36 antigen 125
cellular Flice-inhibitory protein (cFLIP) 123
cellulitis, stasis dermatitis 268
ceramide-based creams/emollients 90, 92, 100, 163
ceramides 133, 135–6
cerebrovascular hemiplegia 144
cetirizine 90, 155
cheeks 45, 46
cheilitis 48, 49
    angular 71, 331
child abuse cases 363–4
child custody 363–4
childhood AD 42, 43
    and adult hand dermatitis 243–4
    clinical presentation 50–4
    differential diagnosis 61–74
childhood infections 146

children, pityriasis alba 303
Chinese 33, 351
Chinese medicine 12
chromate 226
chromium 233
chronic dermatitis 40–1, 124–5
    hands 243–4
ciclopirox olamine 177, 286
claudin-1 109, 136
climate 207, 352–3
clindamycin 168
clinical presentation
    adolescents/young adults 54–6
    adult AD 54–6
    childhood AD 50–4
    infantile AD 39, 42–3, 45–50
    nonessential features 57–60
clobetasol propionate 181
clobetasone butyrate 164
clocortolone pivalate 182
clothing 92, 155
    infants 88
coal tar 285, 286
cobalt 226, 233
Coca, Arthur F 21
collagen deposition 125, 293
collarettes of scale 40
collodion membrane 354
colophony resin 227
compression therapy 273–4
computed tomography (CT) 333–4
conjunctivitis 212–13
construction workers 228
contact allergens 247–8, 273
contact dermatitis 65–6, 247
    acute 289
    adults 74
    association with AD 251–2
    hands 224–6
    See also allergic contact dermatitis (ACD); irritant
        contact dermatitis (ICD)
corneal transplantation 213
corneocytes 108, 109, 132–3, 160
corneodesmosomes 137
cornified envelope 132–3, 160–1
corticosteroids
    adverse effects/cautions 66, 89, 188, 194
    approved for infants 89
    causing cataract and glaucoma 218–21
    erythroderma 319
    interactions 194
    legal issues 360–1, 362
    mechanism of action 189, 194
    rebound phenomenon 218
    systemic 102, 103, 187–8, 194
    topical 86, 88–9, 100, 164, 181–3, 253, 319
        hand dermatitis 237
        ICD 253
        potency 181–2
        seborrheic dermatitis 286
        stasis dermatitis 273
costs, economic 80, 244
counseling 274
cow dander 228
cowhage 94

cow's milk 154
'cradle cap' 276, 280
creatinine 189, 198
Crohn's disease 34
CTCL, See cutaneous T-cell lymphoma
Cushing syndrome 89
cutaneous lymphocyte antigen (CLA) 113, 116
cutaneous T-cell lymphoma (CTCL) 294, 310, 317, 319, 320
    adults 76
    children 72
    HIV 346, 349
cutting oils 243
cyclosporine (ciclosporin) 188–9, 195
    adverse effects 189, 195
    erythroderma 319
    eye disease 213
    hand dermatitis 240
    interactions 195
    mechanism of action 195
    monitoring guidelines 198
    primary immunodeficiency 337
    pruritus of AD 102–3
    skin absorption 138
    USP modified (Neoral) 189
    USP (Sandimmune) 189
cytokine, eosinophil-attracting 142
cytokines 113–16
    anti-inflammatory 36
    eosinophil-attracting 142
    and itch 121
    'proallergic' 140
    Th2 116–17, 166

500-Dalton rule 138
'dandruff' 275, 285
De Morbis Cutaneis (Turner) 16
Dead Sea 207, 208
β-defensins 130, 132, 160, 165–6, 250
definitions 26
    standardization 25
delayed-type hypersensitivity (DTH) 248–9
dendritic cells (DCs) 125–6, 144
    langerin-positive 249
    See also Langerhans cells
dendritic herpetic keratitis 175
Denmark 29, 30, 31, 81, 228, 233, 242
Dennie–Morgan folds 45, 46, 47, 50
dental abnormalities 332
depigmentation 54
dermatology, legal aspects 357
dermatomyositis 47, 281, 310
dermatophyte infections
    adults 75
    children 64
    HIV/AIDS 346
    role in AD 171
    stasis dermatitis 269
dermicidin 130, 139
desmocollin-1 160
desmogleins 160
desonide 92, 164, 182
desoximetasone 181, 182
desquamation 161, 334
    abnormal 316, 351

detergents 155, 162
developing countries 30, 32–3
Di George syndrome 318
diabetes mellitus, type 1 337
diagnostic criteria 27–8, 44
    Hanifin and Rajka 44
    UK working party 27
diaper area 82, 89, 280
diathetic tendency 108
dicloxacillin 168
diet
    elimination 152
    erythroderma 319
    historical treatment of AD 22
    infant 35, 154
    maternal 154
dietary allergies 37, 91, 112, 151–2
differential diagnosis
    adult AD 61, 74–6
    infant and childhood AD 61–74, 282
diflorasone diacetate 181
dihydrofolate reductase 196, 241
dinitrochlorobenzene 251
diphenhydramine 90
direct immunofluorescece (DIF) 283
'dirty neck' appearance 42, 43, 51, 354
disability
    benefits and compensation 358–9
    defined 360
    workplace discrimination 360
discoid eczema, See nummular dermatitis
disease classification 27–8
disease severity 32
DNA vaccines 254
DOCK8 gene 329–30, 334
Down syndrome 281
doxepin 101, 183
doxycyline 168
DRESS syndrome 313–14, 320
drug hypersensitivity syndrome 313
drug interactions
    corticosteroids 194
    cyclosporine 195
    methotrexate 192
drug reactions
    causing erythroderma 313–14, 315, 317
    clinical features 300
    histopathology 302
    HIV/AIDS 346, 349
    nummular dermatitis-like eruptions 260–2
dry skin, See xerosis
dust mite 34–5, 36–7, 108, 112, 127, 137, 152
dyshidrotic eczema (pompholyx) 60, 232–3, 241, 300–1

E-cadherin 122, 123, 124
ear (external), seborrheic dermatitis 278–9
ecchymoses, stasis dermatitis 268
'eczema'
    derivation and evolution of term 11, 13–14
    use/misuse of term 11, 289
eczema craquelé 263
'eczema death' 16
eczema herpeticum 85, 172–5, 177, 221
eczema molluscatum 172
'eczema rubrum' 15

eczema vaccinatum 85–6, 176
edema, peripheral 316, 317
efalizumab 193
eggs 37, 152
elderly
    hand dermatitis 224, 234
    nummular dermatitis 263
emollients 87–8
    ceramide-based 90, 92, 100, 163
    hand dermatitis 235
    and pruritus 100, 101
empiricks 16
Employee Retirement Income and Security Act (ERISA) 359
employment law 358–60
β-endorphins 98
environmental factors 33, 36, 80
    house dust mite 34–5, 36–7, 108, 112, 127, 137, 152
envoplakin 161
eosinophil cationic protein (ECP) 141, 142
eosinophil major basic protein (MBP) 141, 142
eosinophil-derived neurotoxin (EDN) 141, 142
eosinophilia, HIV infection 342
eosinophilic folliculitis 346, 349
eosinophils 141–2, 250, 292, 342
Epiceram 163, 356
epidermal differentiation complex 352
epidermal tight junctions 108, 109, 136
epinastine 97
erythema toxicum neonatorum 307–8
erythroderma 309
    associated disease/malignancies 318
    causes 309–14
    clinical features 316–17
    epidemiology 315
    evaluation 315
    histopathology 302, 317
    neonatal and pediatric 314–15
    Omenn syndrome 334, 335
    prognosis and sequelae 320–1
    systemic complications 315, 317
    treatment 319–20
etanercept 242
ethambutol 315
Ethiopia 30
ethnicity 32–3, 79, 212, 234, 298
European counteis 30
excimer laser 202, 204
excoriations 46
exfoliative dermatitis
    histopathology 302, 317
    See also erythroderma
extensor surface involvement 52, 53
extracellular polysaccharide substance (EPS) 138
extrinsic atopic dermatitis (EAD) 108, 148
eye, anatomy 211–12
eye disorders
    blepharitis 216–18
    cataracts 214–15
    corticosteroid-induced 218–21, 361
    eczema herpeticum 174, 175
    incidence 212
    keratoconjunctivitis 212
    keratoconus 213
    periorbital dermatitis 218
    pigmentation change 50, 57

retinal detachment 215–16
uveitis 216
Wiskott–Aldrich syndrome 326
eye rubbing 213
eyebrow
loss of lateral 48
seborrheic dermatitis 277
eyelid
AD 45, 47, 55, 216–18
eczema herpeticum 175
molluscum contagiosum 173
seborrheic dermatitis 217

facies
childhood atopic dermatitis 50
leonine 312, 313
stereotypic in hyper-IgE syndrome 330–1
famciclovir 175
family law 363–4
family size 33, 80, 146
farm environment 36
Fas receptor 122–3
fatty acids 283–4
FcεR1 receptor 116, 125, 149
fetal predictors 34–5, 80, 81
fever, with erythroderma 315
fibrin cuffs 271–2
fibronectin-binding protein (FBP) 166
fibrosis, dermal 271–2
filaggrin 134, 155, 160, 166, 351
filaggrin gene (FLG) mutations 34, 58, 81, 108, 110, 134–5,
147, 162, 351, 352
fingertip unit 180
fingertips 60
Finland 30
fish 152
fissuring
infra-auricular 48
Sézary syndrome 309
flexures
dermatitis 52, 53, 343–4
sparing 353
fluocinolone acetonide 182
fluocinonide 181
flurandrenolide 182
fluticasone propionate 89, 92, 182, 219
follicular eczema, histopathology 298–9
folliculitis, eosinophilic 346, 349
food allergies 37, 91, 112, 151
allergen avoidance 154
diagnosis 152
food products 228
food service workers 223, 228, 244
foot dermatitis 58
Forkhead box protein 3 (FOXP3) gene 120, 337, 338–9
formaldehyde 66, 227
fragrance mix 233
free amino acids 160
free fatty acids (FFA) 133, 163
fungal infections 170–1
stasis dermatitis 268–9
See also dermatophyte infections; Malassezia spp.
fungid reactions 290
fusidic acid 168

gastrin-releasing peptide receptor (GRPR) 94
gender 32, 224, 233, 234–5, 267
genetics
AD 34, 58, 81, 162
hand dermatitis 234
hyper-IgE syndrome 329–30
Omenn syndrome 335
Wiskott–Aldrich syndrome 328
geographic variation 32–3, 79, 145
German Infant Nutritional Intervention (GINI) 79
Germany 29, 30
gestational age 81
Gianotti–Crosti syndrome 305
giardiasis 262
glaucoma, corticosteroid-induced 220–1, 361
glioma 34
gloves
latex rubber 228–9
prevention of hand dermatitis 235, 245
glucocorticoids
systemic 240
See also corticosteroids
glucosylceramide 133
glycyrrhetinic acid (GA) 163–4, 184
GM-CSF, See granulocyte-macrophage colony-stimulating
factor
Goddard, JA 16
Golgi apparatus 160, 161
gp120 protein 342
graft-versus-host disease (GVHD) 310, 317, 335
granulocyte-macrophage colony-stimulating factor (GM-CSF)
120, 140, 248
Greece, Ancient 12
Green, Jonathan 14
Grenz ray therapy 238–9
Grover disease 307
gut microflora 35, 154

HAART, See highly-active antiretroviral therapy
hair-shaft defects 68, 69
hairdressers 228, 243
halcinonide 181
'halo eczema' 256
halobetasol propionate 181
hand dermatitis
atopic 58, 232, 234
child 52, 53
chronicity and prognosis 243–4
clinical features 226–8
clinical variants 224
contact 224–6
epidemiology 223
evaluation components 225
financial impact 244
frictional 231
HIV/AIDS 233
hyperkeratotic 230–1
nummular 231
and occupation 228, 242–3
outcome studies 242
prevention and lifestyle management 235, 236
risk factors 233–5

treatment 237–43
vesicular 232–3
Hanifin and Rajka criteria *44*
hapten–atopy hypothesis 146
Hardy, Alfred 12, 16
Hassall corpuscles 113
Haxthausen, Holgen 20
hayfever 34, 149
'headlight sign' 45, 46, 82
healthcare costs 80, 244
healthcare workers 228–9
heavy metals 260, *261*
Hebra, Ferdinand 17, 18, 19
Helicobacter pylori 262
heliotherapy *202*, 207
hemopoietic stem cell transplantation 328, 329, 336, 339
hemosiderin deposition 267–8, 272
henna, black 65
herpes simplex virus 85, 174
Hertoghe's sign 48
HIES, *See* hyper-IgE syndrome
highly-active antiretroviral therapy (HAART) 233
Highman, Walter James 17–18
Hill, W 139
Hippocratic humoralist doctrine 16
histamine 97, 98, 142–3
histamine H$_1$ receptor antagonists 97
histamine receptors 97, 143
histamine-sensitive C-nerve fibers 94
histiocytosis X (Langerhans cell histiocytosis) 282
histopathology 290–4
    allergic contact dermatitis 296–7
    atopic dermatitis 111–12, 294–6
    dyshidrotic eczema 300–1
    erythema toxicum neonatorum 307–8
    erythroderma 317–18
    follicular eczema 298–9
    Gianotti–Crosti syndrome 305
    ichthyosis vulgaris 353
    irritant contact dermatitis 297–8
    miliaria 308
    pityriasis alba 303
    pityriasis rosea 303–4
    polymorphous eruption of pregnancy 306–7
    seborrheic dermatitis 283, 299–300
    small-plaque parapsoriasis 305–6
    stasis dermatitis 272, 303
    transient acantholytic dermatosis (Grover disease) 307
historical figures 12
HIV/AIDS
    atopy 342
    cutaneous manifestations 341
    dermatophytosis 348
    diagnosis of AD 343–4
    differential diagnosis of AD 344–50
    erythroderma 310, 315, 318
    hand dermatitis 233
    IgE elevation and eosinophilia 342–3
    malnutrition 349
    photosensitive reactions 347–8
    pruritic papular disorders 350
    seborrheic dermatitis 280–1, 283, 284, 345
    treatment of AD 350
holidays 207
Hong Kong 29

hospitalization, erythroderma 319
house dust mites 34–7, 108, 112, 127, 137, 152
    elimination 155
human β-defensin 2 (HBD2) 130, 132, 165–6, 174, 250
human β-defensin 3 (HBD3) 130, 132, 166, 174
human papillomavirus 86
human rights 364
humidity 352–3
'humors' 16
hyaluronic acid 123–4, 163, 164
Hyde, James Nevins 21
hydration 86–7, 134–5, 162–3, 252–3, 356
hydrocortisone 23, 92, 164, *182*
α-hydroxy acids 356
hygiene hypothesis 36–7, 80, 145–6
Hylatopic Plus 163
hyper-IgE syndrome (HIES) *324–5*, 329–34
hyperhidrosis, palmar 233, 300
hyperkeratosis 230–1, 293
hyperknesis, punctate 96
hyperlinear palms/soles 353
hyperpigmentation 42, 43, 51, 56
hypertension, systemic 274
hypoalbuminemia 317
hypopigmentation 56, 258, 278–9

ichthyosis 314, 351
    acquired 354, *355*
    lamellar 354, 355
    X-linked 354
ichthyosis vulgaris 34, 58–9, 70–1, 108, 111, 155
    clinical features 352–3
    differential diagnosis 354, *355*
    epidemiology 352
    genetics 352
    management 356
    pathophysiology 351–2
id reaction 290
immune disorders/deficiency 314
    association with AD 157
    congenital 67
    and infectious disease 80, 146
    See also named immune disorders; primary
        immunodeficiency diseases (PIDs)
immune dysregulation, polyendocrinopathy, enteropathy,
    X-linked syndrome (IPEX) *324*, 337–9
immune reconstitution inflammatory syndrome 233
immunobiologics 193–4, 237, 319
immunoglobulin, intravenous (IVIG) 337
immunoglobulin A (IgA) 285
immunoglobulin E (IgE) 149
    atopic dermatitis 111–12
    contact dermatitis 249–50
    dermatophytes 171
    erythroderma 318
    FcεR1 receptor *116*, 125, 149
    HIV/AIDS 342
    hyper-IgE syndrome 332
    infantile AD 282
    recombinant monoclonal antibody 150, 193–4, 334
    S. aureus superantigens 166
immunoglobulin G (IgG) 285
immunotherapy 156, 254
impetiginization 167–9

'impetigo' 14
'impetigo sparsa' 14
incontinentia pigmenti 308
indinavir 343
infantile atopic dermatitis
    associated disorders 77–8
    clinical features 39, 42–3, 45–50, 82–4
    complications 84–6
    course 48
    differential diagnosis 61–74, 282
    factors to record in history 84, 91
    historical 14–15
    onset 77
    pathogenesis 81
    treatment 86–91
infantile seborrheic dermatitis
    causes 283
    clinical features 280
    differentiation from AD 282, 283
    treatment 285–6
infants, feeding 35, 154
infections
    associated with AD 34
    childhood 146
    HTLV-1 infective dermatitis 72–3
    and immune disorders 80, 146
    in primary immunodeficiency diseases 325, 326, 328
    role in AD 36, 80
    S. aureus, See Staphylococcus aureus
    secondary in infantile AD 84–6
    viral 34, 85–6, 172–5
    yeasts 170–1, 284–5
inflammatory dendritic epidermal cells (IDECs) 111–12, 125, 148, 149
infliximab 193, 319
innate immune system 129–32
inosine monophosphate dehydrogenase 196
'inside–outside' hypothesis 110
intercellular adhesion molecule-1 (ICAM-1) 136
interferon-α2b 260, 261
interferon-γ (IFN-γ) 35, 115, 116, 118, 125, 140, 249–50, 337
    therapy 193, 197
interleukins 97–8, 114–15
interleukin-1 receptor antagonist (IL-1R) 121, 285
interleukin-1α (IL-1α) 121, 248, 285
interleukin-1β (IL-1β) 121
interleukin-2 (IL-2) 97, 249
interleukin-4 (IL-4) 114, 117, 124, 128, 166, 249
interleukin-5 (IL-5) 114, 117, 128, 249
interleukin-6 (IL-6) 333
interleukin-8 (IL-8) 97, 285
interleukin-10 (IL-10) 36, 114, 119, 126, 166, 249, 333
interleukin-11 (IL-11) 125
interleukin-12 (IL-12) 114, 250
interleukin-13 (IL-13) 115, 116, 124, 128, 166, 332
interleukin-17 (IL-17) 120, 125, 333
interleukin-18 (IL-18) 115, 121, 140, 166
interleukin-21 (IL-21) 333
interleukin-22 (IL-22) 115, 120, 333
interleukin-23 (IL-23) 237
interleukin-25 (IL-25/IL-17E) 115, 121
interleukin-31 (IL-31) 93, 97, 115, 121
interleukin-33 (IL-33) 121

International Study of Asthma and Allergies in Childhood (ISAAC) 25, 32
intertrigo, streptococcal 281
intraocular lens implantation 218
intraocular pressure 220, 221
intrinsic (atopiform) dermatitis 108, 125, 128–9, 148, 346
involucrin 285
ionizing radiation 238–9
iontophoresis 242
irritant contact dermatitis (ICD) 36, 65, 247
    adults 74
    association with AD 252
    children 65–6
    diagnosis 252
    hands 224
    histopathology 297–8
    immunology 248–51
    pathogenesis 248
    treatment 252–4
irritants 36, 248
    avoidance 155
ISAAC, See International Study of Asthma and Allergies in Childhood
isotretinoin 263
itch–scratch cycle 93, 99–100
itch-specific receptors 93–4
'itchy skin' (alloknesis) 96
itraconazole 286

Japan 29, 30, 31
Japanese patients 298, 330
Jewish patients 12
jin yin chuang 12
Job syndrome (hyper-IgE syndrome) 329–34
juvenile plantar dermatitis 66, 67

Kaposi, M 17
Kaposi varicelliform eruption 85, 172–5
keratin K1/K10 285
keratinocyte-derived factors 140
keratinocytes 159–60
    apoptosis 122–3, 160
    cytokines 120–1
    neural mediators 93
keratoconjunctivitis 212–13
keratoconus 213
keratolytics 102, 273, 285, 356
keratosis pilaris 58–9
Kerley, CG 22
ketoconazole 286
ketotifen 90
kitchen workers 223
KOALA study 79
Koebner phenomenon 72, 74
kwashiorkor 71, 349

laboratory studies 84
lactic acid 356
Lactobacillus 154
lamellar body 133, 161
Langerhans cell histiocytosis (histiocytosis X) 282
Langerhans cells (LCs) 111, 112, 125, 144, 291, 292
    contact dermatitis 248–9, 249–50
langerin-positive dermal dendritic cells 249
laser, excimer 202, 204

latex allergy 228–9
  legal issues 360, 363
laundry detergents 155
leather contact dermatitis 65
Leider, Morris 21
Leiner disease 276, 281
'leonine' facies 312, 313
'leopard skin' appearance 70
'lepra' 12
leprosy 116, 262
lesion morphology 40–2
leukemias, causing erythroderma 312–13, 315
'lichen agrius' 15–16
lichen nitidus 72, 74
lichen planus 72, 76, 310
lichen simplex chronicus (LSC) 75, 102, 124–5, 260, 293
lichen spinulosus 74, 76
lichenification 40–1, 55, 56, 57
  childhood AD 54
  HIV/AIDS 341, 343–4
  nummular dermatitis 260
  pathophysiology 124–5
  stasis dermatitis 268
lichenoid papules 41, 52, 53
lichenoid photoeruption 347
lifestyle management, hand dermatitis 235, 236
lifestyle, westernized 33, 145
linoleic acid 163, 164, 283
lip-licker's dermatitis 48, 49, 51
lipids
  epidermal 132–3, 135–6, 160, 161
  skin care agents 163
lipodermatosclerosis 269, 274
liver function 192, 197, 198
loricrin 132, 161
lupus erythematosus 281, 310
lymphadenopathy 83
lymphocytes, exocytosis 292, 293, 294, 295
lymphoma
  risk with azathioprine 190
  risk with calcineurin inhibitors 183
  See also cutaneous T-cell lymphoma (CTCL)

macrophage migration inhibitory factor (MIF) 142
magnetic resonance imaging, functional (fMRI) 94–5
Majocchi granuloma 348
major basic protein (MBP) 141
Malassezia spp. 86, 171, 177, 284–5
  M. furfur 171, 284
  M. globosa 284
  M. sympodialis 56, 284
  restricta 284
malignancy
  associations with AD 34
  erythroderma 312–13, 318
  risk and azathioprine 190
  risk and calcineurin inhibitors 183, 237
  risk and phototherapy 208
  Wiskott–Aldrich syndrome 328
malnutrition 71, 349
manual labor workers 230–1
Marat, Jean Paul 12
Mas-related, G-protein-coupled receptor member A (MRGPRA) 93
mast cells 96, 97, 126–7, 142–3, 259, 264

chymase 143
maternal factors 34–5, 79–80
matrix metalloproteases 125
maxacalcitol 237
medical device creams 163–4, 184, 185
medical malpractice 360–1
melanoma, misdiagnosis 361
menthol 101–2
mercury 13
metalloproteases 123
metals 233, 260, 261
  causing nummular dermatitis-like eruptions 260, 261
  nickel 65–6, 226, 232–3, 248, 251
methotrexate 191–2, 319
  adverse effects/cautions 192, 196, 241
  hand dermatitis 241
  interactions 196
  mechanism of action 196
  monitoring guidelines 197
  nummular dermatitis 264
  pruritus of AD 103, 104
5-methoxypsoralen (5-MOP) 206
methylchloroisothiazolinone/methylisothiazolinone (MCI/MI) 66, 226, 237
methylprednisolone aceponate 89
'Meyerson phenomenon' 256
microabscesses 291
migrant studies 33
miliaria 138, 308
milk
  cow's 152, 154
  See also breast milk
Milton, John Laws 18
Mimyx 163, 184
mirtazapine 103, 104
moisturizers 86–8, 162–4
  ceramide-containing 90, 92, 100, 163
  hand dermatitis 235, 236
  keratolytic 88
  newer formulations 163–4
  and pruritus 100, 101
  stasis dermatitis 273
mold exposure 362
molluscum contagiosum 86, 172
molluscum dermatitis 66, 67, 86
mometasone furoate 182
mononuclear infiltrate 111
morbidity 32
Morris, Sir Malcolm 19
'mournful facies' 50
mouse models 121, 125
mucanain 94, 97
mucin, tear film 212
Mucuna pruriens 94
Munro microabscesses 283
mupirocin 168
muscarinic receptors 99
mycophenolate mofetil (MMF) 189, 190–1
  adult dosages 240
  adverse effects 196
  children 103
  hand dermatitis 240–1
  interactions 196
  mechanism of action 196
  monitoring guidelines 198

pruritus of AD *103*, 104
mycosis fungoides (MF)
    clinical features 72, 76, 262
    erythrodermic 309, 310, 312
    HIV infection *346*, 349
myelotoxicity 241
Mysticus 12

nail abnormalities 71, 319, 320–1
naltrexone 105
napkin dermatitis 276
National Psoriasis Foundation 192
'natural moisturizing factor (NMF) 134–5, 160
nausea, systemic therapies 190, 192
neck, 'atopic dirty' 42, 43, 51, 354
neomycin 217, 273
neonate
    erythema toxicum neonatorum 307–8
    erythroderma 314–15
    See also infantile AD
nerve growth factor (NGF) 96, 98, 143–4
nerves 143–4
Netherton syndrome 67–9, 314, 333
'neurodermatitis' 19–20
neurological compromise 263
neurological disease 281, 286
neuropeptide-Y 144
neurotransmitters 98–9
neurotrophins 96, 143–4
New England Medical Monthly 11
New Zealand *30*
NGF, *See* nerve growth factor
nickel 65–6, 226, 232–3, 248, 251
Nigeria 39
nipple dermatitis 58–60
nitric oxide 218
nitrofurazone 233
NMF, *See* 'natural moisturizing factor
non-Hodgkin lymphoma 190, 349
Norway *31*, 32
nucleotide-binding oligomerization domain (NOD) family 129
nummular dermatitis
    clinical associations 259
    clinical presentation 40, 41, 64, 256–8, 289
    differential diagnosis 75, 260–2
    epidemiology 255
    first description 255, 289
    hands 231, *238*
    laboratory and histological findings 259
    pathogenesis 263–4
    treatment 264
nurse practitioners 23
nutrition 35, 71, 282
    See also diet; food allergies

oatmeal 162–3, 285
occupational disease
    hand dermatitis 228, 233
        financial impact 244
        outcomes 242–3
        prevention/management 235, *236*
    legal aspects 358–60
odontogenic infection *262*
ointment vehicles 88–9, 92, 163, 273
omalizumab 150, 193–4, 334

Omenn syndrome *324–5*, 334–7
oncostatin M receptor (OSMR) gene 93
opioid agonists/antagonists *103*, 104–5
opioid receptors 98
oral/perioral disease 48, 49, 51, 262, 326–7
orbital hyperpigmentation 50, 57
'outside–inside' hypothesis 108, 110, 159
over-the-counter products 273
OX40-ligand 126
oxygen by-products 205, 214

palmitic acid 163
N-palmitoylethanolamine 163, 184
palmoplantar dermatitis 58
palms, hyperlinear 353
papain 97
papular acrodermatitis of childhood (Gianotti–Crosti syndrome) 305
papular eruptions, infantile AD 48, 49
papulovesicles 256, 258
PAR-2, *See* protease activated receptor 2
parakeratosis 283
parapsoriasis, small-plaque 305–6
Parkinson disease 281, 286
paronychia 71
patch testing 117, 137–8, 150–1
    contact dermatitis 226, 252
pathogen associated molecular patterns (PAMPs) 129
pathogenesis 108–10, 159–62
pathophysiology
    acute lesions 122–4
    biphasic model 118
    chronic lesions 124–5
    T lymphocytes and cytokines 113–21
patient education 99–100, 180, 235
patient information sheet 180
pattern recognition receptors (PRRs) 129
peanuts 152
pentoxyfylline 274
perinatal factors 79–80
perioral dermatitis 48, 49, 51
periorbital dermatitis 218
periplakin *161*
periumbilical papules 52, 53
peroxisome proliferator activated receptor γ (PPARγ) 319
personal hygiene products 66
petechiae 326, 327
petrolatum-based moisturizers 163–4, 235
pH, epidermal 99, 136–7, 162, 166
phases of AD 42–3
p-phenylenediamine 226, 233
phenylketonuria 68
phospholipase 162
photo(chemo)therapy
    in children 208
    excimer laser 204
    extracorporeal photopheresis 206–7
    first studies 201
    hand dermatitis 239–40
    malignancy risk 208
    pruritus of AD 105
    PUVA 206
    recommendations *201*
    stapylococcal infections 168–9
    UVA/UVB combined *202*, 203

UVA1 204–5, 209
UVB 202, 203–4, 209, 239–40
worsening of AD 209
photographic chemicals 226
photopheresis, extracorporeal 206–7
photosensitivity reactions 346, 347–8
pigmentation changes
    nummular dermatitis 256, 258
    seborrheic dermatitis 278–9
    stasis dermatitis 267–8, 273
pimecrolimus 89–90, 100, 164
    adverse effects/cautions 100–1, 174–5, 183, 237
    contact dermatitis 253
    hand dermatitis 237
    HIV/AIDs patient 350
pityriasis alba 57, 303
pityriasis lichenoides chronica 70, 304
pityriasis lichenoides et varioliformis acute (PLEVA) 304
pityriasis rosea 262, 303–4
pityriasis rosea gigantea of Darier 304
pityriasis rubra pilaris 68, 70, 310, 314, 317, 320
pityriasis versicolor 280
pityrosporum folliculitis 280
Pityrosporum ovale 284
plantar dermatitis, juvenile 66, 67
plaques 40, 41, 256–7, 289
platelet dysfunction 326
pneumatoceles 333
Pneumocystis jiroveci infections 328, 349
polidocanol 101, 102
pollution 37
pompholyx 60, 232–3, 241
    histopathology 300–1
    treatment 241
'porrigo larvalis' 15, 16
potassium dichromate 233
pramoxine 101, 102
prednicarbate 182
prednisone 188
pregnancy, polymorphous eruption 306–7
prematurity 81
preservatives 237, 251, 273
prevalence 28–32
    increase in 33
    variation of estimates 25
prevention 153–6
    primary 153–5
    secondary 155
    tertiary 155–6
primary immunodeficiency diseases (PIDs) 323
    hyper-IgE syndrome 324–5, 329–34
    IPEX 324–5, 337–9
    Omenn syndrome 324–5, 334–7
    warning signs 326
    Wiskott–alrich syndrome 324–5, 326–9
prisoners' rights 364
probiotics 154
product liability 362–3
profilaggrin 134, 160, 162, 351
propylene glycol 356
prostaglandin D$_2$ 99
prostanoids 99
protease inhibitors 108, 343
protease-activated receptor 2 (PAR2) 94, 97, 130
proteases 97, 99, 162

protein gene product 143
protein–energy malnutrition 71
'prurigo diathésique eczémato-lichénienne' 20, 108
prurigo nodularis 56, 344, 346
pruritic urticarial papules and plaques of pregnancy (PUPPP) 306–7
pruritus 39
    mediators 96–9, 121
    pathophysiology 93–6
    prevalence in AD 93
    skin barrier dysfunction 99
    treatments 99–105, 183
pseudo-CTCL 346, 349
pseudo-Kaposi sarcoma 272
Pseudomonas aeruginosa 333
psoralen plus UVA (PUVA) 168, 202, 206–7, 209
    hand dermatitis 239
    pruritus of AD 105
psoriasiform changes 230
psoriasiform epidermal hyperplasia 125, 291
psoriasis
    children 63
    differentiation diagnosis 63, 231, 260–1, 281, 283
    erythroderma 310, 311, 316, 319, 321
    HIV infection 345–7
    methotrexate therapy 192
    phototherapy 203
psychological disorders 281, 343
psychological therapies 105
purine nucleotide synthesis 196
purpura 268, 326
pustules 167
PUVA, See psoralen and ultraviolet light
pyrrolidone carboxylic acid 139
pyruvic acid 356

quality of life, hand dermatitis 242
quaternium-15 226

radiation therapy 238–9
    malpractice claims 360
radioallergosorbent testing (RAST) 152, 282, 342
RAG-1/RAG-2 genes 335
ragweed 217
Rayer, Pierre 13–14
renal function 197, 198
rete ridges 293
retinal detachment 215–16
retinoids 241, 356
'ringworm' 64
risk factors for AD 34–5
    infantile AD 79–80
rituximab 193, 339
RNase mitochondrial RNA-processing (RMRP) gene 336
roentgenotherapy 22
Romania 29

salicylic acid 101, 102, 273, 285, 356
salt-water baths 207
sarcoidosis 310
scabies
    adults 75
    children 66
    erythroderma 310, 311
    HIV/AIDS 346, 348–9

treatments 262
scale
    collarettes 40
    ichthyosis 351, 352–3
scalp involvement
    differential diagnosis 64, 83
    erythroderma 321
    infants 46, 83
    seborrheic dermatitis 278, 280
Scandinavia, infantile AD 81
Schamberg, Jay 22
'school chair sign' 54
scratching 124–5
scurfy 338
sebaceous glands 275
'seborrhea' 275
seborrhea capitis 276
seborrheic dermatitis 275
    adults 74
    associations 280–1
    children 62, 83
    classification 275
    clinical features 217, 276–81, 299
    differential diagnosis 83, 281–2
    erythroderma 314
    etiology 283–5
    histopathology 283, 299–300
    HIV infection 345, 346
    infantile 275, 276, 280, 281, 282, 285
    treatment 285–6
seborrheic keratoses 321
sebum 283–4
selenium sulfide 285
serine proteases 137
serotonin 96
severe combined immunodeficiency (SCID) 334–5
sexual abuse 364
Sézary cells 312
Sézary syndrome 309, 310, 312, 313, 315
shampoos
    product liability 362
    seborrheic dermatitis 285, 286
shea butter 163
shock 315
'shoreline' nails 319
siderophages 272
signal transducer and activator of transcription 3 (STAT3)
    gene 329, 332, 333, 334
Singapore 29, 39
sirolimus 339
skeletal abnormalities 332
skin barrier 129, 132–3, 159–62
    function assessment 162
    repair 90, 155, 162–4, 356
skin barrier dysfunction 81, 108, 109, 224
    antigen presentation 137
    HIV-infected patient 342–3
    and pruritus 99
    water loss 132–5
skin care, infants 86–8
skin hydration 86–7, 134–5, 162–3, 252–3, 356
skin injury, sites of previous 259
skin testing 150–1
Skin-Cap 361
skinfolds 83

SLS, See sodium lauryl sulfate
small proline-rich proteins (SPRs) 161
smallpox vaccine 176
smoking 37, 79, 233
soaps 136–7, 155, 162, 252
Social Security benefits 358–9
socioeconomic factors 33, 79, 80
sodium hypochlorite 168, 169, 350
sodium lauryl sulfate (SLS) 251, 252
sodium pump (Na+/K+ ATPase) 220
soles 58
South Africa 30
soybean trypsin inhibitors 88
sphingomyelin 133, 136
sphingomyelinase 135–6
sphingosine 136, 139, 166
sphingosophosphorylcholine (SPC) 136
spinal cord injury 263
splenectomy 329
spongiosis 40, 111, 283, 290, 291, 292
    pathophysiology 122–4
staphylococcal scalded skin syndrome 314
Staphylococcus aureus 165–9
    abscess 73
    HIV 350
    infantile AD 84, 90–1
    methicillin-resistant (MRSA) 84, 90, 167–8
    nummular dermatitis 259
    pathogenic role 166
    skin colonization 36, 130, 132, 139–40, 165–9, 333
    superantigens 156, 166
    treatment of infections 90–1, 168–9
Staphylococcus epidermidis 138
stasis dermatitis
    clinical features 267–8, 303
    complications 268–70
    diagnosis 273
    differential diagnosis 303
    histopathology 272, 303
    pathophysiology 271–2
    prevalence 267
    treatment 273–4
STAT 3, See signal transducer and activator of transcription 3
    (STAT3) gene
stearic acid 163
stem cell transplantation 328, 329, 336, 339
steroid rebound 218
sterols 163
stocking erythroderma 268
stockings, compression 273–4
strait-jacket treatment 22
stratum corneum 108, 109, 132–3
    'bricks-and-mortar' model 159–60, 351
    crosstalk with cutaneous nerve fibers 99
stratum corneum chymotryptic enzyme (SCCE) 136
stratum granulosum 108, 109, 111, 136, 160, 161
streptococci, β-hemolytic 168, 170
Streptococcus pyogenes 170
'Strophulus confertus' 15–16
subacute eczema 40
substance P 124, 143, 264
Suetonius 12
sulfamethoxazole–trimethoprim 168, 328, 348
sulfur 285
Sulzberger, MB 11, 21, 22–3, 107

Sulzberger–Garbe syndrome 290
'summoner' 12
sunlight exposure 207
superantigens 91, 156, 166
surfactants 162
sweat glands 99, 138
sweat/sweating 98, 138, 166
Sweden 12, 33, 243, 244
sympathectomy, thoracic 233, 300
systemic treatments
    azathioprine 190
    corticosteroids 187–8, *194*
    cyclosporine 188–9
    immunobiologics 193, 193–4, 237, 319
    infantile AD 91
    methotrexate 191–2, *196–7*, 319
    monitoring guidelines *197–8*
    mycophenolate mofetil 189, 190–1, *196*

T cells 113–16
    CD3+ 263–4
    CD4+ 111, 249
    CD4+:CD8+ ratio 264
    CD8+ 111, 119, 249
    CD25+ 120
    contact dermatitis 248–50
    regulatory (Treg) 119–20
    T helper 1 (Th1) 113, 116, 117, 249, 250
        super-Th1 140
    T helper 2 (Th2) 116–17, 126–7, 148–9
    T helper 17 (Th17) 120, 149, 249, 332–3
T lymphocytic virus type 1 (HTLV-1) dermatitis 72
T-cell peptide epitopes 254
T-cell receptor (TCR), 'mimic peptides' 254
tacrolimus 85, 89–90, 100
    adverse effects/cautions 100–1, 174–5, 183, 237, 319
    contact dermatitis 253
    eye disorders 213, 221
    hand dermatitis 237
    HIV/AIDS patients 350
    skin barrier function 163, 164
    topical, skin absorption 138
Taiwan *31*
Talbot, Fritz 23
tape stripping 137
tar products 23, 183, 253, 264, 285, 286
Tat protein 342
tazarotene 237, 356
tear film, abnormalities 212
tears, artificial 213
teeth, retained deciduous 332
telmestine 184
terbinafine 286
terminology, historical 15–16, 107
Thailand *31*
thigh, dermatitis 54
thiopurine methyltransferase (TPMT) 104, 190
thiuram mix 226
thrombocytopenia 327
thromboxane A$_2$ 99
thromboxane protein (TP) receptors 99
thymic stromal lymphopoietin (TSLP) 113, 121, 126, 127–8, 140, 148
thymus 113

thymus- and activation-regulated chemokine (TARC) *116*
thyroid disease, autoimmune 337
tight junctions 108, *109*, 136
Tilbury Fox, W 17
tinea infections 64, 171, 269, 348
tissue inhibitor of metalloprotease (TIMP-1) 125
tobacco smoke 37, 79
'toilet seat dermatitis' 54
toll-like receptors (TLRs) 129, 147, 251
    TLR-4 226, 248
topical treatments
    calcineurin inhibitors 89–90, 100–1, 163, 174–5, 183, 253, 273, 319
    corticosteroids 88–9, 100, 181–3
    fingertip unit 180
    historical 22–3
    infants 88–91, 92
    medical device creams 184, 185
    paradigm 185
    skin barrier repair 162–4
tort law 360–3
toxic shock syndrome 315
trabecular meshwork 220
tramcinolone acetonide 188
tranquilizers 22
transepidermal water loss (TEWL) 132, 252, 343
    measurement 162
    reduction 162–4
transforming growth factor-β (TGF-β) 36, 119, 125, 140
transglutaminases *160*, *161*, 162
transient receptor potential cation channel subfamily M member 8 (TRPM8) 101–2
transient receptor potential cation channel subfamily V member 1 (TRPV1) receptors 101
treating physician rule 358–9
treatment
    historical 22–3
    permutational paradigm 179
    See also systemic treatments; topical treatments *and specific treatment modalities*
The Treatment of Eczema in Infants and Children (Hill) 139
tretinoin 356
triamcinolone, petrolatum-based ointment 237
triamcinolone acetonide *182*, 264
Trichophyton infections 64
trichorrhexis invaginata 68–9
trimethoprim–sulfamethoxazole 168, 328, 348
trunk involvement
    infantile AD 48, 49
    seborrheic dermatitis 278–9
tryptase 97
TSLP, *See* thymic stromal lymphopoietin (TSLP)
tuberculid rections 290
tumor necrosis factor-α (TNF-α) 126, 248, 274, 296, 318
    antibody 193
'tunnel' hypothesis 143
Tunnessen, Walter 82
Turkey *29*
Turner, Jonathan 16
twin studies 34, 234
tyrosine kinase 2 (*Tyk2*) gene 329–30
tzaarat 12

Ulrich, Dr 22
ultraviolet light therapy

in children 208
hand dermatitis 239–40
PUVA 168, *202*, 206–7, 209
staphylococcal infections 168–9
UVA1 *202*, 204–5, 209
UVB *202*, 203–4, 209, 239–40
umbilicus, seborrheic dermatitis 278–9
United Kingdom (UK) *30*, 32, 228
United States (USA), prevalence of AD *29*, *30*, 79
Unna boot 273
Unna, PG 13, 18
urban/rural gradient 33
urbanization 80
urea-containing creams 356
urocanic acid 137, 139
urticaria, contact 228–9
ustekinumab 237–8, 319
uveitis 216

vaccines 253–4
vagal nerve stimulation 99
valaciclovir 175
Van Harlingen, A 16–17
varicose veins 267
variola 176
vasoactive intestinal peptide (VIP) 264
venous hypertension 271
venous insufficiency 267, 271
    management 273–4
venous ulceration 270
vesicles, Langerhans cells 291, 292
Veterans' benefits 359–60
viral infections 34, 85–6, 172–5
visual loss 213, 220
vitamin D_3 derivatives 237
vitiligo 54
Vitis vinifera 184

Walzer, Abraham 21
warts, viral 34, 86
WASP gene mutations 328
western lifestyle 33, 145
wet dressing, open 253
wet work 233, 244
wet-wrap dressings *101*, 102, 320
White, Dr JC 18, 22
Willan, Robert 13
Wilson, Sir Erasmus 14–15
Wiskott–Aldrich syndrome 67, 282, 323, *324*, 326–9
    clinical presentation *324–5*, 326–8
    diagnosis 328
    management 328–9
    pathophysiology 328
woods, tropical 226
workers' compensation 358
wrists *52*, *53*

X-linked ichthyosis 354
X-linked immune dysregulation, polyendocrinopathy,
    enteropathy (IPEX) *324–5*, 337–9
xerosis 50, 56, 64
    HIV/AIDS 342–3, *344–5*, *346*
    nummular dermatitis 259, 263
    stasis dermatitis 273

yeast infections 170–1, 284–5

zinc deficiency 164, 282
zinc pyrithione 286
zinc transporter gene (*Zip4*) 71

Printed and bound by CPI Group (UK) Ltd, Croydon, CR0 4YY

23/10/2024

01778251-0014